Bovine Tuberculosis: Causes, Symptoms and Treatment

Bovine Tuberculosis: Causes, Symptoms and Treatment

Edited by Owen Collins

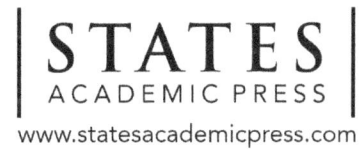

| STATES |
ACADEMIC PRESS
www.statesacademicpress.com

States Academic Press,
109 South 5th Street,
Brooklyn, NY 11249, USA

Visit us on the World Wide Web at:
www.statesacademicpress.com

ISBN: 978-1-63989-758-2

Cataloging-in-Publication Data

Bovine tuberculosis : causes, symptoms and treatment / edited by Owen Collins.
    p. cm.
Includes bibliographical references and index.
ISBN 978-1-63989-758-2
1. Tuberculosis in cattle. 2. Tuberculosis in cattle--Etiology. 3. Tuberculosis in cattle--Treatment.
4. Tuberculosis in cattle--Diagnosis. I. Collins, Owen.
SF808 .B68 2023
636.208 999 5--dc23

Table of Contents

Preface..IX

Chapter 1 **Whole Genome Sequencing for Determining the Source of** *Mycobacterium*
bovis **Infections in Livestock Herds and Wildlife in New Zealand**...........................1
Marian Price-Carter, Rudiger Brauning, Geoffrey W. de Lisle, Paul Livingstone,
Mark Neill, Jane Sinclair, Brent Paterson, Gillian Atkinson, Garry Knowles,
Kevin Crews, Joseph Crispell, Rowland Kao, Suelee Robbe-Austerman,
Tod Stuber, Julian Parkhill, James Wood, Simon Harris and Desmond M. Collins

Chapter 2 **The Distribution of Bovine Tuberculosis in Cattle Farms is Linked to Cattle**
Trade and Badger-Mediated Contact Networks in South-Western
France, 2007–2015...14
Malika Bouchez-Zacria, Aurélie Courcoul and Benoit Durand

Chapter 3 **Roll-Back Eradication of Bovine Tuberculosis (TB) from Wildlife in**
New Zealand: Concepts, Evolving Approaches and Progress.................................26
Graham Nugent, Andrew M. Gormley, Dean P. Anderson and Kevin Crews

Chapter 4 **Negotiated Management Strategies for Bovine Tuberculosis: Enhancing Risk**
Mitigation..37
Ruth A. Little

Chapter 5 **Exploring the Fate of Cattle Herds with Inconclusive Reactors to**
the Tuberculin Skin Test...49
Lucy A. Brunton, Alison Prosser, Dirk U. Pfeiffer and
Sara H. Downs

Chapter 6 **Persistent Spillback of Bovine Tuberculosis from White-Tailed Deer to Cattle in**
Michigan, USA: Status, Strategies and Needs...59
Kurt C. VerCauteren, Michael J. Lavelle and Henry Campa III

Chapter 7 **Validation of a Real-Time PCR for the Detection of** *Mycobacterium tuberculosis*
Complex Members in Bovine Tissue Samples..72
Victor Lorente-Leal, Emmanouil Liandris, Elena Castellanos, Javier Bezos,
Lucas Domínguez, Lucía de Juan and Beatriz Romero

Chapter 8 **TB Control in Humans and Animals in South Africa: A Perspective on**
Problems and Successes...81
Christina Meiring, Paul D. van Helden and Wynand J. Goosen

Chapter 9 **Modeling as a Decision Support Tool for Bovine TB Control**
Programs in Wildlife..88
Graham C. Smith and Richard J. Delahay

Chapter 10 *Mycobacterium caprae* Infection of Red Deer in Western Austria–Optimized
use of Pathology Data to Infer Infection Dynamics..96
Annette Nigsch, Walter Glawischnig, Zoltán Bagó and Norbert Greber

Chapter 11 **Development and Evaluation of a Serological Assay for the Diagnosis of
Tuberculosis in Alpacas and Llamas**..114
Jose A. Infantes-Lorenzo, Claire E. Whitehead, Inmaculada Moreno,
Javier Bezos, Alvaro Roy, Lucas Domínguez,
Mercedes Domínguez and Francisco J. Salguero

Chapter 12 **Impact of Genetic Selection for Increased Cattle Resistance to Bovine
Tuberculosis on Disease Transmission Dynamics**..121
Kethusegile Raphaka, Enrique Sánchez-Molano, Smaragda Tsairidou,
Osvaldo Anacleto, Elizabeth Janet Glass, John Arthur Woolliams,
Andrea Doeschl-Wilson and Georgios Banos

Chapter 13 **Wild Animal Tuberculosis: Stakeholder Value Systems and
Management of Disease**..135
Eamonn Gormley and Leigh A. L. Corner

Chapter 14 **Evaluation of Three Commercial Interferon-γ Assays in a Bovine
Tuberculosis Free Population**..153
Giovanni Ghielmetti, Patricia Landolt, Ute Friedel, Marina Morach,
Sonja Hartnack, Roger Stephan and Sarah Schmitt

Chapter 15 **Mycobacterial Infection of Precision-Cut Lung Slices Reveals Type 1
Interferon Pathway is Locally Induced by *Mycobacterium bovis*
but not *M. tuberculosis* in a Cattle Breed**..163
Aude Remot, Florence Carreras, Anthony Coupé, Émilie Doz-Deblauwe,
Maria L. Boschiroli, John A. Browne, Quentin Marquant, Delphyne Descamps,
Fabienne Archer, Abraham Aseffa, Pierre Germon,
Stephen V. Gordon and Nathalie Winter

Chapter 16 **Human-to-Cattle *Mycobacterium tuberculosis* Complex Transmission**..179
Jason E. Lombard, Elisabeth A. Patton, Suzanne N. Gibbons-Burgener,
Rachel F. Klos, Julie L. Tans-Kersten, Beth W. Carlson, Susan J. Keller,
Delora J. Pritschet, Susan Rollo, Tracey V. Dutcher, Cris A. Young,
William C. Hench, Tyler C. Thacker, Claudia Perea, Aaron D. Lehmkuhl and
Suelee Robbe-Austerman

Chapter 17 **Enhanced Detection of *Mycobacterium bovis*-Specific T Cells in
Experimentally-Infected Cattle**..190
Paola M. Boggiatto, Carly R. Kanipe and Mitchell V. Palmer

Chapter 18 **Whole Genome Sequencing Links *Mycobacterium bovis* from Cattle,
Cheese and Humans**..200
Alejandro Perera Ortiz, Claudia Perea, Enrique Davalos, Estela Flores Velázquez,
Karen Salazar González, Erika Rosas Camacho, Ethel Awilda García Latorre,
Citlaltepetl Salinas Lara, Raquel Muñiz Salazar, Doris M. Bravo,
Tod P. Stuber, Tyler C. Thacker and Suelee Robbe-Austerman

Chapter 19 **Evaluation of P22 ELISA for the Detection of *Mycobacterium bovis*-Specific Antibody in the Oral Fluid of Goats**..214
Javier Ortega, José A. Infantes-Lorenzo, Javier Bezos, Álvaro Roy,
Lucia de Juan, Beatriz Romero, Inmaculada Moreno, Alberto Gómez-Buendía,
Irene Agulló-Ros, Lucas Domínguez and Mercedes Domínguez

Chapter 20 **A Defined Antigen Skin Test for Diagnosis of Bovine Tuberculosis in Domestic Water Buffaloes (*Bubalus bubalis*)**..222
Tarun Kumar, Mahavir Singh, Babu Lal Jangir, Devan Arora, Sreenidhi Srinivasan,
Devender Bidhan, Dipin Chander Yadav, Maroudam Veerasami,
Douwe Bakker, Vivek Kapur and Naresh Jindal

Chapter 21 **Genotypic Characterization of *Mycobacterium bovis* Isolates from Dairy Cattle Diagnosed with Clinical Tuberculosis**..228
Elizabeth Hortêncio de Melo, Harrison Magdinier Gomes, Philip Noel Suffys,
Márcia Quinhones Pires Lopes, Raquel Lima de Figueiredo Teixeira,
Ícaro Rodrigues dos Santos, Marília Masello Junqueira Franco, Helio Langoni,
Antonio Carlos Paes, José Augusto Bastos Afonso and Carla Lopes de Mendonça

Permissions

List of Contributors

Index

Preface

The purpose of the book is to provide a glimpse into the dynamics and to present opinions and studies of some of the scientists engaged in the development of new ideas in the field from very different standpoints. This book will prove useful to students and researchers owing to its high content quality.

Bovine tuberculosis is an infectious disease that occurs in cattle and is primarily caused by Mycobacterium bovis. It is a zoonotic disease affecting the respiratory system of cattle. It affects domestic animals such as equines, sheep, goats, dogs, cats or pigs; and wild animal species such as antelopes, deer or boars. It is a source of infection for humans as well. The traces of bovine tuberculosis can be found in the lungs and throat of the affected cattle. The bacteria causing the disease are transmitted through the breath or discharge from mouth or nose of the affected cattle. The disease can spread in cattle through the placenta before birth, infected milk, and environmental contamination. The symptoms of bovine tuberculosis usually appear after months or years and include weakness, loss of appetite, weight-loss, intermittent hacking cough, and large prominent lymph nodes. There is no treatment available for this disease and the only way to be protected from this disease is through prevention. The other healthy members of the herd should not be exposed to the infected member. This book unravels the recent studies on the causes, symptoms and treatment of bovine tuberculosis. It will serve as a reference to a broad spectrum of readers.

At the end, I would like to appreciate all the efforts made by the authors in completing their chapters professionally. I express my deepest gratitude to all of them for contributing to this book by sharing their valuable works. A special thanks to my family and friends for their constant support in this journey.

Editor

Whole Genome Sequencing for Determining the Source of *Mycobacterium bovis* Infections in Livestock Herds and Wildlife in New Zealand

Marian Price-Carter [1]*, Rudiger Brauning [2], Geoffrey W. de Lisle [1], Paul Livingstone [3], Mark Neill [4], Jane Sinclair [5], Brent Paterson [6], Gillian Atkinson [7], Garry Knowles [8], Kevin Crews [4], Joseph Crispell [9], Rowland Kao [10], Suelee Robbe-Austerman [11], Tod Stuber [11], Julian Parkhill [12], James Wood [13], Simon Harris [12] and Desmond M. Collins [1]

[1] AgResearch, Hopkirk Research Institute, Palmerston North, New Zealand, [2] AgResearch, Invermay Agricultural Centre, Mosgiel, New Zealand, [3] TBfree NZ, Wellington, New Zealand, [4] TBfree NZ, Christchurch, New Zealand, [5] TBfree NZ, Hamilton, New Zealand, [6] TBfree NZ, Dunedin, New Zealand, [7] TBfree NZ, Palmerston North, New Zealand, [8] Aquaculture Veterinary Services Ltd., Clyde, New Zealand, [9] University College Dublin School of Veterinary Medicine, Dublin, Ireland, [10] Royal (Dick) School of Veterinary Studies and Roslin Institute, University of Edinburgh, Edinburgh, United Kingdom, [11] Diagnostic Bacteriology Laboratory, National Veterinary Services Laboratories, U.S. Department of Agriculture, Animal and Plant Health Inspection Service, Veterinary Service, Ames, IA, United States, [12] Wellcome Sanger Institute, Wellcome Genome Campus, Cambridge, United Kingdom, [13] Department of Veterinary Medicine, University of Cambridge, Cambridge, United Kingdom

*Correspondence:
Marian Price-Carter
marian.price-carter@agresearch.co.nz

The ability to DNA fingerprint *Mycobacterium bovis* isolates helped to define the role of wildlife in the persistence of bovine tuberculosis in New Zealand. DNA fingerprinting results currently help to guide wildlife control measures and also aid in tracing the source of infections that result from movement of livestock. During the last 5 years we have developed the ability to distinguish New Zealand (NZ) *M. bovis* isolates by comparing the sequences of whole genome sequenced (WGS) *M. bovis* samples. WGS provides much higher resolution than our other established typing methods and greatly improves the definition of the regional localization of NZ *M. bovis* types. Three outbreak investigations are described and results demonstrate how WGS analysis has led to the confirmation of epidemiological sourcing of infection, to better definition of new sources of infection by ruling out other possible sources, and has revealed probable wildlife infection in an area considered to be free of infected wildlife. The routine use of WGS analyses for sourcing new *M. bovis* infections will be an important component of the strategy employed to eradicate bovine TB from NZ livestock and wildlife.

Keywords: *Mycobacterium bovis*, molecular fingerprint, whole genome sequencing, New Zealand, bovine tuberculosis control, epidemiology

INTRODUCTION

Efforts to control bovine tuberculosis (TB) in domestic livestock in New Zealand (NZ) are driven by the zoonotic risk of the causative agent *Mycobacterium bovis* and its possible impacts on international trade (1, 2). Although in many countries bovine TB has been controlled successfully with test and slaughter strategies and movement restriction, control is particularly challenging in countries like NZ in which there is a wildlife reservoir of infection (1, 3). In Britain and Ireland the Eurasian badger harbors and spreads *M. bovis*, in France the wild boar, in Michigan and Minnesota in the USA, deer, and in NZ the brush-tail possum, [reviewed in (4)]. Effective control under these circumstances involves not only test and slaughter and movement control but also knowledge and control of the infection status in wildlife (3, 5). The challenges imposed in different parts of the world by these varied sources have been reviewed (6). Despite the challenging circumstances imposed by its wildlife reservoir, the control of bovine TB in NZ has recently been re-evaluated and there are now ambitious goals of achieving TB free livestock and wildlife by 2026 and 2040, respectively (2, 7).

Molecular methods provide a means to detect and characterize the spread of pathogens in both domestic livestock and in wildlife populations (3–5, 8). Studies in NZ that employed an early DNA fingerprinting assay that compared the restriction pattern of DNA digests (Restriction Endonuclease Analysis REA typing) of *M. bovis* isolates, demonstrated that livestock and wildlife in the same regions tended to share the same types and thus helped to define the role of wildlife in the spread of bovine TB in New Zealand (1, 9, 10). REA typing was used routinely for over 20 years to efficiently guide wildlife control measures and to aid in tracing the sources of infections that resulted from movement of livestock (10). In other parts of the world, comparison of the direct repeat region of the *M. bovis* chromosome by a process called spoligotyping, and a more sensitive PCR based method that compares repeated sequences at different sites in *M. bovis* genomes, [Variable Number Tandem Repeat (VNTR)] have been used for monitoring the genotypes of isolates from wildlife and livestock, providing insight into the types and spread of *M. bovis* (10–14). Because VNTR was simpler to perform and interpret than REA and was almost as discriminating, the REA method was replaced in NZ by VNTR in 2012 (15). VNTR fingerprint typing is routinely employed in NZ to determine the source of new livestock infections and the types carried by wildlife. In many cases VNTR clearly identifies the regional source of new infections, but it is of less use in cases where the same type is widespread in one or more regions of the country.

Recent advances in DNA sequencing have facilitated the routine comparisons of entire bacterial genomes [whole genome sequencing (WGS)] for determining the source of bacterial infections and this technology shows promise in aiding bovine TB control including situations that are complicated by wildlife reservoirs (4, 16–22). The single nucleotide polymorphism (SNP) lineages that result from WGS are far superior to the "types" that come from comparing a small number of sites in

Spoligo or VNTR typing analyses. There are typically tens to hundreds of SNPs common to a major branch, and 10 s of SNPs common to sub-clusters in each branch. Because so many more similarities and differences are considered in comparisons of lineages, there is less chance for misinterpretation of the relationship between isolates than when typing by VNTR (18, 23). In addition, these lineages provide information about shared common ancestors that is not always obvious by VNTR and spoligotyping. When coupled with knowledge of how quickly these bacteria accumulate new SNPs, this information can provide temporal clues about the arrival and divergence of types, which can greatly aid epidemiological investigations.

The rigor of WGS for elucidating phylogenetic relationships in NZ cycles was demonstrated with an analysis (24) performed on 296 NZ genomes that were available at the time. Four clades were identified and shown to have significant clustering by both REA type and by region but to lack significant clustering by host. These results verified the regional localization of types and rapid switching between wildlife and livestock hosts that was suggested by REA typing. With the extra resolution provided by WGS there were numerous instances where isolates that had identical REA types could now be distinguished. Analysis by a Bayesian approach (Bayesian Evolutionary Analysis by Sampling Trees BEAST) (25) on a subgroup for which there were an adequate number of wildlife and livestock isolates from one clade, that were spread over time, indicated that although there was significant variation, *M. bovis* in infected animals in NZ was accumulating mutations in a clocklike manner at a rate of 0.53 (2.5% Lower: 0.22, 97.5% Upper: 0.94) events per genome per year. The most recent common ancestor (MRCA) to this group was estimated to have been circulating in 1859 (2.5% Lower 1525 97.5% Upper 1936) which agreed with the time when *M. bovis* was likely to have been introduced into NZ in cattle imported directly and indirectly (via Australia) from the UK (26). This study provided convincing evidence that the enhanced resolution from WGS had potential to aid in more precisely determining whether new infections were from persistence or the introduction of infection into NZ livestock and wildlife populations.

Through partnership and contracted work with TBfree and collaborations with Wellcome Sanger Institute, the Wellcome Trust University of Glasgow, United States Department of Agriculture (USDA), Animal Health and Veterinary Laboratories Agency (AHVLA), Landcare Research and Massey University, we have developed a database with over 700 WGS entries of important NZ *M. bovis* types, and a data processing method that identifies robust SNPs that differ from a reference genome and compares these SNPs to those detected in other isolates. This information has helped to precisely define the lineage of NZ *M. bovis* types and has facilitated accurate determination of the source of new infections. Our WGS database has been enriched in recent years by characterizing additional isolates from recent herd breakdowns and outbreaks and the characterization by the WGS of REA and VNTR types that were once prevalent in NZ. Here we demonstrate the suitability of WGS for routine surveillance with three investigations into NZ. *M. bovis* outbreaks in which genetic relatedness of the isolates were determined by

---

Abbreviations: : *M. bovis*, *Mycobacterium bovis*; *M. tuberculosis*, *M. tuberculosis*; NZ, New Zealand; WGS, Whole Genome Sequencing; VNTR, Variable Number Tandem Repeat; REA, Restriction Enzyme Analysis; BEAST, Bayesian Evolutionary Analysis by Sampling Trees; AHVLA, Animal Health and Veterinary Laboratories Agency; USDA, United States Department of Agriculture; NZGL, New Zealand Genomics Limited; UK, United Kingdom; CTAB-N-cetyl-N,N,N-trimethyl ammonium bromide; BWA, Burrows, Wheeler Aligner; OTGO, Otago; CNI, Central North Island; WC, West Coast; PPD, purified protein derivative; Bo, bovine; Po, possum; Pi, pig; Ce, cervine; Fe, ferret; ML, Maximum Likelihood.

comparing these novel SNP lineages to others in the database. The benefits of WGS over REA and VNTR typing methods in each case are discussed.

MATERIALS AND METHODS

The AgResearch *M. bovis* archive has over 8000 NZ isolates that were cultured between 1985 and 2018, from livestock and wildlife suspected of *M. bovis* infection during the post-mortem examination performed as part of routine surveillance. Conventional microbiological tests [described in (27)] were used to positively identify *M. bovis* infection. The WGS database has been assembled by characterizing isolates from the archive selected to provide a representative sample of the *M. bovis* population circulating in cattle and wildlife across NZ between 1985 and 2018. Most isolates that were characterized by WGS were previously either REA typed (10) or VNTR typed (15) and in some cases were typed by both methods. Culture and DNA isolation was performed either at the AgResearch Wallaceville or the AgResearch Hopkirk sites in level 3 containment facilities, adhering to the biosafety guidelines for these procedures outlined in the AgResearch containment facility manual. A total of 783 isolates; 417 bovine, 112 ferret, 106 possum, 72 pig, 67 cervine, 3 feline, 2 stoat, 1 hedgehog, and 1 human isolate were characterized by WGS. Selected isolates were cultured in Tween albumin (TAB) media from frozen stock and DNA was prepared by CTAB extraction essentially as described in (28). DNA submitted for sequencing at the New Zealand Genomic Limited facility at Massey University in NZ (NZGL) and the United States Department of Agriculture (USDA) was additionally purified by digestion with 20 mg/ml RNAse after lysozyme treatment, and with a phenol chloroform isoamyl alcohol extraction after incubation in N-cetyl-N,N,N-trimethyl ammonium bromide (CTAB). DNA library preparation and genome sequencing were performed either at the USDA facility in Ames Iowa USA, at the NZGL facility at Massey University in NZ, or at The Wellcome Trust Glasgow facility in the UK, on an Illumina MiSeq instrument, with 2 X 250 bp paired-end reads or at the Wellcome Sanger Institute (Cambridge, UK) on an Illumina HiSeq instrument with 2×150 bp paired-end reads.

Raw genomic data were trimmed using the DynamicTrim algorithm (v2.0, default settings) in SolexaQA software (29) and mapped to the original UK reference genome (NC_002945.3, AF2122/97) (30) using the Burrows-Wheeler Aligner (BWA)-MEM algorithm (v0.7.9a-r786 with -M setting) in the BWA alignment tool (31). From the resulting alignments, reads that mapped to more than one location in the genome (SAM flags >= 256) were removed. Results were further processed with SAM tools software (32) (v0.1.19-44428cd with settings view -q 30; then rmdup -S) to remove low quality mappings and PCR duplicates. Indels and non A/C/T/G reference alleles were ignored, bcftools (v0.1.19-44428cd, with setting view -N -I -cvg). Subsequently a minimum alignment quality of 80, a minimum total depth per SNP of 10, a maximum reference allele count per SNP of 2, a maximum FQ value of −55, and a

reference to alternative allele ratio of at least 0.9 was enforced. Multiinter from the bedtools suite (v2.17.0) was used to generate a final list of potential genomic differences. SNPs detected in regions that are not well characterized by this methodology, (33) such as PE PGRS regions, IS elements, and poorly covered regions were excluded from the analyses via VCF software (34) (v0.1.12b). Poorly covered regions were defined by comparing 344 genomes with an average coverage of 45X or higher. Regions from which SNPs were excluded and also individual SNPs that were excluded from all of the genomes because they were poorly covered in some of the genomes are listed in **Supplementary File 1**. SNPs that were determined to be of high quality when detected in genomes with 45X or higher coverage and detected but filtered from more poorly covered genomes were added back to the filtered VCF files of the poorly covered genomes. The remaining core SNPs were processed together to produce concatenated alignments, which were compared in order to define the phylogenetic relationship of the isolates. A *Mycobacterium caprae* genome (strain 09-0454) is included as an out-group to root these comparisons. Average coverage and *in silico* spoligotyping were determined with vSNP software / https://github.com/USDA-VS/vSNP using the recently amended UK reference NC_002945.4 (35).

The relationship between isolates that are shown here were determined by BioNJ phylogenetic trees with 100 replicates, using a Jukes and Cantor model with SeaView 4 software (36) and also with RAxML software (37) (version raxmlHPC-PTHREADS-SSE3) with 1000 replicates using a GTRGAMMAI model. BioNJ and RAxML Phylogenetic trees were compared side by side using Phylo.io software (38) and were displayed and colored for other Figures using FigTree v1.4.2 software (39). Distance matrices were generated from concatenated SNP sequences with the Muscle Aligner (40) in the Geneious software package and were colored using the color scale formatter in Excel or alternatively with an R script that uses R's Gplot package to create heat maps via the heatmap.2() function. Global distributions of the four major NZ spoligotypes were obtained with the similarity search tool at the Pasteur-Guadeloupe website http://www.pasteur-guadeloupe.fr:8081/SpolSimilaritySearch/ (41).

RESULTS

A total of 782 *M. bovis* genomes were used here as a basis for comparison of NZ breakdowns and outbreaks. The alignment length for this selection of isolates was 8261 sites. Metadata, coverage statistics and the *in silico* spoligotyping results for these isolates are listed in the spreadsheet in **Supplementary File 2**. The time span for these isolates is 30 years from 1988 to 2018 and includes representatives of important types from throughout the North and South Island. The relationship of prevalent NZ *M. bovis* types is illustrated by the SNP phylogeny that was generated by maximum likelihood analysis in **Figure 1** and is compared to a phylogeny determined by the BioNJ distance method in **Supplementary File 3**. Several genomes from overseas *M. bovis* isolates, including the PPD strain AN5, and three isolates from the USDA elite collection (05_8628, 94_5053, and 12_1874) are included to aid with these comparisons. The 4 distinct branches that were initially detected (24) were also evident in this larger group, and each clade was shown here to share more recent common ancestors with overseas isolates than with other NZ isolates. The same relationship was evident by a BioNJ distance analysis, perhaps reflecting the clonal, primarily non-recombining nature of NZ *M. bovis* evolution (see **Supplementary File 3a**). As was seen in the initial characterization (24) of a subset of these isolates, WGS results for this larger group of isolates corroborate findings from previous REA and VNTR typing studies which revealed that distinct types predominate in different parts of NZ (9, 10, 15).

In silico spoligotyping revealed that most of the NZ isolates in the database have spoligotypes that were common in the UK when cattle were imported into NZ in late 1860s (42), 34% were SB0130 and 41% were SB0140. Two other prevalent spoligotypes that were characterized extensively were SB1504, (121 isolates 15%) a type that is endemic in the Marlborough North Canterbury region of the South Island and SB1031 (23 isolates 3%) a type that is endemic in Southland in the South Island (see the map presented in **Figure 2B**) and was once prevalent in Australia (43). The Global distribution of these types is illustrated in the **Supplementary File 4**. Although SB0130, SB0140 and SB1031 have been isolated in other parts of the world (43), SB1504 has so far only been detected in NZ, suggesting either that it evolved from a different type just prior to becoming established in NZ or that other global sources of this type have not yet been discovered.

The phylogenetic relationship and geographical source of the three outbreaks investigations that will be discussed below are described in the phylogeny in **Figure 2A** and map in **Figure 2B**. Infections that were investigated were from (A) Mt. Cargill in Otago, (B) South Westland in the South Island, and (C) Waiuku in the Central North Island (CNI).

Mt. Cargill Outbreak

An investigation of isolates from the Mt. Cargill region of the South Island was carried out to aid in determining the source of this recent infection, which appeared to have spread throughout the Mt. Cargill region within 1–2 years. We analyzed three groups of isolates: (i) isolates from recently infected cattle (9 isolates), farmed deer (2 isolates) and wildlife (14 isolates) in the region; (ii) a selection of isolates (5 cattle, 5 wildlife) from the AgResearch strain archive that had come from sources within 15 km of the outbreak; and (iii) a group of recent cattle isolates with similar types (AgR1665 type VNTR104, AgR1689 type VNTR135 and AgR1669 VNTR27) to those found in the Mt. Cargill region that had come from outside Mt. Cargill. All isolates were characterized by WGS in order to determine if this outbreak was from local wildlife reinfection, or from introduction of a different type into the region. Also shown in the accompanying figures are the relationship of these outbreak investigation isolates to previously characterized Otago isolates (AgR96, AgR707,

AgR703, AgR726, AgR734, AgR51, AgR76, and AgR53) in the WGS database.

Results of this investigation are shown in (a) SNP Table and (b) the Phylogram (C) the Map in **Figure 3**. When WGS data for Mt Cargill outbreak isolates was compared to WGS data for the other isolates that were characterized for this investigation, the Mt. Cargill outbreak isolates (boxed in purple in **Figure 3a**) shared their most recent common ancestors with livestock and wildlife isolates from more than 20 km north of Mt Cargill and were more distantly related to the other examined types that were prevalent in the nearest known wildlife/domestic stock cases from west of Mount Cargill. The closest known relative to the outbreak was a 2012 isolate (AgR1665) from Waikouaiti (see the SNP table in **Figure 3a**). AgR1665 was missing one SNP that was common to the outbreak isolates, a C to T change at position 4328907 in the reference genome, but had the 11 others that were common to the outbreak cluster. Using the mutation rate estimate from Crispell et al. [0.53 (2.5% Lower: 0.22, 97.5% Upper: 0.94)] this suggests that this likely precursor and the Mt. Cargill outbreak lineage diverged from a common ancestor approximately 2 (3–7) years prior to when the 2012 precursor isolate was detected. The next closest known relatives were several wildlife isolates from northern Otago (AgR707, AgR96, and AgR1673). Mt Cargill isolates shared 10 common SNPs with these wildlife isolates. The Mt. Cargill and North Otago wildlife isolates shared 2 SNPs with recently characterized isolates from Northern Otago (AgR1717 and AgR1666, boxed in yellow in the phylogenetic tree in **Figure 3b** and indicated by yellow symbols on the map in **Figure 3c**). Both groups had acquired numerous SNPs (>20) since diverging from their common ancestor. These results provide evidence to suggest that this type had prevailed in Northern Otago for many years. **Supplementary File 3b** compares the relationship of these isolates by maximum likelihood and BioNJ distance analyses, and the conclusions drawn about the relationship of these isolates was the same regardless of the phylogenetic method used for the analysis perhaps because of the many SNPs that were common to the outbreak isolates and their closest known relatives. Although these results did not rule out the possibility that the infection was circulating undetected in the Mt Cargill region previous to the outbreak, our WGS comparison of outbreak isolates to common wildlife and livestock types suggest that this infection is more likely to have moved into Mt. Cargill from wildlife or livestock from the north than to have come from local wildlife. A direction of the spread of this infection based on these data is indicated by the arrows on the map in **Figure 3c**.

Although in most cases VNTR types of these isolates correlated well with SNP sub-clusters, since the closest relative, a 2012 Waikouaiti cattle isolate (AgR1665) had a slightly variant VNTR type (see the VNTR104 types tabulated in **Figure 3b**), if the Mt. Cargill outbreak investigation was based solely on VNTR results the relevance of this isolate to the outbreak would be much less evident than it is from the SNP lineage. This tree also illustrates how the SNP lineage determined by WGS defines the relationship between early isolates that were originally characterized only by REA to later isolates that were originally

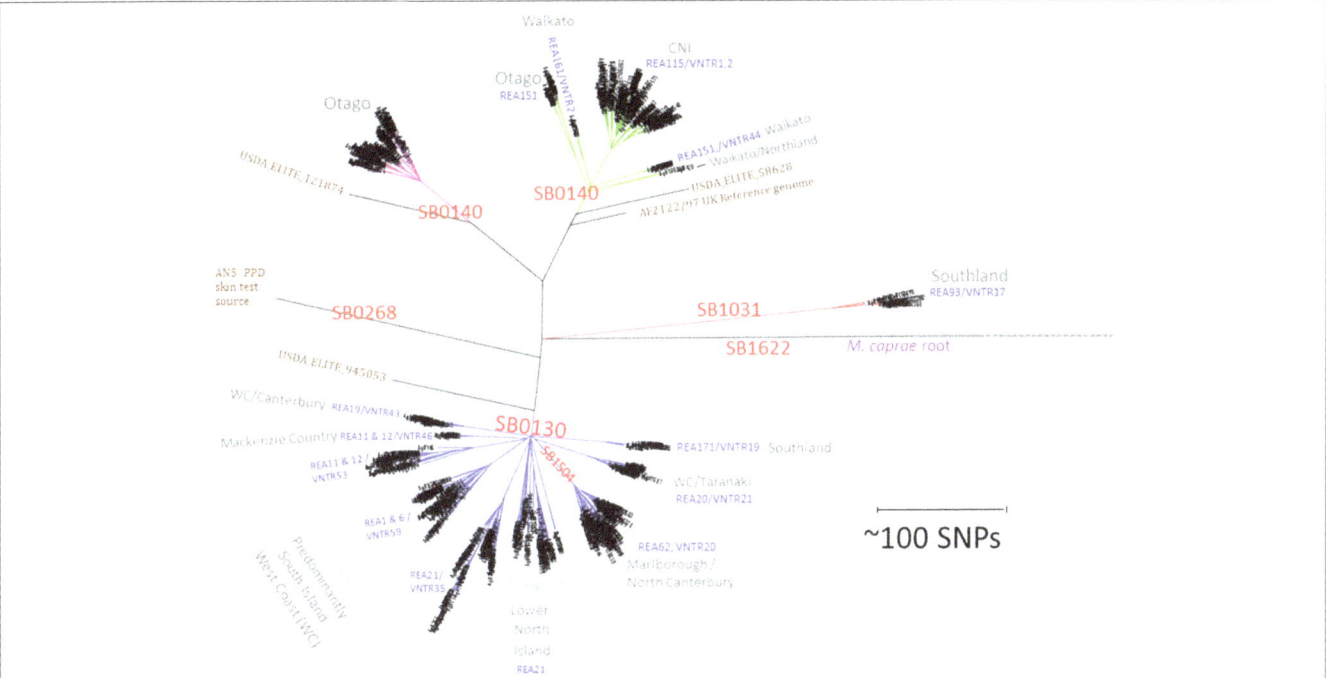

FIGURE 1 | NZ *M. bovis* types. Radial Maximum Likelihood (ML) Phylogram illustrating the relationship of NZ *M. bovis* isolates in the NZ WGS database. The scale bar indicates the approximate distance in SNPs between isolates. "SB" numbers labeled in red are internationally recognized spoligotypes based on differences in the DR/CRISPR region. The REA and VNTR types listed in blue text are the predominant REA type(s) and or VNTR types in the indicated cluster and they are predominant in regions listed in gray. Overseas isolates that are included for comparison are labeled in brown: the UK reference (AF2122/97), the UK strain commonly used as a source of PPD (AN5) and 3 USDA ELITE strains (58628, 945053, and 121874). The branches in the four NZ clusters are colored differently to highlight the distinction from other branches.

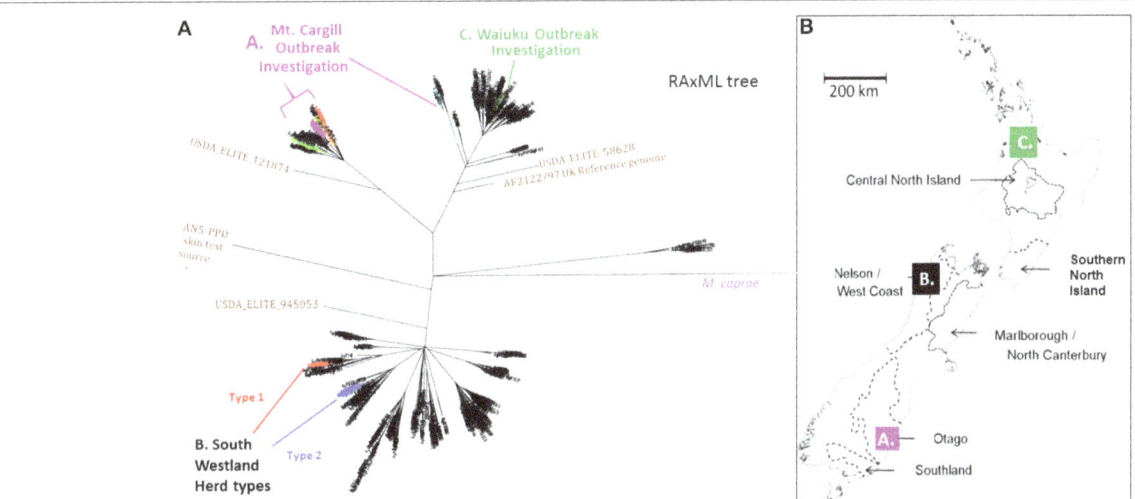

FIGURE 2 | (A) NZ *M. bovis* Radial ML Phylogram illustrating the Phylogenetic relationship of the isolates that will be discussed in more detail below. (A) Mt. Cargill investigation isolates-These isolates cluster in the Otago clade and are colored the same as in the boxed sub-groups in Phylogram in **Figure 3a**. (B) South Westland breakdown types- The two types isolated from the herd in South Westland and the closest relatives (shown in SNP tables in **Figure 4B**) are colored differently; the breakdown type 1 isolate clusters in the VNTR53 group and it and its closest known relatives are colored red, the breakdown type 2 isolates clusters in the VNTR59 subgroup and it and its closest known relatives are colored blue. (C) Waiuku outbreak- isolates cluster in the CNI clade and outbreak isolates described in the SNP table in **Figure 6B** are colored green. **(B)** Map of NZ indicating vector risk areas (shaded regions) and illustrating geographical source of the isolates from the three outbreak investigations described below. Colored squares on the map indicate the regions of the discussed outbreak investigations. The three different investigations that will be discussed below are indicated by letters and color in the Phylogram in **(A)** and the map in **(B)**.

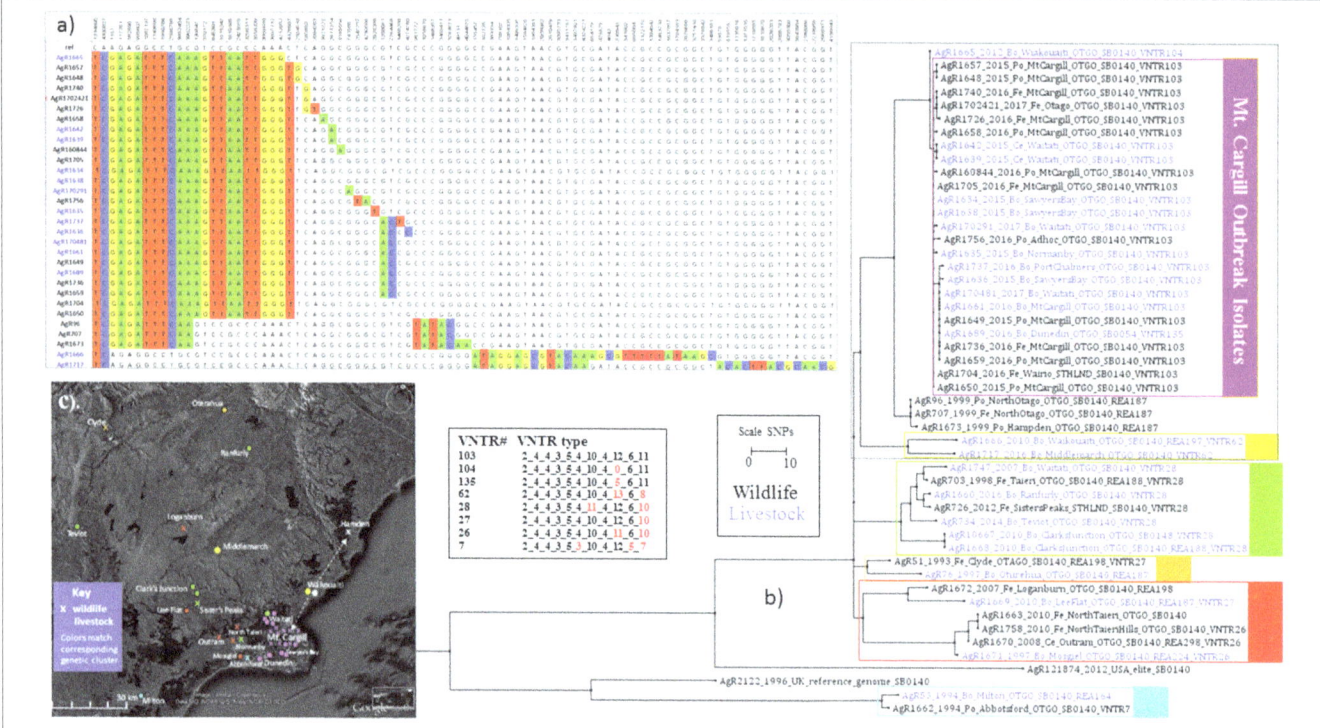

FIGURE 3 | Mt. Cargill Outbreak Investigation. Genetic and spatial relationship of *M. bovis* isolates from southeast Otago. **(a)** SNP table and Phylogram for selected isolates from the Otago cluster. The SNP table illustrates SNP differences in outbreak isolates and their closest known relatives. Chromosomal positions in genomic reference NC_002945.3 are listed across the top. The DNA base found at the indicated chromosomal position in the reference is listed in the next line. DNA bases in the table are colored to indicate differences from the reference genome. **(b)** Square ML Phylogram. The scale bar indicates the distance in SNPs between isolates displayed in the phylograph. Livestock metadata in the tree (_Bo_ for bovine _Ce_ for cervine) is colored blue and wildlife metadata (_Po_ for possum, _Fe_ for ferret), is colored black. The numbers for the listed VNTR types are the number of repeats at the 11 loci as described in Price-Carter et al. (15): Miru40_EtrD_EtrC_EtrE_NZ2_ QUB18_QUB11a_QUB26_DR2_DR1_QUB3232. Red numbers in this VNTR table indicate differences from the outbreak type VNTR103. **(c)** Map of sources of isolates shown in the phylogenetic tree in **(b)**. Symbols on the map indicate the approximate regional sources and are colored to match the genetic cluster of the isolate as indicated by the boxes in **(b)**. The arrows on the map in **(c)** indicate the proposed direction of the spread of this infection based on WGS results.

characterized only by VNTR, which can be very helpful when trying to understand the source of new infections.

South Westland TB Infected Herd

Results from the investigation into the findings of TB cases in a previously disease free dairy herd located in South Westland, West Coast, South Island are shown in **Figures 4, 5** and **Supplementary Files 3c,d,** and **5**). The herd had two separate findings of bovine tuberculosis approximately 5 months apart. There was a clear herd skin test between the two animals being identified at slaughter. Both TB cases were considered to be anergic animals (infected but not detectable through our standard testing procedures) as they were not identified as infected until they were inspected at slaughter, and both animals had been repeatedly TB skin tested before and after leaving their herd of origin.

These isolates were two distinct VNTR types; the first TB case (AgR738) was identified as type VNTR59, and the second case TB case (AgR744) was identified as type VNTR53 (see **Figures 4A,B** and **Supplementary File 5**). The Phylogram in **Figure 4A** illustrates the phylogenetic relationship of the isolates of these two types to others of these types in the

database. This Phylogram was determined by ML analysis. The same relationship was evident by BioNJ analysis (see **Supplementary Files 3c,d**). The distinguishing SNPs in the SNP tables in **Figure 4B** provide a more detailed comparison of the differences between these TB isolates and their closest relatives. WGS clearly demonstrated the close relationship between the isolates and those from historic cases linked to the original locations of these animals. Animal movements were traced using information collected at the time of the epidemiological investigation. Animal identification and movement records were scrutinized as well as gathering information directly from farmers at that time. Although the two types that were detected in this herd could be distinguished from each other by VNTR assay, WGS analysis has allowed these to be compared to other isolates and confirm the most likely transmission pathway (see the square Phylograms in **Supplementary File 5**).

WGS clearly narrowed the list of likely suspects in each case. The isolate from the first TB case (AgR738) was identical or nearly identical by WGS to isolates from a recent outbreak up the coast in the Kowhitirangi and Arahura regions (see the SNP table **Figure 4B**). All of these outbreak isolates appeared to share

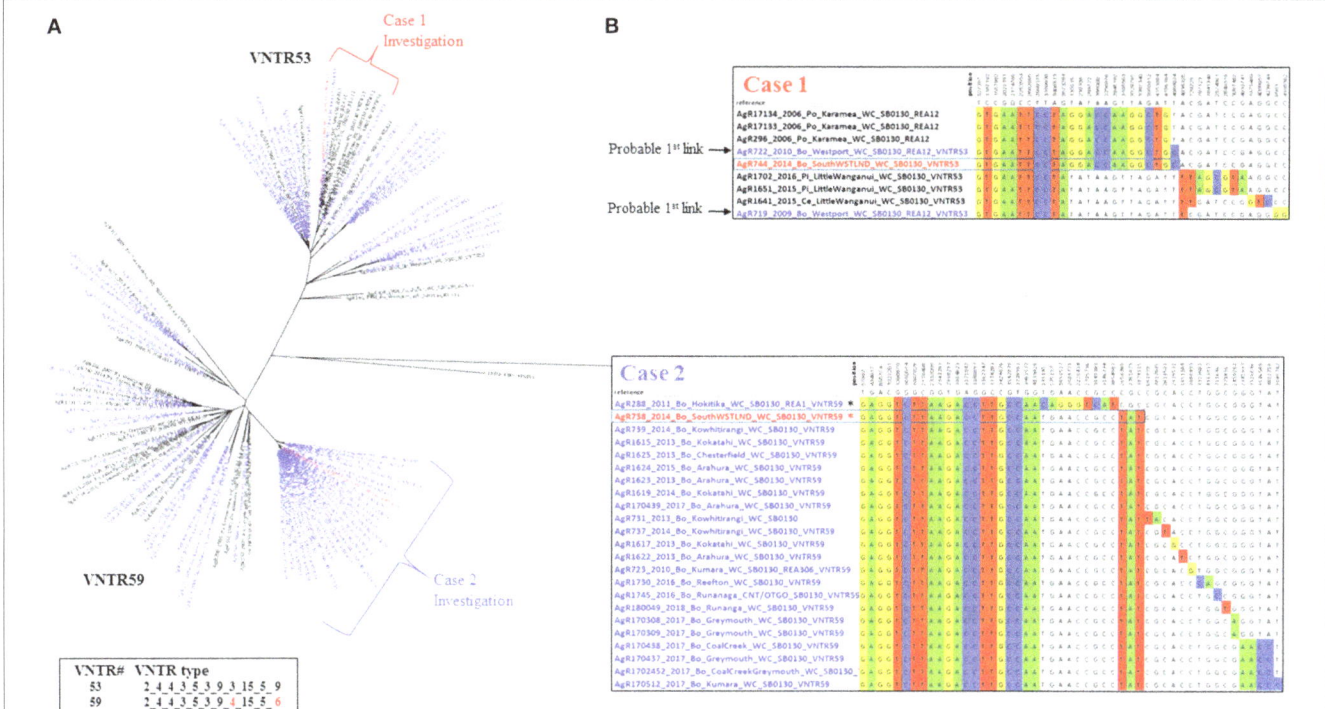

FIGURE 4 | Multiple South Westland herd infections. **(A)** Radial ML Phylogram illustrating the genetic relationship of the two types of *M. bovis* isolates detected during a South Westland breakdown investigation, to other type VNTR59/REA1/REA6 and VNTR53/REA11/REA12 *M. bovis* isolates in the database. Metadata for isolates from this herd are colored red, other livestock metadata are colored blue and wildlife metadata black. Brackets indicate close relatives of the breakdown isolates and are also described in the SNP table in **(B)**. Also shown are the two different VNTR types, with numbering as described in the legend for **Figure 3**. **(B)** SNP tables illustrating the relationship of each type to its closest relatives. The coloring and numbering in this tables is as described in **Figure 3**. SNPs detected in the case 1 and in case 2 isolates are boxed within the table. The asterisk in the case 2 table indicates an isolate (AgR288) that was ruled out as a possible source of infection by this investigation.

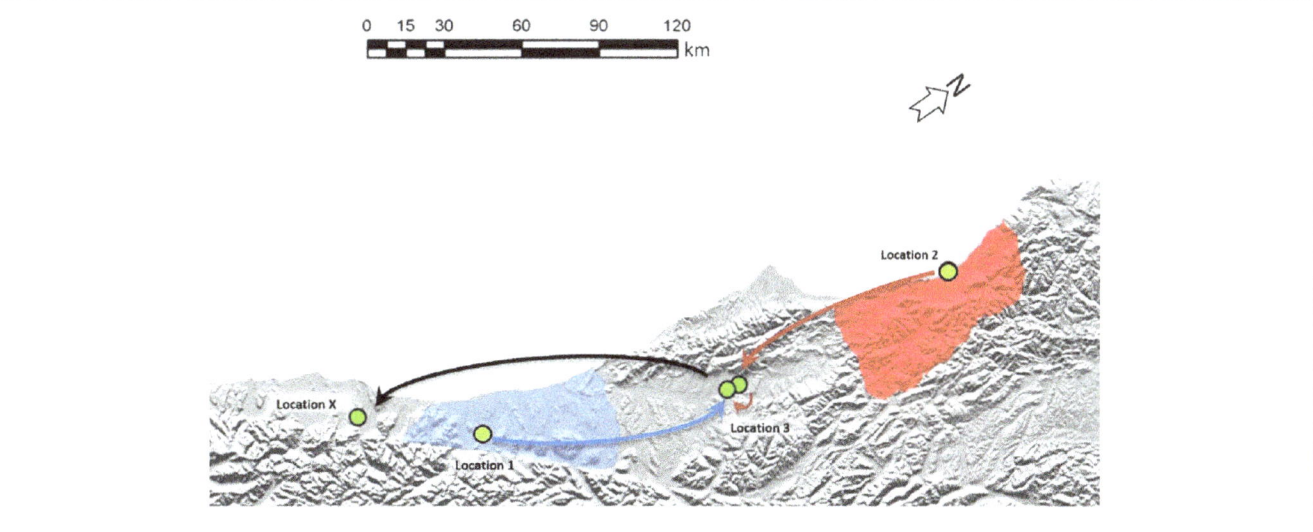

FIGURE 5 | Two separate origins of TB in a South Westland Herd. Cattle movements that led to these two types of infection in the South Westland herd are indicated by arrows. Green circles indicate approximate locations where these animals resided. Shaded areas on the map indicate regions where VNTR53/REA11/REA12 (red) and VNTR59/REA1/REA6 (blue) are endemic in wildlife populations. TB case 1 moved from Location 1 to location 3 before moving to Location X (from where it was identified as TB positive at routine slaughter). TB case 2 was moved from its herd of origin in location 2 to a farm near Location 3 before moving to location 3 and then on to Location X from where it was identified as being infected. The region described here is indicated by the black box in the map in **Figure 2A**.

a recent common ancestor with AgR288, a 2011 cattle beast isolate from a Hokitika farm, and this was thought to be a likely original source, but this isolate was ruled out as a source for the outbreak by WGS, since it was missing the 3 SNPs that are common to the outbreak and had additional SNPs not found in the outbreak isolates (**Figure 4B**). By WGS, the isolate from the second TB case (AgR744) was identical to AgR722, a livestock isolate from Westport, over 170 km from Location X and shared a recent common ancestor with several wildlife isolates (AgR296, AgR17133, AgR17134) from Karamea (location 2) which is over 250 km from Location X (see SNP tables in **figure 4B** and the map in **Figure 5**). Although all four locations on which the animals resided are within a formal Movement Control Area (MCA) where all stock over 12 months of age are to be tested annually AND all stock that are moved are to be TB tested within the 60 days preceding the movement, these results suggests that this infection has most likely resulted from the long distance movement of infected livestock.

Waiuku Outbreak Investigation

The investigation of the *M. bovis* outbreak that began in Waiuku, Central North Island clearly illustrated the close relationship of epidemiologically linked livestock isolates and demonstrated their more distant relationship to other types from the Central North Island (see the Phylogram in **Figure 6A**). The relationship of isolates in the green colored portion of the Phylogram in **Figure 5A** was compared by maximum likelihood and BioNJ methods (**Supplementary File 3e**) and found to be nearly identical by both methods.

There were two cycles of infection associated with this outbreak, the first occurred between 2007 and 2010 and the second in 2013 (see **Figure 7a**). When compared by WGS, there were 10 SNPs detected that were common to both early and later outbreak isolates (see the SNP table in **Figure 6B**) suggesting that both outbreaks were from the same source of infection rather than from two different types introduced into the area. This infection was spread to herds in other regions of the Central North Island (**Figure 7**). Although no infection was detected from the likely source of this spread (black box in **Figure 7a**), isolates from infected animals that had been moved from this herd shared the 10 SNPs that were common to this outbreak (6b).

The relationship of Waiuku outbreak isolates to the closest known wildlife isolates in the database, recent pig isolates from Hauturu (AgR16102 and AgR730),Tihoi (AgR17003411) and Hauhungaroa (AgR1704532) as well as a possum isolate from 2001 (AgR1795) from Taumaranui, are also shown in the SNP table in **Figure 6B**. These results indicate that these wildlife isolates share a common ancestor with the outbreak isolates but they do not have the 10 outbreak specific SNPs and have acquired 13-15 SNPs that were not detected in the outbreak isolate genomes indicating that they are not closely related.

By combining epidemiological investigation with SNP lineage comparisons, far more insight is gained than was possible by VNTR or REA typing. A good example of this is provided by a SNP detected in isolates from livestock in Waiuku that were not known to be linked by movement but were farmed within 4 km of one another (AgR508, AgR546, and AgR548, boxed in black in the SNP table in **Figure 6B** and circled in the transmission path diagram in **Figure 7**) suggesting perhaps that despite extensive surveillance, there may have been either a wildlife vector for this Waiuku infection, or alternatively that there was undocumented herd movement occurring.

Distance of Epidemiologically Linked Isolates

Genetic pairwise distances are the number of SNPs that differ when two isolates are compared. **Table 1** compares pairwise distances for the epidemiologically linked isolates discussed above and the heat map in **Figure 8** and in **Supplementary File 6** show pairwise distances for all of the isolates illustrated for the three discussed investigations. Mt. Cargill isolates were collected over a period of 5 years and differed from one another by 0-5 SNPs. AgR 738, the case 2 isolate from the South Westland herd and its 22 close relatives from the Kowhitirangi outbreak were collected over a period of approximately 5 years, and differed from one another by 0–7 SNPs. The 12 Waiuku outbreak isolates were collected over a period of 6 years and differed from one another by 0–9 SNPs. The New Zealand *M. bovis* mutation rate determined by Crispell et al. (24) (0.53 with a range 0.22–0.94) was closest to that estimated for human tuberculosis by Walker et al. (44) (0.5 with a range of 0.3–0.7), and the pairwise distances of epidemiologically linked isolates shown in **Table 1** are within the 12 SNP limit for epidemiological linkage determined by Walker and colleagues for *Mycobacterium tuberculosis*. These groups of isolates differ from unlinked isolates of the same types by 10's of SNPs and from isolates from other branches of the phylogenetic tree by hundreds of SNPs (see heat maps is **Figure 8** and the more detailed versions in **Supplementary File 6**).

DISCUSSION

Results of our current investigation demonstrated the same overall relationship of types described previously, since by WGS isolates cluster into the same groups that were determined by REA and VNTR analysis, but with the much finer resolution provided by WGS there is increased ability to rule out likely sources of infection. *In silico* spoligotyping confirmed that at least three of the four detected clades were likely to have been imported along with British sources of cattle in the middle to late 1800s. The regional clustering of types determined with REA and VNTR methods was corroborated since livestock and wildlife from the same region clustered. The Mt. Cargill and South Westland investigations illustrated how WGS leads to better definition of the source of new infections by ruling out potential sources, and all three investigations have led to the confirmation of epidemiological sourcing of infection. In addition, the Waiuku investigation indicated probable wildlife infection in an area considered to be free of infection.

The neighbor joining method is often considered useful for getting a quick approximate idea of genetic relationships because it is based principally on genetic distances, and does not incorporate the more accurate models of sequence evolution that are exploited in maximum likelihood analysis. The strikingly

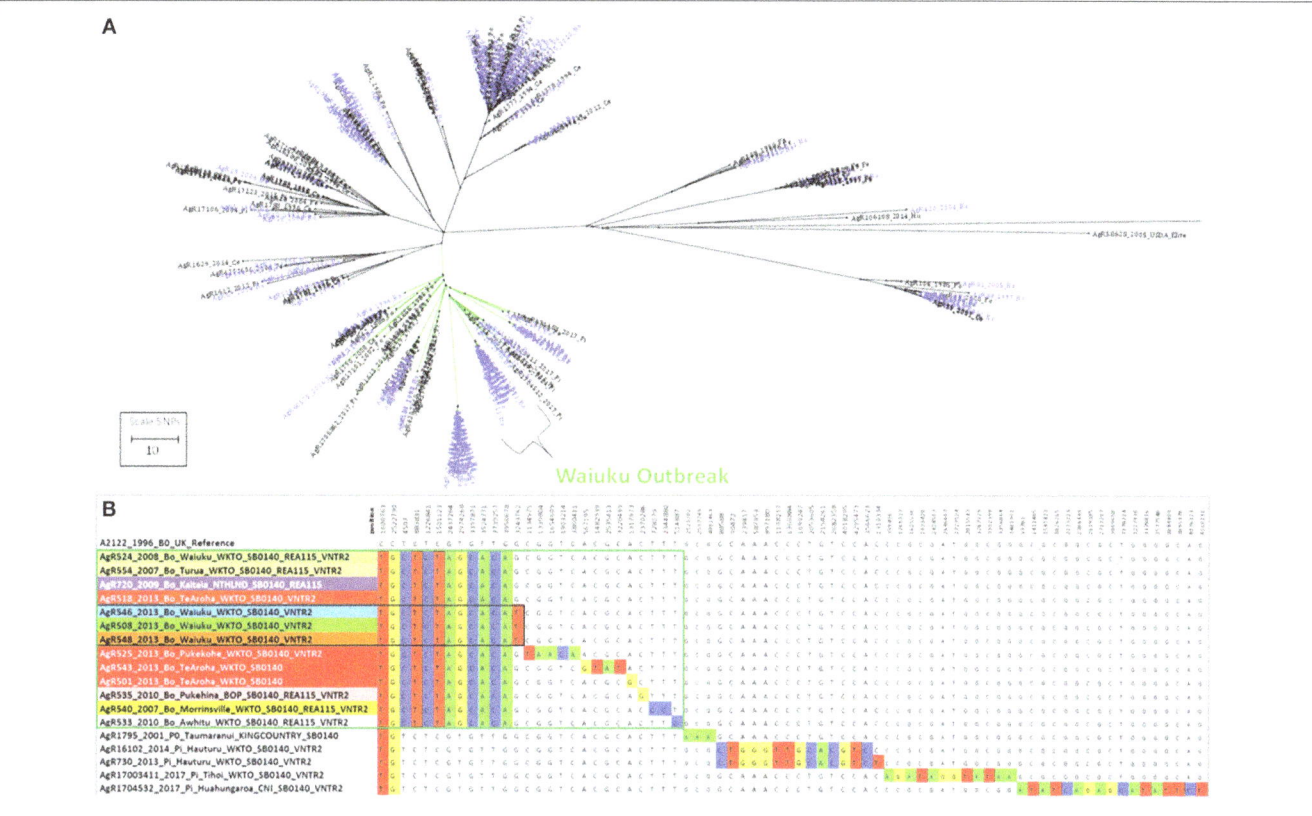

FIGURE 6 | Genetic relationship of Waiuku outbreak Isolates. **(A)** Radial ML Phylogram illustrating the genetic relationship of *M. bovis* isolates from the Waiuku outbreak to other livestock and wildlife isolates in the Central North Island cluster. Livestock metadata are colored blue and wildlife metadata black. Waiuku isolates are indicated by the bracket. The green colored branch indicates the isolates that are compared in **Supplementary File 3e**. **(B)** The relationship of isolates from the Waiuku outbreak is illustrated in a SNP table with DNA bases in the table colored to indicate differences from the reference genome. Metadata for isolates from different herds that were characterized by WGS are shaded differently. Waiuku outbreak isolates characterized for this investigation are boxed in green. Isolates that are boxed in black were not known to be linked by movement but were from farms within 4 km of one another.

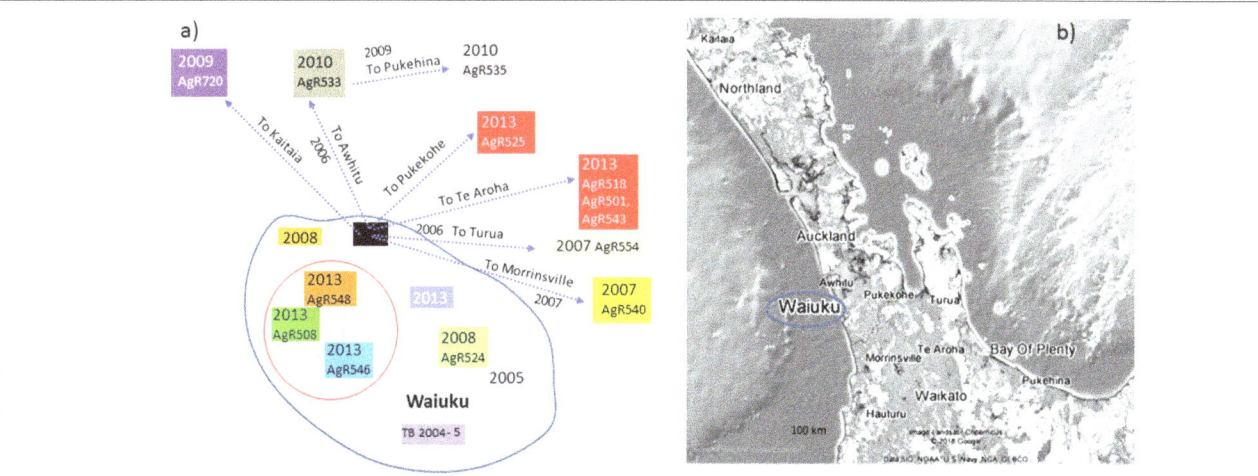

FIGURE 7 | Waiuku outbreak Transmission path. **(a)** The direction of spread deciphered from epidemiological investigation, **(b)** a map illustrating the geographical sources of the characterized isolates. Isolates that have been characterized by WGS are colored to match the genomic data shown in the SNP table in **Figure 6B**. Colored boxes without AgR numbers represent isolates that were not characterized by WGS. Isolates that are circled in red were not known to be linked by movement but were from farms within 4 km of one another.

TABLE 1 | Pairwise genomic distances of epidemiologically linked isolates.

Outbreak	Number of isolates	Time span	Approx. # years	Pairwise distance (SNPs)	Hosts	VNTR
Mt. Cargill	26	2012–2017	5–6	0–5	cattle, deer, possum	103
Kowhitirangi	23	2013–2018	5–6	0–7	cattle	59
Waiuku	12	2007–2013	6–7	0–9	cattle	2

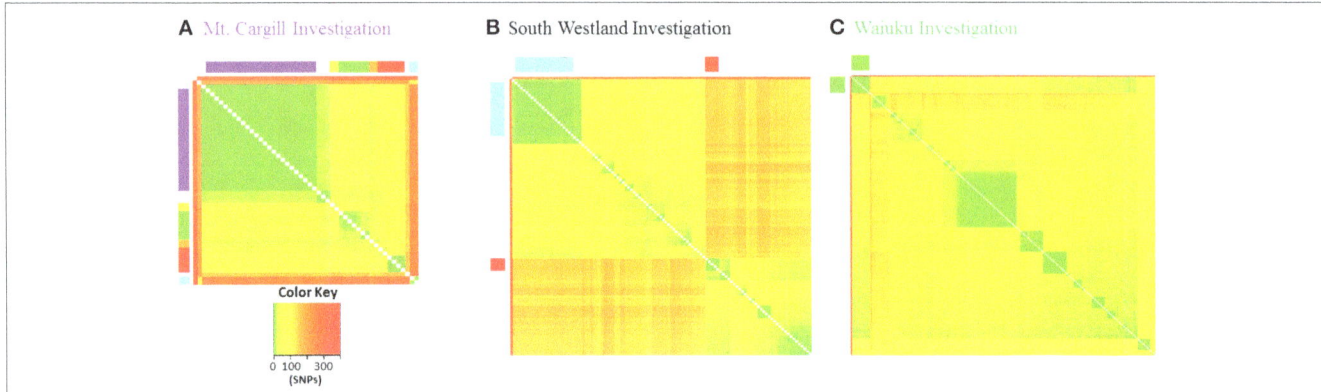

FIGURE 8 | Pairwise genetic distance heat maps. Distance in SNPs between pairs of isolates is illustrated by the different colors as indicated in the color key. **(A)** Mt. Cargill outbreak isolates are in the same order as in the Phylogram in **Figure 3** and colors along the outside of the plot correspond to those in the Phylogram and also to those in the more detailed distance plots in **Supplementary File 6**. **(B)** VNTR53 and VNTR59 isolates. Close relatives of South Westland breakdown type 1 are indicated by red squares and type 2 by the blue rectangles along the outside of the plot. Isolates are in the same order as in the more detailed distance plots in **Supplementary File 6**. **(C)** CNI branch isolates. Waiuku outbreak isolates are indicated by the green squares along the outside of the plot.

similar relationships determined for NZ *M. bovis* isolates by the maximum likelihood, neighbor joining distance methods and SNP tables, suggest that when analyzed by our WGS method, *M. bovis* in NZ cycles of animal infection appears to be evolving in a manner that is well described by incremental changes in genetic distance-clonal evolution. These results are in agreement with the evolutionary mechanism suggested in Smith et al. (45) where it was noted that these bacteria do not tend to carry or incorporate foreign DNA and that their genomes evolve primarily by deletions and the acquisition of SNPs.

The numerous SNPs that are shared by and distinguish members within and between groups give a much more robust indication of the relationship of isolates than our previous typing methods. In most cases the same REA and VNTR types tended to be grouped into one WGS cluster, but in several situations WGS revealed flaws in the apparent relationship of types determined by the other molecular methods. Several instances of homoplasy (the detection of the same REA or VNTR type in distantly related WGS clusters) were revealed during the course of our characterization of NZ types. For example, although most VNTR types tended to cluster into only one sub-group in the Otago branch, type VNTR27 isolates cluster in several different groups (see the phylogenetic tree in **Figure 3b**). This clustering of unrelated types has been described in other comparisons of WGS to VNTR typing (23, 46, 47). There were also several instances where types tended to switch back and forth within a subgroup, (see REA types 11 and 12 and REA types 1 and

6 in the tree in **Supplementary Figure 5**), as was observed by Trewby et al. (18).

Although WGS is far superior to our previous typing methods there are factors that limit the usefulness of WGS data for epidemiological investigations. *M. bovis* accumulates mutations in a clocklike manner, but the fixation of new changes into the population is slow and highly variable over short times. For an example see the SNP table in **Figure 6B**. Waiuku outbreak strains isolated within a year of one another varied by 0–5 SNPs. This variability has been noted in other *M. bovis* (16) and *M. tuberculosis* studies (48), and can make it difficult to determine whether the transmission is occurring within the herd or from local wildlife reinfection. This high variability over short times also makes it difficult to use Bayesian techniques such as BEAST for reconstructing recent local transmission pathways since there is not enough of a consistent temporal signal. Because the *M. bovis* lifestyle switches between an active systemic infection and a localized (difficult to detect) latent infection the time of infection is not necessarily close to the time of isolation. This makes it more difficult to determine when a new infection was introduced. When sampling disease with a wildlife reservoir the data may represent a low proportion of the total infection and it can therefore be difficult to draw valid conclusions about the direction of transmission. This influence of sampling bias was clearly illustrated in our previous work (24). In the current study, the finding of no close links between wildlife and Waiuku livestock may be because this type evolved in livestock populations and therefore there is no transmission linkage with wildlife but it could also be because the wildlife source was not sampled. This same factor weakens the conclusion drawn in the Otago study; although our analyses seem to indicate the infection in Mt Cargill came into the area in infected livestock, because of uneven sampling we cannot be 100% certain that the infection had not spread from an undetected local wildlife source.

The phylogeny in **Figure 1** illustrates that NZ types share common ancestors with types isolated in other parts of the world [also see **Supplementary File 4** and (43)]. We noted previously (24) that NZ strains tended to accumulate mutations at a faster rate than their UK relatives and surmised that the enhanced mutation rate may be the result of the larger amount of bacterial growth in possums, the major wildlife reservoir. Teasing apart these types of differences may be helpful for understanding transmission pathways in other bovine TB cycles.

CONCLUSION

As the NZ epidemic diminishes, accuracy and high resolution becomes even more important for the identification of true sources. By ruling out possible sources of infection the enhanced resolution provided by WGS will likely reduce expenditure on the monitoring of herd infections and of wildlife monitoring and control. The routine use of WGS analyses for determining the source of *M. bovis* infections will be an important component of the strategy employed to eradicate bovine TB from NZ.

AUTHOR CONTRIBUTIONS

MP-C coordinated sequencing and data processing and drafted and revised the manuscript. DC, MP-C, GdL, and PL designed the analysis. RB developed data processing python scripts for mapping filtering and labeling genomic data. RB and MN developed figures. MN and JS shared results of epidemiological investigations, MN drafted a section of the manuscript, DC, GdL, PL, MN, JS, GK, GA, and KC were involved with selection of the isolates and interpretation of results. DC, GD, MP-C, and BP were involved with typing of isolates. JP, SH, and JW provided 200 sequences from Wellcome Sanger. RK provided 100 sequences from Wellcome Trust Glasgow. SR-A and TS shared reference genomes, helped with data filtering and data presentation. TS helped with installing and running vSNP software. DC, GdL,

RB, BP GA RK SR-A JP, and JC critically reviewed and helped revise drafts of the manuscript. JP and MN helped with responses to reviewers.

ACKNOWLEDGMENTS

We would like to acknowledge the efforts of Maree Joyce, Melissa Surry, Gary Yates, Brian Moonsamy, Rebecca Terry, and Kwang Subharat for help with re-culturing these isolates from the strain archive, Maree Joyce, Justine Jacobs, and Kwang Subharat for help with DNA extraction, Richard Fong from NZGL, Doug Harris from Wellcome Sanger, Julie Galbraith from Glasgow University and Patrick Camp from the USDA for DNA library preparation and sequencing, Hannah Trewby for help with data interpretation, Josephine Bryant for initial characterization of the Wellcome Trust Sanger isolates, Nigel French for funding the sequencing of 5 NZ *M. bovis* genomes and Noel Smith for sequencing 3 NZ *M. bovis* genomes and the reviewers of this manuscript for their very helpful suggestions for improvements and clarification.

SUPPLEMENTARY MATERIAL

Supplementary File 1 | SNPs excluded from the analysis. Numbers indicate regions or individual positions in UK reference version NC_002945.3 for which SNPs were excluded from all isolates.

Supplementary File 2 | Isolate metadata, coverage statistics, *in silico* Spoligotype data and metadata explanations.

Supplementary File 3 | Comparison of RaxML and BioNJ phylogenies. **(a)** NZ *M. bovis* tree. The four clades identified in **Figure 1** with differently colored branches are boxed in the same color in this Figure. **(b)** Mt. Cargill outbreak investigation- all isolates shown in the Phylogram in **Figure 3a** are compared. Outbreak isolates are boxed in red. **(c-d)** South Westland investigation isolates are indicated by the red arrow, **(c)** case 1. **(d)** case 2. **(e)** Waiuku investigation. The scale indicates the level of relatedness between plots.

Supplementary File 4 | Global distribution of NZ spoligotypes. Coloring in these plots reflects the relative abundance of this type in the indicated region.

Supplementary File 5 | Square ML Phylogram illustrating the relationship of West Coast types considered for the South Westland investigations. Breakdown isolate metadata is colored red, livestock metadata is colored blue and wildlife metadata is colored black.

Supplementary File 6 | Distance Matrices. Closely related isolates are colored green, more distant isolates yellow, then orange with the most distinct isolates colored red. Color bars indicate the corresponding cluster in **Figures 3**, **4** and **6**.

REFERENCES

1. Livingstone PG, Hancox N, Nugent G, de Lisle GW. Toward eradication: the effect of *Mycobacterium bovis* infection in wildlife on the evolution and future direction of bovine tuberculosis management in New Zealand. *N Z Vet J.* (2015) 63 (Suppl. 1):4–18. doi: 10.1080/00480169.2014.971082

2. Livingstone PG, Hancox N, Nugent G, Mackereth G, Hutchings SA. Development of the New Zealand strategy for local eradication of tuberculosis from wildlife and livestock. *N Z Vet J.* (2015) 1:98–107. doi: 10.1080/00480169.2015.1013581

3. Buddle BM, de Lisle GW, Griffin JF, Hutchings SA. Epidemiology, diagnostics, and management of tuberculosis in domestic cattle and deer in New Zealand

in the face of a wildlife reservoir. *N Z Vet J.* (2015) 63 (Suppl.):19–27. doi: 10.1080/00480169.2014.929518

4. Kao RR, Price-Carter M, Robbe-Austerman S. Use of genomics to track bovine tuberculosis transmission. *Rev Sci Tech.* (2016) 35:241–58. doi: 10.20506/rst.35.1.2430

5. de Lisle GW, Bengis RG, Schmitt SM, O'Brien DJ. Tuberculosis in free-ranging wildlife: detection, diagnosis and management. *Rev Sci Tech.* (2002) 21:317–34. doi: 10.20506/rst.21.2.1339

6. Fitzgerald SD, Kaneene JB. Wildlife reservoirs of bovine tuberculosis worldwide: hosts, pathology, surveillance, and control. *Vet Pathol.* (2013) 50:488–99. doi: 10.1177/0300985812467472

7. TBfree. (2018). *TB Eradication Strategy Overview.* Available online at: https://www.tbfree.org.nz/strategy-overview.aspc

8. Blanchong JA, Robinson SJ, Samuel MD, Foster JF. Application of genetics and genomics to wildlife epidemiology. *J Wildlife Manage.* (2016) 80:593–608. doi: 10.1002/jwmg.1064

9. Collins DM, De Lisle GW, Gabric DM. Geographic distribution of restriction types of *Mycobacterium bovis* isolates from brush-tailed possums (*Trichosurus vulpecula*) in New Zealand. *J Hyg.* (1986) 96:431–8. doi: 10.1017/S0022172400066201

10. Collins DM. Advances in molecular diagnostics for *Mycobacterium bovis*. *Vet Microbiol.* (2011) 151:2–7. doi: 10.1016/j.vetmic.2011.02.019

11. Durr PA, Clifton-Hadley RS, Hewinson RG. Molecular epidemiology of bovine tuberculosis. II Applications of genotyping. *Rev Sci Tech.* (2000) 19:689–701. Available online at: http://www.ncbi.nlm.nih.gov/pubmed/11107612

12. Durr PA, Hewinson RG, Clifton-Hadley RS. Molecular epidemiology of bovine tuberculosis. I. *Mycobacterium bovis* genotyping. *Rev Sci Tech* (2000) 19, 675–688. Available online at: http://www.ncbi.nlm.nih.gov/pubmed/11107611

13. Skuce RA, Neill SD. Molecular epidemiology of *Mycobacterium bovis*: exploiting molecular data. *Tuberculosis* (2001) 81:169–75. doi: 10.1054/tube.2000.0270

14. Gormley E, Corner LA, Costello E, Rodriguez-Campos S. Bacteriological diagnosis and molecular strain typing of *Mycobacterium bovis* and *Mycobacterium caprae*. *Res Vet Sci.* (2014) 97 (Suppl.):S30–43. doi: 10.1016/j.rvsc.2014.04.010

15. Price-Carter M, Rooker S, Collins DM. Comparison of 45 variable number tandem repeat (VNTR) and two direct repeat (DR) assays to restriction endonuclease analysis for typing isolates of *Mycobacterium bovis*. *Vet Microbiol.* (2011) 150:107–14. doi: 10.1016/j.vetmic.2011.01.012

16. Biek R, O'Hare A, Wright D, Mallon T, McCormick C, Orton RJ, et al. Whole genome sequencing reveals local transmission patterns of *Mycobacterium bovis* in sympatric cattle and badger populations. *PLoS Pathog.* (2012) 8:e1003008. doi: 10.1371/journal.ppat.1003008

17. Glaser L, Carstensen M, Shaw S, Robbe-Austerman S, Wunschmann A, Grear D, et al. Descriptive epidemiology and whole genome sequencing analysis for an outbreak of bovine tuberculosis in beef cattle and white-tailed deer in northwestern minnesota. *PLoS ONE* (2016) 11:e0145735. doi: 10.1371/journal.pone.0145735

18. Trewby H, Wright D, Breadon EL, Lycett SJ, Mallon TR, McCormick C, et al. Use of bacterial whole-genome sequencing to investigate local persistence and spread in bovine tuberculosis. *Epidemics* (2016) 14:26–35. doi: 10.1016/j.epidem.2015.08.003

19. Bruning-Fann CS, Robbe-Austerman S, Kaneene JB, Thomsen BV, Tilden JD, Ray JS, et al. Use of whole-genome sequencing and evaluation of the apparent sensitivity and specificity of antemortem tuberculosis tests in the investigation of an unusual outbreak of *Mycobacterium bovis* infection in a Michigan dairy herd. *J Am Vet Med Assoc.* (2017) 251:206–16. doi: 10.2460/javma.251.2.206

20. Sandoval-Azuara SE, Muñiz-Salazar R, Perea-Jacobo R, Robbe-Austerman S, Perera-Ortiz A, López-Valencia G, et al. Whole genome sequencing of *Mycobacterium bovis* to obtain molecular fingerprints in human and cattle isolates from Baja California, Mexico. *Int J Infect Dis.* (2017) 63:48–56. doi: 10.1016/j.ijid.2017.07.012

21. Ghebremariam MK, Hlokwe T, Rutten VPMG, Allepuz A, Cadmus S, Muwonge A, et al. Genetic profiling of *Mycobacterium bovis* strains from slaughtered cattle in Eritrea. *PLoS Negl Trop Dis.* (2018) 12:e0006406. doi: 10.1371/journal.pntd.0006406

22. Lasserre M, Fresia P, Greif G, Iraola G, Castro-Ramos M, Juambeltz A, et al. Whole genome sequencing of the monomorphic pathogen *Mycobacterium bovis* reveals local differentiation of cattle clinical isolates. *BMC Genomics* (2018) 19:2. doi: 10.1186/s12864-017-4249-6

23. Ahlstrom C, Barkema HW, Stevenson K, Zadoks RN, Biek R, Kao R, et al. Limitations of variable number of tandem repeat typing identified through whole genome sequencing of *Mycobacterium avium* subsp. *paratuberculosis* on a national and herd level. *BMC Genomics* (2015) 16:161. doi: 10.1186/s12864-015-1387-6

24. Crispell J, Zadoks RN, Harris SR, Paterson B, Collins DM, de-Lisle GW, et al. Using whole genome sequencing to investigate transmission in a multi-host system: bovine tuberculosis in New Zealand. *BMC Genomics* (2017) 18:180. doi: 10.1186/s12864-017-3569-x

25. Drummond AJ, Suchard MA, Xie D, Rambaut A. Bayesian phylogenetics with BEAUti and the BEAST 1.7. *Mol Biol Evol.* (2012) 29:1969–73. doi: 10.1093/molbev/mss075

26. Binney BM, Biggs PJ, Carter PE, Holland BR, French NP. Quantification of historical livestock importation into New Zealand 1860-1979. *N Z Vet J.* (2014) 62:309–14. doi: 10.1080/00480169.2014.914861

27. de Lisle GW, Kawakami RP, Yates GF, Collins DM. Isolation of *Mycobacterium bovis* and other mycobacterial species from ferrets and stoats. *Vet Microbiol.* (2008) 132:402–7. doi: 10.1016/j.vetmic.2008.05.022

28. van Soolingen D, Hermans PW, de Haas PE, Soll DR, van Embden JD. Occurrence and stability of insertion sequences in *Mycobacterium tuberculosis* complex strains: evaluation of an insertion sequence-dependent DNA polymorphism as a tool in the epidemiology of tuberculosis. *J Clin Microbiol.* (1991) 29:2578–86.

29. Cox MP, Peterson DA, Biggs PJ. SolexaQA: at-a-glance quality assessment of Illumina second-generation sequencing data. *BMC Bioinformatics* (2010) 11:485. doi: 10.1186/1471-2105-11-485

30. Garnier T, Eiglmeier K, Camus JC, Medina N, Mansoor H, Pryor M, et al. The complete genome sequence of *Mycobacterium bovis*. *Proc Natl Acad Sci USA*. (2003) 100:7877–82. doi: 10.1073/pnas.1130426100

31. Li H. Aligning sequence reads, clone sequences and assembly contigs with BWA-MEM. *arXiv:1303.3997v2 [q-bio.GN]* (2013).

32. Li H, Handsaker B, Wysoker A, Fennell T, Ruan J, Homer N, et al. The sequence alignment/map format and SAMtools. *Bioinformatics* (2009) 25:2078–9. doi: 10.1093/bioinformatics/btp352

33. Ford C, Yusim K, Ioerger T, Feng S, Chase M, Greene M, et al. *Mycobacterium tuberculosis*–heterogeneity revealed through whole genome sequencing. *Tuberculosis* (2012) 92:194–201. doi: 10.1016/j.tube.2011.11.003

34. Danecek P, Auton A, Abecasis G, Albers CA, Banks E, DePristo MA, et al. The variant call format and VCFtools. *Bioinformatics* (2011) 27:2156–8. doi: 10.1093/bioinformatics/btr330

35. Malone KM, Farrell D, Stuber TP, Schubert OT, Aebersold R, Robbe-Austerman S, et al. Updated reference genome sequence and annotation of *Mycobacterium bovis* AF2122/97. *Genome Announc.* (2017) 5:e00157–17. doi: 10.1128/genomeA.00157-17

36. Gouy M, Guindon S, Gascuel O. SeaView version 4: a multiplatform graphical user interface for sequence alignment and phylogenetic tree building. *Mol Biol Evol.* (2010) 27:221–4. doi: 10.1093/molbev/msp259

37. Stamatakis A. RAxML version 8: a tool for phylogenetic analysis and post-analysis of large phylogenies. *Bioinformatics* (2014) 30:1312–3. doi: 10.1093/bioinformatics/btu033

38. Robinson O, Dylus D, Dessimoz C. Phylo.io: interactive viewing and comparison of large phylogenetic trees on the web. *Mol Biol Evol.* (2016) 33:2163–6. doi: 10.1093/molbev/msw080

39. Rambaut A. *Fig Tree Tree Figure Drawing Tool* (2014). Available online at: http://tree.bio.ed.ac.uk/software/figtree/

40. Edgar RC. MUSCLE: multiple sequence alignment with high accuracy and high throughput. *Nucleic Acids Res.* (2004) 32:1792–7. doi: 10.1093/nar/gkh340

41. Couvin D, Zozio T, Rastogi N. SpolSimilaritySearch - a web tool to compare and search similarities between spoligotypes of *Mycobacterium tuberculosis* complex. *Tuberculosis* (2017) 105:49–52. doi: 10.1016/j.tube.2017.04.007

42. Smith NH. The global distribution and phylogeography of *Mycobacterium bovis* clonal complexes. *Infect Genet Evol.* (2012) 12:857–65. doi: 10.1016/j.meegid.2011.09.007

43. Milian-Suazo F, Garcia-Casanova L, Robbe-Austerman S, Canto-Alarcon GJ, Barcenas-Reyes I, Stuber T, et al. Molecular relationship between strains of *M. bovis* from Mexico and those from countries with free trade of cattle with Mexico. *PLoS ONE* (2016) 11:e0155207. doi: 10.1371/journal.pone.0155207

44. Walker TM, Ip CL, Harrell RH, Evans JT, Kapatai G, Dedicoat MJ, et al. Whole-genome sequencing to delineate *Mycobacterium tuberculosis* outbreaks: a retrospective observational study. *Lancet Infect Dis.* (2013) 13:137–46. doi: 10.1016/S1473-3099(12)70277-3

45. Smith NH, Gordon SV, de la Rua-Domenech R, Clifton-Hadley RS, Hewinson RG. Bottlenecks and broomsticks: the molecular evolution of *Mycobacterium bovis. Nat Rev Microbiol.* (2006) 4:670–81. doi: 10.1038/nrmicro1472

46. Jajou R, de Neeling A, van Hunen R, de Vries G, Schimmel H, Mulder A, et al. Epidemiological links between tuberculosis cases identified twice as efficiently by whole genome sequencing than conventional molecular typing: a population-based study. *PLoS ONE* (2018) 13:e0195413. doi: 10.1371/journal.pone.0195413

47. Roof I, Jajou R, Kamst M, Mulder A, de Neeling A, van Hunen R, et al. Prevalence and characterization of heterogeneous VNTR clusters comprising drug susceptible and/or variable resistant *Mycobacterium tuberculosis* complex isolates in the Netherlands from 2004-2016. *J Clin Microbiol.* (2018) doi: 10.1128/JCM.00887-18. [Epub ahead of print].

48. Bryant JM, Schürch AC, van Deutekom H, Harris SR, de Beer JL, de Jager V, et al. Inferring patient to patient transmission of *Mycobacterium tuberculosis* from whole genome sequencing data. *BMC Infect Dis.* (2013) 13:110. doi: 10.1186/1471-2334-13-110

The Distribution of Bovine Tuberculosis in Cattle Farms is Linked to Cattle Trade and Badger-Mediated Contact Networks in South-Western France, 2007–2015

Malika Bouchez-Zacria[1], Aurélie Courcoul[2] and Benoit Durand[2]*

[1] Epidemiology Unit, Paris-Sud University, Laboratory for Animal Health, French Agency for Food, Environment and Occupational Health and Safety (ANSES), Maisons-Alfort, France, [2] Epidemiology Unit, Paris-Est University, Laboratory for Animal Health, French Agency for Food, Environment and Occupational Health and Safety (ANSES), Maisons-Alfort, France

Correspondence:
Benoit Durand
benoit.durand@anses.fr

Bovine tuberculosis (bTB), mainly caused by *Mycobacterium bovis*, can affect domestic and wild animals as well as humans. Identifying the major transmission mechanisms in an area is necessary *for* disease control and management. In this study, we aimed *to evaluate* the involvement of different types of contact in *M. bovis* transmission between cattle farms of south-western France between 2007 and 2015. We analyzed an empirical contact network of cattle farms as nodes, with known infection status and molecular types (16 circulated during the study period of which 14 affected only cattle and two both badgers and cattle). Edges were based on cattle trade data (T-edges) and on spatial neighborhood relationships between farms, either direct (P-edges) or badger-mediated, when two farms neighbored the same badger home range (B-edges), or two distinct but neighboring badger home ranges (D-edges). Edge types were aggregated so that the contact network contained only unique edges labeled by one or several edge types. The association between the contact network structure and bTB infection status was assessed using a non-parametric test, each molecular type being considered a marker of an independent epidemic. Using a logistic regression model, we estimated the contribution of each edge type to the probability for an edge originating from an infected farm to end at another infected farm. A total number of 1946 cattle farms were included in the study and were linked by 54,243 edges. Within this contact network, infected farms (whatever the molecular type) always belonged to the same component, suggesting the contact network may have supported bTB spread among those farms. A significant association between the pattern of bTB-infected farms and the structure of the contact network was observed when all the molecular types were simultaneously considered. The logistic regression model showed a significant association between *M. bovis* infection in direct neighbors of infected farms and the connection by T-, B- and D-edges, with odds-ratios of 7.4, 1.9, and 10.4, respectively. These results indicate a multifactorial *M. bovis* transmission between cattle farms of the studied area, with varying implication levels of the trade, pasture and badger networks according to the molecular type.

Keywords: bovine tuberculosis, network analysis, cattle herds, badger-cattle interface, cattle trade, pastures

INTRODUCTION

Since its discovery by Theobald Smith in the late 1800's (1) *Mycobacterium bovis*, the main agent of bovine tuberculosis (bTB) has been found in a wide variety of domestic and wild animal hosts, as well as in humans (2, 3). In Europe, the main host of *M. bovis* is cattle (4–6), but sheep (7), pigs (8) and goats (9) can be affected too. Wildlife species found infected on this continent include red deer (*Cervus elaphus*) (10, 11), roe deer (*Capreolus capreolus*) (12), red fox (*Vulpes vulpes*) (13–16), wild boar (*Sus scrofa*) (17, 18) and badger (*Meles meles*) (19–21).

Different routes may allow *M. bovis* transmission between wild and domestic hosts. The largest part of *M. bovis* shedding seems to occur through aerosols (respiratory tract secretions) and to a lesser extent through saliva, urine, feces (20, 22, 23), milk in cattle (24) and even wound exudates in badgers (20). Therefore close contacts (e.g., nose to nose) between infected individuals and susceptible ones can allow the transmission of *M. bovis*. However, several studies have shown that *M. bovis* may survive outside a host in a favorable environment for several months (24–26), allowing transmission through indirect contacts. *M. bovis* transmission between cattle can also involve different susceptible species either wild (27) or domestic [although the implication of other domestic species than cattle remains unclear regarding cattle transmission (24)]. At the herd level, several risk factors of bTB have been identified such as larger herd sizes, neighborhood with other herds, cattle movements, farm management practices such as grazing, dispersion of slurry on pastures or the share of water points (24, 28–31). Environmental risk factors have also been studied, with certain environmental conditions favoring the survival and persistence of *M. bovis* (such as shade, moisture or even some soil types) that foster *M. bovis* transmission (24–26). A third category of risk factors involves wildlife interactions, especially with badgers, wild boars and deer. For the latter two species, the sharing of feed or water on pastures appears to be a risk factor of *M. bovis* indirect transmission (23, 32, 33). The transmission between badgers and cattle seems a bit more complex, with uncertain direct contacts on pastures (34–36) and/or inside farm buildings (37). This interspecies transmission could occur on pastures through the shedding of the mycobacteria in urine and feces of infected badgers (24), and in respiratory tract secretions and feces of infected cattle (6, 29).

BTB molecular types are stable (38, 39) and can be used to trace independent epidemics (4). In France, while the officially bTB-free status was obtained in 2000, *M. bovis* infection has persisted in several regions. In 2014, 46% of incident outbreaks were detected in south-western France, with a national number of 105 cattle herds newly detected infected (40). Molecular typing methods spoligotyping (39) combined to MLVA (Multiple Loci Variable Number of Tandem Repeats, VNTR Analysis) based on MIRU-VNTR [Mycobacterial Interspersed Repetitive Unit–VNTR; (4, 38)] have allowed identifying 16 molecular types in this area between 2007 and 2015 from cattle isolates, two of which were shared between cattle and wildlife (4). Because spoligotype and MIRU-VNTR are considered stable markers (at least at a time horizon of several years), these 16 molecular types allow identifying 16 independent epidemics spreading in the same area during the same time period.

An effective way of representing the structure of contacts between hosts of an infectious disease consists in building networks (41), with epidemiological units as nodes, to which an infection status is associated. Edges linking nodes represent the contacts between epidemiological units that may allow the transmission of the disease agent. Regarding *M. bovis* transmission between cattle in France and in light of the above, nodes can represent cattle farms and edges may represent direct or indirect contacts between them. Two types of direct contacts may be featured by edges between farms: (i) contacts due to the trade of live cattle (42, 43) and (ii) contacts due to pasture neighborhood between cattle belonging to different farms but with nose to nose contacts over the fence (31, 44, 45). Besides, indirect contacts between cattle farms due the presence of wildlife may also be represented by edges. Concerning the badger, a known susceptible species to *M. bovis* infection (21, 40), the spatial organization of social groups with stable home ranges around setts (46, 47) allows us to represent indirect contacts with cattle based on the spatial intersection between farm pastures and home ranges (48).

The aim of our study was to analyze *M. bovis* transmission between cattle farms in a south-western area of France using contact networks and molecular types as infection status information. We built different networks featuring possible direct and indirect contacts between cattle farms and analyzed the association between their structure and the observed pattern of infected farms.

MATERIALS AND METHODS

Cattle Data

The study population was made up of the 1946 farms having reported cattle between January 2007 and March 2016 (end of the 2015 herd skin-testing period) and owning at least one pasture included in a 2,735 km^2 study area, an area straddling the border of *Pyrénées-Atlantiques* and *Landes* French departments (**Figure 1**). Pastures were defined as land parcels used by cattle for grazing according to the *"Relevé Parcellaire Graphique"* (RPG) of 2013 provided by the French Ministry of Agriculture. Two pastures were considered neighbors if the minimal distance between their borders was less than 3 m. Farm sizes (number of bovine females over two years old) and types (dairy, beef, fattening, mixed, small and other herds) were obtained from the French cattle tracing system (*"Base de Données Nationale d'Identification"* denoted below BDNI) (**Table 1**).

BTB surveillance data were provided by the French Ministry of Agriculture. Herd skin-testing was performed each year in the study area in communes (the smallest French administrative subdivision) where infected farms had been detected the previous year, as well as in the neighboring ones, using either single intradermal comparative tuberculin tests (SICTT) (in all dairy farms or in farms located in the communes with confirmed infected farms) or single intradermal tuberculin tests (SITT) (in all the other situations), both performed in

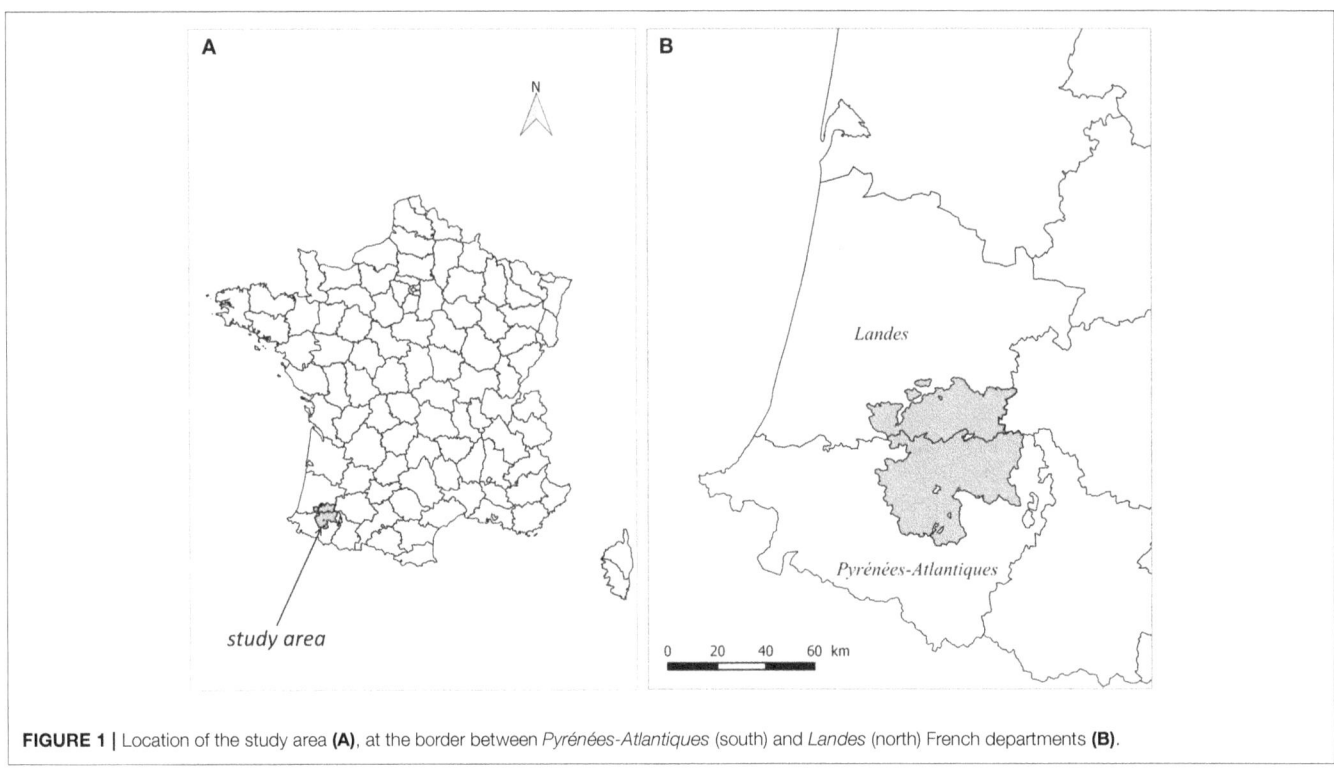

FIGURE 1 | Location of the study area **(A)**, at the border between *Pyrénées-Atlantiques* (south) and *Landes* (north) French departments **(B)**.

TABLE 1 | Description of cattle farms included in the study population.

Farm type	Number of farms	Number of pastures (*)		Herd size (**)		Percentage of farms detected infected (***)
		mean	SD	mean	SD	
Beef	922	9.5	6.5	54.6	34.2	4.2 (*n* = 39)
Dairy	294	8.6	6.0	74.4	43.1	3.7 (*n* = 11)
Fattening	57	7.5	5.8	32.1	28.4	5.2 (*n* = 3)
Mixed	30	12.3	6.5	93.6	32.8	3.3 (*n* = 1)
Other	259	6.3	4.8	21.1	22.9	3.9 (*n* = 10)
Small	384	4.6	3.9	6.7	4.2	1.3 (*n* = 5)
All	1946	7.9	6.1	43.6	39.0	3.5 (*n* = 69)

*, pastures included in the study area; **, number of females of more than 2 years old; ***, at least once over the study period

the cervical region. In the other communes of the study area, herd testing was biennial in *Landes* department, and triennial in *Pyrénées-Atlantiques* department. *M. bovis* infection was confirmed by polymerase chain reaction (PCR) and/or bacterial culture (either following a positive skin test or the detection of a suspect lesion during routine meat inspection at a slaughterhouse) (40) in 69 cattle farms of the study area during the study period; all the cattle of these farms were subsequently slaughtered and molecular typing was performed on each bovid found infected (with a mean of four cattle per farm detected infected during the study period). Molecular typing results were provided by the National Reference Laboratory (NRL) (Anses, Maisons-Alfort). The combination of spoligotyping and MLVA based on MIRU-VNTR allowed identifying 16 distinct molecular types (**Table 2**). A unique molecular type was identified in all of the 69 detected

infected farms, except two where several molecular types were identified.

A farm was classified infected by a given molecular type if this type had been detected at least once in the farm during the study period. Because of the geographic differences in the frequency of skin testing, having detected *M. bovis* earlier in a given farm than in another one does not imply that the former had been infected earlier than the latter. For this reason, the detection dates could not be taken into account.

Badger Data

Two thousand four hundred and 25 badger setts were identified and geolocalised by hunters in the study area, between 2013 and 2015. Around those setts, considered as main setts (i.e., hosting a social group), we defined badger home ranges using a two-step procedure: (i) a Dirichlet tessellation was first built

TABLE 2 | Number of cattle farms detected infected per molecular type during the study period and within the study area.

Molecular types	Number of farms	First and last year of detection
SB0120b	1	2007
SB0120c	2	2009–2011
SB0121a	1	2012–2013[d]
SB0121b	1	2011
SB0121c[b]	1	2012
SB02065[b]	1	2012
SB0295[b]	1	2012
SB0821[a,c]	44	2007–2015
SB0823[c]	1	2010
SB0825[b]	1	2012
SB0827[b]	1	2012
SB0832[a]	13	2012–2015
SB0851	1	2011
SB0853	1	2009
SB0867[b]	1	2012
SB0928	4	2007–2012

[a] molecular types found both in cattle and badgers.
[b] molecular types found in the farm where six molecular types were identified.
[c] molecular types found in the farm where two molecular types were identified.
[d] the same farm as in 2012 (recontamination).

around all setts [in which the perpendicular bisectors of each segment between two adjacent setts delineate the home range around one given sett, thus assuming that boundaries were located halfway between neighboring main setts (47)] and (ii) to avoid unrealistically home range large sizes, a home range was defined as the intersection of a tile with a 1,000 m-radius buffer area drawn around the setts (48). Two setts were considered neighbors if the corresponding home ranges were adjacent. A sett and a farm were considered neighbors if one of the farm pastures intersected with the badger home range.

BTB surveillance data were provided by the French Ministry of Agriculture. In the study area, bTB surveillance in badgers was performed according to the "Sylvatub" surveillance network, which started in 2012 in the study area (49). Surveillance protocol included badger trapping (i) within a 1.5 km-radius around confirmed infected farms, (ii) within a 2 km radius around setts with confirmed infected badgers and (iii) in communes at less than 5 km of communes where confirmed infected farms were located (one badger per sett). Trapping was performed using stopped restraints (https://www.plateforme-esa.fr/filedepot_download/35377/100) and snares were checked the morning after the day they were set up within the 2 h following sunrise, in order to limit the stress of trapped badgers. Trapped badgers were culled by head shot except in a minority of cases where they were found already dead (due to trap related injuries that sometimes occurred when snares were placed on sloping terrain, with no possible alternative). Road-killed badgers were also considered. Stopped restraints used for trapping were placed near sett entrances, those setts being considered as the sett of the trapped animals. Where badgers were found dead along roads, hunters reported the most probable sett according to

their knowledge of the area (48). All the trapped and road-killed badgers were tested for *M. bovis* infection. Among 401 analyzed badgers (4.5% were road-killed badgers), 11.2% were detected infected (45 animals, one was a road-killed badger), of which 39 harbored the SB0821 molecular type and 6 the SB0832 molecular type, both molecular types having also been found in cattle (**Table 2**). All the badgers trapped could be attributed to 113 distinct setts, of which 33.6% hosted at least one infected badger (32 setts with at least one badger detected infected by SB0821 and 6 by SB0832). Road-killed badgers were attributed to five distinct setts. For four of these setts, the analysis of road-killed badgers did not provide additional information as they had also been subjected to trapping measures. For the fifth sett, the analysis of one road-killed badger allowed the detection of infection (SB0821 molecular type), not revealed by trapping. Setts with at least two badgers tested negative were considered as uninfected ($n = 75$). All the remaining setts, either with only one badger tested negative or without analyzed badger were considered of unknown status.

Contact Network

A contact network was built using farms of the study population as nodes, and four types of edges (**Figure 2**):

- A trade edge (denoted T-edge below) from farms i to farm j represented the sale of one or several cattle by farm i to farm j during the study period, at one or several occasions;
- A pasture neighborhood edge (denoted P-edge below) between farms i and j represented the fact that a pasture owned by i and another one owned by j were neighbors;
- A simple badger-mediated edge (denoted B-edge below) between farms i and j represented the fact that both farms were neighbors of a given sett;
- A second level badger-mediated edge (denoted D-edge below) between farms i and j represented the fact that (i) farm i was neighbor of a sett k_1, (ii) farm j was neighbor of a sett k_2, and (iii) the setts k_1 and k_2 were themselves neighbors.

To avoid duplicated edges, the types of edges (T, P, B and D) were aggregated at the edge level. The full contact network thus contained only unique edges labeled by one or several edge types (**Table 3**). Because the T-edges are directed, each undirected P-, B- and D-edge was transformed into two symmetric directed edges. The full contact network was thus a directed network.

Subnetworks were extracted from the full contact network by restricting the edges to those of specific types (**Table 3**). These subnetworks are termed below T-network, P-network, B-network and D-network. Similarly, we used edge types to split the full contact network in three non-overlapping subnetworks:

- the cattle-specific network incorporated edges labeled T, P or T-P, thus representing only contacts induced by cattle breeding practices;
- the badger-specific network incorporated edges labeled B, D or B-D, thus representing only badger-mediated contacts;
- the mixed network incorporated all the remaining edges, thus representing the co-occurrence of cattle-specific and badger-mediated contacts.

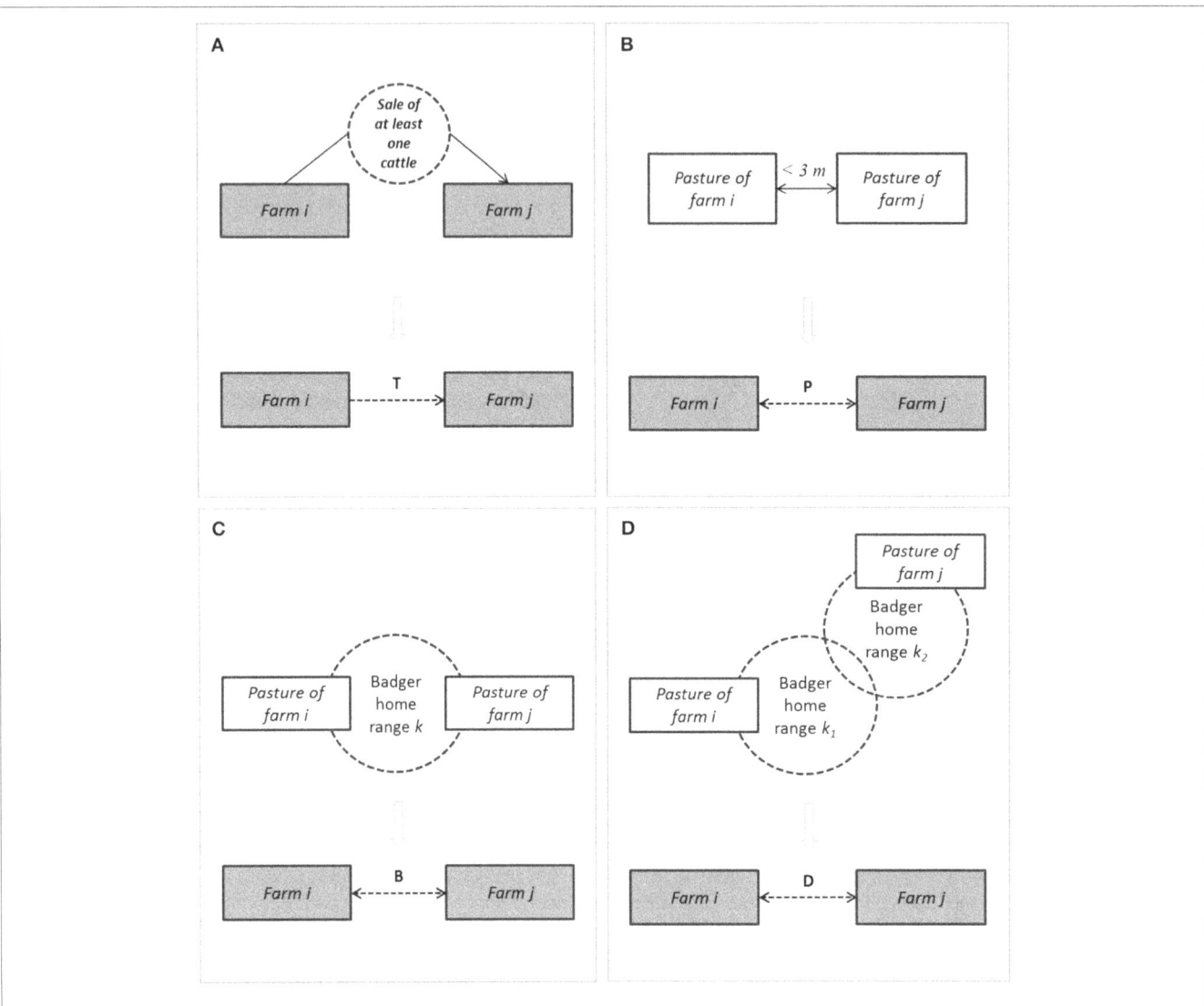

FIGURE 2 | Schematic representation of the four types of edges between cattle farms in the contact network **(A)**, trade edge (noted T); **(B)**, pasture neighborhood edge (noted P); **(C)**, simple badger-mediated edge (noted B); **(D)**, second level badger-mediated edge (noted D).

Statistical Analysis

Each of the 16 molecular types of *M. bovis* identified in the study area was considered as a marker of an independent epidemic. For a given molecular type, the contact network may be considered as supporting *M. bovis* transmission between two farms only if a path exists in the network between these farms. The transmission tree rooted on a detected infected farm should then be entirely located in a single component of the network. The contact network may then be considered as supporting the spread of a given molecular type if most of the farms infected by this molecular type are located in the same component of the contact network. We thus first computed, for each molecular type identified in more than one farm, the number of components in which these infected farms were located (50). For the same subset of molecular types, we also computed, for each infected farm, the length of the shortest path to another farm where the same molecular type was detected.

To evaluate whether the observed pattern of bTB infected farms may have resulted from transmission processes in the contact network, we used the k-test proposed by VanderWaal et al. (51). This permutation-based test is based upon the calculation of the k-statistic: the mean number of infected cases among the neighbors of an infected node (the approach is easily extended to neighborhoods of order >1). The observed value of this statistic is then compared to the distribution of the same statistic obtained by randomly reallocating the location of cases, thus simulating a possible pattern of cases under the null hypothesis of an absence of association between bTB case location and network structure. The empirical p-value of the k-test is then the proportion of permutations for which the k-statistic is greater than the observed one. We adapted this test to a multi-type epidemic by redefining the k-statistic as the mean number of cases among the neighbors of a node, which were infected by the same molecular type as that node.

TABLE 3 | Label of edges in the different networks of contacts between cattle farms in the study area..

Edge label	Full contact network	T-network	P-network	B-network	D-network	Cattle-specific network	Badger-specific network	Mixed network
T	▨	▨				▨		
P	▨		▨			▨		
B	▨			▨			▨	
D	▨				▨		▨	
TP	▨	▨	▨			▨		
TB	▨	▨		▨				▨
TD	▨	▨			▨			▨
PB	▨		▨	▨				▨
PD	▨		▨		▨			▨
BD	▨			▨	▨		▨	
TPB	▨	▨	▨	▨				▨
TPD	▨	▨	▨		▨			▨
TBD	▨	▨		▨	▨			▨
PBD	▨		▨	▨	▨			▨
TPBD	▨	▨	▨	▨	▨			▨

T, trade edge type; P, pasture neighborhood edge type; B, simple badger-mediated edge type; D, second level badger-mediated edge type; edge labels with several letters correspond to combinations of edge types; gray cells indicate the presence of the label within the network.

The k-test was first performed on the full contact network. It was then applied on the cattle-specific, badger-specific and mixed subnetworks; and this, for two groups of molecular types: those observed in cattle only and those observed in cattle and in badgers. Seven tests were thus performed and the Bonferroni correction was applied. Ten thousand permutations were used to compute the empirical p-value.

To further analyse the association between edge types and bTB occurrence, we focused on edges originating from infected farms. A binary status was assigned to each of these edges, with a value of 1 when the destination node was infected by the same molecular type as the originating node, and 0 otherwise. The association between this status and the edge type was then assessed using a case-control design: cases were edges having a status of 1, and controls the edges having the status 0. Four binary explicative variables were defined, based on the types labeling the edge: T, P, B, and D. In addition, we took into account the size (number of bovine females over the age of 2 years) of the edge originating and destination farms, herd size being a well-known risk factor for bTB detection in cattle farms (24). We thus modeled the probability for an edge starting from a detected infected farm to end at a farm detected infected by the same molecular type, using a logistic regression model including six independent variables: four binary variables (presence/absence of the T, P, B and D edge type) and two quantitative variables (sizes of the originating and destination farms). We checked the absence of multicollinearity using variance inflation factors (VIF) with a threshold of 10 (52). Odds ratios (OR) and their associated 95% confidence intervals were computed. Finally, attributable risk fractions (AF) were computed for each edge type.

The definition of badger-mediated edges was based upon the neighborhood between pastures and one (B-edges) or two (D-edges) badger home ranges. For some of the corresponding setts, the trapping results allowed defining an infection status: setts were considered as (i) infected when at least one trapped badger had been found infected with an identified molecular type and (ii) uninfected when at least two trapped badgers had been tested negative and no occupant badger had been found infected [for more details, see (48)]. Based on these data, we finally used a Fisher exact test to analyze the association between the status of B- or/and D-edges and the infection status of the corresponding setts.

Dirichlet tessellations were computed using the deldir package (53) and buffers using the sp package (54). Network analyses were carried out using the igraph package (55) and variance inflation factors were computed using the car package (56). Attributable risk fractions were finally computed using the AF package (57). All those cited packages were used in R 3.3.2 (58).

RESULTS

Within the full contact network, the most frequent edge type was the combination of B- and D-edges, followed by single D-, T-, and B-edges. The P-edge type was less frequent alone than in combination with the other types (**Figure 3**).

The largest weak component of the full contact network incorporated 99.8% of the study population. Regarding the four edge-type-specific networks, the proportion of nodes included in the largest component was higher in trade and badger related networks (94.4% for the T-network, 94.7% for the B-network and 93.6% for the D-network) than in the pasture network (50.4%) (**Table 4**) (a more detailed analysis of networks topology is given in Supplementary Tables 2–4 and Supplementary Figures 1, 2).

For each of the 16 molecular types, the farms where the type had been observed were always located in the same component of

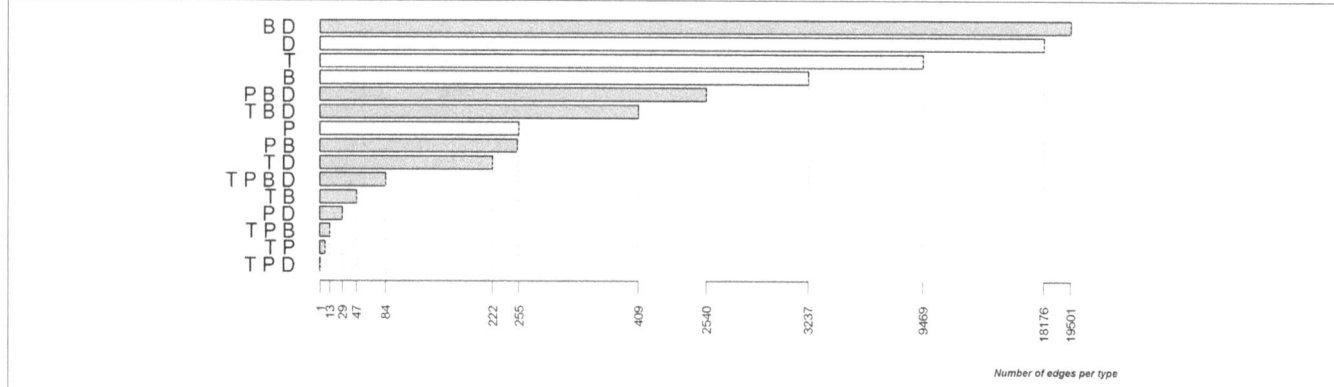

FIGURE 3 | Distribution of the different types and combinations of types for the edges of the full contact network between cattle farms in the study area between 2007 and 2015 (T, trade edge; P, pasture neighborhood edge; B, simple badger-mediated edge; D, second level badger-mediated edge; edges having only one type are in light gray and combinations of several types are in gray).

TABLE 4 | Description of the full contact network and of the four edge-type specific networks.

Indicator	Full contact network	T-network	P-network	B-network	D-network
Number of nodes (size)	1946	1946	1946	1946	1946
Number of edges	54243	10252	3182	26084	40962
Number of components	5	107	716	93	117
Biggest component size	1942	1837	980	1842	1822
Second biggest component size	1	2	23	6	4
Number of components with one farm	4	103	608	86	112

TABLE 5 | Distribution of detected infected farms in the components of the full contact network and in the four edge-type-specific networks for the molecular types identified in more than one farm.

	Number of components containing detected infected farms				
Molecular types	Full contact network	T-network	P-network	B-network	D-network
SB0120c	1	1	1	1	1
SB0821(*)	1	2	15	1	2
SB0832(*)	1	1	3	1	1
SB0928	1	1	3	1	1

*, molecular types found both in badgers and cattle; see **Table 2** for more details.

the full contact network. This was also the case for the B-network, but not for the T-, P-, and D- networks (**Table 5**).

Four molecular types were observed in at least two detected infected farms (**Table 2**). For 87% of these farms, the path to the closest farm detected infected by the same molecular type was made of a single edge. It included one intermediary cattle farm in 11% of cases (**Figure 4** and Supplementary Table 2). This result suggests a prominence of *M. bovis* transmission between an infected farm and its direct neighbors in the full contact network.

We computed the proportion of shortest paths made of a single edge between farms infected (i) by molecular types found only in cattle and (ii) by molecular types found both in badgers

and cattle. The difference between these two proportions was not significant (Fisher exact test: $p = 0.13$).

Using k-tests, a significant association was observed between the pattern of bTB detected infected farms and the structure of the full contact network (observed k-statistic: 2.3; distribution obtained by randomly reallocating the location of cases: mean $= 0.39$, $SD = 0.12$; $p < 7.14^*10^{-3}$, threshold after Bonferroni correction) (**Figure 5**). No significant association was observed for the cattle-specific network, neither for the molecular types observed in cattle only, nor for those found both in cattle and badgers. Conversely, a significant association was observed between the pattern of farms detected infected by molecular types shared between badgers and cattle and the structure of the badger-specific network ($p < 7.14^*10^{-3}$). Finally, the structure of the mixed network was significantly associated with the pattern of bTB-infected farms for both groups of molecular types ($p = 0.006$ and $p < 7.14^*10^{-3}$ respectively) (**Table 6**).

The four edge types were included in the logistic regression model as no significant multicollinearity was detected. T-, B-, and D-edge types were significantly associated to the probability of being a case with an OR of 7.13 for the T-edge type (95% CI: [3.39–15.06]), 1.89 for the B-edge type (95% CI: [1.32–2.76]) and 10.44 for the D-edge type (95% IC: [4.38–26.66]). The size of the destination farm of the edge was also significantly associated to the probability of being a case. Regarding edge types, attributable risk fractions were 84% for the D edge type, 32% for the B edge type, and 12% for the T edge type (**Table 7**).

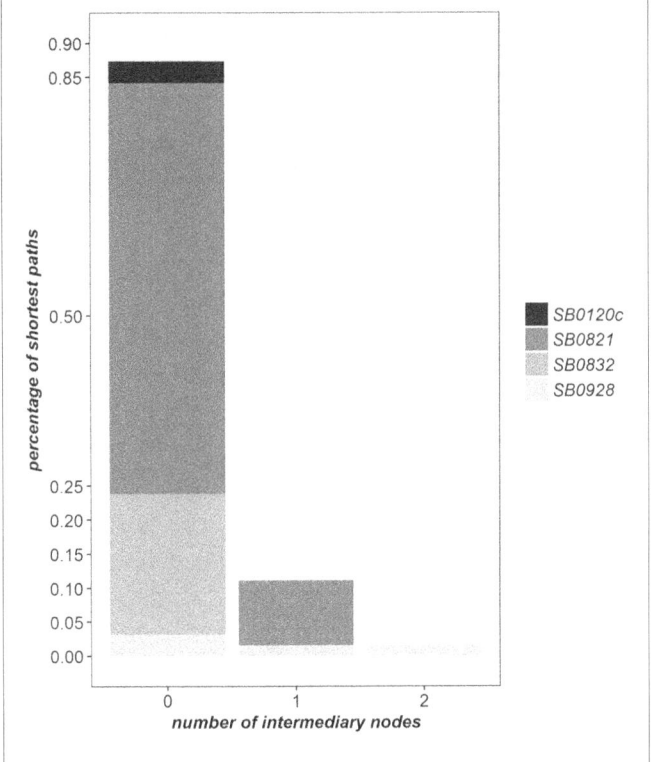

FIGURE 4 | Distribution of the shortest path lengths in the full contact network between pairs of farms detected infected by the same molecular type (only the four molecular types found in at least two farms are considered).

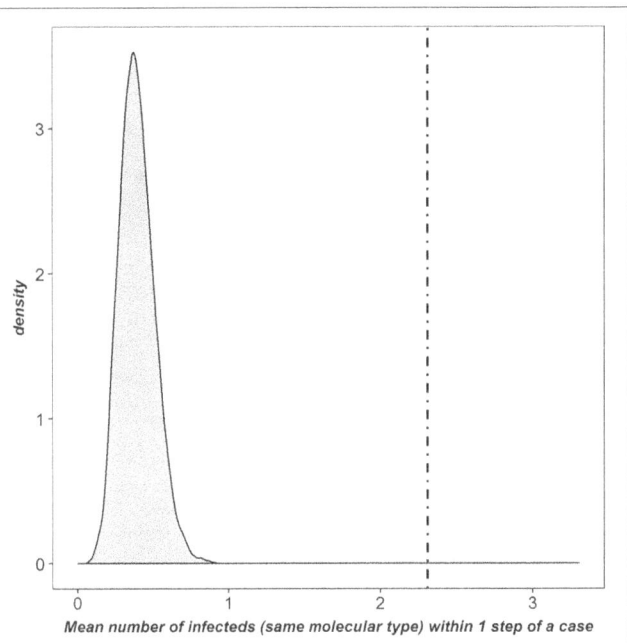

FIGURE 5 | Graphical representation of the k-test results for the full contact network [*dot-dashed line:* k-statistic computed in the observed network; *gray density plot:* distribution obtained by randomly reallocating the location of cases; this last distribution was clearly lower than the k-statistic observed ($p < 7.14*10^{-3}$, threshold after Bonferroni correction)].

Among edges representing badger-mediated transmission (i.e., B- and D-edges), the infection status of badger setts involved (one sett regarding B-edges and at least one of the two setts regarding D-edges) was known for 264 edges (5%) originating from a farm infected by one of the two molecular types shared between badgers and cattle. Among them, 44 were case edges (i.e., the destination farm had also been found infected by the same molecular type) of which 38 (86%) were supported by positive badger setts; and 220 were control edges of which 102 were supported by positive badger setts (46%). These differences were significant (Fisher exact test: $p < 0.0001$) with an associated OR of 7.3 [95% CI: (2.9–21.9)].

DISCUSSION

The objective of this study was to provide a better understanding of *M. bovis* transmission mechanisms between cattle farms in south-western France using networks which represented the direct and indirect contacts that may allow *M. bovis* transmission among farms of this area between 2007 and 2015.

Four types of edges were represented because of their potential involvement in *M. bovis* transmission between cattle farms and we assumed that they represented the main transmission mechanisms in the study area. Cattle movements due to trade are a known *M. bovis* transmission route in Great Britain (59, 60), but also in France (42). The neighborhood with an infected farm

through adjoining pastures (allowing over the fence contacts between herds) has also been identified as a potential risk factor for the *M. bovis* transmission between French cattle farms (31). The intersection of badger home ranges with cattle pastures and between each other's was considered a proxy for badger-mediated transmission, considering the territoriality of badgers (36) and the ability of *M. bovis* to survive in the soil (25, 26). BTB surveillance measures in badgers were not homogeneous among setts of the study area, as they were dependent on bTB detection in the cattle farms in their vicinity. For this reason, although the location of setts was known, we did not model badger setts as nodes in the contact network (we would have been unable to attribute an infection status to each of them). Instead of that, sett location data were used to represent badger-mediated contacts between farms by specific edges, based on neighboring badger home ranges. Two types of badger-mediated contacts were thus modeled by edges. B-edges represented a situation in which two farms neighbored the same badger home range: farm to farm *M. bovis* transmission through such edges thus only assumed cattle to badger and badger to cattle transmission. Conversely, D-edges represented a situation in which two farms neighbored two distinct but neighboring badger home ranges: farm to farm transmission through such edges thus also assumed badger to badger transmission in animals from neighboring setts. Because the epidemiological unit of this study was the farm, P-, B-, and D-edges were built based on the aggregation of pastures of each cattle farm. In the study area, cattle are often moved from one pasture to another one belonging to the same farm,

TABLE 6 | Results of the *k*-tests for the cattle-specific, the badger-specific and for the mixed subnetworks of the full contact network, for the molecular types only found in cattle only and for those found both in badgers and cattle.

Molecular types found in	Networks	*p*-value	Observed networks	Reallocated networks	
			k-statistic	Mean k-statistic	SD k-statistic
Cattle only	Cattle-specific	1	0.00	0.002	0.01
	Badger-specific	0.07	0.11	0.008	0.03
	Mixed	0.006*	0.11	0.0008	0.01
Badger and cattle	Cattle-specific	0.027	0.23	0.09	0.06
	Badger-specific	0*	2.28	0.39	0.13
	Mixed	0*	0.46	0.03	0.03

*significant difference after Bonferroni correction ($p < 7.14 \cdot 10^{-3}$); SD, standard deviation.

TABLE 7 | Logistic model of the probability of an edge starting from a detected infected cattle farm to join another detected infected cattle farm and with the same molecular type according to the type of edge.

Variable	Parameter estimate	OR (95% CI)	P-value	AF (SD)
Intercept	−5.02	0.01 [0.00–0.02]	<0.0001	-
T edge type	1.96	7.13 [3.39–15.06]	<0.0001	12% (6.2)
P edge type	0.30	1.35 [0.77–2.27]	0.26	3% (7.4)
B edge type	0.64	1.89 [1.32–2.76]	<0.0001	32% (8.6)
D edge type	2.34	10.44 [4.38–26.66]	<0.0001	84% (6.9)
Size of the destination farm	−0.0045	0.956 [0.910–0.996] (*)	0.049	-
Size of the originating farm	0.002	1.02 [0.99–1.06] (*)	0.19	-

OR, Odds ratio; CI, Confidence Interval; AF, Attributable Risk Fraction; SD, Standard Deviation.
(*) Odds-ratio corresponding to an increase of ten animals.

e.g., when rotational grazing is used, we thus assumed that this simplification was meaningful.

The frequency of testing cattle was different in the different parts of the study area and this could have biased our results. However, testing was performed each year in communes where infected herds had been detected, and was also performed reactively in farms identified by contact tracing from these herds, based on cattle trade data and on pasture neighborhood. For these reasons, farms directly connected (in the full contact network) to a herd detected infected were considered having been submitted to similar testing regimens, both for B and D edge types (as in most cases the connected farms were located in the same commune), and for the T and P edge types (because of contact tracing). As only edges originating from herds detected infected were considered in the *k*-tests and in the logistic regression model, the corresponding results should not have been biased by geographic variations of the frequency of testing in the study area.

Taking into account the molecular types of isolates allowed considering 16 independent epidemics, of which 12 appeared restricted to a single farm, and 14 to less than 10 farms. All of these 14 molecular types affected only cattle. This predominance of molecular types found in a single cattle farm (75%) was in line with a previous study carried out in France between 1979 and 2000 in which a large majority of molecular types (84%) were found at a low frequency (less than 10 farms). This result has been interpreted as the sign of a poor spread of these

strains (61), which could be traces of older epidemics that would have spread prior to 2007, but without significant transmission afterwards. Indeed, in our study, the 14 molecular types found in less than 10 farms were all detected not later than 2012 (**Table 2**).

Farms detected infected by a given molecular type were always located in the same large weak component of the full contact network that contained 99.8% of farms, whereas it was not the case for three of the edge-type-specific networks: the T-, P-, and D- networks. This indicated that, although the T-, P-, and D-edge-type-specific networks could not alone have supported the spread of bTB infection within the study area (contrary to the B-network), the strong connectivity resulting from the union of the four networks into the full contact network provided a structure that might enable the spread of the *M. bovis* infection in the study area. This result is in line with multifactorial mechanisms of bTB spread previously suggested by other studies (24, 29). As an example in Great Britain, dynamic modeling of cattle taking into account farm environment helped understanding *M. bovis* transmission routes (62). Prominent identified routes of *M. bovis* transmission were moving infected cattle between farms and reinfection from an environmental reservoir. The conclusion of this study was that control measures should simultaneously address several transmission routes to be effective.

Using *k*-tests, a significant association was observed between the pattern of bTB-infected farms and the structure of the full contact network. Moreover, the structures of the badger-specific and mixed networks were significantly associated with the pattern of farms detected infected by molecular types shared between badgers and cattle. This result was expected and confirmed that badger-mediated edges could be viewed as paths for the interspecies *M. bovis* transmission. In addition, the structure of the mixed network was significantly associated with the pattern of bTB-infected farms for molecular types found only in cattle, whereas it was not the case for the cattle-specific network. We could assume that the spread of cattle molecular types would be more efficient when direct contact (trade and/or pasture neighborhood) are associated with indirect badger-mediated contacts. In addition, we should be cautious about the cattle specificity of these molecular types, as these molecular types may be (or have been) present in the badger population without being observed, because of the relatively low sensitivity of bTB surveillance in the badger population.

Considering edges originating from detected infected farms, we used a case-control design and a logistic model to analyse the relationship between the types of an edge and the detection of the same molecular type at the originating and destination farm of the edge (case edges) or at the originating farm only (control edges). Because the detection dates could not be considered in the study to infer dates of infection, the co-occurrence of the same molecular type at both ends of case edges does not model the transmission of *M. bovis* through the edge, although the edges of the full contact network represent possible transmission paths for the bacteria and case edges thus represent possible transmission events. The largest odds-ratio was attributed to the D edge type, followed by the T edge type. This predominance of badger-mediated edges reflects the specific situation of the study area, where molecular types shared between badgers and cattle were predominant (84% of detected infected farms **Table 2**), and the predominant effect of the D edge type suggests a probable spread of *M. bovis* between badgers from neighboring setts, and not only between badgers and cattle. However, B and D edges were defined based on a geographic representation of home ranges, with a maximal distance of 1,000 m to the sett. This distance threshold, the Dirichlet tessellation used to model home ranges, and the fact that some setts may have been unoccupied, are three elements that may have led to an underestimation of home range size, and to an overestimation of the role of the D edge type.

The T edge type was also associated with a putative transmission of *M. bovis* ($AF = 12\%$). This result is in agreement with a previous French study conducted at the national scale, according to which the population attributable risk fraction of bTB infection had been estimated at 12% [5–18%] for cattle trade (42), often allowing long distance bTB spread.

In a previous study conducted in France, pasture neighborhood was found significantly associated with the farm infection status (31). However, in the present study, the P edge type was not significantly associated with *M. bovis* transmission when using the case-control design. This may be first explained by the fact that some of farmers of the study

area use rotational grazing, with some pastures left unoccupied for grass re-growth. Furthermore, P-edges were defined based on a direct neighborhood between pastures (<3 m). This short distance does not allow other opportunities of direct contacts between cattle, such as the wandering of livestock, to be represented.

The badger-specific edges (B and D edge types) were defined based on sett locations, one or two setts being associated to each. For some of these setts, an infection status could be determined based on bTB surveillance data. We showed that this infection status was significantly associated with the fact that the sett as well as the originating and the destination farms had all been found infected by isolates of the same molecular type ($OR = 7.3$; 95% CI:[2.9-21.9]). This result supports an actual badger-mediated transmission through these types of edges. Nevertheless, wild boars have also been found infected with *M. bovis* within the study area. Indeed, among 548 analyzed wild boars between 2011 and 2015, 15 (2.7%) were found infected. The corresponding molecular types found in these wild boars were the two molecular types shared between badgers and cattle. Therefore we cannot exclude the role of this wild species that we could not consider in this study because of a lack of field data that would have allowed its spatial organization (captured through radio tracking, for example) to be represented. Not considering wild boars in our analyses could have led to an over-estimate of the role of B and D edge types in *M. bovis* transmission between cattle farms.

Other indirect contacts through herd practices could also have contributed to the predominance of the D edge type. Indeed, this type of edge created links between farms without direct contacts at pasture but being in a kind of vicinity. As examples, the sharing of material or the loan of animals could create links between farms that may overlap the D edges. However, no data were available to investigate this assumption. Its confirmation or refutation would require supplementary investigation.

In conclusion, this study supports the multifactorial nature of *M. bovis* transmission between cattle farms within the *Pyrénées-Atlantiques–Landes* area, France from 2007 to 2015. The largest part of bTB spread seemed to be due to badger-mediated contacts, however cattle trade played a significant role. Consequently, to be truly effective, control measures should not focus on a single type of contact but ought to act on the different mechanisms we raised.

AUTHOR CONTRIBUTIONS

MB-Z, AC, and BD conceived and designed the study. MB-Z prepared the data for the analysis. MB-Z and BD performed the analysis. MB-Z wrote the manuscript. MB-Z, AC, and BD revised the manuscript. All the authors approved the submitted version of the manuscript.

ACKNOWLEDGMENTS

The authors thank the French Ministry of Food, Agriculture and Forest, Directorate General for Food (DGAl) and by the

University of Paris-Sud, which both funded MB-Z's PhD grant. The authors also warmly thank Pierre Jabert (DGAl), Christian Peboscq (*Pyrénées-Atlantiques* Departmental Federation of Hunters-FDC 64), and all the hunters of the *Pyrénées-Atlantiques* and *Landes* for the census of badger setts in the study area.

REFERENCES

1. Malone KM, Gordon SV. "Mycobacterium tuberculosis complex members adapted to wild and domestic animals." ln: *Strain Variation in the* Mycobacterium Tuberculosis *Complex: its Role in Biology, Epidemiology and Control Advances in Experimental Medicine and Biology.* Cham: Springer (2017). p. 135–54.

2. de la Rua-Domenech R. Human *Mycobacterium bovis* infection in the United Kingdom: incidence, risks, control measures and review of the zoonotic aspects of bovine tuberculosis. *Tuberc Edinb Scotl.* (2006) 86:77–109. doi: 10.1016/j.tube.2005.05.002

3. Good M, Bakker D, Duignan A, Collins DM. The history of *in vivo* tuberculin testing in bovines: tuberculosis, a "One Health" issue. *Front Vet Sci.* (2018) 5:59. doi: 10.3389/fvets.2018.00059

4. Hauer A, De Cruz K, Cochard T, Godreuil S, Karoui C, Henault S, et al. Genetic evolution of *Mycobacterium bovis* causing tuberculosis in livestock and wildlife in France since 1978. *PLoS ONE* (2015) 10:e0117103. doi: 10.1371/journal.pone.0117103

5. Guta S, Casal J, Napp S, Saez JL, Garcia-Saenz A, Perez de Val B, et al. Epidemiological investigation of bovine tuberculosis herd breakdowns in Spain 2009/2011. *PLoS ONE* (2014) 9:e104383. doi: 10.1371/journal.pone.0104383

6. Phillips CJC, Foster CRW, Morris PA, Teverson R. The transmission of *Mycobacterium bovis* infection to cattle. *Res Vet Sci.* (2003) 74:1–15. doi: 10.1016/S0034-5288(02)00145-5

7. Muñoz Mendoza M, Juan L de, Menéndez S, Ocampo A, Mourelo J, Sáez JL, et al. Tuberculosis due to *Mycobacterium bovis* and *Mycobacterium caprae* in sheep. *Vet J.* (2012) 191:267–9. doi: 10.1016/j.tvjl.2011.05.006

8. Bailey SS, Crawshaw TR, Smith NH, Palgrave CJ. *Mycobacterium bovis* infection in domestic pigs in Great Britain. *Vet J.* (2013) 198:391–7. doi: 10.1016/j.tvjl.2013.08.035

9. Napp S, Allepuz A, Mercader I, Nofrarías M, López-Soria S, Domingo M, et al. Evidence of goats acting as domestic reservoirs of bovine tuberculosis. *Vet Rec.* (2013) 172:663. doi: 10.1136/vr.101347

10. Queirós J, Vicente J, Alves PC, de la Fuente J, Gortázar C. Tuberculosis, genetic diversity and fitness in the red deer, Cervus elaphus. *Infect Genet Evol.* (2016) 43:203–12. doi: 10.1016/j.meegid.2016.05.031

11. Zanella G, Bar-Hen A, Boschiroli M-L, Hars J, Moutou F, Garin-Bastuji B, et al. Modelling transmission of bovine tuberculosis in red deer and wild boar in Normandy, France. *Zoonoses Public Health* (2012) 59(Suppl. 2):170–8. doi: 10.1111/j.1863-2378.2011.01453.x

12. Lambert S, Hars J, Réveillaud E, Moyen J-L, Gares H, Rambaud T, et al. Host status of wild roe deer in bovine tuberculosis endemic areas. *Eur J Wildl Res.* (2017) 63:15. doi: 10.1007/s10344-016-1071-4

13. Martín-Atance P, Palomares F, González-Candela M, Revilla E, Cubero MJ, Calzada J, et al. Bovine tuberculosis in a free ranging red fox (*Vulpes vulpes*) from Doñana National Park (Spain). *J Wildl Dis.* (2005) 41:435–6. doi: 10.7589/0090-3558-41.2.435

14. de Lisle GW, Mackintosh CG, Bengis RG. *Mycobacterium bovis* in free-living and captive wildlife, including farmed deer. *Rev Sci Tech Int Off Epizoot.* (2001) 20:86–111. doi: doi: 10.20506/rst.20.1.1262

15. Millán J, Jiménez MA, Viota M, Candela MG, Peña L, León-Vizcaíno L. Disseminated bovine tuberculosis in a wild red fox (*Vulpes vulpes*) in southern Spain. *J Wildl Dis.* (2008) 44:701–6. doi: 10.7589/0090-3558-44.3.701

16. Zanella G, Durand B, Hars J, Moutou F, Garin-Bastuji B, Duvauchelle A, et al. *Mycobacterium bovis* in wildlife in France. *J Wildl Dis.* (2008) 44:99–108. doi: 10.7589/0090-3558-44.1.99

17. Richomme C, Boadella M, Courcoul A, Durand B, Drapeau A, Corde Y, et al. Exposure of wild boar to *Mycobacterium tuberculosis* complex in France since 2000 is consistent with the distribution of bovine tuberculosis outbreaks in cattle. *PLoS ONE* (2013) 8:e77842. doi: 10.1371/journal.pone.0077842

18. Gortázar C, Vicente J, Gavier-Widén D. Pathology of bovine tuberculosis in the European wild boar (*Sus scrofa*). *Vet Rec.* (2003) 152:779–80. doi: 10.1136/vr.152.25.779

19. Balseiro A, Rodríguez O, González-Quirós P, Merediz I, Sevilla IA, Davé D, et al. Infection of Eurasian badgers (*Meles meles*) with *Mycobacterium bovis* and *Mycobacterium avium* complex in Spain. *Vet J.* (2011) 190:e21–5. doi: 10.1016/j.tvjl.2011.04.012

20. Corner LAL, Murphy D, Gormley E. *Mycobacterium bovis* infection in the Eurasian badger (*Meles meles*): the disease, pathogenesis, epidemiology and control. *J Comp Pathol.* (2011) 144:1–24. doi: 10.1016/j.jcpa.2010.10.003

21. Payne A, Boschiroli ML, Gueneau Eric, Moyen J-L, Rambaud T, Dufour B, et al. Bovine tuberculosis in "Eurasian" badgers (*Meles meles*) in France. *Eur J Wildl Res.* (2013) 59:331–9. doi:10.1007/s10344-012-0678-3

22. Neill SD, Bryson DG, Pollock JM. Pathogenesis of tuberculosis in cattle. *Tuberculosis* (2001) 81:79–86. doi: 10.1054/tube.2000.0279

23. Naranjo V, Gortázar C, Vicente J, de la Fuente J. Evidence of the role of European wild boar as a reservoir of *Mycobacterium tuberculosis* complex. *Vet Microbiol.* (2008) 127:1–9. doi: 10.1016/j.vetmic.2007.10.002

24. Broughan JM, Judge J, Ely E, Delahay RJ, Wilson G, Clifton-Hadley RS, et al. A review of risk factors for bovine tuberculosis infection in cattle in the UK and Ireland. *Epidemiol Infect.* (2016) 144:2899–926. doi: 10.1017/S095026881600131X

25. Barbier E, Rochelet M, Gal L, Boschiroli ML, Hartmann A. Impact of temperature and soil type on *Mycobacterium bovis* survival in the environment. *PLoS ONE* (2017) 12:e0176315. doi: 10.1371/journal.pone.0176315

26. Fine AE, Bolin CA, Gardiner JC, Kaneene JB. A study of the persistence of *Mycobacterium bovis* in the environment under natural weather conditions in Michigan, USA. *Vet Med Int.* (2011) 2011:765430. doi: 10.4061/2011/765430

27. Gortázar C, Ruiz-Fons JF, Höfle U. Infections shared with wildlife: an updated perspective. *Eur J Wildl Res.* (2016) 62:511–25. doi: 10.1007/s10344-016-1033-x

28. Griffin JM, Martin SW, Thorburn MA, Eves JA, Hammond RF. A case-control study on the association of selected risk factors with the occurrence of bovine tuberculosis in the Republic of Ireland. *Prev Vet Med.* (1996) 27:75–87. doi: 10.1016/0167-5877(95)00548-X

29. Humblet M-F, Boschiroli ML, Saegerman C. Classification of worldwide bovine tuberculosis risk factors in cattle: a stratified approach. *Vet Res.* (2009) 40:50. doi:10.1051/vetres/2009033

30. Kaneene JB, Bruning-Fann CS, Granger LM, Miller R, Porter-Spalding BA. Environmental and farm management factors associated with tuberculosis on cattle farms in northeastern Michigan. *J Am Vet Med Assoc.* (2002) 221:837–42. doi: 10.2460/javma.2002.221.837

31. Marsot M, Béral M, Scoizec A, Mathevon Y, Durand B, Courcoul A. Herd-level risk factors for bovine tuberculosis in French cattle herds. *Prev Vet Med.* (2016) 131:31–40 doi:10.1016/j.prevetmed.2016.07.006

32. Palmer MV, Thacker TC, Waters WR, Gortázar C, Corner LAL. *Mycobacterium bovis*: a model pathogen at the interface of livestock, wildlife, and humans. *Vet Med Int.* (2012) 2012:236205. doi:10.1155/2012/236205

33. Delahay RJ, Smith GC, Barlow AM, Walker N, Harris A, Clifton-Hadley RS, et al. Bovine tuberculosis infection in wild mammals in the South-West region of England: a survey of prevalence and a semi-quantitative assessment of the relative risks to cattle. *Vet J.* (2007) 173:287–301. doi: 10.1016/j.tvjl.2005.11.011

34. O'Mahony DT. *Badger-cattle Interactions in the Rural Environment - Implications for Bovine Tuberculosis Transmission. TB & Brucellosis Policy Branch, Department of Agriculture and Rural Development, Northern Ireland* (2014). Available online at: https://www.dardni.gov.uk/publications/badger-cattle-interactions-rural-environment-implications-bovine-tuberculosis

35. Böhm M, Hutchings MR, White PCL. Contact networks in a wildlife-livestock host community: identifying high-risk individuals in the transmission of bovine TB among badgers and cattle. *PLoS ONE* (2009) 4:e5016. doi: 10.1371/journal.pone.0005016

36. Woodroffe R, Donnelly CA, Ham C, Jackson SYB, Moyes K, Chapman K, et al. Badgers prefer cattle pasture but avoid cattle: implications for bovine tuberculosis control. *Ecol Lett.* (2016) 19:1201–8. doi: 10.1111/ele.12654

37. Payne A, Chappa S, Hars J, Dufour B, Gilot-Fromont E. Wildlife visits to farm facilities assessed by camera traps in a bovine tuberculosis-infected area in France. *Eur J Wildl Res.* (2015) 62:33–42. doi: 10.1007/s10344-015-0970-0

38. Allix C, Walravens K, Saegerman C, Godfroid J, Supply P, Fauville-Dufaux M. Evaluation of the epidemiological relevance of variable-number tandem-repeat genotyping of *Mycobacterium bovis* and comparison of the method with IS6110 restriction fragment length polymorphism analysis and spoligotyping. *J Clin Microbiol.* (2006) 44:1951–62. doi: 10.1128/JCM.01775-05

39. Aranaz A, Liébana E, Mateos A, Dominguez L, Vidal D, Domingo M, et al. Spacer oligonucleotide typing of *Mycobacterium bovis* strains from cattle and other animals: a tool for studying epidemiology of tuberculosis. *J Clin Microbiol.* (1996) 34:2734–40. Available online at: http://jcm.asm.org/content/34/11/2734.short

40. Cavalerie L, Courcoul A, Boschiroli M-L, Réveillaud E, Gay P. Bovine tuberculosis in France in 2014: a stable situation. *Bull Épidémiologique Anim Health Nutr.* (2015) 71:4–11. Available online at: http://www.bovinetb.info/docs/bovine-tuberculosis-in-france-in-2014-a-stable-situation.pdf

41. Wang XF, Chen G. Complex networks: small-world, scale-free and beyond. *IEEE Circuits Syst Mag.* (2003) 3:6–20. doi: 10.1109/MCAS.2003.1228503

42. Palisson A, Courcoul A, Durand B. Role of cattle movements in bovine tuberculosis spread in France between 2005 and 2014. *PLoS ONE* (2016) 11:e0152578. doi: 10.1371/journal.pone.0152578

43. Dubé C, Ribble C, Kelton D, McNab B. Estimating potential epidemic size following introduction of a long-incubation disease in scale-free connected networks of milking-cow movements in Ontario, Canada. *Prev Vet Med.* (2011) 99:102–11. doi: 10.1016/j.prevetmed.2011.01.013

44. Palisson A, Courcoul A, Durand B. Analysis of the spatial organization of pastures as a contact network, implications for potential disease spread and biosecurity in livestock, France, 2010. *PLoS ONE* (2017) 12:e0169881. doi: 10.1371/journal.pone.0169881

45. Dommergues L, Rautureau S, Petit E, Dufour B. Network of contacts between cattle herds in a French area affected by bovine tuberculosis in 2010. *Transbound Emerg Dis.* (2012) 59:292–302. doi: 10.1111/j.1865-1682.2011.01269.x

46. Bodin C, Benhamou S, Poulle M-L. What do European badgers (*Meles meles*) know about the spatial organisation of neighbouring groups? *Behav Processes* (2006) 72:84–90. doi: 10.1016/j.beproc.2006.01.001

47. Roper TJ. *Badger*. London: Collins (2010).

48. Bouchez-Zacria M, Courcoul A, Jabert P, Richomme C, Durand B. Environmental determinants of the *Mycobacterium bovis* concomitant infection in cattle and badgers in France. *Eur J Wildl Res.* (2017) 63:74. doi: 10.1007/s10344-017-1131-4

49. Sylvatub. *Surveillance de la tuberculose bovine dans la faune sauvage en France : Dispositif SYLVATUB - Bilan fonctionnel et sanitaire 2014-2015.* Plateforme ESA (2015). Available online at: https://www.plateforme-esa.fr/filedepot_download/36412/1100

50. Robinson SE, Everett MG, Christley RM. Recent network evolution increases the potential for large epidemics in the British cattle population. *J R Soc Interface* (2007) 4:669–74. doi: 10.1098/rsif.2007.0214

51. VanderWaal K, Enns EA, Picasso C, Packer C, Craft ME. Evaluating empirical contact networks as potential transmission pathways for infectious diseases. *J R Soc Interface* (2016) 13:20160166. doi: 10.1098/rsif.2016.0166

52. Dohoo I, Martin W, Stryhn H. *Veterinary Epidemiologic Research*. 2nd Edn. Charlottetown: VER Inc. (2009).

53. Turner R. *deldir: Delaunay Triangulation and Dirichlet (Voronoi) Tessellation. R Package Version 0.1-14.* Available online at: https://CRAN.R-project.org/package=deldir (2017).

54. Pebesma EJ, Bivand RS. *Classes and methods for spatial data in R. R News 5 (2),* Available online at: https://cran.r-project.org/doc/Rnews/. (2005).

55. Csardi G, Nepusz T. The igraph software package for complex network research. *InterJ Complex Syst.* (2006) 1695:1–9. Available online at: http://www.necsi.edu/events/iccs6/papers/c1602a3c126ba822d0bc4293371c.pdf

56. Fox J, Weisberg S. *An {R} companion to applied regression, 2nd Edn.* Thousand Oaks CA: Sage. Available online at: http://socserv.socsci.mcmaster.ca/jfox/Books/Companion. (2011).

57. Dahlqwist E, Sjölander A. *AF: Model-Based Estimation of Confounder-Adjusted Attributable Fractions. R package version 0.1.4.* Available online at: https://CRAN.R-project.org/package=AF. (2017).

58. R Development Core Team. *R: A Language and Environment for Statistical Computing. R Foundation for Statistical Computing, Vienna* (2016). Available online at: http://www.R-project.org.

59. Clegg TA, Blake M, Healy R, Good M, Higgins IM, More SJ. The impact of animal introductions during herd restrictions on future herd-level bovine tuberculosis risk. *Prev Vet Med.* (2013) 109:246–57. doi: 10.1016/j.prevetmed.2012.10.005

60. Gopal R, Goodchild A, Hewinson G, Domenech R de la R, Clifton-Hadley R. Introduction of bovine tuberculosis to north-east England by bought-in cattle. *Vet Rec.* (2006) 159:265–71. doi: 10.1136/vr.159.9.265

61. Haddad N, Ostyn A, Karoui C, Masselot M, Thorel MF, Hughes SL, et al. Spoligotype diversity of *Mycobacterium bovis* strains isolated in France from 1979 to 2000. *J Clin Microbiol.* (2001) 39:3623–32. doi: 10.1128/JCM.39.10.3623-3632.2001

62. Brooks-Pollock E, Roberts GO, Keeling MJ. A dynamic model of bovine tuberculosis spread and control in Great Britain. *Nature* (2014) 511:228–31. doi: 10.1038/nature13529

Roll-Back Eradication of Bovine Tuberculosis (TB) from Wildlife in New Zealand: Concepts, Evolving Approaches and Progress

Graham Nugent[1]*, Andrew M. Gormley[1], Dean P. Anderson[1] and Kevin Crews[2]

[1] Manaaki Whenua – Landcare Research, Lincoln, New Zealand, [2] OSPRI, Christchurch, New Zealand

*Correspondence:
Graham Nugent
nugentg@landcareresearch.co.nz

The New Zealand government and agricultural industries recently jointly adopted the goal of nationally eradicating bovine tuberculosis (TB) from livestock and wildlife reservoirs by 2055. Only Australia has eradicated TB from a wildlife maintenance host. Elsewhere the disease is often self-sustaining in a variety of wildlife hosts, usually making eradication an intractable problem. The New Zealand strategy for eradicating TB from wildlife is based on quantitative assessment using a Bayesian "Proof of Freedom" framework. This is used to assess the probability that TB has been locally eradicated from a given area. Here we describe the framework (the concepts, methods and tools used to assess TB freedom and how they are being applied and updated). We then summarize recent decision theory research aimed at optimizing the balance between the risk of falsely declaring areas free and the risk of overspending on disease management when the disease is already locally extinct. We explore potential new approaches for further optimizing the allocation of management resources, especially for places where existing methods are impractical or expensive, including using livestock as sentinels. We also describe how the progressive roll-back of locally eradicated areas scales up operationally and quantitatively to achieve and confirm eradication success over the entire country. Lastly, we review the progress made since the framework was first formally adopted in 2011. We conclude that eradication of TB from New Zealand is feasible, and that we are well on the way to achieving this outcome.

Keywords: bovine tuberculosis, eradication, TB, possums, disease freedom, wildlife surveillance

INTRODUCTION

In 2016 the New Zealand government and agricultural industries jointly adopted the ambitious goal of nationally eradicating bovine tuberculosis (TB) from livestock and from all wildlife reservoirs by 2055 (1, 2). *Mycobacterium bovis*, the cause of TB, undoubtedly first arrived in New Zealand with imported cattle in the 1800s (3). By the mid-1900s it had spread into wildlife, and the disease became widely established in a highly susceptible and ubiquitous maintenance host, the introduced brushtail possum (*Trichosurus vulpecula*) (4), from which it often spills over to a number of other wildlife hosts, including feral pigs and wild deer (5) and feral ferrets (6).

Although diagnostic testing and removal of test-positive animals, coupled with slaughterhouse carcass inspection and livestock movement control to prevent further outbreaks, has reduced TB levels in livestock in many developed countries (7), the disease has been difficult to fully eradicate, especially in countries where TB is also independently cycling in wildlife reservoirs, such as badgers in Great Britain, wild boar and red deer in Spain, African buffalo and other species in South Africa, cervids (white tailed deer and elk) in North America, and brushtail possums in New Zealand (8). An exception is the successful eradication of TB from introduced water buffalo in Australia, where the "wildlife host" was a semi-domesticated or feral bovid with much the same TB epidemiological dynamics as cattle (9).

The main wildlife host in New Zealand (the brushtail possum) is very different from cattle: it is a small, nocturnal, and predominantly arboreal marsupial that is widespread and can occur at high densities (>20/ha) (4). Although it is a comparatively rapidly fatal disease for individuals, high-density possum populations can independently maintain TB (10) and can readily transmit TB to cattle (11). As a result of TB becoming widespread in possums in some parts of New Zealand in the 1970s, management of TB in New Zealand since then has therefore necessarily involved not only conventional management of the disease in livestock (12) but also efforts to break the TB cycle in possums though severe reductions in local possum density ("control") (3). In this review we first very briefly summarize the c. 50-year history of TB management in New Zealand since it became both a livestock and wildlife problem, and then describe the key concepts and tools that have recently been developed to help achieve and confirm the new (2016) goal of national TB eradication.

We then focus more specifically on the concept of roll-back eradication. TB is established in wildlife in four main areas of New Zealand, which in total covered about 40% of the country in 2011. As the name implies, roll-back eradication entails locally eradicating TB from wildlife at the fringes of those four main areas and, over time, shrinking the size of each area from the outside in.

The key tool underpinning this concept is a Bayesian "Proof of Freedom" (PoF) framework, which is used to quantify the probability that TB is absent from possums in a specific area (P_{free}). When that probability is considered high enough, an area is declared free of TB in wildlife and active management of TB in wildlife there ceases, with the management resources redirected to other areas where possums (and other wildlife) are still likely to be infected.

The PoF framework utilizes a number of information streams, including assessments of how effective efforts to reduce (control) possum densities have been, and infection surveillance data, not only from possums themselves but also from other TB hosts that can be infected by possums. We describe the background to the PoF framework (the concept of combining theoretical prediction of P_{free} with empirical TB-possum surveillance data), and how it was first implemented in 2011. We then summarize recent innovations, as follows:

i. Simultaneous use of possum control efficacy data as well as TB surveillance data for updating the prior probability of freedom (13)
ii. Use of livestock as additional sources of data (sentinels) for detecting TB in wildlife (14)
iii. Use of decision theory to determine the optimal "stopping threshold" probability for declaring a particular local area free of TB (15)
iv. A description of how the progressive roll-back based on local areas can be scaled up to eventually confirm eradication success over the entire country (16).

Lastly, we review actual roll-back progress since 2011, and assess the likely accuracy of the P_{free} estimates given the lack (thus far) of any "post-freedom" failures (i.e., local re-emergence of TB in wildlife).

The review is based largely on the published work of the authors and our colleagues within Manaaki Whenua—Landcare Research, and builds on the comprehensive set of reviews about the epidemiology and management of TB in New Zealand wildlife in a 2015 special issue of the *New Zealand Veterinary Journal*. However, we also cite four reports documenting research that has not yet been published; these are available online via the DOIs appended to their citations.

We use "eradication" to refer to the complete or absolute absence of *M. bovis* from New Zealand livestock and wildlife, with negligible chance of re-invasion (except perhaps in human immigrants). Declaration of national eradication will signal the end of the programme. The term "TB freedom" is used in this paper specifically to denote a lesser but still high level of confidence that *M. bovis* is actually absent from wildlife in a given local area, either because wildlife there were never infected or because the disease has been eradicated. An area designated as free of TB can contain infected livestock if that infection is known to have not been caused by wildlife. The declarations of local-area freedom in wildlife therefore differ conceptually from the international standard for declaring national TB freedom in bovids and cervids, which explicitly permits a low level of continued infection in livestock (17). We also note that, for convenience, the term "disease" is used throughout this paper to encompass the presence of subclinical *M. bovis* infection as well as the presence of actual symptoms of disease (**Appendix**).

MANAGEMENT OF TB IN NEW ZEALAND

Since about 1995, management of TB in New Zealand has been conducted by a non-government agency (OSPRI, formerly TBFreeNZ, and even earlier the Animal Health Board). OSPRI represents a public–private partnership between government and the agricultural industries, and is responsible for implementing a formal National Pest Management Plan (NPMP) for TB (18). The initial NPMP in the mid-1990s aimed simply to try to prevent TB spreading further in wildlife. Then, in revisions in 2004 and 2011, it adopted more ambitious goals of not only reducing TB levels in livestock but also locally eradicating TB from possums and other wildlife (18, 19). By 2016 the national cattle herd TB annual period prevalence had been reduced to 0.09% (20), below the 0.2% threshold stipulated by the OIE (17) for declarations of whole-country TB freedom.

That success led to a fourth iteration of the NPMP, which adopted not only an ultimate goal of national eradication by 2055, but also intermediate goals of disease elimination from farmed livestock by 2026, and TB freedom in wildlife by 2040 (21). The long, 39-year timeline to eradication reflects the immensity of the problem: by 2004 TB was believed to be potentially established in wildlife in 10.5 million ha of New Zealand (c. 40% of the country), which encompassed not only farmed areas but also large tracts of remote, mountainous, and/or heavily forested lands, often occupied by high densities of possums (3). The scale of the problem was such that it was never economically feasible to immediately apply possum control over the whole of the affected area, so the eradication campaign has been, of necessity, centred on progressive reduction or "roll-back" of the areas thought to contain infected wildlife, termed vector risk areas (VRAs).

THE CONCEPT OF ROLL-BACK ERADICATION

The progressive roll-back concept is based on local TB management units within the VRAs, called vector control zones (VCZs), of which there were about 700 in 2011, with a typical size of 10,000–15,000 ha (but ranging from <1,000 ha to one of over 100,000 ha). The history of possum population control, livestock surveillance (herd test-and-cull and slaughterhouse inspection), and wildlife TB surveillance (necropsy) is recorded for each VCZ, and after 5–20 years of management an effort is made to quantitatively assess the probabilities that both livestock and wildlife are free of TB. When those probabilities are considered high enough, the VCZ is declared free of TB, and most of the management resources (funding) for that VCZ are then shifted to still-possibly-infected VCZs.

The broad theory and concepts underpinning this local PoF approach for wildlife are described in detail by Anderson et al. (22), but, briefly, are as follows.

- The effectiveness of possum control is assessed by field monitoring of possum relative abundance (or by inference from the known typical effectiveness of the control techniques)
- A spatially explicit model of TB dynamics in possums (23). is then used to predict the probability that TB could still be present given that level of control.
- Using Bayesian logic, this "prior" probability is then updated with empirical TB surveillance data. These data are based on necropsies of possums, or of spill over hosts (such as pigs) that act as sentinels of TB in possums, to calculate a "posterior" probability of TB freedom P_{free} (22); that is, the probability of TB freedom given negative surveillance.
- Decisions on whether or not to declare the area free are then based on the estimated posterior probability.

The approach was first developed and used formally in 2011, and 174 VCZs totalling 2.05 million ha were declared free using this process in the subsequent 7 years (Crews, OSPRI, unpubl. data).

THE INITIAL (2011) POF FRAMEWORK FOR POSSUMS
The TB Freedom Concept
The original concept underpinning the PoF framework for roll-back eradication (24) was simply that local management units (i.e., VCZs) can be quantitatively declared free of TB in possums (i.e., at some arbitrarily specified minimum level of confidence, usually, thus far, 95%) if:

(i) There is sufficient theoretical evidence (prediction) indicating that enough control has been applied to break the TB cycle in possums
(ii) This prediction was backed up by empirical field surveillance data indicating a low probability of continued TB presence in possums.

For this, Bayes' rule was formulated as:

$$P_{free} = \frac{Prior}{1 - (SS(1 - Prior))}$$

where P_{free} is the estimate of the "posterior" P_{free} required for decision-making, Prior is the measure of belief that an area is free of TB in wildlife based on historical control effort, and SS is a measure of surveillance sensitivity (formally defined below) describing how much effort has been made to find TB in possums without success. This simplified version of Bayes theorem assumes perfect specificity; i.e., surveillance is always negative when TB is not present in possums.

In operational terms, this usually translated into conducting intensive possum control for at least 5 (and often 10 or more) years and then implementing 2–3 years of field surveillance in an effort to detect any remaining TB in the residual possum population (25).

Theoretical Prediction of TB Freedom Based on Control Effectiveness
Because VCZs vary greatly in topography, habitat, possum density and TB history, the number of years of control (duration) and efficacy of control (percentage reduction in possum density) result in wide variation in control histories between VCZs, which is amplified by frequent changes in funding priorities. Prediction of whether a given control history is likely to have succeeded in eradicating TB is based on early modeling indicating TB has very little chance of persisting in possum populations that reduced to well below 40% of carrying capacity for 10–15 years (26). This was subsequently supported by field data (11), and a spatially explicit individual-based version of the Barlow model (the "SPM") (23).

The SPM includes parameters representing both possum population dynamics (e.g., birth rates, mortality, density dependence, dispersal) and the epidemiological dynamics of TB in possums (e.g., transmission rates, TB-induced mortality). It is used within the PoF framework to simulate the effect of population control on reducing TB prevalence (23). To initialize these simulations, TB managers summarize the "control history" for the VCZ of interest, using (as far as possible) field measurements of the relative abundance of possums, most commonly a standardized index of trapping success (25). For un-monitored control operations, conservative estimates of control efficacy are assumed based on monitored outcomes at similarly managed sites. At least 100 simulations of the control history are then run with the SPM, with the prevalence of TB 30 years before the first control operation usually assumed to be 2.5% (based on the 2–5% prevalence typically recorded in unmanaged long-infected possum populations (4). The proportion of simulations in which TB is predicted to disappear is then used as a Bayesian "prior" P_{free} at the end of the series of control operations.

When the PoF framework was initially implemented, many of the VCZs being assessed had been under some form of possum control for more than two decades due to the strategic goal of the previous NPMP being one of ongoing TB suppression rather than eradication. When those long control histories were simulated in the SPM, the model would often predict eradication in every simulation (i.e., $P_{free} = 1.0$). As the predicted P_{free} exceeded the desired >95% minimum level of confidence, such VCZs could have been declared free on the basis of the model predictions alone, but TB managers required additional supporting empirical data from surveillance.

Requirement for Empirical Possum-TB Surveillance

The reason TB managers required additional information is that there is uncertainty about the accuracy of the SPM predictions. Not all SPM parameters have been formally validated, so it was accepted that some were likely to be wrong; for example, it was originally assumed that infected possums lived for about a year after becoming infected (23), but recent evidence indicates a much shorter duration of infection (27). Further, the accuracy of the control histories is often suspect as a result of data gaps. It was therefore decided by OSPRI that, as an operating principle, declarations of freedom would always require a minimum level of empirical post-control surveillance. To achieve this, a default maximum-permissible prior P_{free} of 0.9 was prescribed; in other words, if the SPM predicted (based on simulations of the duration and intensity of historical possum control) a prior of >0.90, it would be reduced to 0.90. In addition, at that time a posterior P_{free} of 0.95 was prescribed as the desired threshold ("stopping rule") for declaring a VCZ free of possum TB. The gap between the maximum-permissible prior ($\leq$0.90) and the stopping rule (0.95) meant that some surveillance was always needed.

The empirical TB surveillance required under this operating principle is obtained through necropsy surveys of possums or sentinel species. The surveys aim to quantify the surveillance sensitivity (SS), or the probability of detecting a TB-positive animal if the disease were actually present in a specified number of possums [the design prevalence, P^*; (28)]. In principle, P^* should be set at one possum if the goal is confirming TB absence at the time of the survey. If the prior P_{free} is predicted to be at (or above) the maximum permitted level (0.95), and $P^* = 1$, then 53% of the possum populations would need to be tested (with perfect test sensitivity) to increase the posterior P_{free} to the 0.95 stopping rule for declaring local Tb freedom. More pragmatically P^* is now routinely set at 2, on the assumption that possum

densities in the surveillance phase will almost always be well below the disease maintenance threshold, so TB is much more likely to die out rather than persist. That reduces the amount of field surveillance required by about 40%.

Once surveillance has been completed (and assuming no TB has been found in possums), the SPM-predicted prior P_{free} is updated annually using the surveillance sensitivity data obtained that year. If the posterior P_{free} exceeds the 0.95 stopping rule, the VCZ can be declared free of TB. If not, further surveillance is usually undertaken. However, in recognition that both the prior and the SS estimates are based on assumptions that may not all be valid, other qualitative factors (such as historical levels of infections, infection in neighboring VCZs, ease of remedying false declaration) are taken into consideration.

Possum-TB Surveillance in Practice—Alternative Sampling Units

(i) Possums as the sampling unit: The amount of surveillance required under the maximum-prior and stopping-rule settings above is large, usually equating to the equivalent of necropsying at least a third of the residual low-density possum population. Surveys of TB prevalence in possums had traditionally been conducted by capturing possums in leg-hold traps set for three or more nights, necropsying them, and conducting mycobacterial culture of tissues most likely to be infected, an approach believed to detect TB in about 95% of infected possums (29). Given negative surveillance (no TB detected), the SS could in theory then be calculated as a joint function of diagnostic test sensitivity and the proportion of the population sampled. However, the latter requires a precise estimate of local possum population size, which would be prohibitively expensive to routinely obtain. In addition, because surveys are usually conducted when possum densities are very low, much of the trapping effort results in empty traps. Such empty traps would not contribute to a conventional SS calculation based on number of possums necropsied, but failure to capture a possum at a particular site indicates a high probability that possums (and therefore TB) are absent from that site.

(ii) Traps and detection devices as the sampling unit: To circumvent the problem of not knowing possum population size, and to make use of the information provided by empty traps, a novel spatially explicit data-modeling approach to disease surveillance was developed (22), in which a VCZ is divided into 1 ha grid cells, and the cell rather than the individual possum is used as the sampling unit. Using data from all set traps (empty and captures), and estimated parameters for other studies on possum home range size and probabilities of trapping, this method estimates a VCZ-level SS (22).

To describe how this is done, assume that a trap is placed within the home range of a TB-infected possum, and that if that infected possum is captured it is necropsied and tested for TB. The probability of detecting TB given that TB is present (SS) is the product of (1) the probability of trapping the infected possum, and (2) the probability that the diagnostic test (mycobacterial culture) returns a positive result. By considering the trapping and diagnostics as two independent "tests" conducted in series, this allows us to include traps that do not capture possums (22, 30); i.e., the product can be applied to the trap whether or not it captures a possum, provided a diagnostic test is always performed whenever a possum is captured. This spatially explicit approach to estimating SS readily accounts for non-random sampling (so it does not require representative sampling).

A further extension of the ability to use empty traps (rather than possums) as sampling units involves the use of detection devices to reduce the trapping effort required. The detection devices [peanut-butter-lured chewcards (31)] are far lighter and easier to deploy than traps, and do not need to be checked daily, so they are used to cheaply identify the few small areas where possums are still present. Traps are then deployed only at those positive detection sites, and all possums captured are necropsied and tested for TB. The probability of detecting TB in this system (given TB presence) is the serial product of the probability of detection, the probability of capturing a possum in traps set at detection sites, and the probability of a positive diagnostic test. Although deploying traps only at detection sites results in a lower SS than if traps were deployed everywhere, the much lower cost of deploying chewcards and trapping only at detection sites makes this approach more cost effective, but still only affordable in readily accessible areas.

(iii) Spill-over hosts as the sampling unit: The high cost of direct possum surveillance led to the use of other spill-over host species as sentinels for TB presence in possums (32). By making data-based assumptions about sentinel home range size and the probability of a sentinel becoming infected when its home range overlaps with that of an infected possum, the surveillance sensitivity provided by these sentinels can also be estimated in a similarly spatially explicit way (22). Pigs, in particular, are highly sensitive sentinels because they very readily become infected in the presence of infected possums (33), have homes ranges that are much larger than those of possums (34), and survive in an infected state for far longer than possums (35). So where pigs can be readily obtained, surveying pigs can sometimes provide much cheaper possum-TB surveillance than would surveying possums themselves.

RECENT INNOVATIONS

Combining Surveillance and Final Control

One shortcoming of the sequential "control-then-survey" approach outlined above is that it is only affordable in easily accessible farmland. There are many less accessible areas within VRAs where ground-based control and subsequent surveillance would be prohibitively expensive. Aerial poisoning provides an affordable alternative to ground control of possums in these areas (25), and sentinel pigs can sometimes provide the required level of surveillance at an affordable cost, but there are many areas where they do not.

A new approach for such difficult areas partially reverses the control-then-survey paradigm by conducting surveillance in conjunction with a final aerial control operation (13). That final operation will have been preceded by one or more earlier aerial poisoning operations, so the prior P_{free} (as predicted by the SPM) will already be high at the time of the final operation. A low level of direct possum TB surveillance is undertaken within a mark-recapture framework, involving trapping and marking (radio-collaring) and releasing possums just before the control operation and then, after the aerial poisoning, recapturing possums by searching for, recovering, and necropsying the killed possums.

Provided no TB is detected, the likelihood of no TB being detected in the survey for each possible number of TB possums in the population (i.e., 0, 1, 2, 3,..., up to N: the pre-control population size) is calculated (**Figure 1A**). The efficacy of the control operation is determined from the percentage of radio-collared possums killed, and from that the probability that at least one TB possum would have survived if 0, 1, 2, 3,..., N infected possums were actually present (**Figure 1B**). The two probability distributions are then combined to estimate the probability that any infected possum could have survived undetected for each possible prevalence value (**Figure 1C**). Despite never knowing the number of TB possums in the population before surveillance and final control, we can use the maximum of the curve in **Figure 1C**, which corresponds to the worst-case scenario. The inverse of this can be further combined with the prior P_{free} to calculate the posterior P_{free}.

The concept was successfully demonstrated in the Hauhungaroa Range in 2016/17 (13). This c. 80,000 ha area historically had some of the highest recorded levels of TB infection in wildlife, with almost all pigs and at least a third of the wild deer infected in the 1990s (4, 5). By 2016 all parts of the area had been under intensive control for 10–22 years, and the estimated P_{free} was 0.9. About 7% of the possum population ($N =$ c. 4000) was necropsied, with no TB detected. Control efficacy was extremely high, with 99.6% of 241 radio-collared possums killed, resulting in a <4% probability that any infected possum would have survived undetected, which when combined with the prior $P_{free} = 0.9$ results in a posterior $P_{free} > 0.99$ (**Figure 1C**).

The main advantage of this approach is the greatly reduced amount of surveillance needed, although that is partially offset by the need to obtain precise estimates of control efficacy (% kill) and the proportion of the population sampled. The other main advantage is that it enables faster declarations of freedom.

Balancing Control and Surveillance Effort and Optimizing the Stopping Rule

The total costs of possum control and possum-TB surveillance depend on a number of factors (such as possum carrying capacity, ease of access, etc.), most of which have wide cost ranges. We modelled and compared management options to demonstrate that the optimal balance between the two activities necessary to achieve and verify eradication of TB from New Zealand wildlife varied greatly between VCZs (36). This work provided managers with a simple cost- and risk-evaluation framework they could use to identify the most expedient and economical ways of achieving

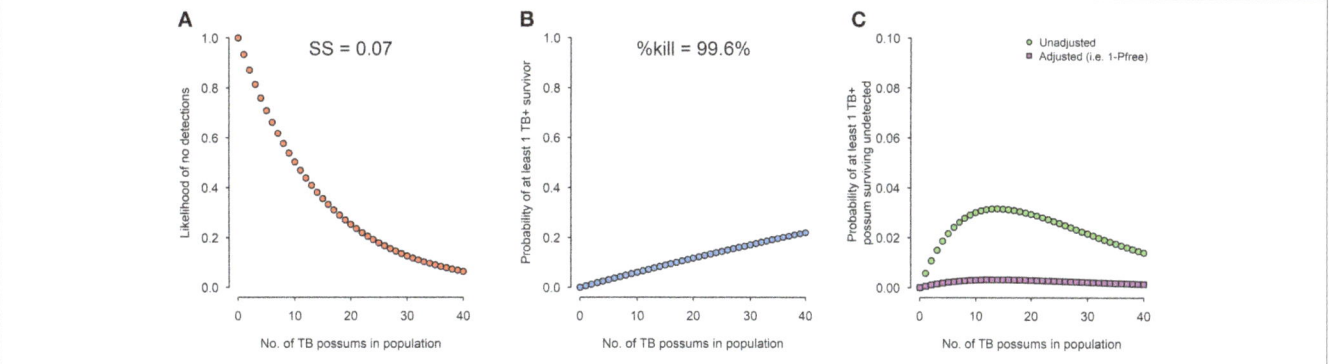

FIGURE 1 | For the range of 0–40 TB possums in the population before surveillance and final control, **(A)** surveillance sensitivity (the likelihood of no detections) from a survey of 7% of the population with 95% diagnostic sensitivity; **(B)** TB survival probability (probability of at least one TB+ survivor) given a recorded control efficacy (% kill) of 99.6%; and **(C)** the probability of at least one TB possum surviving undetected which is shown both unadjusted (i.e., based solely on the evidence from the 2016/17 operation) and adjusted by the prior probability of freedom derived from the history of previous control, and is the complement of P_{free}.

and quantitatively verifying TB eradication from possums in a particular VCZ.

The initial stopping rule (posterior $P_{free} > 0.95$) was chosen subjectively by TB managers and their stakeholders (e.g., farming organizations, governmental funding bodies) to represent what they considered to be an "acceptable" level of risk of disease persistence. Our recent decision-theory modeling (15) indicates how the choice of stopping rule could be better optimized for each VCZ by explicitly including costs of surveillance and potential re-control costs.

If the posterior P_{free} are accurate, and if all VCZs are declared free as soon as they reach 0.95, it follows that 5% of VCZs will be falsely declared free of TB. TB managers therefore expect that in up to 5% of declared-free VCZs, TB will re-emerge in possums after possum control ceases, but will possibly not be detected for many years: where that occurs, potentially expensive re-control will obviously be required.

A higher stopping rule will result in a lower *expected cost* of re-control (the actual cost of re-control multiplied by the probability of incurring that cost). However, the cost of surveillance to achieve that higher target will increase. Conversely a lower stopping rule will result in a higher expected cost of re-control (due to an increased chance of incurring the actual re-control cost), but a lower surveillance cost due to stopping earlier. The optimal stopping rule for a VCZ will be the one that minimizes the total expected cost (expected costs of surveillance and re-control combined).

Our analysis of the total expected costs indicates that where surveillance is relatively expensive compared with re-control, it will usually be more cost-effective to stop earlier than 0.95 at an increased risk of incorrect declaration [**Figure 2A**; (15)]. Conversely, where re-control is much more expensive than surveillance, it should be better to carry out more surveillance and choose a stopping threshold that is higher than 0.95 in order to mitigate the risk of incurring expensive re-control (**Figure 2B**).

This analysis has been used to develop a decision-support framework that provides guidance on how to optimize the economics of TB eradication, with the aim of eliminating the

inefficiencies arising from relying on a single, predetermined, arbitrary stopping rule. Further work is now underway to see how best to include socio-political costs (the loss of credibility associated with incorrectly declaring an area free of TB), and therefore the risk profiles of decision-makers (risk averse vs. risk takers).

Livestock as Sentinels

Having expanded TB-possum surveillance options from surveying possums themselves to using data from traps and detection devices, and/or using spill-over hosts as possum-TB sentinels, we next explored the option of also using livestock as sentinels. Livestock are tested annually within all VCZs (and at longer intervals in areas designated as being free of TB in wildlife), and all livestock sent to slaughter are subject to rigorous inspection. The primary purpose of this testing and inspection is to determine TB levels in the livestock, but the same data can be used (at very little extra cost) to assess the likelihood TB is present in sympatric possums.

This might, at first sight, seem problematic because cattle are themselves maintenance hosts, so the occurrence of TB in a herd could be caused by recrudescence of latent in-herd infection or transfer of infection between herds by livestock movement rather than by transmission from wildlife. Identifying between-farms movement of livestock as the cause of a new outbreak in livestock (and therefore ruling out wildlife as the source) is facilitated by New Zealand's National Animal Identification and Tracing system, which is also managed by OSPRI. If, however, there is no detection of TB in livestock within a VCZ for many years, that obviously indicates there is no transmission from any source, including from possums.

We therefore developed an analytical technique to objectively use livestock as sentinels for TB in possums as an additional source of possum-TB surveillance information. For this, the spatially explicit modeling approach used to estimate SS from point-source data [i.e., the known kill locations of wildlife sentinels; (22)] was adapted to take into account the fact that the location of an individual cow or deer (and therefore the negative

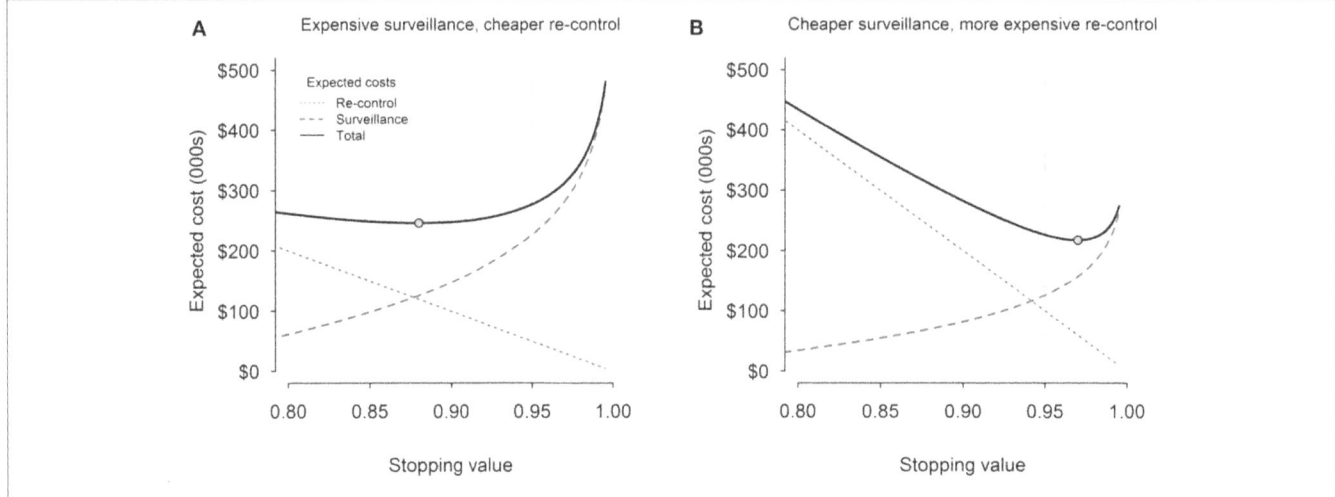

FIGURE 2 | Cost of surveillance (red dashed line), expected cost of re-control (blue dotted line), and total combined expected cost (black solid line) for **(A)** expensive surveillance and cheaper re-control; and **(B)** cheaper surveillance and expensive re-control. The gray circles indicate the point associated with the minimum total expected cost. The vertical dashed gray line indicates the current default stopping threshold of 0.95.

result of any TB test or slaughterhouse inspection) could not be localized to a single point. Instead, the surveillance data for the herd as a whole have to be spread evenly over the entire area in which they were grazed (14).

Because the probability of an individual cow becoming infected by a single infected possum somewhere on the same farm is believed to be very low (24), the SS provided by testing or inspection of a single cow is inevitably low. However, that poor individual sensitivity is offset by a large amount of livestock testing and slaughterhouse inspection data, available at very little cost because livestock are intensively surveyed annually within VRAs to confirm (or not) that the herds themselves remain free of TB (12). Thus, ongoing negative surveillance outcomes from livestock surveillance provide very-low-cost surveillance of TB in possums, reducing the amount of wildlife surveillance required.

Although not yet implemented, we envisage that in VCZs where herds were clear of TB before the end of the control phase, the livestock data will also be taken into account in identifying the prior P_{free}. In addition, we believe the use of livestock as possum-TB sentinels will provide a crucial low-cost form of "post-freedom assurance surveillance," particularly for on- and near-farm areas. The aim of such assurance surveillance is to provide the earliest possible detection of local eradication failure (i.e., persistence and re-emergence of TB in possums). It typically relies on passive (unfunded) rather than active (planned and funded) surveys. A key point is if TB does re-emerge, the numbers of infected possums will progressively increase over time, which will substantially increase the sensitivity of livestock surveillance in detecting the presence of TB.

Scaling Up From VCZs to National Eradication

To date, the roll-back eradication process has focused on achieving and declaring TB freedom at the VCZ level. This is done in a spatially strategic way to minimise the risk of

reinvasion into VCZs previously declared free of TB. It may be tempting to simplistically conclude that the entire country will be free of TB once all VCZs have been declared free in this way. However, the declarations are probabilistic rather than certain. Given the 0.95 stopping rule used, there is a probability of up to 0.05 that the VCZ declared free was still infected. This error rate is compounded across all c. 800 VCZs so that the overall probability of total eradication from the country will be very close to zero (e.g., $0.95^{800} \approx 0$). This is not a bad result, because the bioeconomic optimisation modeling indicates that it is economically sensible to take some risks and be prepared to fail in some of the VCZs and have to re-initiate control and surveillance in them (**Figure 2**).

To account for this failure rate across VCZs in the context of the goal of declaring eradication from the entire country, the operational and decision processes can be divided into two stages (16). Stage I ("achieving freedom") covers the initial efforts to eliminate TB from a given VCZ and the operational decision to declare that VCZ free of possum TB. Stage II (the "assurance" phase) requires (as noted above) ongoing but very-low-cost surveillance to either (i) quickly detect TB in cases where the declaration of freedom was false, or (ii) provide broad-scale SS data that can be used to calculate a probability of eradication at the level of whole regions, whole islands, or the whole country.

As outlined above, continued TB testing of livestock and slaughterhouse inspection is likely to provide such quantifiable assurance surveillance in on- and near-farm areas. Away from farmland there is currently mostly only limited passive and unquantified surveillance provided by recreational or commercial hunters, who might notice and report infection in any grossly infected pig or deer or ferret they kill, so consideration may need to be given to encouraging and quantifying the sensitivity of this kind of surveillance (or to funding low-intensity surveillance of sentinels and possums in high-risk areas with limited or no such passive surveillance).

Once all VCZs in a region, an island or the nation have been declared free, and TB is no longer being detected in them, the Stage II surveillance sensitivities across all VCZs will be aggregated to calculate a whole-area probability of eradication. Only when that exceeds some very high threshold (e.g., 0.99) will we be able to confidently declare that TB has been eradicated from New Zealand.

PROGRESS TOWARD ERADICATION

In the 7 years since the PoF framework was first formally adopted, 174 VCZs have been declared free, with all but 15 of those declarations based at least partly on the estimated posterior P_{free} (OSPRI, unpubl. data). A majority of these are farmed areas, and given the roll-back approach, most are at the former fringes of the VRAs where TB was generally not as well established in possums as in more central parts of VRAs. Nonetheless, the total does include several of the worst-affected forest areas in which TB was long established in wildlife at high levels, including the Hauhungaroa Range mentioned above. In total, over 2.05 million ha has now been declared free using the PoF framework, about 20% of the total area designated VRA in 2011.

By 2018 these 174 VCZs had been free for an average of 3.8 years, equating to 694 years of VCZ freedom. If TB was still present in a declared-free VCZ, we expect that it would re-emerge and be detected (on average) within 4–5 years of being declared free (at least where high numbers of cattle are TB tested and/or slaughtered annually). If so, and if up to 5% of declarations were false, we would have expected the detection of re-emergent TB in 5–10 VCZs by now. There have been none (OSPRI, unpubl. data).

The lower-than-expected failure rate partly reflects the fact that many of the VCZs were not declared free until the posterior P_{free} was substantially above the 0.95 stopping rule (**Figure 3**). This is largely because until recently the PoF process was very largely retrospective: control and surveillance were conducted according to a fixed standard schedule (25), and only on completion of that were the data analyzed. That resulted, in many instances, in far more surveillance being done than was strictly necessary. To help avoid that in future, we have developed an online decision-support tool (https://landcare.shinyapps.io/JESS), which enables managers to determine, for any given prior P_{free}, the minimum amount of surveillance needed to reach the stopping rule.

A second possible reason for the low failure rate is the conservative setting, by OSPRI, of a maximum prior P_{free} of 0.90 even when the SPM predicts that a given control history would have eradicated TB in 100% of simulations. If the model predictions were accepted as accurate, the posterior P_{free} estimates would have been higher (and therefore the expected failure rate lower).

Another possible reason for the low failure rate is that the SPM may be predicting that eradicating TB from possums is more difficult than it actually is, biasing the prior P_{free} estimates low. A converse point is that the low failure rate provides some validation of the SPM predictions: if the SPM was falsely providing overly optimistic predictions of the probability of

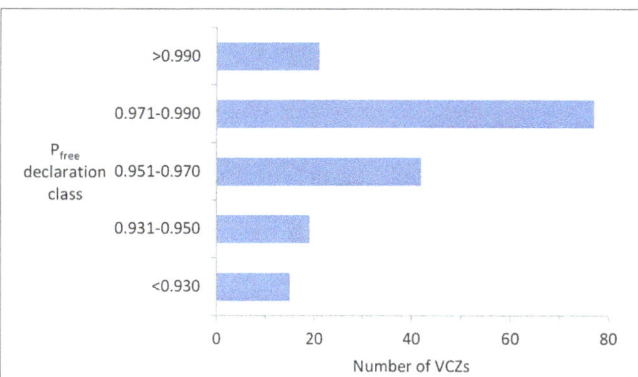

FIGURE 3 | Frequency distribution of the number of VCZs declared free between 2011 and 2018 in relation to the Pfree estimates (calculated using a design prevalence of 2, and grouped into five classes) at the time of declaration. The "Pfree declaration class <0.930" represents VCZs declared free on a largely qualitative basis rather than a quantitative one.

eradication, there would have been more failures observed than expected.

There are some indications that the SPM was indeed biased when applied to areas in which possum carrying capacity was well below average. In such areas the SPM often predicted TB would not persist even without control, despite evidence that TB had actually been detected in possums in some such areas (Crews, OSPRI, unpubl. data). To remedy that mismatch between model prediction and reality, the SPM has been revised by changing the possum–possum contact-rate function from one based on distance between home range centres to a more realistic one based on home range overlap (37), resulting in a greater amount of control being needed than previously for the model to predict eradication in areas of poor possum habitat.

Whatever the reason, there is evidence that the prior P_{free} estimates being used are conservative. In 2015, key TB managers were asked to subjectively assign prior P_{free} estimates for all VCZs in which TB surveys of possums had recently been conducted (38). There were 133 surveys in VCZs that had been under possum control for many years and that had prior P_{free} estimates in the range 0.70–0.95. Using conventional probability theory, the surveillance sensitivity estimates from these surveys were used to determine the probability that those surveys would have detected TB if it were actually present as frequently as the managers' prior P_{free} suggested it should be. Collectively, these 133 surveys should have resulted in 13 detections of infected possums if the P_{free} estimates were accurate, but again there were no detections. The implication is that there was far less infection in long-managed populations than managers believed, based on their experience with the PoF framework.

DISCUSSION

The evolution of the TB eradication programme in New Zealand (3) is the product of an adaptive management (39) effort in which management decisions are evidence based, and new research questions and developments are shaped by management outcomes and needs. New Zealand's TB management agency, OSPRI, has historically funded, and continues to fund, robust and innovative science to support their desire for evidence-based decision-making. There is a strong focus on continual improvement, with a constant appetite for exploring new methodologies in order to achieve TB freedom ever more cost-effectively and ever more quickly.

A key factor in the continued success of the components of the "TBfree" programme that are specifically aimed at eliminating TB in wildlife has been the strong partnership and close working relationships over more than two decades between the end-user (OSPRI) and researchers at New Zealand's main terrestrial environment research institute (Manaaki Whenua—Landcare Research). This relationship, and the research findings that have flowed from it, has resulted in wide-ranging changes in operational strategies and activities. In particular, the PoF framework has become an integral part of TB management, with the posterior P_{free} increasingly recognized as the ultimate management performance metric. We believe that the challenges and successes of this collaborative experience will be instructive for other countries aiming to manage or eradicate TB from very large areas.

With less than a quarter of the area believed to contain infected wildlife declared free so far, there is clearly still an immense amount of management (and research) to be done. However, the success and progress to date, as well as the development and implementation of new methodologies and smarter decision-making tools, means that New Zealand is well on the way to eliminating TB in both livestock and wildlife, and is well on track to achieve the goal of disease eradication by 2055.

AUTHOR CONTRIBUTIONS

GN, AG, and DA reviewed and summarized their own bodies of work and collectively integrated those summaries into the overall review. KC (and other OSPRI staff) provided data on eradication progress, and also reviewed the whole document.

ACKNOWLEDGMENTS

We acknowledge the insight and guidance provided over the last decade by Dr. Paul Livingstone, former Eradication and Research Manager at OSPRI. We also acknowledge the contributions of numerous colleagues and co-workers in both Manaaki Whenua—Landcare Research and OSPRI in helping develop, test, and implement the new theory, tools, and systems summarized in this review.

REFERENCES

1. TB Free NZ (2016). *Approval of Funding for TB Eradication Plan Welcomed*. Available online at: https://tbfree.org.nz/approval-of-funding-for-tb-eradication-plan-welcomed.aspx (Accessed May 31, 2018).

2. Crews K, Nugent G. *Proving Freedom from TB: The Pathway to Eradication*. DairyNZ Technical Series (2018).

3. Livingstone P, Hancox N, Nugent G, De Lisle G. Toward eradication: the effect of *Mycobacterium bovis* infection in wildlife on the evolution and future direction of bovine tuberculosis management in New Zealand. *N Z Vet. J.* (2015) 63:4–18. doi: 10.1080/00480169.2014.971082

4. Nugent G, Buddle B, Knowles G. Epidemiology and control of *Mycobacterium bovis* infection in brushtail possums (*Trichosurus vulpecula*), the primary wildlife host of bovine tuberculosis in New Zealand. *N Z Vet J.* (2015) 63:28–41. doi: 10.1080/00480169.2014.963791

5. Nugent G, Gortázar C, Knowles G. The epidemiology of *Mycobacterium bovis* in wild deer and feral pigs and their roles in the establishment and spread of bovine tuberculosis in New Zealand wildlife. *N Z Vet J.* (2015) 63:54–67. doi: 10.1080/00480169.2014.963792

6. Byrom A, Caley P, Paterson B, Nugent G. Feral ferrets (*Mustela furo*) as hosts and sentinels of tuberculosis in New Zealand. *N Z Vet J.* (2015) 63:42–53. doi: 10.1080/00480169.2014.981314

7. Olmstead AL, Rhode PW. An impossible undertaking: the eradication of bovine tuberculosis in the United States. *J Econ Hist.* (2004) 64:734–72. doi: 10.1017/S0022050704002955

8. Corner LA. The role of wild animal populations in the epidemiology of tuberculosis in domestic animals: how to assess the risk. *Vet Microbiol.* (2006) 112:303–12. doi: 10.1016/j.vetmic.2005.11.015

9. More SJ, Radunz B, Glanville R. Lessons learned during the successful eradication of bovine tuberculosis from Australia. *Vet Rec.* (2015) 177:224. doi: 10.1136/vr.103163

10. Morris R, Pfeiffer D, Jackson R. The epidemiology of *Mycobacterium bovis* infections. *Vet Microbiol.* (1994) 40:153–77. doi: 10.1016/0378-1135(94)90053-1

11. Caley P, Hickling G, Cowan P, Pfeiffer D. Effects of sustained control of brushtail possums on levels of *Mycobacterium bovis* infection in cattle and brushtail possum populations from Hohotaka, New Zealand. *N Z Vet J.* (1999) 47:133–42. doi: 10.1080/00480169.1999.36130

12. Buddle B, De Lisle G, Griffin J, Hutchings S. Epidemiology, diagnostics, and management of tuberculosis in domestic cattle and deer in New Zealand in the face of a wildlife reservoir. *N Z Vet J.* (2015) 63:19–27. doi: 10.1080/00480169.2014.929518

13. Nugent, G, Sweetapple P, Yockney I, Morriss G. *TB Freedom in the Hauhungaroa Range: A Large-Scale Test of a New Surveillance Approach*. Landcare Research Contract Report (unpubl.). Lincoln: Landcare Research (2017). doi: 10.7931/dl1t7035.3

14. Anderson D, Gormley A, Bosson M, Livingstone P, Nugent G. Livestock as sentinels for an infectious disease in a sympatric or adjacent-living wildlife reservoir host. *Prevent Vet Med.* (2017) 148:106–14. doi: 10.1016/j.prevetmed.2017.10.015

15. Gormley A, Anderson D, Nugent G. Cost-based optimization of the stopping threshold for local disease surveillance during progressive eradication of tuberculosis from New Zealand wildlife. *Transbound Emerg Dis.* (2018) 65:186–96. doi: 10.1111/tbed.12647

16. Anderson D, Gormley A, Ramsey D, Nugent G, Martin P, Bosson M, et al. Bio-economic optimisation of surveillance to confirm broadscale eradications of invasive pests and diseases. *Biol Invas.* (2017) 19:2869–84. doi: 10.1007/s10530-017-1490-5

17. OIE. *Terrestrial Animal Health Code, Chapter 8.11: Infection with Mycobacterium Complex*. Office International des Epizooties (World Organisation for Animal Health) (2018). Available online at: http://www.oie.int/index.php?id=169&L=0&htmfile=chapitre_bovine_tuberculosis.htm (Accessed September 14, 2018).

18. Livingstone P, Hancox N, Nugent G, Mackereth G, Hutchings S. Development of the New Zealand strategy for local eradication of tuberculosis from wildlife and livestock. *N Z Vet J.* (2015) 63(Suppl. 1):98–107. doi: 10.1080/00480169.2015.1013581

19. Hutchings S, Hancox N, Livingstone P. A strategic approach to eradication of bovine TB from wildlife in New Zealand. *Transbound Emerg Dis.* (2013) 60:85–91. doi: 10.1111/tbed.12079

20. OSPRI. *Annual Report 2015/2016*. Wellington: OSPRI New Zealand (2016). Available online at: https://www.ospri.co.nz/assets/Uploads/

Documents/OSPRI-Annual-Review-201516.pdf (Accessed August 8, 2018).

21. OSPRI *Annual Report 2016/2017*. Wellington: OSPRI New Zealand (2017). Available online at: https://www.ospri.co.nz/assets/Uploads/Documents/OSPRI-Annual-Report-201617.pdf (Accessed August 8, 2018).

22. Anderson D, Ramsey D, Nugent G, Bosson M, Livingstone P, Martin P, et al. A novel approach to assess the probability of disease eradication from a wild-animal reservoir host. *Epidemiol Infect.* (2013) 141:1509–21. doi: 10.1017/S095026881200310X

23. Ramsey DS, Efford MG. Management of bovine tuberculosis in brushtail possums in New Zealand: predictions from a spatially explicit, individual-based model. *J Appl Ecol.* (2010) 47:911–9. doi: 10.1111/j.1365-2664.2010.01839.x

24. Nugent G, Ramsey D, Caley P. *Enhanced Early Detection of TB Through Use and Integration of Wildlife Data Into the National Surveillance Model.* Landcare Research Contract Report (unpubl.). Lincoln: Landcare Research (2006). doi: 10.7931/dl1t7035.4

25. Warburton B, Livingstone P. Managing and eradicating wildlife tuberculosis in New Zealand. *N Z Vet J.* (2015) 63:77–88. doi: 10.1080/00480169.2014.981315

26. Barlow N. Control of endemic bovine TB in New Zealand possum populations: results from a simple model. *J Appl Ecol.* (1991) 28:794–809. doi: 10.2307/2404208

27. Nugent G, Yockney I, Whitford J, Cross ML. Mortality rate and gross pathology due to tuberculosis in wild brushtail possums (*Trichosurus vulpecula*) following low dose subcutaneous injection of *Mycobacterium bovis*. *Prevent Vet Med.* (2013) 109:168–75. doi: 10.1016/j.prevetmed.2012.09.008

28. Cannon R. Demonstrating disease freedom: combining confidence levels. *Prevent Vet Med.* (2002) 52:227–49. doi: 10.1016/S0167-5877(01)00262-8

29. Lugton IW. *The Contribution of Wild Mammals to the Epidemiology of Tuberculosis (Mycobacterium bovis) in New Zealand: A Thesis Presented in Partial Fulfilment of the Requirements for the Degree of Doctor of Philosophy at Massey University* (1997). Palmerston North: Massey University.

30. Gardner IA, Stryhn H, Lind P, Collins MT. Conditional dependence between tests affects the diagnosis and surveillance of animal diseases. *Prevent Vet Med.* (2000) 45:107–22. doi: 10.1016/S0167-5877(00)00119-7

31. Sweetapple P, Nugent G. Chew-track-cards: a multiple-species small mammal detection device. *N Z J Ecol.* (2011) 153–62.

32. Nugent G. Maintenance, spillover and spillback transmission of bovine tuberculosis in multi-host wildlife complexes: a New Zealand case study. *Vet Microbiol.* (2011) 151:34–42. doi: 10.1016/j.vetmic.2011.02.023

33. Nugent G, Whitford J, Young N. Use of released pigs as sentinels for *Mycobacterium bovis*. *J Wildlife Dis.* (2002) 38:665–77. doi: 10.7589/0090-3558-38.4.665

34. Yockney I, Nugent G, Latham M, Perry M, Cross M, Byrom A. Comparison of ranging behaviour in a multi-species complex of free-ranging hosts of bovine tuberculosis in relation to their use as disease sentinels. *Epidemiol Infect.* (2013) 141:1407–16. doi: 10.1017/S0950268813000289

35. Nugent G, Whitford J, Yockney I, Cross M. Reduced spillover transmission of *Mycobacterium bovis* to feral pigs (*Sus scofa*) following population control of brushtail possums (*Trichosurus vulpecula*). *Epidemiol Infect.* (2012) 140:1036–47. doi: 10.1017/S0950268811001579

36. Gormley AM, Holland EP, Barron MC, Anderson DP, Nugent G. A modelling framework for predicting the optimal balance between control and surveillance effort in the local eradication of tuberculosis in New Zealand wildlife. *Prevent Vet Med.* (2016) 125:10–8. doi: 10.1016/j.prevetmed.2016.01.007

37. Barron MC, Nugent G, Latham MC. *Improved Modelling of TB Persistence in Possum Populations.* Landcare Research Contract Report (unpubl.). Lincoln: Landcare Research (2017). doi: 10.7931/dl1t7035.1

38. Latham MC, Nugent G. *Evaluating Assessments of TB Freedom in Possums: How Close Are We?* Landcare Research Contract Report (unpubl.). Lincoln: Landcare Research (2016). doi: 10.7931/dl1t7035.2

39. Walters CJ. *Adaptive Management of Renewable Resources.* New York, NY: Macmillan Publishers Ltd (1986).

APPENDIX: LIST OF ABBREVIATIONS AND DEFINITIONS USED IN THE TEXT

Assurance surveillance	Possum-TB surveillance undertaken after an area has been declared free, usually using unplanned, low-cost, "passive" methods (hunter observations from possums, deer and pigs, and livestock testing or slaughterhouse inspection data collected for other purposes).
Control	Reduction in possum density by lethal trapping or poisoning.
Control	efficacy Effectiveness of possum population reduction (% kill).
Control history	Summary of the duration (span of years) and intensity (control effectiveness or efficacy).
Disease	A term of convenience used to encompass the presence of subclinical *M. bovis* infection as well as the presence of actual symptoms of disease.
Eradication	Complete or absolute removal of *M. bovis* infection from all animals in an area with negligible chance of re-establishment.
Freedom	High but not absolute probability of absence of *M. bovis* infection from all animals in a specified area at a specific time.
Max prior	Maximum permissible prior: a subjective precautionary prescription of the maximum value that can be ascribed to the prior (defined below).
NPMP	National Pest Management Plan: a national plan required under New Zealand biosecurity legislation, first developed in the mid-1990s and revised and updated in 2005, 2011, and 2016.
P_{free}	Probability of absence of *M. bovis* infection from possums in a specified area at a specific time.
PoF	Proof of Freedom: a Bayesian belief-updating framework in which a quantitative estimate of the belief (confidence) that an area is free of TB at a given time (the "prior") is updated at a later time by the new information gathered between the two times to produce a new estimate (the posterior). The updating takes into account the possibility of re-introduction of new infection.
Posterior	A quantitative probabilistic estimate of the belief (confidence) that an area is free of TB at a given time that is derived by updating an initial prior belief with new empirical evidence of TB absence.
Prior	A quantitative probabilistic estimate of the belief (confidence) that an area is free of TB at a given time
P_*	Design prevalence: the specified surveillance target.
Re-control	Additional control required when an area is falsely declared free of TB, resulting in eventual to re-emergence of the disease and a need to again reduce possum densities in a further effort to break the TB cycle in possums.
Sentinels	Spill-over hosts of TB that can become infected by transmission from possums, but which do not independently maintain the infection, either because they are largely end hosts (pigs, deer, and ferrets in most places), or because they are subject to effective TB management (livestock).
SPM	Spatial Possum Model: an individual-based, spatially explicit simulation model of the eco-epidemiological dynamic of TB in possums, which is used to predict the likely effect of historical possum control on TB prevalence in possums.
SS	Surveillance sensitivity: the probability of finding an *M. bovis* infected animal in a particular survey sample of possums or sentinels if n TB possums were actually present in the area surveyed, with n/N (the population size) being the design prevalence P_*.
Stopping rule	The desired or prescribed level of confidence required before an area can be declared free of wildlife TB.
Surveillance	Empirical survey of animal disease status (through necropsy and mycobacterial culture of wild animals, or TB testing and/or slaughterhouse inspection of livestock).
TB	Bovine tuberculosis, caused by infection with *Mycobacterium bovis*.
TB possum	A possum with *M. bovis infection*.
VCZ	Vector control zones: formally defined areas, typically of 10,000–20,000 ha, used for planning possum control and surveillance, and forming the primary spatial management unit.
VRA	Vector risk area: an area considered to have a non-zero probability of containing infected wildlife (see https://ospri.co.nz/our-programmes/tbfree/about-the-tbfree-programme/wildlife-and-pest-management/vector-risk-areas/). "Vector free" areas (all of the non-VRA land) can contain infected livestock provided there is high confidence that the infection originated in other livestock elsewhere.

4

Negotiated Management Strategies for Bovine Tuberculosis: Enhancing Risk Mitigation in Michigan and the UK

Ruth A. Little*

Department of Geography, University of Sheffield, Sheffield, United Kingdom

*Correspondence:
Ruth A. Little
ruth.little@sheffield.ac.uk

Bovine tuberculosis (bTB) is an epidemiologically, politically, and socially complex disease. Across multiple international contexts, policy makers have struggled to balance the competing demands of wildlife and agricultural interests in their efforts to create workable and effective disease management strategies. This paper draws comparative lessons between the cases of Michigan in the USA and the UK to exemplify some of the challenges of developing an effective strategy for the long-term control of endemic disease, particularly reflecting on efforts to "responsibilise" cattle producers and engage them in proactive activities to mitigate transmission risks on their own farms. Using qualitative data derived from 22 stakeholder interviews, it is argued that the management of bTB in Michigan has important lessons for the UK on the role of human dimensions in influencing the direction of disease control. The management of endemic bTB relies on the actions of individuals to minimise risk and, in contrast to the predominantly voluntary approach pursued in the UK, Michigan has shifted the emphasis towards obtaining producer support for wildlife risk mitigation and biosecurity via a mix of regulatory, fiscal, and social interventions. Whilst the scale of the bTB challenge differs between these two contexts, analysis of the different ideological bases for selecting management approaches offers interesting insights on the role of negotiated outcomes in attempts to adaptively manage a disease that is characterised by complexity and uncertainty.

Keywords: bovine tuberculosis, risk mitigation, biosecurity, human dimensions, responsibilisation

INTRODUCTION

Bovine tuberculosis (bTB) is principally a disease of cattle, but there are several places worldwide where free-ranging wildlife are reservoirs of infection, namely brushtail possums in New Zealand, European badgers in the United Kingdom, wood bison and elk in Canada, African buffalo in South Africa and white-tailed deer in the United States (1). Where the disease has become established, it can have considerable economic consequences for livestock keepers and poses challenges for national governments and agencies in devising a workable and socially acceptable eradication plan. The ultimate rationale for intervention is based on the potential threat *Mycobacterium bovis* poses to public health (2); however, the proximate driver for expenditure on bTB management is the potential economic effect of trade restrictions on milk and meat products (3, 4) and the wider ecological concerns associated with potential disease spread into new regions and ecosystems.

The case for eradication has been contested based upon cost benefit criteria and the relative importance of the risk posed to human health [see (5–7)], but it remains the declared goal for many international control programmes [see, for example, (4, 8)].

Experiences from around the world exemplify the challenges faced by disease managers in constructing a coherent, cost-effective, and workable strategy for eradication. Multiple ecological and epidemiological challenges remain [see (9, 10) for a review], but socio-economic and political factors also have a key role to play in influencing the outcomes of disease control strategies; including, the cost-effectiveness of the policies, political will to implement management programmes and the social acceptability of individual control measures. The UK is perhaps the foremost example of the difficulties involved in constructing a control regime under conditions of intense socio-political scrutiny. A primary point of contention has been the decision to cull badgers in England, which are considered to have important cultural associations for the general public [see (11, 12)]. Vigorous debate on the role of badger culling in the control of bTB has resulted in policies that have been considered to lack coherence (13) and a situation where the devolved administrations pursue their own control policies, with differing approaches to addressing the disease in their wildlife populations (14, 15)[1]. This has resulted in what Allen et al. [(10), p. 110] considers this to be part of "the current impasse in bTB control" across Britain and Ireland, with multi-factorial problems inhibiting the national eradication programmes.

Socio-economic and political factors have been highlighted as determinants of success in analyses of international control programmes. For example, Professor Ian Boyd, The Chief Scientific Adviser to the UK government's Department for Environment, Food and Rural Affairs (DEFRA) described bovine tuberculosis as a "sociological problem," stressing the importance of human dimensions in influencing disease outcomes. Similar claims have been made in review papers on the complexity of bTB control (16) and in studies of eradication attempts in the US (1), Australia (17), and New Zealand (18, 19). These determinants tend to focus on three separate, but interconnected factors: the effectiveness of political decision-making; social acceptability of the policies; and the attitudes and actions of affected stakeholders.

This paper focuses on the experience of bTB control in the US state of Michigan to provide a comparison for current and future policy developments in the UK. Whilst the scale of the problem in Michigan is different to the UK, there are interesting comparators in terms of socio-economic and political factors influencing the perceived success of efforts to achieve effective disease control. For example, Carstensen et al. (1) reported, "public tolerance" and political will were considered to exert significant influence on the control measures available to disease managers in the US. The authors also cite a series of temporal, social, economic, and logistical factors that shaped public and stakeholder attitudes towards aggressive disease control strategies, the limitations that these factors placed on management options and the subsequent implications for bTB eradication from the wildlife reservoirs in the USA. Carstensen et al. (1) concluded that, in comparison to the response to a notable outbreak of bTB in Minnesota in 2006, which successfully prevented the self-sustaining establishment of the disease in wildlife, Michigan has lacked the leadership to initiate more "aggressive" bTB management strategies in both cattle (via, for example, buy-out options for herds in areas of high bTB risk) and wildlife (through substantial reduction in deer numbers via intensive culling).

Without the will to institute more "aggressive" responses to controlling the disease in cattle and wildlife populations, the management of bTB often requires a negotiated management response, based upon the level of funding available and the buy-in from the thousands of individual disease managers (e.g., farmers, hunters, and the like) tasked with controlling the disease over a sustained period. As Miller (20) notes, management of diseases at the livestock–wildlife interface often require long-term engagement using a combination of altered livestock husbandry practices, active disease suppression in wildlife, and prevention of transmission using mitigation techniques. Considerable attention has been given to the development of interventions designed to mitigate the risk of bTB disease transmission between cattle and wildlife [see (21, 22)]. Generally, the research concludes that risk mitigation interventions such as deer exclusion fences have great potential but the challenge lies in farmers modifying their husbandry practices and behaviours (20) including maintaining the integrity of fences and keeping gates closed (23, 24). Risk mitigation measures that rely on stakeholder adoption of preventative behaviours [see (25)], therefore, pose challenges for risk managers in formulating measures that will incentivize positive responses.

Similar issues can be observed in the UK relating to the adoption of preventative biosecurity measures at the farm level. Whilst biosecurity is cited as a key part of the Defra's 25 year Strategy to Achieve Officially Bovine Tuberculosis Free Status for England (2014), multiple challenges remain regarding farmers' adoption of measures to reduce the risk of bTB transmission between cattle and between cattle and wildlife. Farmers can be reticent to implement measures because of the limited evidence surrounding the efficacy of many of the interventions (9, 26, 27); the perceived impracticality of implementing measures on their own farms (28), particularly relating to badger exclusion and isolation of bought in cattle, and the uncertain benefits that will accrue in reducing their risk of a bTB breakdown as opposed to the costs of modifying feed and water sources, installing fences to reduce contacts with neighboring herds or establishing isolation facilities for newly bought in animals. Whilst farmers acknowledge the theoretical importance of biosecurity as a preventative measure, this does not always result in taking action to reduce risks on farm (29–31). Such reluctance to act may be associated with farmers' often-reported "fatalistic" belief that there is little that they can proactively do to prevent a bTB breakdown or that "luck" rather than their own actions has more

---

[1]Animal health is a devolved issue in the United Kingdom. England, Wales, Scotland, and Northern Ireland each have the ability to develop and implement their own control policy for bovine tuberculosis, which is currently subject to oversight and audit by the Food and Veterinary Office of the European Commission. It should be noted that Scotland has been Officially Tuberculosis Free (OTF) since September 2009.

of an influence on the likelihood of the disease entering their herds (32–34).

Currently, the majority of biosecurity measures outlined in Defra's 25 year Strategy are voluntary, with some additional requirements for farms within badger culling areas and for "persistent" bTB herds. Improving biosecurity on and off farm is stated as an important management goal within Defra's Strategy. As the literature indicates, risk managers will need to formulate measures to address the apparent disjuncture between the acknowledged importance yet under-implementation of risk mitigation measures on farm. Using Michigan as a case study, the objectives of this study were to investigate management approaches, policies and interventions designed to engage farmers in adopting and sustaining preventative bTB biosecurity measures and qualitatively assess their impact in contributing to disease control.

The paper will outline some of the comparative lessons that can be learned from Michigan in their attempts to enhance the on-farm risk mitigation element of their disease management strategies and the policies considered most effective in encouraging proactive disease management at the farm level.

METHODOLOGY

The research focused on stakeholder perspectives on eradication efforts, assessing the relative merits of different policy interventions aimed at disease management and appraising the key factors affecting efforts to achieve bTB eradication. The research approach was based upon 22 in-depth face to face interviews conducted at the end of 2014. Non-probabilistic, purposive sampling [akin to (25, 35)] was used to select interviewees with individuals identified based upon their roles as "experts" and "key stakeholders" involved in the development or implementation of bTB policies in Michigan. This research was part of a wider study that included a further set of interviews in Minnesota; the results of which was not reported here. Interviewees were stratified into the following three broad categories: agency professionals involved in bTB management in cattle or wildlife (wildlife managers, programme coordinators, field veterinarians, and communications specialists); university academic and extension personnel; and cattle producer and wildlife stakeholders involved in implementing management practices on the ground. Interviews were conducted in the State capital and in the Modified Accredited Zone (MAZ) in the northeastern lower peninsula (NELP) of Michigan, concentrating on the counties of Alcona, Alpena, Montmorency, and Oscoda Counties.

The research was designed to be a qualitative, in-depth assessment of bTB management approaches in Michigan. As indicated by Naylor et al. [(36), p. 286] "interviewing is the method most often adopted to explore potentially sensitive and controversial issues… and are often commended as a research method for their flexibility and ability to explore difficult issues in a comprehensive and sensitive manner." Unlike the standardised and structured approaches of farmer attitude surveys or Q-Methodology [e.g., (35, 37, 38)] the interviews

were semi-structured and discussions were based around a set of themes within an interview guide; this approach has been used in equivalent qualitative studies on bTB and biosecurity [see (32)]. The interview guide consisted of questions relating to the participant's role in bTB control; overview of the factors influencing the relative success of bTB control (including identifying effective policies and interventions); identification of key stakeholders and their positive or negative contribution to disease management; modes of risk communication and the challenges and successes encountered in promoting "best practice" in disease mitigation; and lessons learnt from their experience of managing bTB in Michigan[2]. Each interview was tailored to the expertise and knowledge of the interviewee and so the focus of each discussion was context specific. However, all interviewees were asked about and responded to questions on policies and interventions that were considered to be effective in encouraging disease managers (e.g., farmers and hunters) to adopt positive disease management practices. The results of which are reported here.

Interviews were digitally recorded (with the participants' informed consent) and later fully transcribed. The data was manually coded in order to develop an empirically grounded coding framework, guided by the key research questions. This involved an iterative and in-depth process of "careful reading and re-reading of the data" [(39), p. 258], beginning with an informal reading of the materials to identify an initial set of high-level thematic codes. The approach followed the conventions of Seidel and Kelle (40) quoted in Basit [(41), p. 144] who "view the role of coding as noticing relevant phenomena; collecting examples of those phenomena; and analyzing those phenomena in order to find commonalities, differences, patterns and structures." Categories were developed via a process "data distillation" (42) to organise the coded data into meaningful overarching themes. The themes were based upon concepts from existing literature and from words and phrases used by the interviewees e.g., notions of responsibility and responsibilisation; social networks and peer example; drivers and incentives. These themes are represented as organising concepts in the results section.

Following a broad introduction to bTB management approaches in Michigan, an overview will be provided of the Wildlife Risk Mitigation project, which was identified as being a key development in efforts to enhance on-farm biosecurity activities.

RESULTS

Management Approaches for bTB in Michigan

On-farm Wildlife Risk Mitigation (WRM) is part of a wider approach to bTB management in Michigan, including surveillance, and control measures aimed at reducing the disease burden in both cattle and wildlife (white-tailed deer). The focus

---

[2]For study replication purposes, the interview guide is included as a **Supplementary Data File**. Full details of the sampling, research approach, and anonymized transcripts can be found within the ReShare UK Data Service repository.

of this paper is WRM, however a brief overview of the control programme is described here.

Michigan was declared free of bTB in cattle and bison in 1979. However, in 1975, and again in 1994, bTB was identified in one wild white-tail deer in the NELP of Michigan. Subsequent testing revealed the disease to be endemic in the white-tail deer population within five of the most north easterly counties of the Lower Peninsula. Since 1995 surveillance and testing has been carried out in the affected area via annual surveillance of hunter harvested deer. To date, the disease has been confirmed in nearly 875 of over 254,000 free-ranging deer tested in Michigan, with 77% of bTB-positive deer found in a core area— Deer Management Unit 452—in the NELP of Michigan, where the counties of Alcona, Alpena, Montmorency, and Oscoda meet (**Figure 1**). Reduction in deer density within the affected area is a key part of the policy, with enhanced measures introduced over successive seasons designed to maximise legal opportunities for the public to harvest deer. These strategies include liberalised hunting seasons; issuing landowners Deer Management Assistance permits to supplement hunting licences; providing disease control permits to cattle producers and non-agricultural landowners in high prevalence areas; and, most recently, the introduction of the Hunter Access Program, to match hunters in search of places to hunt with agricultural landowners seeking additional deer harvest on their land. Deer baiting and feeding bans are also in operation in some of the affected areas.

Following the identification of bTB positive deer in the 1990s, the reinstatement of cattle testing in the affected area revealed the first infected cattle herd in June 1998. Michigan subsequently lost its bTB free status in June 2000 and state-wide surveillance testing was instituted from 2000 to 2003. The Upper Peninsula regained bTB Free status in 2005 and 57 counties in the Lower Peninsula regained bTB Free status in 2011. Surveillance testing identified a core disease outbreak area in 11 counties in the northeastern tip of the Lower Peninsula; since October 2014, seven more of those counties have been declared bTB Free for cattle, leaving 4 remaining. Annual testing of all livestock (cattle, goats, bison) and captive cervids remains in place in the 4 counties (classified as the MAZ by the US Department of Agriculture's Animal and Plant Health Inspection Service-Veterinary Services Branch[3]), with risk-based testing applied throughout the remainder of the State. In the MAZ, the traceability and movement of livestock is regulated through movement permits obtained from the field offices of the Michigan Department of Agriculture and Rural Development (MDARD), electronic identification of animals and annual herd inventories to reconcile discrepancies between animals on farm and official records. Other policies governing livestock movements and limiting deer-cattle contacts will be covered more fully in the following section.

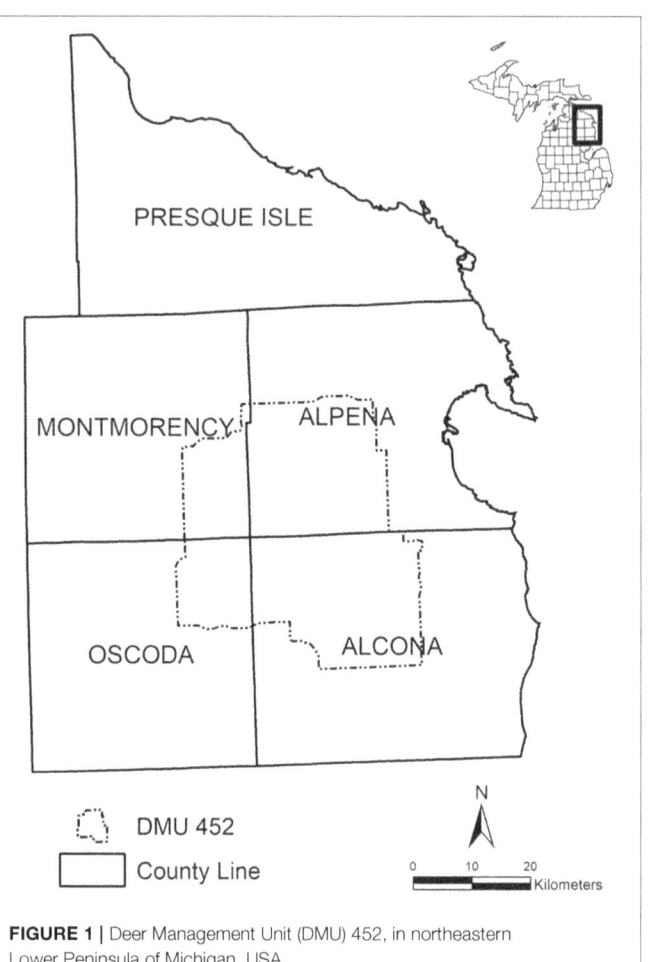

FIGURE 1 | Deer Management Unit (DMU) 452, in northeastern Lower Peninsula of Michigan, USA.

Wildlife Risk Mitigation

WRM is now a key element of the bTB management strategy, particularly concentrating on the commercial farms in and around the MAZ in the NELP of Michigan, identified as at risk for bTB transmission from wildlife. The policy began as a series of small scale activities at Michigan State University (MSU) which, from 2008, formalised into a voluntary initiative developed by MDARD, MSU Extension, United States Department of Agriculture (Veterinary Services, Wildlife Services), and the Natural Resources Conservation Service (NRCS), with some input from industry. The objective of the programme was to assist producers in identifying high risk areas and practices on their holding and develop plans to reduce the risk of cattle-wildlife interactions. The approach was designed to form part of the "safety nets" (44) put in place to control the disease, complementing the surveillance testing and movement restrictions in helping to prevent opportunities for infection; the ultimate aim being to draw down the disease incidence in cattle.

The programme required changes to be made to management practices and farm infrastructure in the endemic area. It relied upon the development of a series of interventions to assist and influence the implementation of risk reduction measures on farm, including the introduction of hoop barns and deer-proof

---

[3]The prevalence of infection a State or zone are classified in five categories: (1) Accredited-free state or zone; (2) Modified Accredited Advanced state or zone; (3) Modified Accredited state or zone; (4) Accreditation Preparatory state or zone; and (5) Non-Accredited state or zone [see (43) for an explanation of the United States bTB accreditation categories].

fencing to protect stored feeds and actions related to cattle accessing feed and water sources. The changes required at farm-level meant that the concept of WRM was controversial from the outset. According to a Michigan policy lead, *"this was probably the most controversial thing that happened in the course of the bTB programme; more so even than testing…there was a tremendous amount of angst and anger about this wildlife risk project."* Producer concerns focused on the practicalities of excluding deer from their property; the cost of implementing the measures and a perceived inadequacy on the part of Department of Natural Resources (DNR) to deal effectively with the disease in wildlife (e.g., through the reduction of deer numbers). Due to the contentious nature of the proposal, the policy making process involved a series of meetings to develop proposals and standards which were an acceptable compromise between what was desired by policy makers and risk managers and what was considered achievable in practice by the agricultural industry. The process was described in the following terms by an individual involved in the development of the scheme:

> *"it's that idea of, okay, if you can't build 20 foot or 12 foot high barbed wire fences all the way round…where are the opportunities to reduce risk most cost effectively? So we got the best available science from [Michigan's bTB Programme] and we started sharing it with our stakeholders, the producers and let them decide."*

The process of negotiation, over a series of three meetings, focused on achieving a balance between an epidemiological ideal and an implementable policy. The process was facilitated by MSU staff as intermediaries and the University published the document.

Implementation

The implementation of the scheme was described by its instigators in terms of a phased approach, based upon the principles of adaptive management [see (45–47)]: phase one was aimed at individuals identified as "early adopters" who were engaged with a prototype version of the WRM intervention; the second phase was an expansion of the programme, designed to appeal to "capable learners"; and the third was regulatory enforcements to draw in those who were "resistant to change." It was also phased in regionally; MDARD concentrated on the outlying areas first, where there was an opportunity to elevate the accreditation status more swiftly (for example, in Michigan's Northwest Region where bTB was not endemic in wild deer) and moved on to the more challenging and higher risk area of the MAZ over time. This incremental approach evolved into an increasingly statutory regime and relied on a number of key push and pull factors designed to maximise participation in the scheme. A combination of one-to-one assistance, co-funding of risk mitigation measures (such as deer fencing) and restrictions placed on market access have been employed to both encourage and enable producer engagement in the scheme, but also to make it challenging for them to stay outside of the system.

The WRM project is designed around a five-step process which aims to bring livestock producers and technical experts together to create a tailored on-farm plan to reduce the risk of infection between cattle and wildlife. Producers are offered an educational meeting before completing an on-farm risk assessment. The risk assessment is conducted between government agency staff and is designed to be both educational (recognising potentially risky areas, and practices on farm) and regulatory, with the implementation of certain mitigation actions being classified as compulsory. Once the WRM Action Plan has been agreed, the producer then indicates a timescale within which they propose to complete the actions. Depending on the risks identified on farm, these actions may include interventions to limit potential infection transfer at sites where cattle are fed (governing where, how often and how much cattle are fed), water sources for cattle and where cattle feed is stored. Each of these sites have been identified as a risk for disease transmission (48, 49) and so require changes to management practices, including fencing off feed and water sources to prevent deer access. Once the plan has been implemented, the work is subject to an annual verification process to check that the interventions and actions are still in place.

As part of the development of the plan, a cost-sharing scheme was introduced to assist cattle producers in implementing the actions. During 2008–2013, over $3.6 m was expended on WRM measures. Government, state and federal funds accounted for $2,637,000 of this figure and a further $1,002,000 was contributed by cattle producers. In the early phases of the scheme, 50% of the cost-share funding came from the state and the USDA, and in the later phases, the bTB programme utilised the USDA, NRCS's Environmental Quality Incentives Programme. The benefit of the latter approach being that mutual aims could be achieved from a single funding allocation and that the conservation office, which already had close historical links to the farming community, could take over the responsibilities for the continuation and annual verification of the scheme.

Drivers and Incentives

The development of the risk assessment and verification process was originally badged as a voluntary approach. However, (dis)incentives were introduced to influence the level of uptake amongst producers. One interviewee described it as, *"incentives on the cattle side were, first of all, it was disincentives, you couldn't move [cattle] if you didn't do it."* Additional testing and restrictions on market access were the primary levers to encourage uptake of the WRM. The policy stipulated that a pre-movement test be carried out on cattle from non-WRM farms, with a further post-movement test 60 to 120 days after purchase being required of the purchaser at their own expense. The rationale for the approach was described by an individual involved in developing the policy as follows:

> *"So the state used to pay for all that [testing] and in these counties we've said okay, you know, you have an hour, you could get a biosecurity plan and you don't have to do this test, but, you know, if you don't want to do that that's fine, you can do this additional test, but you get to pay for it now and then the guy who buys your cows, unless he gets them slaughtered, has to also do a test at his expense. Well that means that the cattle are discounted, because when people go, oh, I got to do a test, well that's going to cost me something, so*

I'm not going to pay quite so much for these cattle and so that has driven some people and we were trying to use market forces to, you know, move people towards doing the right thing."

Through restricting market access and attaching a financial disincentive to the cattle from non-WRM farms, the aim was to shift producers' assessment of the costs and benefits in favour of enrolling in the WRM scheme. The (dis)incentives were strengthened in January 2015, when regulations were introduced stating that all farms in the bTB core area must be wildlife risk mitigated; otherwise, these producers could only send their animals to slaughter.

Social Networks and Peer Example

In addition to perceived economic (dis)benefits, risk managers involved in developing, and refining Michigan's eradication programme employed a series of techniques to influence the social context into which their strategies were being placed. The approach included the use of existing social networks within the locality to promote sign up to the scheme and peer example coupled with "teachable moments" to encourage producer-advocates of the scheme to explain the benefits, particularly following cases of bTB outbreaks where WRM may have been assistive in preventing disease transmission. The rationale being, as summarised by an extension agent, *"peer example, call it, rather than peer pressure, can be very effective."* The use of social networks was seen as a way of dealing with the negative view towards government officials and enlisting more trusted intermediaries to deliver the message on the benefits of the scheme. This approach is exemplified in the following quotes:

"I think other people have said okay yeah if I'm hearing this from my neighbour and my friend I'm not hearing it from the state veterinarian or, you know, some USDA regulator, but I'm hearing it from, you know, my friends and they tend to take it a little bit more seriously, especially if you're seeing that person every day or at church or in a grocery store or at the bar or whatever, so that makes it a little bit more real".

"So one of the things we did, we had I don't know about maybe 45, 46 of these that were still hanging out here in the farms in here that had not done a biosecurity plan and so back in April I made phone calls to people that work on these farms and just trying to ascertain who is the person that might most effectively communicate things in a positive way, where we would get them actually to do something and so actually some of our guys, you know, are relatives to these people or they've cultivated, you know, decent relationships."

The role of these gate keepers within the producer community was important to facilitate wider implementation, using existing social networks to connect government authorities with producers at the farm level. There were also particular individuals that were highly functional in terms of engaging producers and hunters in disease management efforts, be they as an identifiable, visible, and approachable lead of the bTB programme or as key personnel within the areas most at risk from a bTB outbreak. In the words of one policy maker, *"[t]he policies were supporting the risk mitigation, the policies were making sure you had some*

local expertise, it wasn't just coming out of Lansing to talk to people." The division of "distant" government officials in the State Capital of Lansing and the affected communities in the NELP was addressed through convening local meetings, placing the onus on appointing personnel from within the local area and working through MSU extension, which has long-established links with cattle producers via existing research programmes and community outreach.

Sustaining Disease Management Practices

During the development phases, it was recognised that the installation of measures such as deer fencing was only the first part of a successful WRM plan. The second part was the maintenance and continued use of measures by cattle producers, such as keeping gates to feed sources closed. The challenge of sustaining disease management practices at the farm level was described in the following terms:

"How do we get producers to do that, how do we support it, you know, how do we maintain it, because, you know, you can pour a lot of money into fencing and, you know, other mitigation, but if you do it for 1 year and then you say it's too much trouble, you know, to keep the fences maintained and stuff like it doesn't really matter then, so it's not only doing the mitigation, but then maintaining it over time."

To address this challenge, conditions were attached to the grants allocated for co-funding of WRM measures. Producers were required to sign a contract outlining their obligations (e.g., closing gates) and if they were found to be in contravention of those conditions, then the state would be entitled to reclaim the cost-share money and the farm's WRM verification would be withdrawn, with consequent implications for trade and enhanced testing.

Promoting Action and Assessing Impact

WRM began as a controversial policy aimed at enhanced risk mitigation at the farm level. As already noted, the development was controversial because of the implications that the new measures and requirements had for farm management decisions and infrastructure. During interviews, stakeholders reflected on the difficulties involved in introducing and implementing the scheme, but also recognised the perceived benefits that WRM provided in terms of enhanced disease management through reducing risk at the livestock-wildlife interface and the transfer of responsibilities for disease management to producers on their own properties. The following section provides an overview of stakeholder perspectives on the perceived utility and impact of the WRM scheme.

Responsibility

A clear reason for the development of the WRM scheme was to re-centre the responsibility for keeping bTB out of herds back into the hands of the cattle producers. Whilst WRM has been a predominantly government-led scheme (with input from producers and producer organisations), the aim has been to highlight what producers can do on their own holdings to mitigate risk and then, via co-funding and advisory visits, enable them to implement exclusion measures such as barns and deer fences. This represented a step change in the policy. In the words of a field veterinarian:

> "I mean before [WRM] it was just test, test, test, test, test, test, find it, where do we find it? And it wasn't until the wildlife risk programme started that we started having something to say hey, let's do something to help prevent it".

The emphasis on engaging producers in proactive action was driven by a number of considerations: first, the need for producers in the NELP to act in the interest of the rest of the cattle industry in the state of Michigan (to retain interstate market access); and second, the realisation that deer would remain only a partially controllable element of disease transmission due to a perceived—on the part of the cattle industry—lack of social and political will to reduce deer densities. Producers were, therefore, encouraged to look at what they could do on their own holdings to institute some control over the opportunities for transmission within the farm boundaries.

Whilst the aim was to transfer responsibility for mitigating risk to individual producers, the initiative remained government-led. Through the implementation of market-driven interventions, co-funding opportunities and increasingly statutory measures, the onus for compliance came from a regulatory source. Thus, replacing the previous approach of leaving it to individual farmers to assess and institute risk management on farm and relying on peer pressure amongst producers to encourage uptake. When asked about the role of peer pressure, a cattle producer commented:

> "It's not so much peer pressure as it is pressure on the government or those above to make the policies that'll force them into it, yeah, that's more the pressure than me going over. I don't want to go over to my neighbour and tell him you have to do this, you know, I can go over there and nicely tell him why he should do it, but for me to go tell him he has to do it I don't want to do that, I don't want to put myself in that spot either."

Engendering greater responsibility for assessing what was possible on individual holdings and underlining producers' ability to exert some control over their own situations was an important driver. This was, however, coupled with a more top-down approach of imposing market and regulatory conditions to promote and embed management changes across areas most at risk from a bTB breakdown.

Assessing the Impacts

WRM was designed as a management strategy to reduce rather than eliminate risk on farm, placing the emphasis on taking greater control over limiting opportunities for deer-cattle interactions and working with producers to focus on the elements within their control to promote effective management of deer-cattle interactions. In terms of benefits, interviewees cited a greater awareness amongst producers of the risks posed to their own farms and enhanced actions around careful storage of cattle feed, with wider general improvements to biosecurity. Whilst being unable to provide evidence for or quantify the benefits

of WRM, an assumption was shared amongst interviewees that decreasing the risk of contacts would decrease the number of cases. This opinion is exemplified in the following quotes—the first from a member of the USDA's epidemiological research team and the second from a cattle producer in the high risk area of the MAZ:

> "Well if the producers are compliant with their plan it has I believe reduced the wildlife livestock interface quite a bit and it's also made people I think more aware of how the disease transmission could occur and what they need to do to decrease the amount of contact that the cattle have with deer."
>
> "Well the risk mitigation I believe has worked. It's not foolproof, but it has helped. If nothing else has brought it to the people's attention that these are the focus areas that they should focus on, you know, keeping the feed away and that type of thing. It's brought some attention at least that way and I think some people are becoming more receptive to "agriculture's going to have to take some role in this." I mean when this first started Ag kind of stepped back and said this is their [the DNR's] problem; let them deal with it and it'll work out when they work out their problem. Well obviously, we're not going to reach that point, so we have to step up to the plate and do our part too. Now we have different opinions on what our part is, you know, every person has a different opinion what they're willing to do and capable of doing."

Both of these quotes raise the issue of producers' implementation of the stipulated measures, and is indicative of a wider theme of discussion on compliance with the control regime. Producers and those involved in the preparation and verification of individual farm plans, stated that WRM tended to be based upon a negotiation between the ideals envisaged by state agencies and the practicalities of what was considered achievable at the farm level. This process was described by producers as a form of "trading" back and forth to find a plan that was acceptable to both parties. Finding this middle ground for WRM was considered to be more constructive than imposing a set of measures that were deemed unattainable by the producer and which may prompt non-compliance. As one producer commented,

> I'm sure [MDARD] would like us to tighten up a lot of our standards... but then nobody's going to follow through with it.... our standard might not be exactly as high as we want it to be, but if it'll address 50% of the risk and they'll do it 100% of the time; that's better than addressing 90% of the risk and doing it none of the time.

The same producer stated that, if measures were too onerous, there would be a temptation to make sure that the farm seemed compliant for the winter inspection, but that the effort would not be sustained throughout the remainder of the year.

In addition to reporting that the prevailing opinion had become one of grudging acceptance within the industry, the interviewed producers also raised concerns about what they considered to be the negative consequences of WRM. Issues cited included the reduced carrying capacity of farms (due to restrictions on grazing and availability of land for harvesting winter forage in areas considered attractive to and frequented by wild deer) and the negative implications for smaller producers who were less able to absorb the costs of complying with the new management regime. Whilst lower stocking densities and removing smaller producers less able to comply with WRM regulations may have positive benefits for the programme as a whole, the social implications of "it hurts some people" was raised as an issue.

A final point of note was the importance of risk perception in sustaining the momentum of the programme. The perception being that, as the sense of risk associated with tackling bTB decreases, the levels of complacency in sustaining disease management efforts increases. The risk of complacency was considered a high priority when developing a control strategy for a disease where endemic infection in the wildlife population persists. Progress towards eradication ultimately depends on a long-term commitment from multiple stakeholders (including producers, hunters, state agencies, and the federal government) to implement mitigation measures, provide adequate economic and political support for sustained management interventions and sustain the policy direction towards a goal that may take decades to achieve.

DISCUSSION

This paper has highlighted that bTB is an epidemiologically, socially and politically complex disease, creating multiple challenges for disease managers in constructing a coherent, cost-effective and workable strategy for eradication. This complexity is particularly pertinent in countries where the disease has become endemic in cattle and wildlife populations, demanding a long-term, multifactorial approach that is dependent upon a comprehensive set of control measures, sustained political will, adequate funding, stakeholder involvement and acceptance of interventions. Michigan and the UK have been highlighted as examples of how this complexity has played out in practice and underlines the case that the development of bTB management strategies need to be viewed as a social as well as scientific undertaking. This argument is in line with the analysis of Gormley and Corner (50) who point to the key role of stakeholders in bTB eradication programmes around the world and underlines calls for interdisciplinary research [e.g., (51–53)] and the development of viable management solutions based upon socio-technical approaches and interventions.

Enhancing Engagement

Human dimensions have been recognised as a key factor influencing the relative success of management approaches (17, 19, 54) with research efforts focusing on the role of public acceptability of wildlife control measures, the attitudes and actions of stakeholders (38, 55, 56) and the adoption of preventative biosecurity measures at the individual farm level. A central research theme, particularly in the UK, has focused on the adoption of biosecurity interventions and efforts to enhance opportunities to limit disease transmission between cattle and between cattle and wildlife at the farm level. Research has highlighted key reasons for the under-implementation of measures, including fatalism, uncertainty and scepticism on the practicality and efficacy of biosecurity interventions and, consequently, an unclear cost-benefit analysis of spend vs. gain.

Critically, in an endemic disease situation, progress towards eradication will depend upon sustaining risk mitigation efforts over long periods, depending on the cooperation and buy in of producers and key stakeholders. The research reported here sought to provide an analysis of how risk mitigation became embedded within the state of Michigan's eradication programme and uses stakeholder narratives to identify key components that were considered effective in generating change.

The literature review identified a specific challenge for risk managers: formulating measures that incentivise positive and proactive risk management actions from stakeholders (25). The findings presented here identified Michigan's WRM programme as a step change in the state's approach to disease control. Interviewees identified the programme as a means to transfer some of the responsibility to producers to take a more proactive approach towards risk mitigation, first relying on voluntary uptake and then moving to more statutory measures. Social as well as technical processes were developed to address some of the barriers to change identified in the social scientific literature. For example, WRM was used as a tool to shift the uncertain cost-benefit of instituting biosecurity measures through introducing market and regulatory (dis)incentives; "trusted intermediaries" were identified to communicate with producers, recognising the lack of trust and confidence in government agencies to eradicate the disease (57–60) and finally, questions of practicality and efficacy were addressed by working with individual producers to highlight opportunities for change, facilitating their implementation via co-funding and enforcing change where necessary. WRM is essentially a government-led programme with regulatory backing, but the creation of individual farm plans is based upon a negotiation, balancing the epidemiological ideals of risk mitigation with the willingness and ability of producers to institute what are considered to be practical and acceptable interventions on their holdings. Interviewees could not provide evidence of the effectiveness of WRM, but considered it to be successful in changing the management approach towards more actively involving producers in the control strategy for mitigating their own risks.

When drawing comparisons between Michigan and countries with areas affected by endemic bTB such as the UK, there are limitations that should be recognised when offering any "lessons learnt." First, this is a relatively small qualitative study which was designed to be illustrative rather than representative of stakeholder views. Second, the scale of Michigan's bTB problem is very different to that of the UK, with only 5–6 cases per year in the cattle herd and a prevalence of around 2% in the deer population (47). For example, in 2016, 4 beef herds, 1 feedlot, and 1 dairy herd within the MAZ were found to be bTB positive, which was considered a "spike" in incidence of infected herds (54). By comparison, in the same year, there were 3,753 new bTB incidents in England alone (61). Third, as with any international comparison, there is a difference in the political context for decision-making; particularly relevant in this case is the need for the state of Michigan to conform to Federal requirements established by the USDA, which govern the acceptable level of bTB prevalence and is the ultimate arbiter for restricting or enabling interstate trade of cattle. The different pressures applied and the balance established between maintaining a viable cattle industry and eradicating bTB are important contextual factors in guiding the policies pursued in charting a course towards eradication.

Whilst recognising these caveats of generalisability, scale and differing political contexts, the Michigan experience does offer an interesting case study in negotiating the challenges of shifting the focus beyond testing and surveillance towards obtaining producer engagement in WRM and farm biosecurity. Defra's Strategy to Achieve Officially TB Free Status for England similarly recognises the need to engage farmers in reducing their risk through careful cattle purchasing and limiting opportunities for transmission between cattle and between cattle and wildlife. However, the Strategy largely remains split between the application of statutory control measures—including continuous surveillance of cattle herds, removal of bTB test reactors and other cattle suspected of being infected with bTB and movement restrictions for bTB breakdown herds—and a predominantly non-statutory (voluntary) approach towards biosecurity implementation. In recognition of the persistent challenges surrounding biosecurity implementation [see (31)], there are ongoing discussions to identify mechanisms to encourage herd owners to take additional steps to improve their purchasing and biosecurity practices, including linking compensation to membership of herd health schemes such as the Cattle Health Certification Standards (CHeCS) scheme (62) and investigating means to give "earned recognition" to farmers for verifiable good biosecurity practices [see (63–65) for context]. This represents a movement towards rethinking the governance of biosecurity, but remains dependent upon the voluntary enrolment of farmers which, to date, has resulted in limited sign-up to the Bovine TB Herd Accreditation element of the CHeCS cattle health scheme. Clearly, as was the case in Michigan prior to the introduction of WRM, the challenge of achieving sustained farmer engagement remains unresolved and potentially requires a rethink of the socio-technical mechanisms by which this could be achieved.

Responsibilisation

Developing a greater sense of responsibility for biosecurity management is an important theme in both the Michigan case study and in policy narratives in the UK. As reported in the work of multiple social scientists, the "responsibilisation" of a wide range of actors beyond government is a process closely linked to the increasing neoliberalisation of animal health management, shifting the onus on to industry and farmers to manage their own risks through enhanced "biosecure citizenship" (66–69). This reflects wider trends in international policy development towards "empowering" citizens to take greater control of their own individual and community well-being in, for example, making themselves less vulnerable to crime through changing their actions and routines to minimise their potential exposure to risk, or making proactive changes to diet and exercise to mitigate future health risks (70, 71).

Whilst the principle of enhanced responsibility is a common theme between the Michigan and UK policy landscapes, the mechanisms to achieve change are different. As Enticott et al. (27)

report, the UK model of promoting biosecurity has developed within a political context based upon an ideological reluctance to regulate and has increasingly relied upon theories of behaviour change designed to "nudge" farmers towards taking action via the use of social norms and provision of information to guide choices [see also (72, 73)]. Examples include the introduction of ibTB—a publically available web-based interactive map showing the locations of bTB breakdowns and breakdowns resolved in the last 5 years, in England [see (74)]—and the promotion of the principles of risk-based trading to encourage farmers to make "informed" cattle purchasing decisions and reduce the risk of introducing disease via trade (75–77). This strategy is essentially voluntary, based upon improved communications to heighten awareness towards mitigating risks and operates as a "population strategy" [see (27)] using universal biosecurity principles to convey what should be "best practice" rather than considering applications that are more specific to individual farm contexts. Conversely, Michigan has moved towards a mix of regulatory, fiscal and social interventions that attempt to fit the ideals of standardised biosecurity protocols to specific farm contexts on a one-to-one basis (54).

The neoliberal logic of devolving biosecurity governance to industry and individual farmers has been questioned in the social scientific literature, citing farm-level and institutional factors as reasons why enhanced participation is unlikely to occur [see (78)]. For example, the approach assumes that farmers are willing to take on the additional responsibility and associated actions and that they have the knowledge and resources to implement the changes on their own holdings (ibid). Research suggests that this is not the case, as stated concerns for better biosecurity are not being translated into practice [e.g., (28, 31, 35)]. The reasons cited in Higgins et al. (78) include: farmers considering their biosecurity to already be of a satisfactory standard; concerns over the evidence base underpinning biosecurity interventions and the perceived controllability of the disease [see also (79)]; the applicability of universal biosecurity recommendations to individual farms; and the opinion that biosecurity is essentially a "government issue" with suggested biosecurity actions representing an external solution to an externally imposed problem. Taking each of these issues into account, and adding the unclear cost-benefit of biosecurity applications for bTB, there is a clear lack of incentives for taking voluntary action, often leading to uneven application of measures; the result of which is currently an unknown in terms of its effect on the UK bTB disease control regime.

Incentivising and Sustaining Change

The Michigan case study responds to a number of these critiques through creating a clearer rationale for incentivising changes to biosecurity practices. It also answers concerns about the utility of a one-size fits all set of recommendations that runs counter to farmers' view that these measures are impractical to implement and that they do not solve the complexity and uncertainty that are inherently linked to the disease. In a study of the Biosecurity Intensive Treatment Area (ITA), developed by the Welsh Assembly Government in 2006, Enticott et al. (27) highlighted the limitations of universal biosecurity practices and the difficulties of inspiring behavioural change with broad-scale knowledge. Instead, the authors advocated for an approach that matches solutions to individual farms via a more discursive process between farmers and advisors. Much like the conclusions reached in the case study presented here, Enticott et al. [(27), p. 334] state that "whilst some biosecurity interventions may make veterinary sense, without the support of the farmer and the wider social environment there is little point suggesting them for they will be rejected."

Incorporating processes of discussion, negotiation and accommodation to individual farm contexts may introduce concerns about diluting potential management outcomes. However, as Enticott (26) and Higgins et al. (69) suggest, finding a balance between standardisation and negotiation may provide options for progressive and responsive solutions that incorporates the challenging component of social complexity into management responses. As multiple authors and policy makers have stated, people and their actions are critically important factors in influencing the trajectory of bTB control and progress towards eradication. Using existing social scientific evidence on the institutional and farm-level factors that both promote and undermine efforts to enhance biosecurity responses should be the first step in devising, implementing, and evaluating different approaches towards embedding interventions that are capable of creating and sustaining proactive management options for bTB.

CONCLUSION

The aim of this paper was to draw comparative lessons between the cases of Michigan and the UK to exemplify some of the challenges of developing an effective strategy for the long-term control of endemic disease, particularly reflecting on efforts to "responsibilise" cattle producers and engage them in proactive activities to mitigate transmission risks on their own farms. The study was designed to respond to prominent themes in the social scientific literature that identified a range of socio-political and economic factors inhibiting the implementation of risk mitigation measures on farm; an issue that is particularly critical in areas with endemic bTB. The results indicate that in contrast to the predominantly voluntary approach pursued in the UK, Michigan has shifted the emphasis towards obtaining

producer support for wildlife risk mitigation and biosecurity via a mix of regulatory, fiscal, and social interventions. Whilst there is a common goal of transferring responsibility to producers to exert control over their own transmission risks, Michigan's WRM exemplifies a socio-technical approach that goes beyond highlighting what producers can do (through information and communications campaigns) to incentivising and promoting change via market (dis)incentives, co-funding, utilising social networks and tailoring approaches to individual farm contexts.

Neoliberal approaches designed to "responsibilise" cattle producers have been identified as problematic because the approach assumes that farmers are willing to take on the additional responsibility and associated actions and that they have the knowledge and resources to implement the changes on their own holdings. Taking these issues into account, and adding the unclear cost-benefit of biosecurity interventions for bTB, there is arguably a need to create a clearer rationale for incentivising changes to biosecurity practices in the UK. Whilst the scale of the bTB challenge differs between these two contexts, the development of WRM in Michigan offers instructive lessons in creating a clearer rationale for incentivising changes to biosecurity practices and offers interesting insights on the role of negotiated outcomes in attempts to adaptively manage a disease that is characterised by complexity and uncertainty.

ETHICS STATEMENT

This study was carried out in accordance with the recommendations of the University of Sheffield ethical review panel with written informed consent from all subjects. All subjects gave written informed consent in accordance with the Declaration of Helsinki. The protocol was approved by the University of Sheffield ethics committee.

AUTHOR CONTRIBUTIONS

RL collected the data, came up with the concept for the manuscript and drafted the content.

REFERENCES

1. Carstensen M, O'Brien DJ, Schmitt SM. Public acceptance as a determinant of management strategies for bovine tuberculosis in free-ranging US wildlife. *Vet Microbiol.* (2011) 151:200–4. doi: 10.1016/j.vetmic.2011.02.046

2. World Health Organization. *Roadmap for Zoonotic Tuberculosis.* (2017). Available online at: http://apps.who.int/iris/bitstream/10665/259229/1/9789241513043-eng.pdf (Accessed June 29, 2018).

3. Buhr B, McKeever K, Adachi K. *Economic Impact of Bovine Tuberculosis on Minnesota's Cattle and Beef Sector. Michigan Bovine Tuberculosis Bibliography and Database.* (2009). Available online at: http://digitalcommons.unl.edu/michbovinetb/20 (Accessed June 29, 2018).

4. DEFRA. (2014). *The Strategy for Achieving Officially Bovine Tuberculosis Free Status for England. April 2014.* London: Department for the Environment, Food and Rural Affairs.

5. Torgerson P, Torgerson D. Does risk to humans justify high cost of fighting bovine TB? *Nature.* (2008) 455:1029. doi: 10.1038/4551029a

6. Torgerson P, Torgerson D. Benefits of stemming bovine TB need to be demonstrated. *Nature.* (2009) 457:657. doi: 10.1038/457657d

7. Torgerson P, Torgerson D. Public health and bovine tuberculosis: what's all the fuss about? *Trends Microbiol.* (2010) 18:67–72. doi: 10.1016/j.tim.2009.11.002

8. USDA. *Status of Current Eradication Programs. USDA APHIS Status of Current Eradication Programs.* (2017). Available online at: www.aphis.usda.gov/aphis/ourfocus/animalhealth/animal-disease-information/ct_status_of_eradication_programs (Accessed June 29, 2018).

9. Godfray HCJ, Donnelly CA, Kao RR, Macdonald DW, McDonald RA, Petrokofsky G, et al. A restatement of the natural science evidence base relevant to the control of bovine tuberculosis in Great Britain. *Proc R Soc B.* (2013) 280:20131634. doi: 10.1098/rspb.2013.1634

10. Allen A, Skuce R, Byrne A. Bovine tuberculosis in Britain and Ireland–A Perfect Storm? The confluence of potential ecological and epidemiological impediments to controlling a chronic infectious disease. *Front Vet Sci.* (2018) 5:109. doi: 10.3389/fvets.2018.00109

11. Cassidy A. Vermin, victims and disease: UK framings of badgers in and beyond the bovine TB controversy. *Sociol Ruralis.* (2012) 52:192–214. doi: 10.1111/j.1467-9523.2012.00562.x

12. Cassidy A. Badger-human conflict: an overlooked historical context for bovine TB debates in the UK. In: Hill CM, Webber AD, Priston NE, editors. *Understanding Conflicts About Wildlife: A Biosocial Approach.* Vol. 9. New York, NY: Berghahn Books (2017). p. 65–95.

13. Grant W. Intractable policy failure: the case of bovine TB and badgers. *Br J Politics Int Relat.* (2009) 11:557–73. doi: 10.1111/j.1467-856X.2009.00387.x

14. Abernethy DA, Upton P, Higgins IM, McGrath G, Goodchild AV, Rolfe SJ, et al. Bovine tuberculosis trends in the UK and the Republic of Ireland, 1995–2010. *Vet Rec.* (2013) 172:312. doi: 10.1136/vr.100969

15. Spencer A. One body of evidence, three different policies: bovine tuberculosis policy in Britain. *Politics.* (2011) 31:91–9. doi: 10.1111/j.1467-9256.2011.01407.x

16. Pfeiffer DU. Epidemiology caught in the causal web of bovine tuberculosis. *Transbound Emerg Dis.* (2013) 60:104–10. doi: 10.1111/tbed.12105

17. More SJ, Radunz B, Glanville RJ. Lessons learned during the successful eradication of bovine tuberculosis from Australia. *Vet Rec.* (2015) 177:224. doi: 10.1136/vr.103163

18. Livingstone PG, Hancox N, Nugent G, Mackereth G, Hutchings SA. Development of the New Zealand strategy for local eradication of tuberculosis from wildlife and livestock. *NZ Vet J.* (2015) 63:98–107. doi: 10.1080/00480169.2015.1013581

19. Livingstone P, Hancox N. 15 Managing *Bovine tuberculosis*: successes and issues. *Bovine Tuberculosis.* (2018) 225–43. doi: 10.1079/9781786391520.0225

20. Miller RS, Farnsworth ML, Malmberg JL. Diseases at the livestock–wildlife interface: status, challenges, and opportunities in the United States. *Prev Vet Med.* (2013) 110:119–32. doi: 10.1016/j.prevetmed.2012.11.021

21. VerCauteren KC, Lavelle MJ, Hygnstrom S. Fences and deer-damage management: a review of designs and efficacy. *Wildl Soc Bull.* (2006) 34:191–200. doi: 10.2193/0091-7648(2006)34[[191:FADMAR]]2.0.CO;2

22. VerCauteren KC, Lavelle MJ, Phillips GE. Livestock protection dogs for deterring deer from cattle and feed. *J Wildl Manage.* (2008) 72:1443–8. doi: 10.2193/2007-372

23. Lavelle MJ, Henry CI, LeDoux K, Ryan PJ, Fischer JW, Pepin KM, et al. Deer response to exclusion from stored cattle feed in Michigan, USA. *Prev Vet Med.* (2015) 121:159–64. doi: 10.1016/j.prevetmed.2015.06.015

24. VerCauteren KC, Seward NW, Lavelle MJ, Fischer JW, Phillips GE. Deer guards and bump gates for excluding white-tailed deer from fenced resources. *Human-Wildlife Conflicts.* (2009) 3:145–53. Retrieved from: http://www.jstor.org/stable/24875696

25. Riley SJ, Gore ML, Muter BA. *Expert perspectives on bovine tuberculosis management policies in Michigan and Minnesota.* East Lansing, MI: Michigan Agricultural Experiment Station (2010).

26. Enticott G. The spaces of biosecurity: prescribing and negotiating solutions to bovine tuberculosis. *Env Planning A.* (2008) 40:1568–82. doi: 10.1068/a40304

27. Enticott G, Franklin A, Van Winden S. Biosecurity and food security: spatial strategies for combating bovine tuberculosis in the UK. *Geograph J.* (2012) 178:327–37. doi: 10.1111/j.1475-4959.2012.00475.x

28. Gunn GJ, Heffernan C, Hall M, McLeod A, Hovi M. Measuring and comparing constraints to improved biosecurity amongst GB farmers, veterinarians and the auxiliary industries. *Prev Vet Med.* (2008) 84:310–23. doi: 10.1016/j.prevetmed.2007.12.003

29. O'Hagan MJH, Matthews DI, Laird C, McDowell SWJ. Herd-level risk factors for bovine tuberculosis and adoption of related biosecurity measures in Northern Ireland: a case-control study. *Vet J.* (2016) 213:26–32. doi: 10.1016/j.tvjl.2016.03.021

30. O'Hagan MJH, Matthews DI, Laird C, McDowell SWJ. Farmers' beliefs about bovine tuberculosis control in Northern Ireland. *Vet J.* (2016) 212:22–6. doi: 10.1016/j.tvjl.2015.10.038

31. Robinson P. *Behavioural Appraisal of the Recommendations of the TB Strategic Partnership Group* (TBSPG). Belfast: DAERA (Department of Agriculture, Environment and Rural Affairs) (2016).

32. Enticott G, Vanclay F. Scripts, animal health and biosecurity: The moral accountability of farmers' talk about animal health risks. *Health, Risk Soc.* (2011) 13:293–309. doi: 10.1080/13698575.2011.575456

33. Enticott G. Market instruments, biosecurity and place-based understandings of animal disease. *J Rural Studies.* (2016) 45:312–9. doi: 10.1016/j.jrurstud.2016.04.008

34. Naylor R, Courtney P. Exploring the social context of risk perception and behaviour: farmers' response to bovine tuberculosis. *Geoforum.* (2014) 57:48–56. doi: 10.1016/j.geoforum.2014.08.011

35. Heffernan C, Nielsen L, Thomson K, Gunn G. An exploration of the drivers to bio-security collective action among a sample of UK cattle and sheep farmers. *Prev Vet Med.* (2008) 87:358–72. doi: 10.1016/j.prevetmed.2008.05.007

36. Naylor R, Maye D, Ilbery B, Enticott G, Kirwan J. Researching controversial and sensitive issues: using visual vignettes to explore farmers' attitudes towards the control of bovine tuberculosis in England. *Area.* (2014) 46:285–93. doi: 10.1111/area.12113

37. Kristensen E, Jakobsen EB. Danish dairy farmers' perception of biosecurity. *Prev Vet Med.* (2011) 99:122–9. doi: 10.1016/j.prevetmed.2011.01.010

38. Lahuerta-Marin A, Brennan ML, Finney G, O'Hagan MJH, Jack C. Key actors in driving behavioural change in relation to on-farm biosecurity; a Northern Ireland perspective. *Irish Vet J.* (2018) 71:14. doi: 10.1186/s13620-018-0125-1

39. Rice PL, Ezzy D. *Qualitative Research Methods: A Health Focus.* Melbourne, Australia. Oxford: Oxford University Press (1999).

40. Seidel J, Kelle U. Different functions of coding in the analysis of textual data. In: Kelle U, editor. *Computer-Aided Qualitative Data Analysis: Theory, Methods and Practice.* London: Sage (1995). p. 52–61.

41. Basit T. Manual or electronic? The role of coding in qualitative data analysis. *Educ Res.* (2003) 45:143–54. doi: 10.1080/0013188032000133548

42. Tesch R. *Qualitative Research: Analysis Types and Software Tools* Vol. 337. New York, Falmer: Psychology Press (1990).

43. Carneiro PA, Kaneene JB. Bovine tuberculosis control and eradication in Brazil: lessons to learn from the US and Australia. *Food Contr.* (2018) 93:61–9. doi: 10.1016/j.foodcont.2018.05.021

44. Michigan State University Extension. *Wildlife Risk* A* Syst for Bovine, TB. FAS 113.* Lansing, MI: Michigan State University (2010).

45. Enck JW, Decker DJ, Riley SJ, Organ JF, Carpenter LH, Siemer WF. Integrating ecological and human dimensions in adaptive management of wildlife-related impacts. *Wildlife Soc Bull.* (2006) 34:698–705. doi: 10.2193/0091-7648(2006)34[698:IEAHDI]2.0.CO;2

46. Nishi JS, Shury T, Elkin BT. Wildlife reservoirs for bovine tuberculosis (Mycobacterium bovis) in Canada: strategies for management and research. *Vet Microbiol.* (2006) 112:325–38. doi: 10.1016/j.vetmic.2005.11.013

47. O'Brien DJ, Schmitt SM, Fitzgerald SD, Berry DE. Management of bovine tuberculosis in Michigan wildlife: current status and near term prospects. *Vet Microbiol.* (2011) 151:179–87.

48. Berentsen AR, Miller RS, Misiewicz R, Malmberg JL, Dunbar MR. Characteristics of white-tailed deer visits to cattle farms: implications for disease transmission at the wildlife–livestock interface. *Eur J Wildlife Res.* (2014) 60:161–70. doi: 10.1007/s10344-013-0760-5

49. Kaneene JB, Bruning-Fann CS, Granger LM, Miller R, Porter-Spalding BA. Environmental and farm management factors associated with tuberculosis on cattle farms in northeastern Michigan. *J Am Vet Med Assoc.* (2002) 221:837–42. doi: 10.2460/javma.2002.221.837

50. Gormley E, Corner L. Wild animal tuberculosis: stakeholder value systems and management of disease. *Front Vet Sci.* (2018) 5:327. doi: 10.3389/fvets.2018.00327

51. White PC, Ward AI. Interdisciplinary approaches for the management of existing and emerging human–wildlife conflicts. *Wildlife Res.* (2011) 37:623–9. doi: 10.1071/WR10191

52. Olea-Popelka F, Fujiwara PI. Building a multi-institutional and interdisciplinary team to develop a zoonotic tuberculosis roadmap. *Front Public Health.* (2018) 6:167. doi: 10.3389/fpubh.2018.00167

53. Ryan MR, Cleaveland S. Zoonotic diseases: sharing insights from interdisciplinary research. *Vet Rec.* (2017) 180:270–1. doi: 10.1136/vr.j1261

54. VerCauteren KC, Lavelle MJ, Campa H. Persistent spillback of bovine tuberculosis from white-tailed deer to cattle in Michigan, USA: status, strategies and needs. *Front Vet Sci.* (2018) 5:301. doi: 10.3389/fvets.2018.00301

55. Brook RK, Vander Wal E, van Beest FM, McLachlan SM. Evaluating use of cattle winter feeding areas by elk and white-tailed deer: implications for managing bovine tuberculosis transmission risk from the ground up. *Prev Vet Med.* (2013) 108:137–47. doi: 10.1016/j.prevetmed.2012.07.017

56. Cowie CE, Gortázar C, White PC, Hutchings MR, Vicente J. Stakeholder opinions on the practicality of management interventions to control bovine tuberculosis. *Vet J.* (2015) 204:179–85.

57. Enticott G. The ecological paradox: social and natural consequences of the geographies of animal health promotion. *Trans Inst Br Geogr.* (2008) 33:433–46. doi: 10.1111/j.1475-5661.2008.00321.x

58. Garforth C. Livestock keepers' reasons for doing and not doing things which governments, vets and scientists would like them to do. *Zoonoses Public Health.* (2015) 62:29–38. doi: 10.1111/zph.12189

59. Broughan JM, Maye D, Carmody P, Brunton LA, Ashton A, Wint W, et al. Farm characteristics and farmer perceptions associated with bovine tuberculosis incidents in areas of emerging endemic spread. *Prev Vet Med.* (2016) 129:88–98. doi: 10.1016/j.prevetmed.2016.05.007

60. Robinson PA. Farmers and bovine tuberculosis: Contextualising statutory disease control within everyday farming lives. *J Rural Studies.* (2017) 55:168–80. doi: 10.1016/j.jrurstud.2017.08.009

61. DEFRA. *Bovine Tuberculosis in England in 2016. Epidemiological Analysis of the 2016 Data and Historical Trends.* London: Department for the Environment, Food and Rural Affairs (2017).

62. DEFRA. *Government and the Cattle Industry Working Together to Improve Bovine TB Biosecurity: A Progress Report and Next Steps.* London: Department for the Environment, Food and Rural Affairs (2018).

63. Angus A, Booth C, Armstrong G, Pollard SJT. Better evidence for regulatory reform: rapid evidence appraisals. *Report to Defra, ERG*117 (2013).

64. DEFRA. *Farming Regulation Task Force Implementation: Earned Recognition Plan.* London: Department for the Environment, Food and Rural Affairs (2013).

65. Jones G, Gosling JP. *Study on Farm Assurance Scheme Membership and Compliance With Regulation Under Cross Compliance.* Report to Defra, BR0114 (2013).

66. Barker K. Biosecure citizenship: politicising symbiotic associations and the construction of biological threat. *Trans Inst Br Geograph.* (2010) 35:350–63. doi: 10.1111/j.1475-5661.2010.00386.x

67. Donaldson A. Governing biosecurity. In: Dobson A, Barker K, Taylor SL, editors. *Biosecurity: The Socio-Politics of Invasive Species and Infectious Diseases.* Abingdon: Routledge (2013). p. 61–74.

68. Enticott G. Biosecurity and the bioeconomy: the case of disease regulation in the UK and New Zealand. In: Marsden T, Morley A, editors. *Researching Sustainable Food: Building the New Sustainability Paradigm.* London: Earthscan (2014). p. 122–42.

69. Higgins V, Bryant M, Hernández-Jover M, McShane C, Rast L. Harmonising devolved responsibility for biosecurity governance: the challenge of competing institutional logics. *Env Planning A.* (2016) 48:1133–51. doi: 10.1177/0308518X16633471

70. O'Malley P. Responsibilization. In: Wakefield A, Fleming J, editors. *The SAGE Dictionary of Policing.* London: SAGE Publications Ltd. (2009). p. 277–9.

71. Brown BJ, Baker S. *Responsible Citizens: Individuals, Health, and Policy Under Neoliberalism.* London: Anthem Press (2012).

72. Wright BK, Jorgensen BS, Smith LD. Understanding the biosecurity monitoring and reporting intentions of livestock producers: identifying opportunities for behaviour change. *Prev Vet Med.* (2018) 157:142–51. doi: 10.1016/j.prevetmed.2018.07.007

73. Richens I, Houdmont J, Wapenaar W, Shortall O, Kaler J, O'Connor H, et al. Application of multiple behaviour change models to identify determinants of farmers' biosecurity attitudes and behaviours. *Prev Vet Med.* (2018) 155:61–74. doi: 10.1016/j.prevetmed.2018.04.010

74. Enticott G, Mitchell A, Wint W, Tait N. Mapping disease data: a usability test of an internet-based system of disease status disclosure. *Front Vet Sci.* (2018) 4:230. doi: 10.3389/fvets.2017.00230

75. Gibbens N. Bovine TB: implementing risk-based trading. *Vet Rec.* (2013) 173:557–558 doi: 10.1136/vr.f7222

76. Adkin A, Brouwer A, Simons RRL, Smith RP, Arnold ME, Broughan J, et al. Development of risk-based trading farm scoring system to assist with the control of bovine tuberculosis in cattle in England and Wales. *Prev Vet Med.* (2016) 123:32–8. doi: 10.1016/j.prevetmed.2015.11.020

77. Little RA, Wheeler K, Edge S. Developing a risk-based trading scheme for cattle in England: farmer perspectives on managing trading risk for bovine tuberculosis. *Vet Rec.* (2017) 180:148. doi: 10.1136/vr.103522

78. Higgins V, Bryant M, Hernández-Jover M, Rast L, McShane C. Devolved responsibility and on-farm biosecurity: practices of biosecure farming care in livestock production. *Sociol Ruralis.* (2018) 58:20–39. doi: 10.1111/soru.12155

79. Enright J, Kao RR. A few bad apples: a model of disease influenced agent behaviour in a heterogeneous contact environment. *PLoS ONE.* (2015) 10:e0118127. doi: 10.1371/journal.pone.0118127

5

Exploring the Fate of Cattle Herds with Inconclusive Reactors to the Tuberculin Skin Test

Lucy A. Brunton[1]*, Alison Prosser[2], Dirk U. Pfeiffer[1,3] and Sara H. Downs[4]

[1] Veterinary Epidemiology, Economics and Public Health Group, Department of Pathobiology and Population Sciences, Royal Veterinary College, University of London, London, United Kingdom, [2] Data Systems Group, Department of Epidemiological Sciences, Animal and Plant Health Agency, Weybridge, United Kingdom, [3] College of Veterinary Medicine and Life Sciences, City University of Hong Kong, Kowloon Tong, Hong Kong, [4] Epidemiology Group, Department of Epidemiological Sciences, Animal and Plant Health Agency, Weybridge, United Kingdom

Correspondence:
Lucy A. Brunton
lbrunton@rvc.ac.uk

Bovine tuberculosis (TB) is an important animal health issue in many parts of the world. In England and Wales, the primary test to detect infected animals is the single intradermal comparative cervical tuberculin test, which compares immunological responses to bovine and avian tuberculins. Inconclusive test reactors (IRs) are animals that demonstrate a positive reaction to the bovine tuberculin only marginally greater than the avian reaction, so are not classified as reactors and immediately removed. In the absence of reactors in the herd, IRs are isolated, placed under movement restrictions and re-tested after 60 days. Other animals in these herds at the time of the IR result are not usually subject to movement restrictions. This could affect efforts to control TB if undetected infected cattle move out of those herds before the next TB test. To improve our understanding of the importance of IRs, this study aimed to assess whether median survival time and the hazard of a subsequent TB incident differs in herds with only IRs detected compared with negative-testing herds. Survival analysis and extended Cox regression were used, with herds entering the study on the date of the first whole herd test in 2012. An additional analysis was performed using an alternative entry date to try to remove the impact of IR retesting and is presented in the **Supplementary Material**. Survival analysis showed that the median survival time among IR only herds was half that observed for clear herds (2.1 years and 4.2 years respectively; $p < 0.001$). Extended Cox regression analysis showed that IR-only herds had 2.7 times the hazard of a subsequent incident compared with negative-testing herds in year one (hazard ratio: 2.69; 95% CI: 2.54, 2.84; $p < 0.001$), and that this difference in the hazard reduced by 63% per year. After 2.7 years the difference had disappeared. The supplementary analysis supported these findings showing that IR only herds still had a greater hazard of a subsequent incident after the IR re-test, but that the effect was reduced. This emphasizes the importance of careful decision making around the management of IR animals and indicates that re-testing alone may not be sufficient to reduce the risk posed by IR only herds in England and Wales.

Keywords: bovine, tuberculosis, SICCT, inconclusive, tuberculin

INTRODUCTION

Bovine tuberculosis (TB) caused by *Mycobacterium bovis* occurs throughout the world, being particularly prevalent in Africa and South America. In Europe, countries that had not achieved Officially Bovine Tuberculosis Free Status (OTF) status in 2016 included Bulgaria, Croatia, Cyprus, Greece, Ireland, Italy, Portugal, Romania, Spain, and the United Kingdom (1). Bovine TB is one of the most important animal health issues in England and Wales, with prevalence of the disease in some parts of England being the highest in the European Union (2). Control of the disease is based on detection and slaughter of infected cattle using immunological testing of cattle herds, restriction of movement from infected herds and carcase inspection of animals at slaughter. Additional testing may be performed in herds perceived to be at risk, e.g., contiguous to an infected herd, or in animals prior to movement. More rigorous testing is applied to herds in which disease is suspected or confirmed.

In England, Defra's strategy for achieving OTF status for England published in 2014 saw the regionalisation of control measures to take account of the spatial heterogeneity of incidence risk (3). The overall incidence rate for England as a whole was 10.2 per 100 herd years at risk in 2016 (4), but this varied considerably across the High Risk (HRA), Edge, and Low Risk (LRA) areas of England [12.8, 3.4, and 0.3 herd years at risk respectively (5)]. In the HRA and Edge area, herds are tested on an annual basis, with herds in some parts of the Edge area being tested every 6 months, whereas in the LRA, herds are tested every 4 years. Tailored control measures are applied to each area in order to meet the objectives of the eradication strategy, which are to achieve OTF status, and more specifically to reduce incidence in the HRA, stop and reverse the spread of disease in the Edge area, and maintain or further reduce incidence in the LRA.

Wales has tested all herds annually since 2008, and in 2016, the TB incidence rate in Wales was 7.0 per 100 herd years at risk (6). Wales has also moved toward a regional approach to TB eradication, by establishing Low, Intermediate, and High TB Areas defined by disease incidence risk. A number of changes to TB control were introduced in October 2017 as part of the Welsh Government's eradication programme (7). In Scotland, which is officially free of tuberculosis, herd-level risk-based surveillance is used for a more targeted approach to routine tests. Herds defined as low-risk are excluded from routine testing.

The primary test used to detect infected animals is the single intradermal comparative cervical tuberculin (SICCT) test, which is based upon injection of bovine and avian tuberculins alongside one another in the skin of the neck. Cattle infected with *M. bovis* tend to show a greater response to bovine tuberculin than avian tuberculin, distinguishing infection with *M. bovis* from infection with other mycobacteria (8). However, while the test is estimated to have high specificity (nearly 100%) (9), the sensitivity of the test at the animal level when using standard interpretation has been estimated to be around 80% but could be as low as 50% (8, 10).

Inconclusive reactors (IRs) to the skin test are defined in England and Wales as animals that demonstrate a reaction to the bovine tuberculin that is less than 4 mm larger than an avian reaction under standard interpretation of the test, or less than 2 mm larger than an avian reaction under severe interpretation. In 2015, there were 2,785 herds in England in which only IRs were detected and which went on to have a re-test, and 21% of these herds had positive reactors (i.e., an incident) at the re-test (5). In Wales, there were 970 IR-only herds of which 21% had an incident at the re-test (6). Animals in these herds at the time of the IR result may be infected, yet the herds will not usually be subject to movement restrictions unless there is a recent history of TB in the herd. In England, 1,420 IRs were slaughtered in 2016 and 13.4% were found to have visible lesions (4). In Wales, 862 IRs were slaughtered in 2016 and 2.9% had visible lesions (6). This could have implications for efforts to control TB if undetected infected cattle move out of those herds over the 60-days period prior to the re-test. This has been demonstrated in Ireland where Clegg et al. (11) reported that between 11.8 and 21.4% of IRs slaughtered before being re-tested were infected with *M. bovis* at post mortem, compared with between 0.13 and 0.22% of animals with a negative SICCT test.

A change in policy for the management of IRs was introduced in England in November 2017. The policy now requires that all IRs in the HRA and Edge Area with a negative result on re-testing must remain restricted for life to the holding in which they were identified. This also applies to IRs in infected herds in the LRA. In comparison, the Welsh eradication programme aims to remove IRs detected in chronically infected herds, under specific circumstances, alongside any reactors. These proactive approaches to managing the risks of IRs are appropriate in light of current knowledge, yet the factors associated with the fate of IR herds are still not well understood. Analysis of 2016 surveillance data has shown that in the HRA and Edge areas of England, herds with a history of TB had a significantly greater risk of having a confirmed incident at the IR retest (4). However, the association between a herd having an IR-only test result and the time to a subsequent incident has not been explored in England and Wales. To improve our understanding of the risk that IRs represent, this study aims to assess whether there are differences in the time to a subsequent incident in herds with only IRs detected compared with herds that test negative at a whole herd test.

MATERIALS AND METHODS

Study Population and Data Extraction

A retrospective cohort study followed cattle herds in England and Wales between 1st January 2012 and 31st December 2016. Data describing TB testing and incidence for the study period were obtained from the Animal and Plant Health Agency's Sam database. The study population included all unrestricted herds (TB-free) in the high-risk and edge areas of England and Wales that had a whole-herd type test (WHT) in 2012. This included a small number of routine herd tests (5% of all WHT included) which in some cases might not include all animals in the herd. Herd demographic data, information relating to the first WHT in 2012 and the first subsequent incident (test where reactors were disclosed or infected animals detected at slaughter) were obtained. The number of incidents in the 10 years prior to the 2012 WHT, and the annual rolling county-level incidence at the end of 2012 were also obtained. The dataset was prepared using Microsoft SQL Server 2012 and extracted for cleaning and analysis using Stata 14 (Stata Corporation, College Station, TX, USA).

Herds entered the study on the date of their first WHT in 2012. Herds with a positive test result at the first 2012 WHT, or an incident linked to this test, were excluded. The remaining herds were grouped into two cohorts: those with a clear test result at the 2012 WHT ("clear herds") and those that had only IRs detected ("IR only herds"). The outcome was defined as a subsequent incident (i.e., reactors detected at a subsequent test or infected animals detected at slaughter) during the follow-up period. Herds were censored either on the date of the test that disclosed an incident or at the end of the study period, whichever was earlier. Herds lost to follow-up due to the closure of the farm contributed time at risk until the date they were archived in Sam. Time was measured in days, but scaled up to years for the analysis.

The hypothesis being tested was that the hazard of a subsequent incident is different between herds in which IRs have been detected and herds which test negative.

Statistical Analyses

Descriptive analyses were performed to examine the number of herds in each cohort (clear herds or IR only herds), and the number of incidents during the follow-up period. The median survival time in years for each cohort was estimated using the Kaplan-Meier method (12). Differences in survival time between the two cohorts were analyzed using the log-rank statistic.

Cox regression was used to examine the association between first WHT status in 2012 and the hazard of a subsequent incident. Other explanatory variables examined for an association with the hazard of a subsequent incident were herd type, herd size, the season in which the 2012 WHT took place, the number of incidents in the previous 10 years, geographical risk area and annual rolling county-level incidence at the end of 2012. These other explanatory variables were then individually added to a model with first WHT status in 2012 to assess whether they resulted in a change in the hazard ratio for the primary exposure. Herd size, the number of incidents in the previous 10 years and county-level incidence were analyzed as both continuous and categorical variables, and those that resulted in the greatest change in the hazard ratio for first WHT status in 2012 were used in the analysis. Efron's method for dealing with ties was used since there were a large number of tied events in the dataset due to the large number of herds and the resolution of the temporal unit (days). All variables associated with the hazard of a subsequent incident with a $p < 0.20$ in univariable analyses were considered for inclusion in a multivariable model.

The multivariable analysis was performed in a stepwise manner with the variable first WHT status in 2012 ("clear" or "IR only") forced into the model as the primary exposure variable. The outcome variable was occurrence of a subsequent incident. Confounders were then sequentially added to the model in a forward stepwise manner, starting with the variable that resulted in the greatest change in the hazard ratio for first WHT status in the univariable analysis. An interaction between herd type and location was considered. The likelihood ratio test and Akaike's

Information Criterion (AIC) were used to compare models (13). Model fit was assessed using Harrell's C concordance statistic and by plotting the Cox Snell residuals and deviance residuals, as recommended by Dohoo et al. (14).

To test the assumption of proportional hazards, a log-minus-log survival plot was generated for first WHT status adjusted for variables included in the final model. The correlation between the Schoenfeld residuals of each variable and transformed time was assessed using the Chi-squared test. A $p < 0.05$ was taken as evidence against the null hypothesis that the hazards were proportional. In addition, graphs of the scaled Schoenfeld residuals over time were plotted for each variable to look for nonlinear relationships between the residuals and time or influential outliers. Interactions between each of the variables and log time were assessed by extending the model to include time varying coefficients using the tvc command in Stata. Model fit could not be assessed using the Cox-snell and deviance residuals after the inclusion of the time-varying coefficients, so models were assessed using the likelihood ratio test and AIC.

An additional analysis was performed using the date of the first subsequent clear herd test after the first WHT as the entry date, thereby excluding herds that were disclosed as infected at the IR retest. The purpose of this was to try to remove the impact of the IR retesting and ensure that all herds were starting out on comparable testing regimes. The results of this analysis are presented in the **Supplementary Material**.

RESULTS

Descriptive Analysis

There were 30,600 unrestricted herds that had a WHT in 2012, and overall, the median percentage of animals tested per herd at the first WHT in 2012 was 98%. Of the 30,600 herds, 27,289 (89%) tested negative (clear), and 3,311 (11%) only had IRs (IR only) at the first WHT in 2012. Overall, 30% of herds went on to have a subsequent incident within the follow-up period. A greater percentage of IR only herds went on to have a subsequent incident compared with clear herds (63 and 27% respectively) (Z-test to compare two proportions: $p < 0.001$) (**Table 1**).

The percentage of herds that suffered a subsequent incident was greater among herds with three or more incidents in the 10 years prior to the 2012 WHT, dairy herds, and increased with herd size (**Table 1**). In addition, herds appeared to be more likely to have a subsequent incident if they were located in the high-risk area of England and in a county where incidence was greater than the median incidence across all counties at the end of 2012 (**Table 1**). The percentage of herds that had a subsequent incident did not vary with the season in which the 2012 WHT took place. Among IR only herds, 53% of subsequent incidents were disclosed by an IR retest, whereas among clear herds, 19% of subsequent incidents were disclosed by an IR retest (Z-test to compare two proportions: $p < 0.001$). The median number of skin test reactors was lower among incidents disclosed by an IR retest than among incidents disclosed by other tests (0 vs. 1 respectively; Wilcoxon rank-sum test: $p < 0.001$). However, the median numbers of IRs and reactors to the gamma interferon test was zero among incidents disclosed by an IR retest and among incidents disclosed by other tests.

Seven herds were excluded from the analysis as they had an archive date (date herd closed down) that fell before the date of the first WHT in 2012 and they were not tested again within the follow-up period. This left 30,593 herds under observation. There were 9,326 herds with a subsequent incident, which occurred at a median follow-up time of 1.8 years (range: 0.02–4.9), while 21,267 herds were censored at a median follow-up time of 4.5 years (range: 0.03–5.5). There were 3,705 herds lost to follow-up because the business closed down. More clear herds were lost to follow-up (13.1%) than IR only herds (3.8%).

The median survival time among IR only herds was over half that observed for clear herds. Median survival time was also reduced among herds with more than 200 animals, dairy herds, and herds with 3 or more incidents in the previous 10 years (**Table 2**).

TABLE 1 | Number and percentage of herds that had a subsequent incident, stratified by each explanatory variable.

Variable	N	Missing	Herds with a subsequent incident		
			n	%	95% CI[a]
FIRST WHT STATUS IN 2012					
Clear	27,289	0	7,231	26.5	26.0–27.0
IRs Only	3,311		2,095	63.3	61.6–64.9
SEASON IN WHICH 2012 WHT TOOK PLACE					
Spring	9,935	0	2,976	30.0	29.1–30.9
Summer	3,996		1,198	30.0	28.6–31.4
Autumn	7,474		2,253	30.1	29.1–31.2
Winter	9,195		2,899	31.5	30.6–32.5
NUMBER OF INCIDENTS IN THE PREVIOUS 10 YEARS					
0–2	27,639	0	7,376	26.7	26.2–27.2
3 or more	2,961		1,950	65.9	64.1–67.5
GEOGRAPHICAL RISK AREA					
England high-risk	17,145	0	6,595	38.5	37.7–39.2
England Edge	3,311		636	19.2	17.9–20.5
Wales	10,144		2,095	20.7	19.9–21.5
ANNUAL ROLLING COUNTY LEVEL INCIDENCE AT THE END OF 2012					
0–14.6 per 100 herd years at risk	17,431	0	3,983	22.9	22.2–23.5
>14.6 per 100 herd years at risk	13,169		5,343	40.6	39.7–41.4
HERD TYPE					
Beef	23,713	0	6,087	25.7	25.1–26.2
Dairy	6,447		3,189	49.5	48.3–50.7
Other	440		50	11.4	8.7–14.7
HERD SIZE					
0–10	4,941	1,563	453	9.2	8.4–10.0
11–50	8,697		1,755	20.2	19.4–21.0
51–100	5,488		1,802	32.8	31.6–34.1
101–200	5,164		2,336	45.2	43.9–46.6
201–300	2,196		1,218	55.5	53.4–57.5
>300	2,551		1,700	66.6	64.8–68.4

[a]Confidence interval.

There was a difference in the survival functions of the clear and IR only cohorts (**Figure 1**) and this observation was supported by the results of the log-rank test (**Table 3**). Significant differences in survival were also observed between herds grouped according to their TB history, geographical area, county level incidence, production type, and size (**Figures 2B–F**). The survival of herds did not appear to vary according to the season in which their 2012 WHT took place (**Figure 2A**), although the log-rank test indicated there was some evidence of a difference ($p = 0.04$).

Assessment of the Hazard of Subsequent Incidents Among Clear and IR Only Herds

A Cox regression was performed to assess the hazard of a subsequent incident within the two cohorts. There were strong associations between each of the explanatory variables and the hazard of subsequent incidents in the univariable analysis (**Table 4**). Factors found to be associated with increased relative hazard of a subsequent incident were having an IR only test result at the 2012 WHT, having the first 2012 WHT in autumn or winter compared with spring, a recent history of TB, increased county-level incidence, being a dairy herd (compared to a beef herd), and increasing herd size. Herds in the edge area of England, and those in Wales, had a reduced incidence rate when compared to the high-risk area of England. Herds classed as production type

TABLE 2 | Median, minimum, and maximum survival time in the clear and IR only cohorts, and by each explanatory variable.

Variable	Level	Survival time (years)		
		Median	Min	Max
First WHT status in 2012	Clear	4.21	0.02	5.46
	IR	2.07	0.02	5.09
Season in which 2012 WHT took place	Spring	4.63	0.02	4.84
	Summer	4.36	0.05	5.46
	Autumn	4.11	0.02	5.28
	Winter	4.08	0.02	5.08
Number of incidents in the previous 10 years	0–2	4.22	0.02	5.46
	3 or more	2.36	0.02	5.42
Geographical risk area	England high-risk	4.07	0.02	5.28
	England Edge	4.26	0.05	5.46
	Wales	4.31	0.12	5.19
Annual rolling county level incidence at end of 2012	0–14.6 per 100 herd years at risk	4.27	0.04	5.46
	>14.6 per 100 herd years at risk	4.31	0.12	5.19
Herd type	Beef	4.23	0.02	5.46
	Dairy	3.76	0.02	5.22
	Other	4.25	0.18	4.99
Herd size	0–10	4.34	0.03	5.25
	11–50	4.36	0.05	5.42
	51–100	4.25	0.06	5.46
	101–200	4.11	0.02	5.22
	201–300	3.40	0.02	5.15
	>300	2.57	0.02	5.24

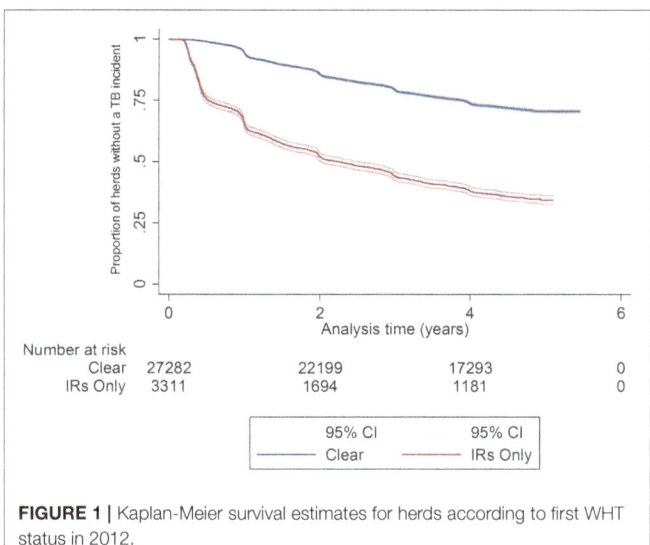

FIGURE 1 | Kaplan-Meier survival estimates for herds according to first WHT status in 2012.

TABLE 3 | Results of the log-rank tests for equality of survivor functions.

Variable	Chi-squared	P-value
First WHT status in 2012	3,008.9	<0.001
Season in which 2012 WHT took place	8.51	0.037
Number of incidents in the previous 10 years	2,635.7	<0.001
Geographical risk area	1,238.86	<0.001
Herd type	1,535.93	<0.001
Herd size	4,388.12	<0.001
Annual rolling county level incidence at end of 2012	1,207.05	<0.001

"other" also had a reduced incidence rate compared with beef herds (**Table 4**).

The initial multivariable Cox regression model included first WHT status in 2012, herd size, the number of incidents in the 10 years before the first WHT in 2012, herd type, county-level TB incidence and geographical risk area. The plot of the Cox-Snell residuals (**Figure 3**) indicated that the model was a poor fit, and the plot of the deviance residuals over time (**Figure 4**) revealed a number of observations that were not well fit by the model, particularly those herds with the shortest survival time. However, the Harrell's C statistic was 0.75 indicating that the model correctly predicted the sequence of two observed failures 75% of the time. Assessment of the proportionality of the hazards using the log-minus-log plot (**Figure 5**) indicated that the ratio of hazards varied over time. The Chi-squared test of the correlation between the Schoenfeld residuals of each variable and transformed time generated a $p < 0.05$ for all variables except local incidence, indicating that the proportional hazards assumption had been violated. The log-minus-log plot illustrated a change in the ratio of hazards around 60 days, which correlated with the timing of IR retests. This indicated that an analysis of the time to a subsequent incident may not be appropriate given the differences in follow-up testing between the cohorts,

and that time varying coefficients should be included to model interactions between the explanatory variables and time.

The final extended Cox regression model contained first WHT status, herd size, recent history of TB, herd type, local incidence and geographical risk area, and included interactions between time and first WHT status, herd size, TB history, risk area and herd type. The relative hazard of having a subsequent incident was 2.7 times greater among herds that were IR only at the 2012 WHT compared with herds that had a clear test result (after adjusting for herd size, testing following the 2012 WHT, recent history of TB, herd type, local incidence and geographical risk area) (**Table 5**). The interaction with time indicated that the increased relative hazard of having a subsequent incident among IR only herds decreased by 63% each year. This means that according to the model, the relative hazard of 2.7 in year one is reduced to 1.34 in year two, and drops to 0.89 by year three. This change in relative hazard over time is presented in **Figure 6**. This shows that the effect disappears (i.e., the relative hazard = 1) by around 970 days, or 2.7 years.

DISCUSSION

Understanding the level of infection that could be present among IRs is important for directing control measures. In Ireland, Clegg et al. (11) found that IRs that passed the IR retest and then moved herds within 6 months were 12 times more likely to have a positive result at the next test, or have lesions detected at slaughter, compared to all animals in Ireland. Our analysis has shown that the time interval before a new TB incident in IR only herds was around half that of herds with a negative whole herd test; and that the hazard of a subsequent incident was 2.7 times greater for IR only herds compared with clear herds after accounting for the influence of traditionally accepted drivers of TB. This difference in hazard decreased over time by 63% per year.

The number of incidents in the 10 years prior to the study was consistently associated with an increase in the hazard of a subsequent incident. This is in agreement with other studies where TB history has been identified as a risk factor for future incidents (15–17). Herd size has frequently been associated with increased disease risk (1, 15, 18, 19), but this association can be difficult to interpret. An effect of increasing herd size may simply reflect changes in other risk factors related to farm management, or it may have implications on the sensitivity and specificity of the test at herd level (20).

Dairy herds located within areas subject to badger culling in England were shown to have a greater risk of TB than beef herds in the same areas (21). It has also been shown in separate analyses for England and Wales that the effect of herd type is reduced after adjusting for herd size and location (4, 6). In this study, there was no difference in the rate of subsequent incidents among dairy compared with beef herds, after adjusting for herd size, location and other factors that were not included in the country-level analyses described above (4, 6). However, the time-varying coefficient for herd type was significant for dairy. This

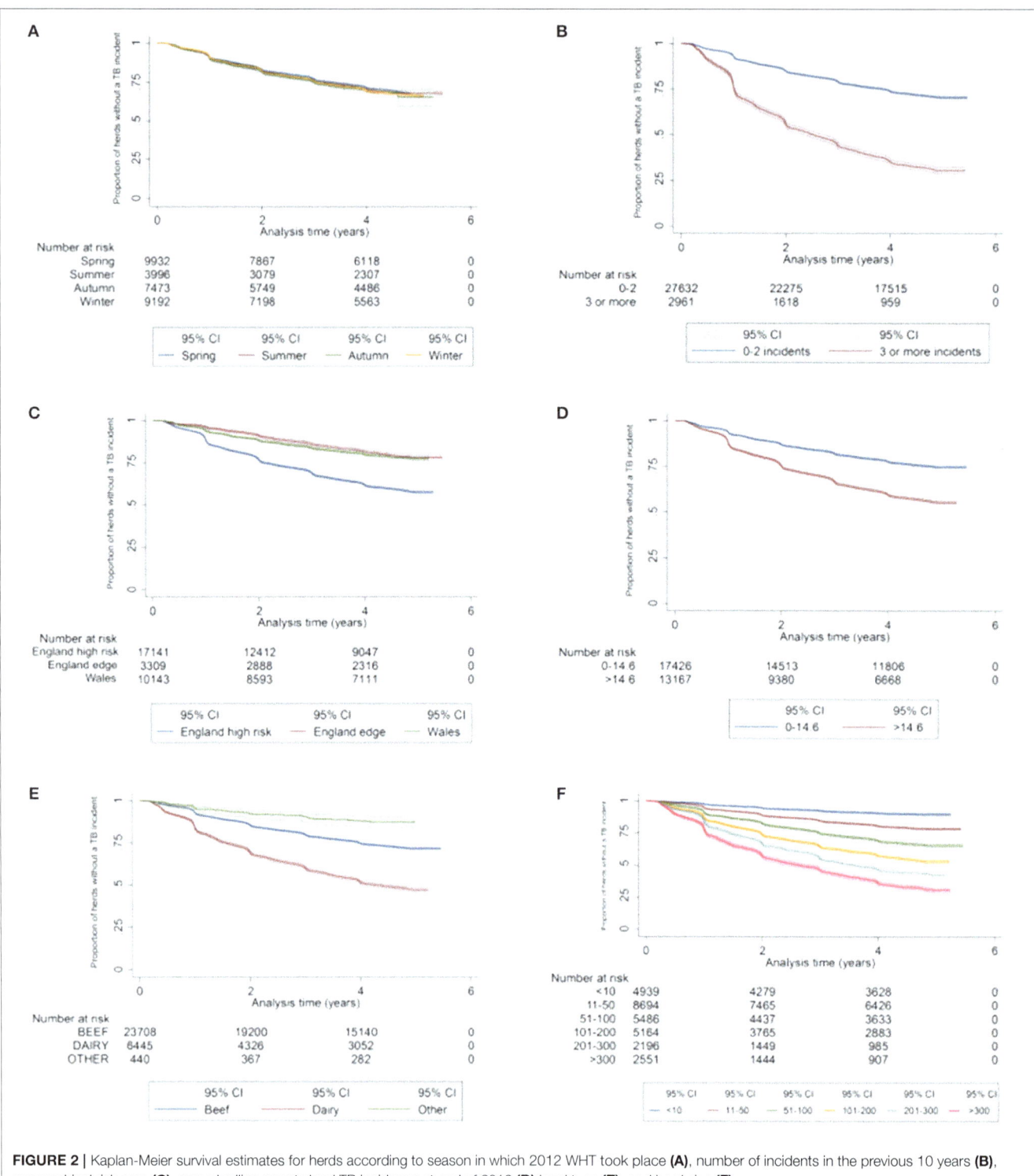

FIGURE 2 | Kaplan-Meier survival estimates for herds according to season in which 2012 WHT took place **(A)**, number of incidents in the previous 10 years **(B)**, geographical risk area **(C)**, annual rolling county level TB incidence at end of 2012 **(D)** herd type **(E),** and herd size **(F)**.

suggests that the hazard of a subsequent incident among dairy herds increases by 14% each year. This may be related to the longer life expectancy of dairy cattle compared to beef cattle, meaning that dairy cattle are at risk of exposure to TB for longer than beef cattle (21, 22). Both O'Hagan et al. (23) and Downs et al. (24) have shown that dairy SICCT reactors are less likely to have visible lesions than beef reactors, which could indicate that infected dairy cattle are detected through SICCT surveillance earlier than beef cattle. Therefore, one might expect IRs from beef herds to pose a higher future risk than IRs from dairy herds.

TABLE 4 | Results of the univariable Cox regression analysis of factors associated with the rate of subsequent incidents.

Variable	Level	HR[a]	95% CI[b]		P-value
First WHT status in 2012	Clear	*1.00*			
	IRs only	3.58	3.41	3.76	<0.001
Season in which first WHT took place	Spring	*1.00*			
	Summer	1.06	0.99	1.13	0.105
	Autumn	1.08	1.02	1.14	0.007
	Winter	1.06	1.01	1.11	0.031
Number of incidents in the previous 10 years	<3	*1.00*			
	3 or more	1.50	1.49	1.52	<0.001
Geographical risk area	England high risk	*1.00*			
	England Edge	0.43	0.40	0.47	<0.001
	Wales	0.47	0.44	0.49	<0.001
Annual rolling county level incidence at end of 2012	0–14.6 per 100 herd years at risk	*1.00*			
	>14.6 per 100 herd years at risk	1.07	1.07	1.07	<0.001
Herd type	Beef	*1.00*			
	Dairy	2.26	2.16	2.36	<0.001
	Other	0.44	0.33	0.58	<0.001
Herd size	1–10	*1.00*			
	11–50	2.21	1.99	2.45	<0.001
	51–100	3.82	3.44	4.23	<0.001
	101–200	5.74	5.19	6.35	<0.001
	201–300	7.71	6.92	8.59	<0.001
	>300	10.49	9.45	11.63	<0.001

[a] Hazard ratio.
[b] Confidence interval.
Ratios in italics represent the reference groups.

Increased county-level incidence was associated with an increased hazard of a subsequent incident, and herds in the edge area of England and in Wales had a reduced hazard compared with herds in the high risk area of England. Olea-Popelka et al. (15) and Green et al. (25) both showed that increased local prevalence of TB is associated with an increased risk of infection. Johnston et al. (26) found regional variation in risk factors for TB incidents, and Brunton et al. (27) reported spatial heterogeneity in the factors associated with the spread of endemic TB. The significant time-varying coefficient for Wales is interesting, and indicates that the hazard for herds in Wales reduces over time. This was not seen for herds in England, so could be related to differing policies on IRs in the two countries.

The TB testing regime in England and Wales is determined by factors such as location, animal movements and disease history. As such, it varies considerably between herds across both cohorts. However, there are also structural differences in the data due to the TB control policy. IRs have a subsequent test following disclosure of IRs, which does not take place in herds where all the cattle tested negative to the whole herd test. This increases the probability of IR-only herds having a subsequent incident compared with herds that tested clear, since increased testing increases the chances of detecting disease. This is further complicated by the fact that animals that have a second IR test

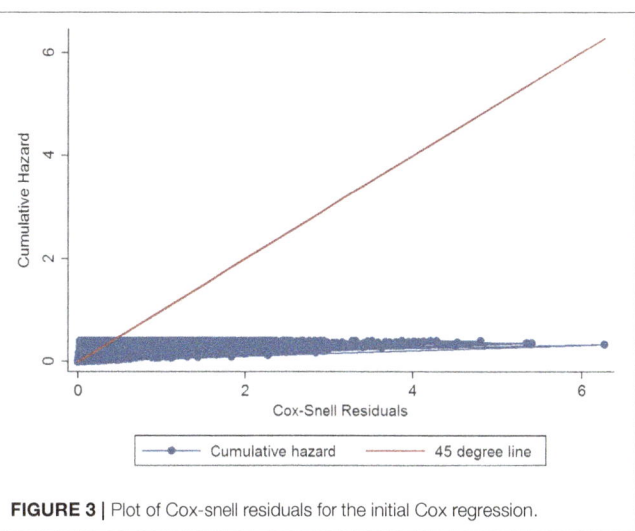

FIGURE 3 | Plot of Cox-snell residuals for the initial Cox regression.

result at the follow up test will automatically be classified as reactors. This means that there is a bias toward detecting cases within the IR only cohort. Unfortunately, the structure of the data did not allow the analysis of individual test data for each herd to explore the impact of this further. Instead, the time-varying coefficients were included to model how the relative hazard of a subsequent incident amongst IR only herds compared with clear herds varied over time. A reduction in the hazard ratio over time was observed, which indicates that the hazard for IR only herds becomes comparable to that of clear herds after around two and a half years. If the effect of re-testing was the only reason that IR only herds had a greater hazard of a subsequent incident, then we would expect the hazard ratio to reach 1.0 after the 60 days retest. The fact that it takes over 2 years to reach 1.0 suggests that the hazard of a subsequent TB incident is still higher among IR only herds than herds that tested negative to a whole herd test once the effect of re-testing has been removed.

An additional analysis was performed to try to remove the impact of the IR re-testing by ensuring that all herds were starting out on comparable testing regimes, and the results of this analysis are presented in the **Supplementary Material**. The results of this additional analysis indicate that there is still a significantly greater hazard of a subsequent incident amongst IR only herds compared with clear herds, but that this is reduced once the effect of re-testing is removed. This aligns with the finding that the hazard ratio is still greater than 1.0 after the 60 days re-test has passed. However, the additional analysis needs to be interpreted cautiously as the sample size for the IR cohort was reduced by almost half (46%) due to missing or inaccurate values within the subsequent clear test variable used as the new entry date. The clear herd cohort was less affected by missing values (15%). This introduces a considerable bias to the additional analysis and makes it difficult to draw firm conclusions from this about the fate of IR only herds compared to clear herds after they get through the IR testing regime.

There is potential for the misclassification of IRs due to the imperfect test for TB. The influence of disease prevalence on the predictive value of the test also introduces the potential for

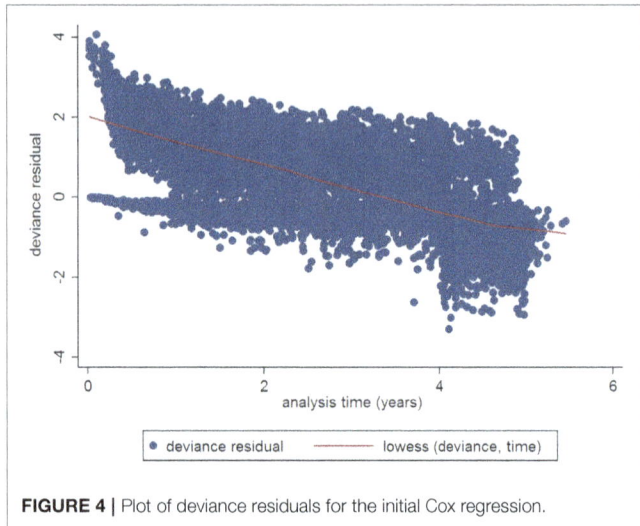

FIGURE 4 | Plot of deviance residuals for the initial Cox regression.

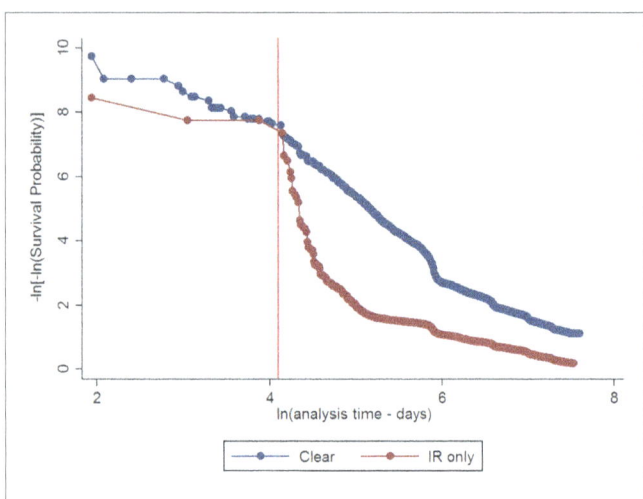

FIGURE 5 | Log-minus-log survival plot for first WHT status adjusted for herd size, the number of incidents in the 10 years before the first WHT in 2012, herd type, county level TB incidence and geographical risk area. A reference line has been added to indicate the change in the HR at 60 days.

TABLE 5 | Multivariable extended Cox regression model of factors associated with a subsequent incident amongst clear and IR only herds, including time varying coefficients.

Variable	Level	HR[a]	95% CI[b]		P-value
MAIN COVARIATES					
First WHT status in 2012	Clear	*1.00*			
	IRs only	2.69	2.54	2.84	<0.001
Herd size	1–10	*1.00*			
	11–50	1.92	1.70	2.17	<0.001
	51–100	3.00	2.66	3.39	<0.001
	101–200	3.93	3.49	4.43	<0.001
	201–300	4.65	4.09	5.30	<0.001
	>300	6.18	5.45	7.02	<0.001
Number of incidents in the previous 10 years		1.19	1.17	1.21	<0.001
Herd type	Beef	*1.00*			
	Dairy	0.98	0.93	1.04	0.547
	Other	0.61	0.45	0.82	0.001
Annual rolling county level incidence at end of 2012	0–14.6 per 100 herd years at risk	*1.00*			
	>14.6 per 100 herd years at risk	1.05	1.05	1.06	<0.001
Geographical risk area	England high risk	*1.00*			
	England Edge	0.90	0.80	1.02	0.088
	Wales	0.80	0.75	0.86	<0.001
TIME-VARYING COEFFICIENTS					
First WHT status in 2012	Clear	*1.00*			
	IRs only	0.37	0.34	0.39	<0.001
Herd size	1–10	*1.00*			
	11–50	1.20	1.05	1.38	0.008
	51–100	1.26	1.10	1.44	0.001
	101–200	1.32	1.16	1.51	<0.001
	201–300	1.46	1.26	1.69	<0.001
	>300	1.40	1.21	1.61	<0.001
Number of incidents in the previous 10 years		1.02	1.01	1.04	0.008
Geographical risk area	England high risk	*1.00*			
	England Edge	1.04	0.93	1.17	0.464
	Wales	0.88	0.83	0.94	<0.001
Herd type	Beef	*1.00*			
	Dairy	1.14	1.07	1.21	<0.001
	Other	0.62	0.44	0.88	0.007

[a] Hazard ratio.
[b] Confidence interval.
Ratios in italics represent the reference groups.

misclassification across risk areas. For example, the low positive predictive value of the test when prevalence is low means that IRs in the low-risk areas may be false positives, while the low negative predictive value of the test when prevalence is high means that IRs in high-risk areas may be false negatives. Even if perfect classification were possible, the nature of IRs is that their infection status is uncertain. They may be uninfected animals that have been exposed to other mycobacteria, or they may be infected animals that do not respond adequately to the test due to factors such as immunosuppression or co-infection (8). This uncertainty makes managing the potential risk that IRs pose challenging, and highlights the need for evidence to understand this risk.

The finding that the hazard of a subsequent incident reduces over time among IR only herds indicates that the policy in England and Wales for dealing with IRs is having an effect. However, these herds still appear to be at greater risk of having an incident after the IR re-testing regime. This could reflect

that the testing is not removing all potentially infected animals from the herd, or there may be other factors which put these herds at a greater risk of having a TB incident that we have yet to understand. This is important information for both policy makers in England and Wales, and those in other countries looking to learn from the English and Welsh experience in tackling bovine TB. The evidence from this analysis suggests

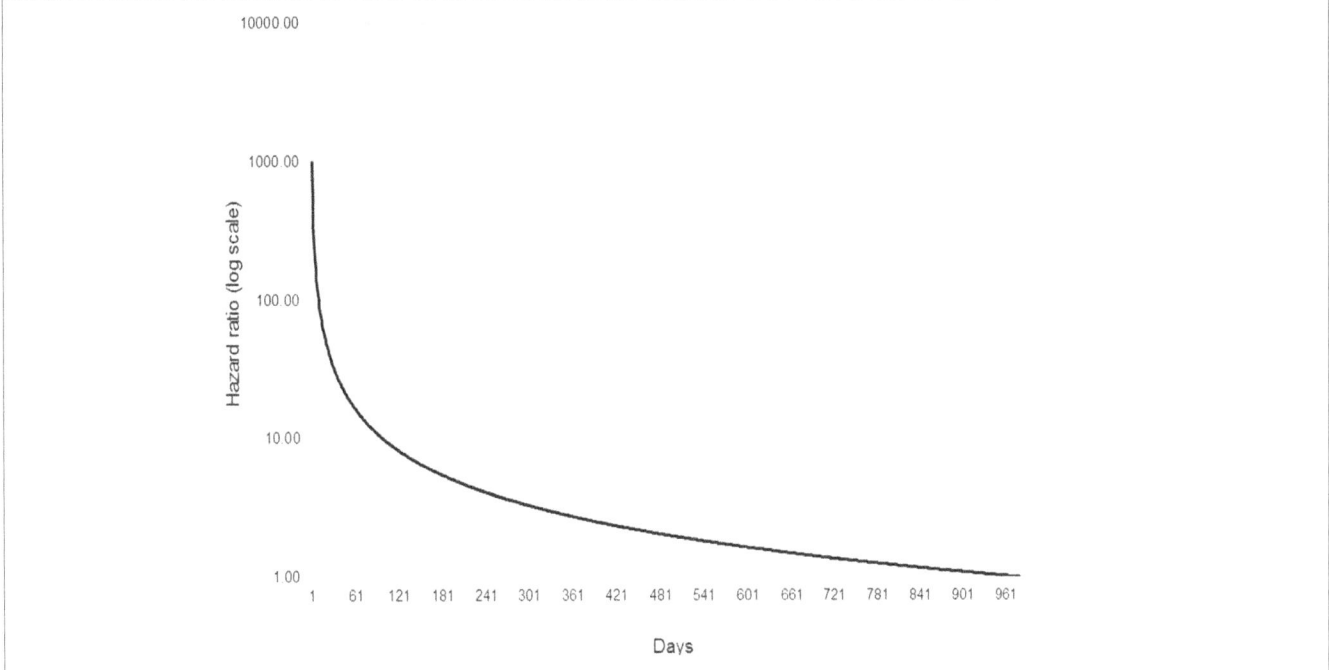

FIGURE 6 | Change in relative hazard over time amongst IR only herds compared with clear herds, adjusted for herd size, the number of incidents in the 10 years before the first WHT in 2012, herd type, county level TB incidence and geographical risk area, and interactions between time and first WHT status, herd size, the number of incidents in the 10 years before the first WHT in 2012, herd type, and geographical risk area.

that the new policy decision in England, restricting IRs with a negative re-test to the herd in which they were detected for life, should help reduce any residual risk associated with an IR for disease spread. This approach has been implemented in Ireland since 2012 (28) following the analysis of the fate of IRs by Clegg et al. (29).

The present study has shown that the hazard of a subsequent TB incident is greater among IR only herds than herds that tested negative to a whole herd test, and that the hazard ratio decreases over time, but remains greater than 1.0 after the IR re-testing regime. This emphasizes the importance of careful decision making around the management of IR animals and indicates that re-testing alone may not be sufficient to reduce the risk posed by IR only herds. Further characterisation of IRs is needed to determine whether the differences observed here are related to management or biological factors. This may be best achieved through an animal-level analysis so that the risk of retaining individual IR animals in a herd in England and Wales can be understood. Our findings correlate with the Irish findings, indicating that the risks of IRs are unlikely to be country and context specific. This provides further evidence of the risk that

IRs pose for the spread of TB, which can support the development of policies in other countries relating to the management of IRs.

AUTHOR CONTRIBUTIONS

LB designed the study, performed the analysis, and drafted the manuscript in part fulfillment of the requirements for the degree of Master of Science in Veterinary Epidemiology at the Royal Veterinary College, University of London. AP generated the dataset and edited the manuscript. DP and SD provided advice on study design and analysis, made additions to the text, and edited the manuscript.

ACKNOWLEDGMENTS

We wish to thank Paul Upton (APHA) for his expertise and assistance in collating the data, and to Professor Glyn Hewinson (APHA) for reviewing the manuscript. We thank Defra for funding data provision and contributions from SD and AP through projects EA3131 and SB4500.

REFERENCES

1. Brooks-Pollock E, Keeling M. Herd size and bovine tuberculosis persistence in cattle farms in Great Britain. *Prev Vet Med.* (2009) 92:360–5. doi: 10.1016/j.prevetmed.2009.08.022

2. EFSA and ECDC. The European Union summary report on trends and sources of zoonoses, zoonotic agents and food-borne outbreaks in 2016. *EFSA J.* (2017) 15:5077. doi: 10.2903/j.efsa.2017.5077

3. DEFRA. *The Strategy for Achieving Officially Bovine Tuberculosis Free Status for England* (2014). Available online at: https://www.gov.uk/government/

uploads/system/uploads/attachment_data/file/300447/pb14088-bovine-tb-strategy-140328.pdf

4. APHA. *Bovine Tuberculosis in England in 2016: Epidemiological Analysis of the 2016 Data and Historical Trends* (2017a). Available online at: https://www.gov.uk/government/uploads/system/uploads/attachment_data/file/660133/tb-epidemiology-england-2016.pdf

5. APHA. *Bovine Tuberculosis in Great Britain: Surveillance Data for 2016 and Historical Trends. Commisioned by: Department For Environment Food and Rural Affairs and Scottish Government and Welsh Government* (2017b). Available online at: https://www.gov.uk/government/uploads/system/uploads/attachment_data/file/660136/tb-epidemiology-2016-suppl.pdf

6. APHA. *Epidemiology of Bovine Tuberculosis in Wales: Annual Surveillance Report for the Period January to December 2016* (2017c). Available online at: http://gov.wales/docs/drah/publications/180216-annual-surveillance-report-2016-en.pdf

7. Welsh Government. *Wales TB Eradication Programme Delivery Plan* (2017). Available online at: http://gov.wales/docs/drah/publications/170809-tb-eradication-programme-delivery-plan-en.pdf

8. De La Rua-Domenech R, Goodchild AT, Vordermeier HM, Hewinson RG, Christiansen KH, Clifton-Hadley RS. Ante mortem diagnosis of tuberculosis in cattle: a review of the tuberculin tests, γ-interferon assay and other ancillary diagnostic techniques. *Res Vet Sci.* (2006) 81:190–210. doi: 10.1016/j.rvsc.2005.11.005

9. Goodchild AV, Downs SH, Upton P, Wood JL, De La Rua-Domenech R. Specificity of the comparative skin test for bovine tuberculosis in Great Britain. *Vet Rec.* (2015) 177:258. doi: 10.1136/vr.102961

10. Nuñez-Garcia J, Downs SH, Parry JE, Abernethy DA, Broughan JM, Cameron AR, et al. Meta-analyses of the sensitivity and specificity of ante-mortem and post-mortem diagnostic tests for bovine tuberculosis in the UK and Ireland. *Prev Vet Med.* (2017) 153:94–107. doi: 10.1016/j.prevetmed.2017.02.017

11. Clegg TA, Good M, Duignan A, Doyle R, Blake M, More SJ. Shorter-term risk of *Mycobacterium bovis* in Irish cattle following an inconclusive diagnosis to the single intradermal comparative tuberculin test. *Prev Vet Med.* (2011a) 102:255–64. doi: 10.1016/j.prevetmed.2011.07.014

12. Kaplan E, Meier P. Nonparametric estimationfrom incomplete observations. *J Am Stat Assoc.* (1958) 53:457–81. doi: 10.1080/01621459.1958.10501452

13. Burnham KP, Anderson DR. *Model Selection and Multi-Model Inference: a Practical Information-Theoretic Approach.* New York, NY: Springer-Verlag (2002).

14. Dohoo I, Martin W, Stryhn H. *Veterinary Epidemiologic Research.* Charlottetown, PE: VER Inc., (2010).

15. Olea-Popelka FJ, White PW, Collins JD, O'Keeffe J, Kelton DF, Martin SW. Breakdown severity during a bovine tuberculosis episode as a predictor of future herd breakdowns in Ireland. *Prev Vet Med.* (2004) 63:163–72. doi: 10.1016/j.prevetmed.2004.03.001

16. Good M, Clegg TA. Duignan A, More SJ. Impact of the national full herd depopulation policy on the recurrence of bovine tuberculosis in Irish herds, 2003 to 2005. *Vet Rec.* (2011) 169:581. doi: 10.1136/vr.d4571

17. Karolemeas K, Mckinley TJ, Clifton-Hadley RS, Goodchild AV, Mitchell A, Johnston WT, et al. Recurrence of bovine tuberculosis breakdowns in Great Britain: risk factors and prediction. *Prev Vet Med.* (2011) 102:22–29. doi: 10.1016/j.prevetmed.2011.06.004

18. Green LE, Cornell SJ. Investigations of cattle herd breakdowns with bovine tuberculosis in four counties of England and Wales using VETNET data. *Prev Vet Med.* (2005) 70:293–311. doi: 10.1016/j.prevetmed.2005.05.005

19. Reilly LA, Courtenay O. Husbandry practices, badger sett density and habitat composition as risk factors for transient and persistent bovine tuberculosis on UK cattle farms. *Prev Vet Med.* (2007) 80:129–42. doi: 10.1016/j.prevetmed.2007.02.002

20. Skuce RA, Allen AR, McDowell SW. Herd-level risk factors for bovine tuberculosis: a literature review. *Vet Med Inter.* (2012) 2012:621210. doi: 10.1155/2012/621210

21. Vial F, Johnston WT, Donnelly CA. Local cattle and badger populations affect the risk of confirmed tuberculosis in British cattle herds. *PLoS ONE* (2011) 6:e18058. doi: 10.1371/journal.pone.0018058

22. Humblet MF, Boschiroli ML, Saegerman C. Classification of worldwide bovine tuberculosis risk factors in cattle: a stratified approach. *Vet Res.* (2009) 40:50. doi: 10.1051/vetres/2009033

23. O'Hagan MJ, Courcier EA, Drewe JA, Gordon AW, Mcnair J, Abernethy DA. Risk factors for visible lesions or positive laboratory tests in bovine tuberculosis reactor cattle in Northern Ireland. *Prev Vet Med.* (2015) 120:283–90. doi: 10.1016/j.prevetmed.2015.04.005

24. Downs SH, Broughan J, Goodchild A, Upton PA, Durr P. Responses to diagnostic tests for bovine tuberculosis in dairy and non-dairy cattle naturally exposed to *Mycobacterium bovis* in Great Britain. *Vet J.* (2016) 216:8–17. doi: 10.1016/j.tvjl.2016.06.010

25. Green DM, Kiss IZ, Mitchell AP, Kao RR. Estimates for local and movement-based transmission of bovine tuberculosis in British cattle. *P Roy Soc B.* (2008) 275:1001–5. doi: 10.1098/rspb.2007.1601

26. Johnston WT, Vial F, Gettinby G, Bourne FJ, Clifton-Hadley RS, Cox DR, et al. Herd-level risk factors of bovine tuberculosis in England and Wales after the 2001 foot-and-mouth disease epidemic. *Int J Infect Dis.* (2011) 15:833–40. doi: 10.1016/j.ijid.2011.08.004

27. Brunton LA, Alexander N, Wint W, Ashton A, Broughan JM. Using geographically weighted regression to explore the spatially heterogeneous spread of bovine tuberculosis in England and Wales. *Stoc Env Res Risk A* 31:339–52. doi: 10.1007/s00477-016-1320-9

28. DAFM. Ireland Eradication Programme for Bovine TB 2017-2018 (2016). Available online at: https://www.agriculture.gov.ie/animalhealthwelfare/diseasecontrol/bovinetb/diseaseeradicationtb/irelanderadicationprogrammeforbovinetb2017-2018/

29. Clegg TA, Good M, Duignan A, Doyle R, Blake M, More SJ. Longer-term risk of *Mycobacterium bovis* in Irish cattle following an inconclusive diagnosis to the single intradermal comparative tuberculin test. *Prev Vet Med.* (2011b) 100:147–54. doi: 10.1016/j.prevetmed.2011.02.015

6

Persistent Spillback of Bovine Tuberculosis from White-Tailed Deer to Cattle in Michigan, USA: Status, Strategies and Needs

Kurt C. VerCauteren[1]*, Michael J. Lavelle[1] and Henry Campa III[2]

[1] National Wildlife Research Center, USDA/APHIS/Wildlife Services, Fort Collins, CO, United States, [2] Department of Fisheries and Wildlife, Michigan State University, East Lansing, MI, United States

*Correspondence:
Kurt C. VerCauteren
kurt.c.vercauteren@aphis.usda.gov

Free-ranging white-tailed deer (*Odocoileus virginianus*) are believed to be a self-sustaining reservoir for bovine tuberculosis (bTB) in northeastern Lower Michigan, USA. Although a comprehensive control program is in place and on-farm mitigation strategies to curtail bTB transmission between cattle and deer have been implemented for over a decade, cattle and deer continue to become infected with the disease. Thus, renewed motivation to eradicate bTB is needed if that is truly the goal. Recurrent detection of bTB in cattle in the region is of mounting concern for state and federal agricultural agencies, producers, and wildlife managers. Current on-farm mitigation efforts include fencing and refined cattle feeding and watering practices. Liberal removal of antlerless deer through hunter harvest and disease control permits (DCPs) issued to cattle producers and agency sharp shooters have also been ongoing. Although these strategies have merit and efforts to reduce prevalence in deer and occurrence of positive farms are elevated, additional actions are needed. Heightened management actions to combat bTB in deer could include deer vaccination programs, strategic habitat manipulations to redistribute deer from farms, and precision removal of deer in proximity to high-risk farms. Foundational research to address development and delivery of vaccine to free-ranging deer is complete. Strategic management and habitat manipulation could reduce and disperse local concentrations of deer while better meeting wildlife, forestry, and agricultural goals. The responses of local deer populations to targeted removal of individuals are generally understood and there is potential to reduce deer activity around agricultural operations while allowing them to persist nearby on natural foods. We summarize the history and progress to date, discuss the realized merit of novel management strategies, and suggest options to rid deer and cattle in Michigan of bTB.

Keywords: bovine tuberculosis, cattle, disease, *Odocoileus virginianus*, transmission, spillback, spillover, white-tailed deer

KEY CONCEPTS

Integrated disease management: employing a variety of proven strategies simultaneously to most efficiently achieve management objectives.

Mitigation measures to protect cattle: specific actions taken to reduce potential for direct and indirect transmission of *M. bovis* from wildlife to cattle.

Management strategies for deer: specific actions designed to reduce potential for maintaining disease within free-ranging deer such as using hunters or professional sharpshooters to reduce deer numbers and eliminating the provisioning of anthropogenic food sources with the intent of attracting and maintaining deer concentrations.

Negative impacts of supplemental feeding and baiting: anthropogenic feeding leads to artificially high and concentrated populations of wildlife which in turn increases disease transmission risk and prevalence.

Setting realistic goals: developing a documented and well-informed formal strategy designed to reach a common and achievable goal.

Public support, political will: varying stakeholder motivations must be considered, reconciled and presented to decision makers so they can empower the pursuit of common goals.

INTRODUCTION

History of Bovine Tuberculosis in Michigan, USA

Bovine tuberculosis (bTB), caused by the *Mycobacterium bovis* (*M. bovis*) bacterium was historically a disease among cattle that spilled over into free-ranging wildlife where it persists (1–3). Bovine tuberculosis is a threat to national and international beef and dairy markets. There are currently more than 13,000 cattle producers maintaining >1.1 million cattle in Michigan. The United States Department of Agriculture (USDA) has 5 levels of zoning regarding bTB status that states, or zones within states, fall into regarding presence of bTB infection in cattle ranging from 1 with no apparent prevalence in cattle and bison (*Bison bison*) to 5 with an unknown or ≥ 0.5% herd prevalence. The 5 levels include: (1) Accredited-free zone ("TB free"), (2) Modified accredited advanced zone (MAAZ), (3) Modified accredited zone (MAZ), (4) Accredited preparatory zone, and (5) Non-accredited zone. Zoning enables agencies to tailor surveillance and management strategies relative to regional disease prevalence and potential risk of spread (4). The continual appearance of bTB in livestock facilities in Michigan annually keeps the zoning status of the state at risk while maintaining producer's ability to engage in national and international markets (5).

Movement of cattle from the MAZ must originate from a bTB accredited-free herd or one that has had a negative whole herd test within the previous 12 months and requires a movement certificate, unless the cattle are being moved directly to slaughter. On March 21, 2018 a new TB Zoning Order was signed into effect by the Michigan Department of Agriculture and Rural Development (MDARD) that established the Enhanced Wildlife Biosecurity Area (EWBA; an area slightly larger than Deer Management Unit (DMU) 452 in the center of the MAZ) (6). Development of the EWBA and increased disease mitigation efforts were an intensified effort to avoid another spike in incidence of infected herds like was seen in 2016 when 4 beef herds, 1 feedlot, and 1 dairy herd within the MAZ were found bTB positive (see **Figure 1**) (5, 7). As such, if the incidence of bTB infected cattle herds continues to rise or fluctuate like it has in recent years, there is a chance that the 4-county MAZ status or even statewide status (TB Free) could be in jeopardy (5).

History of bTB in Deer in Michigan

In 1975 and again in 1994 bTB was detected in white-tailed deer in the northeastern lower peninsula (NELP) of Michigan. After which the Michigan Departments of Natural Resources (MDNR) initiated a surveillance program of testing hunter-harvested deer (8–10) (**Figure 2**). A collaborative effort was initiated in 1996 by Michigan Departments of Agriculture (MDA), Community Health (MDCH), MDNR, the USDA, and Michigan State University (MSU) to manage bTB by initiating the Michigan Bovine Tuberculosis Eradication Program (11). In 1997, bTB was identified in the first positive cattle herd in the core disease outbreak area since 1974 (12) (**Figure 2**). In January 1998, the Governor of Michigan directed the MDCH, MDA, and MDNR to develop a plan for eradicating bTB from Michigan deer (13). In summary, the directive included the following components for the 5-county endemic area: (1) implement a deer feeding ban, (2) develop deer harvest quotas consistent with eradication goals, (3) develop methods for eliminating contact between cattle and deer, (4) continue surveillance and determine actual prevalence and evaluate trends, (5) educate stakeholders on managing deer with the goal of eradicating bTB, and (6) enlist a Coordinator to implement the eradication strategy (13). The directive was prepared based on the prioritization of public health and natural resources and insuring the vitality of agricultural industries.

Cattle are acknowledged to be the original source from which bTB or more specifically, *M. bovis* bacterium were disseminated into the spill-over host, deer, which now spill the pathogen back over to cattle (3, 14). The deer in this area of Michigan, then, are acting as a maintenance or reservoir host sustaining the disease on the landscape (see **Figure 2**) (3). Likelihood of maintaining disease would be increased if there was continued spillover from another reservoir host, such as the original source, cattle. Though considerable attention is paid toward protecting cattle and their feed and water sources from potentially infected wildlife species, it must be emphasized that deer are at risk of infection from cattle as well (3). As bTB-positive livestock operations are identified every year, more novel and aggressive approaches will be required to eradicate bTB from the NELP of Michigan, USA.

The infected deer population of the endemic area contributes to continued infections in cattle (1, 3, 10). This area lies within state-designated DMU 452 which is within a 4-county area consisting of Alcona, Alpena, Montmorency, and Oscoda counties. By 1994, the estimated deer densities where bTB occurred were at or beyond biological carrying capacity (19–23/km^2) and there were high densities maintained largely

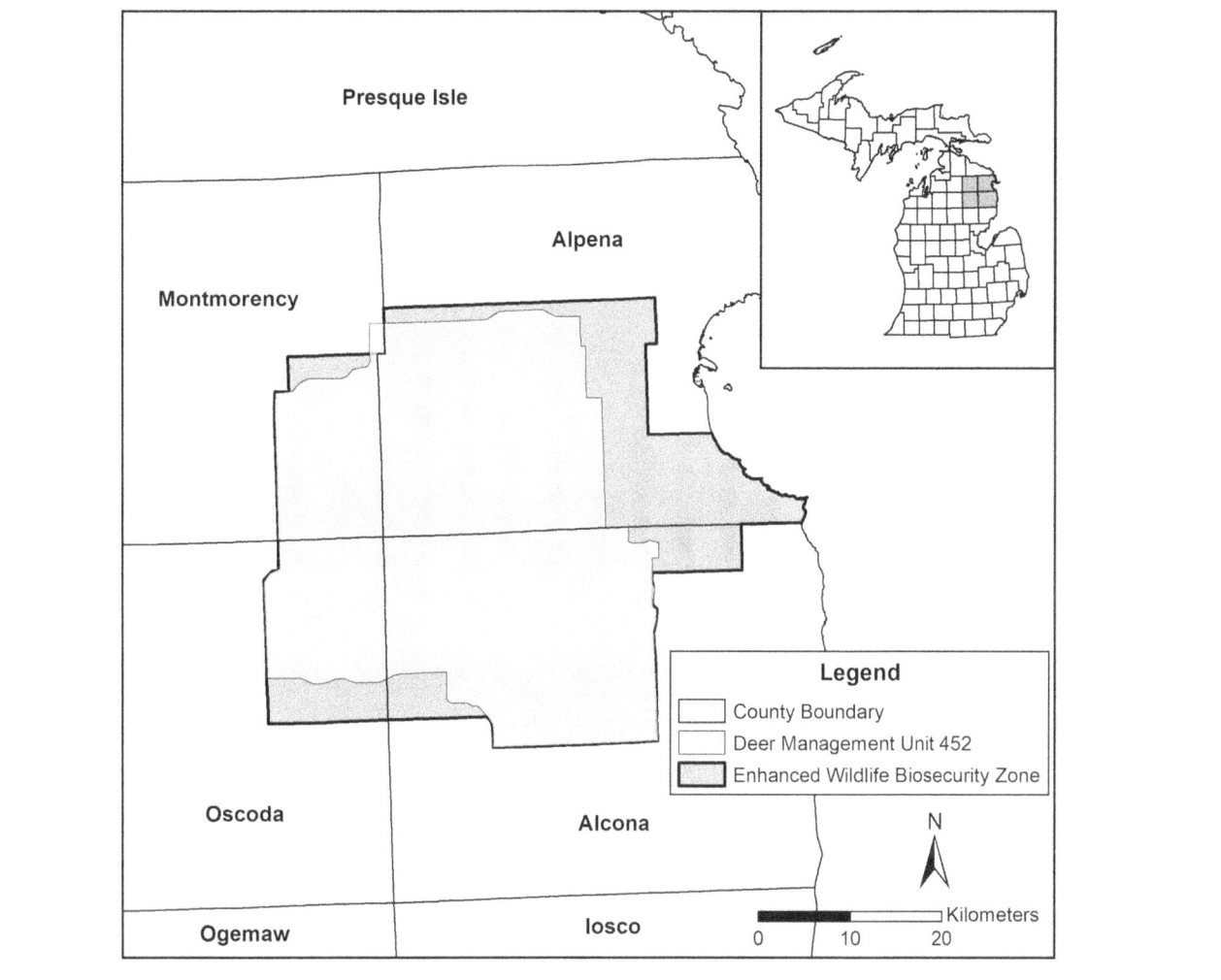

FIGURE 1 | Area of endemic bovine tuberculosis infection in both livestock and wildlife in Michigan, USA, often referred to as the "4-county area" or Deer Management Unit 452 (149,018 ha). The Enhanced Wildlife Biosecurity Zone is an area with increased disease mitigation efforts focused on separating cattle and white-tailed deer (*Odocoileus virginianus*).

through supplemental feeding by hunters and other deer enthusiasts (**Figure 2**) (15). Apparent prevalence rates for bTB in deer in the endemic area as of 2011 ranged from 1.2% (2005) to as high as 4.9% (1995) and has hovered just below 2% over the two decades since (12). Although apparent prevalence rates are an imperfect predictor, they are frequently the best information available to monitor trends in disease (16). From 1994 to 2009 apparent prevalence of bTB in deer correlated with deer population estimates in the endemic area very well (**Figure 2**) (12).

History of Baiting and Feeding Relative to Maintenance of bTB in Deer in Michigan

In general, the bTB endemic area of Michigan consists of several land management types that are relevant to perpetuating the disease and managing the situation: first, several large privately owned parcels of deer habitat are managed exclusively for hunting (17); second, large tracts of public and privately owned

forests exist in multiple successional stages thus providing ample deer habitat components in proximity to one another (18); and third, interspersed agricultural lands consisting of dairies, crops, pastures, and beef cattle operations. The makeup of these agricultural lands provides high quality deer habitat in the region.

Supplemental feeding to sustain and concentrate deer and baiting to attract them to specific locations for hunting purposes were common practices in this area and contributed largely to high deer densities and disease transmission (17, 19–21). Prior to restrictions and bans on feeding and baiting, 72% of non-resident and 87% of resident hunters in the NELP of Michigan used bait while hunting (22), illustrating how prevalent these practices had become. Feeding and baiting helped develop a deer population that ultimately exceeded an estimated 20 deer per km^2 (8). As discussed by 8 baiting and feeding are recognized by natural resources professionals as the primary reasons originally enabling deer to become reservoir hosts for bTB in this area.

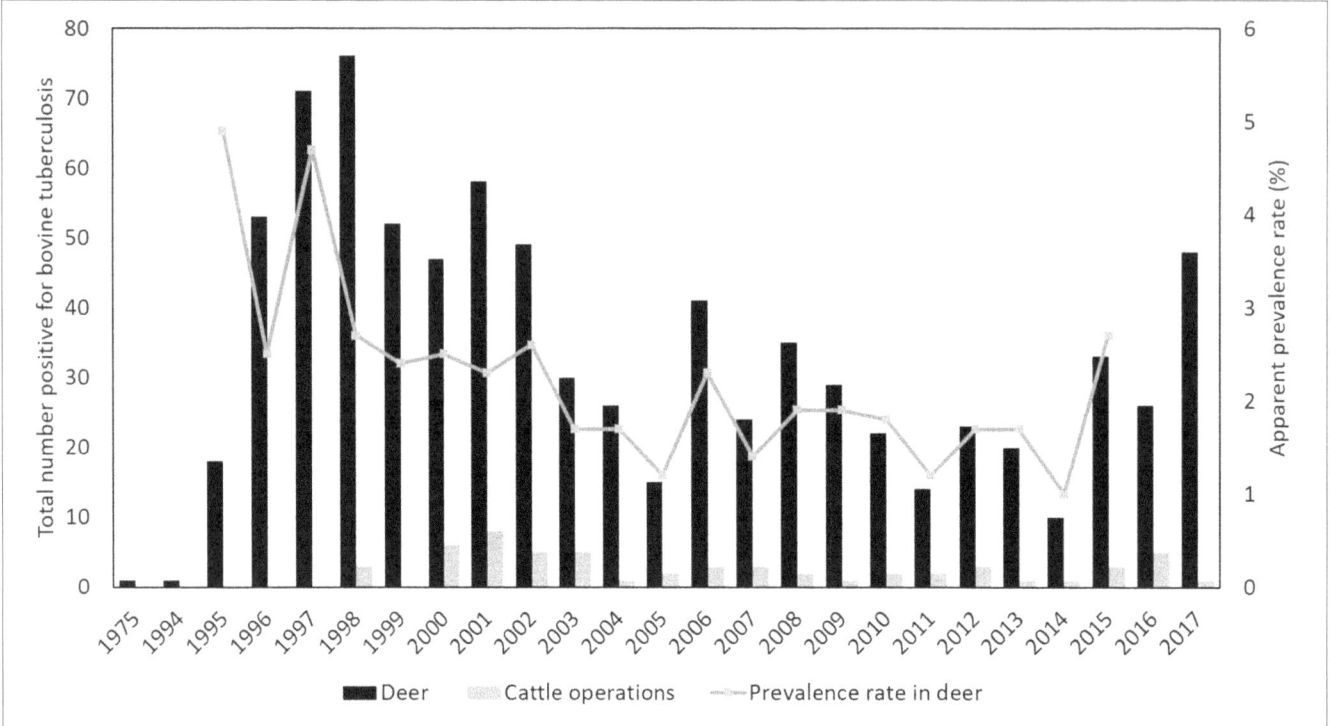

FIGURE 2 | Apparent prevalence rates in white-tailed deer (*Odocoileus virginianus*) as well as numbers of cattle operations and white-tailed deer confirmed positive for infection with *Mycobacterium bovis*.

KEY CONCEPTS IN MOVING FROM MANAGEMENT TOWARD ERADICATION

Approaches to eradicating disease are situational dependent though often include common key components. Components of previous eradication strategies include: (1) implementation of mitigation measures to protect against transmission of *M. bovis* to and from livestock, (2) implementation of management strategies to reduce prevalence in host species including wildlife and livestock; (3) establishment of well-defined goals, plans and policies; and (4) initiation of strategies to build and maintain support of the broad array of stakeholders.

Current Efforts Toward Eradication in Michigan

As in most disease eradication situations, any single strategy alone will rarely eliminate the disease, especially when there are more than a single reservoir host and free-ranging wildlife are involved (23). As such, a combination of strategies need to be implemented in an integrated approach as this will improve efficacy while reducing overall effort and cost (24). In 2008 MDARD initiated the Wildlife Risk Mitigation Project (WRMP) which focused on enrolling and assisting livestock producers in implementing and maintaining an array of measures to reduce risks for transmission of *M. bovis* between deer and cattle on their properties (2, 25–27). Producers were encouraged to participate in the project which entailed education, completing an on-farm assessment of risks, committing to a formal action plan, initiating

the action items within the plan, and passing a verification visit to ensure they implemented the plan (25).

A primary risk of transmission between wildlife and cattle stems from shared resources like food, water, and habitat (19, 27–29). Thus, mitigation measures were directed at protecting resources that are concentrated such as stored cattle feed, watering systems and areas routinely occupied by cattle (2, 26–28). It was also recognized that commonly used farm management practices needed to be evaluated and improved upon. Practices such as the collection of waste slurry from cattle that is then applied to crop fields is questionable especially when there's potential for *M. bovis* to be present (30, 31). This practice often occurs during spring green up when nutritionally stressed deer are dispersing from winter concentration areas in search of nutritious food sources like crop residues and lush new growth emerging in crop fields following snow melt (32).

At the initiation of a plan within the WRMP, landowners meet with an agency wildlife biologist on the farm to assess risk factors for disease transmission. Mitigation measures ranging from strategic feeding practices to constructing feed storage facilities are then recommended based on identified risk factors. The WRMP is a science-based program and the efficacy of many of the recommended mitigation strategies have been supported by research findings including the use of fencing (26, 33) and gates (34, 35) to protect stored feed and feeding areas. Risk mitigation strategies prescribed included, but were not limited to: (1) protecting cattle feed by storing it in buildings or within deer-proof fences with gates closed, (2) feeding cattle daily and away from deer cover, (3) strategically positioning water sources to minimize access and potential contamination by deer, and (4) using disease control permits (DCPs) to reduce antlerless deer numbers on and around farms (5). The majority (545 of 620; 88%) of the farmers in the 4-county MAZ participated in the Program and were subject to annual inspections to insure compliance and maintain their verification (5).

When motivation for deer to access food and water is elevated, such as during late winter, increased vigilance and additional measures to exclude or deter deer may be required (26, 36). The efficacy of mitigation measures is directly related to the motivation of an animal to overcome it and the vigilance of the farmer. Motivation also varies with circumstances relative to season (e.g., severity or length of winter, drought conditions in the summer) and availability of natural foods and water. Producers must be cognizant of these factors, and therefore, when risk is increased, must increase vigilance to maintain an effective level of biosecurity (26, 36, 37). Such mitigation measures and environmental influences are discussed during risk assessments to insure producers understand that wildlife risks are not static and identify factors and scenarios that may increase risk.

Current Efforts: Exclusionary Fences

The use of fencing to exclude deer is an effective means for protecting concentrated resources meant for livestock (2, 26, 33). Numerous fence types exist and fence selection can be based on the predicted level of motivation for deer to breach, the desired longevity, and associated cost (33, 38). In high-biosecurity situations where essentially no deer breaches are acceptable, woven-wire fences ≥ 2.44 m in height are recommended (33, 39). Interestingly, the "weakest link" of a fence is the gate, which obviously must be closed to be effective (26, 34). While this may seem like common sense, in areas where frequent access is needed, livestock producers commonly become lax, leaving gates open, especially during daylight hours. Deer, then, have been documented entering fenced areas of stored feed through open gates in the middle of the day when it was assumed they would not be nearby or active (26).

Current Efforts: Livestock Protection Dogs

Livestock protection dogs (LPDs), traditionally developed and used for reducing the killing of livestock by predators, have also proven effective in keeping deer from directly and indirectly coming in contact with cattle (40). Using specially trained dogs for protecting numerous agricultural resources is becoming more widespread (41, 42). For example, LPDs have proven effective in protecting crops (43), cattle pastures, and feed (40, 44). In the case of transmission of *M. bovis* between cattle and deer in which concerns over indirect transmission through contaminated resources are greatest, LPDs employed to protect stored feed and other resources would be beneficial (40, 44). Although LPDs can effectively repel deer to protect localized areas and livestock, there is a point in which the size of the area or the amount of deer activity exceeds the abilities of a single LPD and either additional LPDs or integrating other measures such as exclusionary fences are needed (33, 44).

Current Efforts: Strategically Locating Feed and Water for Cattle

Currently, 88% of commercial farms in the MAZ are incorporating practices focused on protecting cattle-related resources from wildlife that is potentially harboring bTB (5). Although participation is high, increased emphasis on consistent use and maintenance of mitigation measures is needed (26). Such resources include water, feed, and mineral supplements, all of which are sought by deer and other wildlife and should be a focus of concern regarding the transmission of *M. bovis* (19, 28, 45, 46). Initially, USDA cost-share programs assisted producers in incorporating secure feed storage options including hoop barns and deer-exclusionary fencing to minimize deer access to cattle resources. Refined feeding strategies including limiting provisions to just what a group of cattle will consume that day and constricting the time and duration of availability to just daylight hours can help reduce deer activity in cattle feeding areas (5). Water, though, needs to be available continuously so could be more difficult to protect from contamination by deer (5). Storing and providing cattle resources (feed, supplements, minerals, water, etc.) away from permanent deer habitat and closer to areas of human activity is also recommended.

Current Efforts: Cattle Identification and Tracking

Annual whole-herd testing of cattle for bTB and outfitting cattle with radio-frequency identification (RFID) tags became a requirement for Michigan producers in the endemic area to move live cattle off their farms in 2007. These requirements enable trace-back investigations to locate where and when bTB-infected cattle shared the same space as other cattle, with the goal of identifying other potentially infected animals and premises (29, 37, 47). Although the infection of a herd due to movement of an infected cow into that herd occurs (48), it was presumed to be a lesser risk for cattle producers in Michigan than infected deer (29, 47). Yet recent cases outside of the endemic area and within the accredited-free zone of southern Michigan suggest spread of bTB via infected cattle may actually be increasing (49).

Current Efforts: Reducing Deer Numbers

Population reductions are often considered or used in response to outbreak of disease and involves reducing the density of the host population through strategic lethal removals, usually through culling by professional sharpshooters, or increased recreational hunter harvest (50, 51). Large-scale removals of reservoir species have been implemented and proven effective in some cases (23, 52–55). Though used to a degree in the endemic area of Michigan, these options have proven controversial and have not been wholly accepted by producers, hunters or other publics in Michigan (24, 56).

With the goal of reducing the potential for transmission of *M. bovis* between deer and cattle the MDNR initiated a program in 1998 in which cattle producers could acquire DCPs allowing them to personally address the deer situation on their land by harvesting deer themselves or enlisting the help of sharpshooters with the USDA Wildlife Services (12). Producer use of these permits, though, was low. Only 12% of 6,427 tags were filled in

2008 and deer numbers have since increased as have associated disease prevalence rates (12, 57).

Damage tags or block permits were also available to producers who were experiencing damage to crops by deer, allowing them to harvest deer on their property to alleviate ongoing problems (57, 58). Similar to DCPs, participation was low and lack of local public support was presumed to be the cause (12, 57, 59). Occasionally, negative concerns about these non-traditional deer harvest strategies were voiced by owners of recreational lands adjacent to at-risk farms (12). For example, even when deer density estimates were 8–15/km^2 and crop damage was substantial, only five of 31 alfalfa growers participating in a crop damage project requested permits to control damage on their property and only 42% of issued permits were used. Similarly, red kidney bean growers were issued a total of 88 permits and only 23% were used (60, 61). These data illustrate that even when landowners were faced with substantial amounts of crop damage and provided permits to reduce deer numbers, they were not using them (60, 61).

The MDNR increased the number of available deer tags and the number of hunting seasons, with the focus on removal of antlerless deer, and successfully reduced deer numbers within DMU 452 by 50% from 1995 to 2004 (12, 62). However, deer numbers rebounded rapidly since 2005 to >110,000 and remained steady through 2009 (12). More recently hunting opportunity and harvest potential has been essentially unlimited in DMU 452, though hunters have harvested less than one thousandth of the tags available (i.e., 4,388 deer from 5,575,390 potential tags), demonstrating that demand for opportunity has been saturated (63). Although the MDNR was effective in reducing deer numbers initially, hunters were not overwhelmingly supportive of these actions (22). As a new strategy to address insufficient harvest on farms, it is now a requirement for livestock producers to include and implement a deer reduction component within their EWB Plan, specifically focused on those deer routinely in proximity to farms with cattle (5). As this is a recently enacted requirement, the effects are yet to be seen.

Intensifying Efforts to Reduce Potential Transmission of *M. bovis*

Nearly 20 years ago it was stated that "The measures of apparent bovine TB prevalence have decreased by half since 1997, providing hopeful preliminary evidence that eradication strategies are succeeding" (15), but bTB still persists in Michigan. Ongoing and increased efforts to reduce the persistence of *M. bovis* continue; however, the rate of cattle operations being identified as positive for bTB fluctuates at levels that put the accredited-free status of Michigan in jeopardy (>3 positive herds detected/year) (5). Despite extensive efforts prescribed by the previous WRMP, bTB-positive herds continue to be identified each year, thus new approaches are needed if the goal is still to eliminate the disease. To this end the EWB Project was initiated to involve more thorough on-the-ground assessments of properties housing cattle by an "EpiTeam," similar to what is used following the detection of positive cattle. Each team includes a MDARD veterinarian, a USDA or Alpena Conservation District wildlife biologist, a MSU Extension cattle specialist, and a local producer (5). Each assessment results in an action plan (now entitled "Enhanced Wildlife Biosecurity Plan") that needs to be implemented on the ground by the producer, similar to how the WRMP was implemented from 2008 to present. Producers must implement and maintain all prescribed mitigation measures relating to high-risk areas on their farms by December 31, 2019 or will lose their ability to sell cattle other than directly to slaughter (6).

Intensified Efforts: Targeted Deer Removals

All existing 130 commercial cattle producers in the EWB Area require a deer removal component that enables sharpshooters to remove deer from in and around farms and pastures. For example, in Dressel's (32) study up to 13 deer were removed from a single landowner's property. Action plans in the EWBP are designed to eliminate deer whose home range includes farms and deter others from establishing ranges in proximity to farms (5). The frequency of visitation to highly-desirable resources such as stored feed and agricultural crops may be a learned behavior that could be curtailed by removing mature does or entire family groups of offending deer (64). It has been documented that fawns can learn movement patterns from adult does and that it is typically a few specific deer in a given area that will share space and time with cattle or frequent stored feed areas (27, 36, 37). As such, targeted removal of offending individuals may curb present and future visitation of farms by deer. Research has shown deer frequent farms the most often during: January through mid-April; and Mid-July through August (26, 36), thus these periods are when removal efforts should be focused.

Intensified Efforts: Strategic Habitat Manipulations

Wildlife management consists of three components: (1) the biota or populations, (2) the habitats or ecosystems organisms need to persist, and (3) the people or stakeholders that live in the ecosystems and interact with the wildlife resource (65). To date, bTB research and management practices have been directed primarily at two components, namely the biota (i.e., deer) by reducing numbers through recreational hunting and targeted deer removals and the people (i.e., hunters, producers) by manipulating harvest regulations, deer baiting, and feeding practices, and how producers store and protect feed and water resources. Historically, the third component of wildlife management, the species' habitat, has not been factored into bTB management strategies. Perhaps because, as Felix et al. (66) suggested, "managers may lack sufficient understanding of long-term spatial and temporal links between habitat supply and population response." There has, though, been an extensive amount of research on why and how forest management practices can be used to enhance or reduce quality of deer habitat [e.g., (67, 68)] and potentially influence the distribution of deer across a landscape (18).

The Alpena-Montmorency Conservation District of Michigan has recently initiated a cost-share program that may assist in influencing deer movement patterns, potentially away from stored feed, water sources and livestock concentrations, by initiating habitat improvements for deer through forest management activities. This new program, if implemented strategically could stimulate deer to redistribute themselves away from agricultural areas to other, naturally occurring vegetation types. The program also includes incentives that encourage data collection and the liberal harvest of antlerless deer (69).

The quality and distribution of a species' habitat is a primary driver influencing the spatial and temporal distribution of species [e.g., (70)], including deer [e.g., (18, 71)] and elk [e.g., (72, 73)]. Recognizing how habitat quality and its distribution can influence the movement patterns of a species, a strategy could be to use this basic ecological principle as a tool to combat bTB in the NELP. An additional step may be to take measures to lessen the quality of habitat for deer on and adjacent to farms, lowering the area's carrying capacity, the desire of deer to be there, and the fitness of deer that persist.

The core of the bTB area, DMU452 is composed primarily of private land (93%) (74) that is dominated by forest cover types. For example, within Alpena County alone, 60% of the area is covered by lowland conifer swamps and northern hardwood forests interspersed among agricultural areas. Much of the forest is relatively later successional stage, especially on private lands. Given that the life requisites of deer in this area include: spring and summer food, thermal cover, and fall and winter food (66), much of the agricultural lands and livestock areas are often under tremendous feeding pressure by deer especially in late-winter through summer (32, 60, 61, 75). A cover type lacking in this area that deer could use extensively for feeding and cover is regenerating deciduous stands (e.g., aspen clearcuts of predominately early age classes) (66). Experimenting with forest management practices as a method to manipulate how deer use the landscape has merit.

Habitat management on public lands is a primary activity used by agencies to meet wildlife management objectives and satisfy a diversity of stakeholders, yet it is poorly understood how frequently or what types of management, if any, occur across private lands. The use of landowner incentive or cost-share programs to manipulate forest cover types to improve habitat conditions away from agricultural lands and livestock operations should be investigated for their efficacy in: (1) providing quality habitat, (2) shifting the distribution of deer away from agricultural areas at high risk for transmission of *M. bovis*, (3) reducing crop damage, and (4) meeting economic objectives of landowners for harvesting forest types. Such a habitat-based bTB management and research approach could be initiated and simultaneously integrated with other bTB mitigation practices. The successful management of this complex problem could be enhanced if the habitat for deer were factored into the management equation.

Potential Future Efforts

Original actions to eradicate bTB in Michigan combined with recently emerging science-based strategies have all been insufficient to date, primarily due to waning stakeholder support. Several new strategies and directions are mentioned above and have begun, here we discuss additional potential measures to consider if the collective desire of agencies, stakeholders, and other publics is to eradicate bTB from Michigan.

Potential Future Efforts: Reducing Deer Numbers

As stated by Riley et al. (76), "An assumption in most conventional deer harvest strategies is that adequate demand for and successful use of antlerless deer permits exists to achieve desired deer harvest." As deer densities decline and number of deer encounters are reduced, hunter perception and support, effort, and desire to continue hunting fade and hunters will often transition to other locations or species (77, 78). When hunter harvest is no longer effective in maintaining deer populations at or below goal, additional measures must be contemplated. In such situations "Hunting eventually may become less a recreation and more a community service or civic duty ... Culling may be a more appropriate term for the kind and purpose of hunting under such circumstances" (76). Although recreational hunting is and should remain the primary means for managing white-tailed deer, there are situations in which it may not be safe, feasible, or effective and other means need to be considered (79). Within DMU 452 where deer reductions are needed and current harvest is insufficient, strategies like earn-a-buck or incentivizing hunters by allowing easy donation or profiting from venison may be worth consideration (79–81).

Most (>90%) of the bTB area in Michigan is privately owned (74) which has contributed to challenges in achieving wildlife management goals (9). Although purely speculative, it is uncertain about what the future for large privately-owned "hunt clubs" will be with consistently declining numbers of hunters. Will the owners of these lands want to hunt them in the future or use them simply as family get-aways? How will this affect the local deer population? A decreasing trend in hunters has been well-documented in the US (82, 83) and in Michigan specifically (84, 85). Because of these trends, other approaches might be warranted such as the MDNR purchasing large tracts of hunt clubs or other private lands (farms) to improve access. For example, from January 1998 to November 2018, the MDNR purchased a total of 34,240 ha state-wide with an average of 1,630 ha being purchased annually and the mean amount of land acquired per transaction was 53 ha (K. Wildman, Biologist, MDNR, personal communication, 05 Nov 2018). Non-profit conservation organizations such as the Rocky Mountain Elk Foundation are often partners in purchasing land which the state then manages and oftentimes provides public access for hunting. A local example in northern Michigan was the purchase of the Green Timbers tract in 1982. This property is now attached to the Pigeon River Country State Forest and provides unique walk-in only hunting and other recreational activities (e.g., backpacking, hiking, cross country) for the public. Acquisitions such as this improve the ability of the MDNR to manage the deer population and provide opportunity to its constituents.

Potential Future Efforts: Vaccination Program for Deer

An additional novel tool that could aid eradication of bTB in Michigan is an oral vaccine against bTB for deer. Interest in using a vaccine for bTB in deer is increasing (32, 63, 86). Bacille Calmette-Guerin (BCG) vaccine reduces disease severity by decreasing gross lesions and sites of infection, suggesting potential for reducing transmission and minimizing endemic infection in wildlife (87, 88). Significant progress has been made in demonstrating the safety, efficacy, and feasibility of implementing a vaccination program against bTB for deer (89–92). Researchers modeled vaccination and demonstrated that vaccinating just 50% of the deer would contribute to an 86% probability of eradicating bovine tuberculosis in DMU 452 in 30 years (63). Interestingly, in the presence of recreational baiting it would be highly unlikely to achieve eradication within the next 30 years at the same vaccination rate (63). A vaccination rate higher than 50% could likely be achieved based on an experiment where placebo vaccine baits were effectively delivered to free-ranging deer (32) which would increase the probability of eradication. Of course, implementing a vaccination program while maintaining the use of additional management strategies; restrictions on baiting, liberal recreational harvest, DCPs, and fencing stored feed and other cattle resources would be the most efficient path to eradication (63, 86).

Potential Future Efforts: Novel Diagnostic Tests for bTB

As current live-test methods involve multiple animal handlings, take 48–72 h to produce results, or require specialized laboratory procedures, improved methods are needed for reliable and timely detection of bTB (93, 94). A "trap–test–cull" project was evaluated using a rapid test and live capture of deer, though it was deemed cost-prohibitive (>$1.5 million US annually) and ineffective in reducing prevalence of bTB (95). Recently developed methods that enable the antemortem detection of unique biomarkers of disease suggest improved diagnostics are becoming available. For example, infection by *M. bovis* results in the presence of specific peptides in the blood which can be detected with common laboratory analyses (96). Additionally, the analyses of breath from cattle to detect bTB-specific volatile organic compounds has proven effective in experimental settings and has potential for applications with deer (94). Also, genotyping particular strains of bTB pathogens enable back tracking to determine the source herd of cattle for the disease (97). New tools like these and the support to develop them are desperately needed.

The People Piece

Public support and involvement is essential if complete eradication is the goal. Are Michigan residents accepting of a low level of bTB sustained in their deer herd? It was apparent in 2006 that Michigan hunters felt bTB was not a problem, ranking it considerably lower than "more extensive problems" including too few mature bucks and too few deer in general (12). Are Michigan livestock producers comfortable with the risk that they may have a reactor cow in this year's whole-herd test and that theirs could be the next positive herd? It is clear that Federal and State agricultural agencies are losing tolerance for reoccurring positive cattle farms. As it should be, input from stakeholder groups and various publics have played a large role in political and management decisions regarding bTB in Michigan since 1994 when the second bTB positive deer

in 20 years was found. There is potential that had managers been more empowered or convincing and decision makers more stalwart the bTB situation in NELP may be quite different today. Despite extensive surveys examining strategies used to improve stakeholder appreciation of the situation with bTB in deer (98–101), public and political support has been too little to enable the actions necessary to improve the situation (101). To make better progress going forward, more emphasis must be placed on the human dimensions aspects of the issue by more effectively engaging the diversity of stakeholders associated with this deer-bTB-agricultural industry issue.

Policy Based on Science or Public Demand?

Although state wildlife management agencies are responsible for managing wildlife populations, habitats, and the people who use wildlife resources (65), elected and appointed government officials typically make the underlying decisions driving management actions of agencies (102). In 1996, Michigan voters elected to transfer the responsibility for managing game animals from the MDNR to the 7-member governor appointed Natural Resources Commission (NRC). The NRC was mandated to integrate scientific findings and public input into new policies that the MDNR follows; in turn, the MDNR provides recommendations to the NRC to help them make informed decisions when establishing such policies (20). Policy established by the NRC in 2007 presents the goals of the MDNR as using science-based management practices to maintain a healthy deer population as determined by the carrying capacity of its range and the effects upon native plant communities, crops, and public safety (103). Additionally, they set out to maintain an active educational program to inform the public on practices of deer management for achieving a healthy and vigorous herd (103). Despite these basic, well-intended goals driving policy, public trust (of NELP residents) in the ability of MDNR to set deer hunting rules relative to eradicating bTB was lower than 50% in 2011 (104). This distrust has impacted the ability of MDNR to manage bTB and created backlash by local residents and hunting constituency groups (105).

Tools such as spatial models for forecasting likelihood of disease eradication given various approaches are the types of informative tools needed to aid in establishing goals and creating policy (63). A key strategy for facilitating scientifically based decisions leading to effective management actions lies in providing policy makers with accurate information derived from high quality research while respecting their role of representing those that elected or appointed them (102). Further, educating the general public and earning acceptance and trust are also essential to successful management of healthy wildlife populations and their habitats (15, 22).

Building Widespread Stakeholder Support

Initial efforts by state and federal agencies to eradicate bTB in Michigan were extensive despite minimal public support (106). To be effective and successful, actions initiated by agencies have to be accepted and adopted by citizens including hunters, livestock producers, and wildlife viewers. For example, MDNR initiated strategies to reduce deer numbers through increased availability of hunting licenses and implemented baiting and feeding restrictions (20, 56). Public support and action was needed to harvest additional antlerless deer and to cease baiting and feeding. Although there was a documented 50% decline in apparent prevalence from 1995 to 2004 due to reductions in deer numbers and restricting baiting and feeding (107), deer numbers and prevalence rates have since rebounded. As demonstrated by the incessant reappearance of bTB in deer and cattle, it is apparent public support and involvement are essential for successful eradication or even tempered control (20, 106, 108). It is also apparent that the lucid presentation of specific disease-related risks to one's personal interests are needed to truly bring about action and change (99, 100). Frequently updated information with an emphasis on successes is essential to maintaining or increasing stakeholder support (98).

In addition to insufficient stakeholder support, there has been decreasing financial support to and from federal and state agencies to enable the eradication of bTB from wildlife and livestock in Michigan. This issue has led to fewer personnel and waning awareness and support from most publics. Thus, current and future efforts toward eradicating bTB require maximizing knowledge gained from past efforts to inform next steps for research and management (62). To this end, modeling efforts have helped predict likely outcomes given the tools and resources available to begin answering questions to help optimize and select combinations of strategies to implement (63). Without incorporating new tools and revising strategies, it was predicted that eradicating bTB from Michigan in the next 30 years was unlikely (63, 95).

It has become clear that ongoing strategies for eradicating or even minimizing the transmission of bTB in Michigan have been insufficient, primarily due to lack of sufficient long-term determination of stakeholders. If the Michigan and US goal is to protect the entire country's cattle herd and trade status, increased support and strategies are needed. Further, it is apparent that increased public acceptance and involvement will be required to defeat the challenges associated with the eradication of bTB (56, 107).

Unfortunately, these challenges are deeply rooted in the culture of the area and will not be overcome easily. There are apparent divides and disconnects amongst the interests and demands of various factions of the public (i.e., hunters, cattle producers, policy makers, general public), with public servants from natural resource and agricultural agencies struggling to regain healthy wildlife and livestock populations for them. It seems that through efforts to achieve healthy deer densities in Michigan following the appearance of bTB, public resentment has actually grown (12, 62). Agencies need improvements in public outreach about all aspects of the bTB issue to reverse this trend and garner support for the intentions behind management actions. Given the current popularity and user involvement in social media (i.e., YouTube, Instagram, Podcasts, etc.), it is a new tool that could be used to aid ongoing and future efforts associated with bTB. Although previous efforts to engage and motivate hunters to actively participate in non-traditional deer management actions (i.e., increased harvest of antlerless deer) failed over the long term, significant changes such as providing

extended or alternative seasons and increasing attention on new hunters may improve participation (101). Unfortunately, common trends such as managing for more, larger, and more mature (i.e., older) male deer on the landscape, primarily through imposing antler point restrictions, does not align well with disease management strategies focused on removing more males with an emphasis on older age classes (10).

Optional Approaches Toward Managing bTB in Michigan

Going forward, agencies need to (1) establish long-term, mutually agreed upon objectives, (2) develop well-defined strategies that align with those objectives, and (3) develop and implement practices to evaluate the efficacy of those strategies (109). All options toward managing disease, including no action, need to be considered in establishing objectives (24, 86). First and foremost it needs to be determined what the long-term goal is: status quo, eradicating bTB throughout Michigan, eliminating bTB in deer in Michigan, or eliminating bTB in cattle in Michigan. If the presence of bTB in Michigan truly is acceptable, there is always the option of no additional management action whatsoever, although this may need to be coupled with the buyout of all cattle across the region to eliminate potential for cattle becoming infected. Additionally, compartmentalization could be considered to limit the potential for geographic spread of bTB through the use of significant barriers such as large-scale exclusionary fences for deer (24). It was well-stated by Olmstead and Rhode (110) regarding the interconnectedness of the cattle industry, "Given the benefits from trading in livestock and the contagious nature of the disease, it was more efficient to build a "fence" around the entire country than to create barriers around each and every farm."

If the goal is still to eradicate bTB across Michigan as stated by the Governor in 1998, then the potential exists to make great strides. Actions should include but are not limited to: significantly reducing deer densities with focus on those in the vicinity of cattle operations, eliminating baiting and supplemental feeding, segregating wildlife and cattle/cattle resources, using habitat management to change the spatial distribution of deer, and deploying a vaccine for deer.

If the goal is only to eliminate bTB in cattle, the strategy is relatively straightforward especially if all transmission is occurring only between deer and cattle (111). With cattle being the primary concern, excluding deer from all cattle-related resources with true deer exclusionary fencing (i.e., 2.4-m-h woven wire fence) is needed (24, 26, 39). Where this is not possible, such as a body of water bordered by cover used by deer and cattle pastures, either the deer or cattle must be excluded. Although reliable deer-exclusionary fence is initially expensive and may be considered unsightly, it is effective when maintained and would minimize potential for transmission via indirect and direct contact (24, 26, 33, 38). This level of biosecurity is commonplace in other production animal systems such as within the swine industry (24, 112, 113), especially in areas where the threat of disease transmission is a reality. Permanent deer-proof fences are also commonplace and widely accepted in areas where the captive cervid industry is active, as well as along expansive stretches of highway systems throughout the US where deer-vehicle collisions had been common. These fences are also used around the world in places such as in Africa because they enable managers to achieve extensive and reliable manipulation and protection of various species (33). Given the serious nature of eradicating bTB, reliable management of deer and cattle are needed in Michigan and thus similar measures could be considered.

CONCLUSION

The ongoing situation with bTB in Michigan has been a persistent and expensive management challenge for livestock producers and state and federal agencies for more than a quarter of a century. As biologists and public servants, we may feel ethically committed to ridding the landscape of this disease that impacts the wildlife resource and a primary agricultural industry. But unless the societal and related political support for this exists, perhaps we need to either stand down or double down. The situation in Michigan is a multi-faceted issue with several imposing barriers, ecologically and socially, that are impeding the possibility for progress toward eradicating the disease. The first and foremost challenge is inadequate public concern over the health of the deer population and cattle herd and subsequent lack of political support and action. This challenge obstructs many crucial steps in wildlife management toward eradication, including the banning of baiting and feeding, reducing host populations, and understanding and accepting the severity of the bTB situation across the landscape.

If there was increased public concern about the occurrence of bTB in wildlife, livestock, and humans there would likely be compounded support and participation in actively pursuing eradication. As demonstrated during the era of market hunting, even before the advent of modern hunting tools and technologies (i.e., high-powered rifles and scopes, night vision, remote cameras, helicopters, drones), Americans demonstrated our ability to severely reduce, and in some cases, decimate deer populations when motivated. Conversely and more recently, due to changes in motivators, we have demonstrated our ability to

develop large numbers and concentrations of white-tailed deer. Now we must refocus on maintaining populations of fewer but healthy deer in concert with the limitations of local agricultural goals and available natural vegetation types that can provide deer habitat. In 1949, Aldo Leopold wrote, "A thing is right when it tends to maintain the integrity, stability, and beauty of the biotic community, it is wrong when it tends otherwise" (114). Natural resource professionals can still keep this goal in mind while simultaneously acknowledging and addressing the food production needs of our continually growing and hungry populous.

The toolbox contains much of what is needed to combat bTB in Michigan; including increased hunting license allocations, increased availability of disease permits, financial cost-share programs to increase biosecurity on farms, feeding and baiting bans, the use of educational stakeholder meetings, new novel tools to facilitate diagnosis and surveillance, and even a vaccine for deer or evaluating the use habitat manipulations to redistribute deer. None of these tools will be effective alone, they must be applied aggressively and in unison to complement each other. Progress has been made in understanding and managing livestock-wildlife interactions and the transmission of bTB in the Michigan landscape and recent decisions and new strategies have great potential.

AUTHOR CONTRIBUTIONS

KV, ML, and HC contributed equally in the development of the idea, collection of the data, and preparation of the manuscript. KV fleshed out the original outline. ML drafted the manuscript and continually incorporated and massaged his, KV and HC's thoughts. All authors continually reviewed and edited the manuscript, producing the submitted draft.

ACKNOWLEDGMENTS

We appreciate the assistance and support provided by R. Smith, recently retired MDARD. This research was funded in part by the U.S. Department of Agriculture.

REFERENCES

1. Palmer M. *Mycobacterium bovis* shuttles between domestic animals and wildlife. *Microbe Am Soc Microbiol.* (2008) 3:27.
2. Walter WD, Anderson CW, Smith R, Vanderklok M, Averill JJ, VerCauteren KC. On-farm mitigation of transmission of tuberculosis from white-tailed deer to cattle: literature review and recommendations. *Vet Med Int.* (2012) 2012:616318. doi: 10.1155/2012/616318
3. Palmer MV. *Mycobacterium bovis*: characteristics of wildlife reservoir hosts. *Transbound Emerg Dis.* (2013) 60:1–13. doi: 10.1111/tbed.12115
4. Livingstone P, Ryan T, Hancox N, Crews K, Bosson M, Knowles G, et al. Regionalisation: a strategy that will assist with bovine tuberculosis control and facilitate trade. *Vet Microbiol.* (2006) 112:291–301. doi: 10.1016/j.vetmic.2005.11.016

5. MDARD. *Bovine Tuberculosis Eradication Program Quarterly Update.* Legislative report. Animal Industry Division (2018). Available online at: https://www.michigan.gov/documents/emergingdiseases/MDARD_ LegislativeRptTBProgram_Jan2018_QtrlyUpdate010518_w_attachments_ 610072_7.pdf (Accessed August 27, 2018).
6. MDARD. *Zoning Order, Establishment of Zones for Bovine Tuberculosis* (2018). Available online at: https://www.michigan.gov/documents/ emergingdiseases/MDARD_TB_Zoning_Order_2018_FINAL-_ DIGITALVERSION_wo_signature_619715_7.pdf (Accessed August 27, 2018).
7. MDARD. *Bovine Tuberculosis Eradication Program Quarterly Update.* Legislative report. Animal Industry Division (2017). Available online at: https://www.michigan.gov/documents/emergingdiseases/MDARD_ LegislativeRptTBProgram_Oct2017_QtrlyUpdate100417_602704_7.pdf (Accessed August 27, 2018).

8. Schmitt SM, Fitzgerald SD, Cooley TM, Bruning-Fann CS, Sullivan L, Berry D, et al. Bovine tuberculosis in free-ranging white-tailed deer from Michigan. *J Wildl Dis*. (1997) 33:749–58. doi: 10.7589/0090-3558-33.4.749

9. O'Brien DJ, Fitzgerald SD, Lyon TJ, Butler KL, Fierke JS, Clarke KR, et al. Tuberculous lesions in free-ranging white-tailed deer from Michigan. *J Wild Dis*. (2001) 37:608–13. doi: 10.7589/0090-3558-37.3.608

10. O'Brien DJ, Schmitt SM, Fierke JS, Hogle SA, Winterstein SR, Cooley TM, et al. Epidemiology of *Mycobacterium bovis* in free-ranging white-tailed deer, Michigan USA, 1995–2000. *Prev Vet Med*. (2002) 54:47–63. doi: 10.1016/S0167-5877(02)00010-7

11. Lipe, J. *Proceedings of the 2004 Bovine Tuberculosis Conference* (2004). Available online at: http://digitalcommons.unl.edu/cgi/viewcontent.cgi?article=1004&context=michbovinetb (Accessed August 27, 2018).

12. O'Brien DJ, Schmitt SM, Fitzgerald SD, Berry DE. Management of bovine tuberculosis in Michigan wildlife: current status and near term prospects. *Vet Microbiol*. (2011) 151:179–87. doi: 10.1016/j.vetmic.2011.02.042

13. Engler, J. *Bovine Tuberculosis in Michigan Deer. Executive Directive 1*. Office of the Governor, State of Michigan, Lansing, MI (1998).

14. Daszak P, Cunningham AA, Hyatt AD. Emerging infectious diseases of wildlife-threats to biodiversity and human health. *Science* (2000) 287:443–9. doi: 10.1126/science.287.5452.443

15. Schmitt SM, O'Brien DJ, Bruning-Fann CS, Fitzgerald SD. Bovine tuberculosis in Michigan wildlife and livestock. *Ann N Y Acad Sci*. (2002) 969:262–8. doi: 10.1111/j.1749-6632.2002.tb04390.x

16. O'Brien DJ, Schmitt SM, Berry DE, Fitzgerald SD, Vanneste JR, Lyon TJ, et al. Estimating the true prevalence of *Mycobacterium bovis* in hunter-harvested white-tailed deer in Michigan. *J Wild Dis*. (2004) 40:42–52. doi: 10.7589/0090-3558-40.1.42

17. Garner MS. *Movement Patterns and Behavior at Winter Feeding and Fall Baiting Stations in a Population of White-Tailed Deer Infected with Bovine Tuberculosis in the Northeastern Lower Peninsula of Michigan*. Thesis. Lansing, MI: Michigan State University (2001).

18. Felix AB, Walsh DP, Hughey BD, Campa H, Winterstein SR. Applying landscape-scale habitat-potential models to understand deer spatial structure and movement Patterns. *J Wildl Manag*. (2007) 71:804–10. doi: 10.2193/2006-366

19. Palmer MV, Whipple DL. Survival of *Mycobacterium bovis* on feedstuffs commonly used as supplemental feed for white-tailed deer (*Odocoileus virginianus*). *J Wildl Dis*. (2006) 42:853–8. doi: 10.7589/0090-3558-42.4.853

20. Rudolph BA, Riley SJ, Hickling GJ, Frawley BJ, Garner MS, Winterstein SR. Regulating hunter baiting for white-tailed deer in Michigan: biological and social considerations. *Wildl Soc Bull*. (2006) 34:314–21. doi: 10.2193/0091-7648(2006)34[314:RHBFWD]2.0.CO;2

21. Thompson AK, Samuel MD, Van Deelen TR. Alternative feeding strategies and potential disease transmission in Wisconsin white-tailed deer. *J Wild Manag*. (2008) 72:416–21. doi: 10.2193/2006-543

22. Dorn ML, Mertig AG. Bovine tuberculosis in Michigan: stakeholder attitudes and implications for eradication efforts. *Wild Soc Bull*. (2005) 33:539–52. doi: 10.2193/0091-7648(2005)33[539:BTIMSA]2.0.CO;2

23. White PC, Böhm M, Marion G, Hutchings MR. Control of bovine tuberculosis in British livestock: there is no "silver bullet". *Trends Microbiol*. (2008) 16:420–7. doi: 10.1016/j.tim.2008.06.005

24. Gortazar C, Diez-Delgado I, Barasona JA, Vicente J, De La Fuente J, Boadella M. The wild side of disease control at the wildlife-livestock-human interface: a review. *Front Vet Sci*. (2015) 1:27. doi: 10.3389/fvets.2014.00027

25. Michigan State University Extension. *Wildlife Risk*A*Syst for Bovine TB. FAS 113*. Lansing, MI (2010).

26. Lavelle MJ, Campa HI, LeDoux K, Ryan PJ, Fischer JW, Pepin KM, et al. Deer response to exclusion from stored cattle feed in Michigan, USA. *Prev Vet Med*. (2015) 121:159–64. doi: 10.1016/j.prevetmed.2015.06.015

27. Lavelle MJ, Kay SL, Pepin KM, Grear DA, Campa H, VerCauteren KC. Evaluating wildlife-cattle contact rates to improve the understanding of dynamics of bovine tuberculosis transmission in Michigan, USA. *Prev Vet Med*. (2016) 135:28–36. doi: 10.1016/j.prevetmed.2016.10.009

28. Fine AE, Bolin CA, Gardiner JC, Kaneene JB. A study of the persistence of *Mycobacterium bovis* in the environment under natural weather conditions in Michigan, USA. *Vet Med Int*. (2011) 2011:1–12. doi: 10.4061/2011/765430

29. Okafor CC, Grooms DL, Bruning-Fann CS, Averill JJ, Kaneene JB. Descriptive epidemiology of bovine tuberculosis in Michigan (1975–2010): lessons learned. *Vet Med Int*. (2011) 2011:874924. doi: 10.4061/2011/874924

30. Kellogg RL, Lander CH, Moffitt DC, Gollehon N. Manure nutrients relative to the capacity of cropland and pastureland to assimilate nutrients: spatial and temporal trends for the United States. *Proc Water Environ Fed*. (2000) 16:18–157. doi: 10.2175/193864700784994812

31. McCallan L, McNair J, Skuce R, Branch B. *A Review of the Potential Role of Cattle Slurry in the Spread of Bovine Tuberculosis*. Agri-food and Biosciences Institute, Northern Ireland (2014).

32. Dressel D. *Development of Strategies to Orally Deliver Vaccine for Bovine Tuberculosis to White-Tailed Deer of Northeastern Lower Michigan*. Thesis. Lansing, MI: Michigan State University (2017).

33. VerCauteren KC, Lavelle MJ, Hygnstrom SE. Fences and deer-damage management: a review of designs and efficacy. *J Wildl Manag*. (2006) 34:191–200. doi: 10.2193/0091-7648(2006)34[191:FADMAR]2.0.CO;2

34. VerCauteren KC, Seward NW, Lavelle MJ, Fischer JW, Phillips GE. Deer guards and bump gates for excluding white-tailed deer from fenced resources. *Hum Wildl Conflicts* (2009) 3:145–53.

35. Berentsen AR, Dunbar MR, Misiewicz R. PVC curtains to prevent deer access to stored feed: a pilot study. *Proc Vert Pest Conf*. (2010) 2010:315–8.

36. Berentsen AR, Miller RS, Misiewicz R, Malmberg JL, Dunbar MR. Characteristics of white-tailed deer visits to cattle farms: implications for disease transmission at the wildlife–livestock interface. *Eur J Wildl Res*. (2014) 60:161–70. doi: 10.1007/s10344-013-0760-5

37. Ribeiro-Lima J, Carstensen M, Cornicelli L, Forester J, Wells S. Patterns of cattle farm visitation by white-tailed deer in relation to risk of disease transmission in a previously infected area with bovine tuberculosis in Minnesota, USA. *Transbound Emerg Dis*. (2016) 64:1519–29. doi: 10.1111/tbed.12544

38. VerCauteren KC, Lavelle MJ, Hygnstrom SE. A simulation model for determining cost-effectiveness of fences for reducing deer damage. *Wildl Soc Bull*. (2006) 34:16–22. doi: 10.2193/0091-7648(2006)34[16:ASMFDC]2.0.CO;2

39. VerCauteren KC, Van Deelen TR, Lavelle MJ, Hall WH. Assessment of abilities of white-tailed deer to jump fences. *J Wildl Manag*. (2010) 74:1378–81. doi: 10.1111/j.1937-2817.2010.tb01260.x

40. VerCauteren KC, Lavelle MJ, Phillips GE. Livestock protection dogs for deterring deer from cattle and feed. *J Wildl Manag*. (2008) 72:1443–8. doi: 10.2193/2007-372

41. VerCauteren K, Lavelle M, Landry JM, Marker L, Gehring TM. *Use of Dogs in the Mediation of Conservation Conflicts*. Oxford: Oxford University Press (2014).

42. Zingaro M, Salvatori V, Vielmi L, Boitani L. Are the livestock guarding dogs where they are supposed to be? *Appl Anim Behav Sci*. (2018) 198:89–94. doi: 10.1016/j.applanim.2017.10.002

43. VerCauteren KC, Seward NW, Hirchert DL, Jones ML, Beckerman SF. Dogs for reducing wildlife damage to organic crops: a case study. *Proc Wildl Dam Manag Conf*. (2005) 11:286–93.

44. VerCauteren KC, Lavelle MJ, Gehring TM, Landry JM. Cow dogs: use of livestock protection dogs for reducing predation and transmission of pathogens from wildlife to cattle. *Appl Anim Behav Sci*. (2012) 140:128–36. doi: 10.1016/j.applanim.2012.06.006

45. Fine AE. *The Role of Indirect Transmission in the Epidemiology of Bovine Tuberculosis in Cattle and White-Tailed Deer in Michigan*. Dissertation. Lansing, MI: Michigan State University (2006).

46. Kaneene JB, Hattey JA, Bolin CA, Averill J, Miller R. Survivability of *Mycobacterium bovis* on salt and salt-mineral blocks fed to cattle. *Am J Vet Res*. (2017) 78:57–62. doi: 10.2460/ajvr.78.1.57

47. Grear DA, Kaneene JB, Averill JJ, Webb CT. Local cattle movements in response to ongoing bovine tuberculosis zonation and regulations in Michigan USA. *Prev Vet Med*. (2014) 114:201–12. doi: 10.1016/j.prevetmed.2014.03.008

48. Dunn C. More bovine TB in Huerfano herds. *World J*. (2010) 31.

49. Surveillance Preparedness and Response Services. *Bovine Tuberculosis and Brucellosis Surveillance Results Monthly Reports, Federal Fiscal Year (FY) 2018*. USDA (2018).

50. Carstensen M. *Managing Bovine Tuberculosis in White-Tailed Deer in Northwestern Minnesota: A 2008 Progress Report*. Minneapolis, MN (2009). Available online at: http://digitalcommons.unl.edu/michbovinetb/18/ (Accessed August 24, 2018).

51. Carstensen M, DonCarlos MW. Preventing the establishment of a wildlife disease reservoir: a case study of bovine tuberculosis in wild deer in Minnesota, USA. *Vet Med Int*. (2011) 2011:1–10. doi: 10.4061/2011/413240

52. Radunz B. Surveillance and risk management during the latter stages of eradication: experiences from Australia. *Vet Microbiol*. (2006) 112:283–90. doi: 10.1016/j.vetmic.2005.11.017

53. Cowie CE, Gortázar C, White PC, Hutchings MR, Vicente J. Stakeholder opinions on the practicality of management interventions to control bovine tuberculosis. *Vet J*. (2015) 204:179–85. doi: 10.1016/j.tvjl.2015.02.022

54. Livingstone P, Hancox N, Nugent G, de Lisle G. Toward eradication: the effect of *Mycobacterium bovis* infection in wildlife on the evolution and future direction of bovine tuberculosis management in New Zealand. *New Zealand Vet J*. (2015) 63:4–18. doi: 10.1080/00480169.2014.971082

55. More SJ, Radunz B, Glanville R. Lessons learned during the successful eradication of bovine tuberculosis from Australia. *Vet Rec*. (2015) 177:224. doi: 10.1136/vr.103163

56. O'Brien DJ, Schmitt SM, Rudolph BA, Nugent G. Recent advances in the management of bovine tuberculosis in free-ranging wildlife. *Vet Microbiol*. (2011) 151:23–33. doi: 10.1016/j.vetmic.2011.02.022

57. Butchko PH, Schmitt SM. Bovine tuberculosis in Michigan: the work on the wildlife side. *Proc Vert Pest Conf*. (2004) 2004:202–5.

58. Fritzell Jr P, Dudderar G, Peyton RB. An evaluation of farmer applications of deer damage controls. *Eastern Wildl Damag Cont Conf*. (1997) 8:108–19.

59. Dudderar GR, Haufler JB, Winterstein SR, Gunarso P. GIS: a tool for analyzing and managing deer damage to crops. *Eastern Wildl Damag Cont Conf*. (1989) 4:182–97.

60. Braun KF. *Ecological Factors Influencing White-Tailed Deer Damage to Agricultural Crops in Northern Lower Michigan*. Dissertation. Ann Arbor, MI: Michigan State University (1996).

61. Campa HIII, Winterstein S, Peyton R, Dudderar G, Leefers L. An evaluation of a multidisciplinary problem: ecological and sociological factors influencing white-tailed deer damage to agricultural crops in Michigan. *Trans North Am Wildl Nat Resour Conf*. (1997) 62:431–40.

62. O'Brien DJ, Schmitt SM, Fitzgerald SD, Berry DE, Hickling GJ. Managing the wildlife reservoir of *Mycobacterium bovis*: the Michigan, USA experience. *Vet Microbiol*. (2006) 112:313–23. doi: 10.1016/j.vetmic.2005.11.014

63. Ramsey DS, O'brien DJ, Cosgrove MK, Rudolph BA, Locher AB, Schmitt SM. Forecasting eradication of bovine tuberculosis in Michigan white-tailed deer. *J Wildl Manag*. (2014) 78:240–54. doi: 10.1002/jwmg.656

64. Tosa MI, Schauber EM, Nielsen CK. Localized removal affects white-tailed deer space use and contacts. *J Wildl Manag*. (2016) 81:26–37. doi: 10.1002/jwmg.21176

65. Giles RH *Wildlife Management Techniques*. Washington, DC: The Wildlife Society (1978).

66. Felix AB, Campa H, Millenbah KF, Winterstein SR, Moritz WE. Development of landscape-scale habitat-potential models for forest wildlife planning and management. *Wldlf Soc Bull*. (2004) 32:795–806. doi: 10.2193/0091-7648(2004)032[0795:DOLHMF]2.0.CO;2

67. Verme LJ. Swamp conifer deeryards in northern Michigan their ecology and management. *J For*. (1965) 63:523–9.

68. Byelich JD. *Management for Deer. Aspen: Symposium Proceedings*. USDA Forest Service General Technical Report NC-1. (1972). p. 120–5.

69. Alpena-Montmorency Conservation District. *Deer Habitat Improvement Program* (2018). Available online at: http://www.alpenamontcd.org/deer-habitat-improvement-program-dhip.html (Accessed August 24, 2018).

70. Leopold A. *Game Management*. New York, NY: Charles Scribner's Sons (1933).

71. Van Deelen TR, Campa H III, Hamady M, Haufler JB. Migration and seasonal range dynamics of deer using adjacent deeryards in northern Michigan. *J Wildl Manag*. (1998) 62:205–13. doi: 10.2307/3802280

72. Ruhl J. *Elk Movements and Habitat Utilization in Northern Michigan*. Thesis. Lansing, MI: Michigan State University (1985).

73. Beyer DE. *Population and Habitat Management of Elk in Michigan*. Dissertation. Lansing, MI: Michigan State University (1987).

74. Michigan GIS Open Data (2018). Available online at: https://gismichigan.opendata.arcgis.com/datasets?q=land

75. Sitar K. *Seasonal Movements, Habitat Use Patterns, and Population Dynamics of White-Tailed Deer in an Agricultural Region of Northern Lower Michigan*. Thesis. Lansing, MI: Michigan State University (1996).

76. Riley SJ, Decker DJ, Enck JW, Curtis PD, Lauber TB, Brown TL. Deer populations up, hunter populations down: implications of interdependence of deer and hunter population dynamics on management. *Ecoscience* (2003) 10:455–61. doi: 10.1080/11956860.2003.11682793

77. Frawley BJ. *Factors Affecting the Sale of Antlerless Deer Hunting Licenses in the Northeast Lower Peninsula*. Wildlife Division Report. Michigan Department of Natural Resources, Lansing, MI (2002).

78. Van Deelen TR, Etter DR. Effort and functional response of deer hunters. *Hum Dimens Wildl*. (2003) 8:97–108. doi: 10.1080/10871200304306

79. VerCauteren KC, Anderson CW, Van Deelen TR, Drake D, Walter WD, Vantassel SM, et al. Regulated commercial harvest to manage overabundant white-tailed deer: an idea to consider? *Wildl Soc Bull*. (2011) 35:185–94. doi: 10.1002/wsb.36

80. Thogmartin W. Why not consider the commercialization of deer harvests? *BioScience* (2006) 56:957. doi: 10.1641/0006-3568(2006)56[957:WNCTCO]2.0.CO;2

81. Hildreth AM, Hygnstrom SE, Hams KM, VerCauteren KC. The Nebraska deer exchange: a novel program for donating harvested deer. *Wldlf Soc Bull*. (2011) 35:195–200. doi: 10.1002/wsb.11

82. Winkler R, Warnke K. The future of hunting: an age-period-cohort analysis of deer hunter decline. *Popul Environ*. (2013) 34:460–80. doi: 10.1007/s11111-012-0172-6

83. Tack JLP, McGowan CP, Ditchkoff SS, Morse WC, Robinson OJ. Managing the vanishing North American hunter: a novel framework to address declines in hunters and hunter-generated conservation funds. *Hum Dimens Wildl*. (2018). doi: 10.1080/10871209.2018.1499155. [Epub ahead of print].

84. Frawley BJ. *Michigan Deer Harvest Survey Report 2016 Seasons*. Wildlife Report 3639. Michigan Department of Natural Resources, Lansing, MI (2017).

85. US Fish and Wildlife Service. *2011 National Survey of Fishing, Hunting, and Recreation*. USFWS: Department of Interior (2011). p. 1–56.

86. Gortázar C, Che Amat A, O'Brien DJ. Open questions and recent advances in the control of a multi-host infectious disease: animal tuberculosis. *Mammal Rev*. (2015) 45:160–75. doi: 10.1111/mam.12042

87. Nol P, Palmer MV, Waters WR, Aldwell FE, Buddle BM, Triantis JM, et al. Efficacy of oral and parenteral routes of *Mycobacterium bovis* bacille Calmette-Guerin vaccination against experimental bovine tuberculosis in white-tailed deer (*Odocoileus virginianus*): a feasibility study. *J Wildl Dis*. (2008) 44:247–59. doi: 10.7589/0090-3558-44.2.247

88. Palmer MV, Thacker TC, Waters WR, Robbe-Austerman S. Oral vaccination of white-tailed deer (*Odocoileus virginianus*) with *Mycobacterium bovis* Bacillus Calmette-Guerin (BCG). *PLoS ONE* (2014) 9:e97031. doi: 10.1371/journal.pone.0097031

89. Buddle BM, Wedlock DN, Denis M. Progress in the development of tuberculosis vaccines for cattle and wildlife. *Vet Microbiol*. (2006) 112:191–200. doi: 10.1016/j.vetmic.2005.11.027

90. Palmer MV, Thacker TC, Waters WR. Vaccination of white-tailed deer (*Odocoileus virginianus*) with *Mycobacterium bovis* bacillus Calmette Guerin. *Vaccine* (2007) 25:6589–97. doi: 10.1016/j.vaccine.2007.06.056

91. Nol P, Lyashchenko KP, Greenwald R, Esfandiari J, Waters WR, Palmer MV, et al. Humoral immune responses of white-tailed deer (*Odocoileus virginianus*) to *Mycobacterium bovis* BCG vaccination and experimental challenge with *M. bovis*. *Clin Vaccine Immunol*. (2009) 16:323–9. doi: 10.1128/CVI.00392-08

92. Palmer MV, Thacker TC, Waters WR. Vaccination with *Mycobacterium bovis* BCG strains Danish and Pasteur in white-tailed deer (*Odocoileus virginianus*)

experimentally challenged with *Mycobacterium bovis*. *Zoonoses Public Hlth.* (2009) 56:243–51. doi: 10.1111/j.1863-2378.2008.01198.x

93. Cosgrove MK, Campa H, Schmitt SM, Marks DR, Wilson AS, O'Brien DJ. Live-trapping and bovine tuberculosis testing of free-ranging white-tailed deer for targeted removal. *Wildl Res.* (2012) 39:104. doi: 10.1071/WR11147

94. Ellis CK, Stahl RS, Nol P, Waters WR, Palmer MV, Rhyan JC, et al. A pilot study exploring the use of breath analysis to differentiate healthy cattle from cattle experimentally infected with *Mycobacterium bovis*. *PLoS ONE* (2014) 9:e89280. doi: 10.1371/journal.pone.0089280

95. Cosgrove MK, Campa H, Ramsey DSL, Schmitt SM, O'Brien DJ. Modeling vaccination and targeted removal of white-tailed deer in Michigan for bovine tuberculosis control. *Wildl Soc Bull.* (2012) 36:676–84. doi: 10.1002/wsb.217

96. Wanzala SI, Palmer MV, Waters WR, Thacker TC, Carstensen M, Travis DA, et al. Evaluation of pathogen-specific biomarkers for the diagnosis of tuberculosis in white-tailed deer (*Odocoileus virginianus*). *Am J Vet Res.* (2017) 78:729–34. doi: 10.2460/ajvr.78.6.729

97. Glaser L, Carstensen M, Shaw S, Robbe-Austerman S, Wunschmann A, Grear D, et al. Descriptive epidemiology and whole genome sequencing analysis for an outbreak of bovine tuberculosis in beef cattle and white-tailed deer in northwestern Minnesota. *PLoS ONE* (2016) 11:e0145735. doi: 10.1371/journal.pone.0145735

98. Muter BA, Gore ML, Riley SJ, Lapinski MK. Evaluating bovine tuberculosis risk communication materials in Michigan and Minnesota for severity, susceptibility, and efficacy messages. *Wldlf Soc Bull.* (2013) 37:115–21. doi: 10.1002/wsb.238

99. Triezenberg HA, Gore ML, Riley SJ, Lapinski MK. Perceived risks from disease and management policies: an expansion and testing of a zoonotic disease risk perception model. *Hum Dimens Wildl.* (2014) 19:123–38. doi: 10.1080/10871209.2014.844288

100. Triezenberg HA, Gore ML, Riley SJ, Lapinski MK. Persuasive communication aimed at achieving wildlife-disease management goals. *Wldlf Soc Bull.* (2014) 38:734–40. doi: 10.1002/wsb.462

101. Triezenberg HA, Riley SJ, Gore ML. A test of communication in changing harvest behaviors of deer hunters. *J Wldlf Manag.* (2016) 80:941–6. doi: 10.1002/jwmg.21078

102. Smith CA. The role of state wildlife professionals under the public trust doctrine. *J Wildl Manag.* (2011) 75:1539–43. doi: 10.1002/jwmg.202

103. Michigan Department of Natural Resources. *A Review of Deer Management in Michigan* (2016). Available online at: https://www.michigan.gov/documents/dnr/mi_deer_management_plan_547265_7.pdf (Accessed August 27, 2018).

104. Rudolph BA, Riley SJ. Factors affecting hunters' trust and cooperation. *Hum Dimens Wildl.* (2014) 19:469–79. doi: 10.1080/10871209.2014.939314

105. Holsman RH. Goodwill hunting. Exploring the role of hunters as ecosystem stewards. *Wildl Soc Bull.* (2000) 28:808–16.

106. Dorn ML. *Bovine Tuberculosis in Michigan: Understanding Stakeholder Attitudes Towards the Disease and Eradication Efforts*. Thesis. Lansing, MI: Michigan State University (2003).

107. de Lisle GW, Bengis RG, Schmitt SM, O'Brien DJ. Tuberculosis in free-ranging wildlife: detection, diagnosis and management. *Rev Sci Tech Off Int Epiz.* (2002) 21:317–34. doi: 10.20506/rst.21.2.1339

108. Carstensen M, O'Brien DJ, Schmitt SM. Public acceptance as a determinant of management strategies for bovine tuberculosis in free-ranging U.S. wildlife. *Vet Microbiol.* (2011) 151:200–4. doi: 10.1016/j.vetmic.2011.02.046

109. Wobeser GA. *Investigation and Management of Disease in Wild Animals*. Berlin: Springer Science & Business Media (2013).

110. Olmstead AL, Rhode PW. An impossible undertaking: the eradication of bovine tuberculosis in the United States. *J Econ Hist.* (2004) 64:734–72. doi: 10.1017/S0022050704002955

111. Ramsey DS, O'Brien DJ, Smith RW, Cosgrove MK, Schmitt SM, Rudolph BA. Management of on-farm risk to livestock from bovine tuberculosis in Michigan, USA, white-tailed deer: predictions from a spatially-explicit stochastic model. *Prev Vet Med.* (2016) 134:26–38. doi: 10.1016/j.prevetmed.2016.09.022

112. Amass SF, Clark LK. Biosecurity considerations for pork production units. *J Swine Health Prod.* (1999) 7:217–28.

113. Moore DA, Merryman ML, Hartman ML, Klingborg DJ. Comparison of published recommendations regarding biosecurity practices for various production animal species and classes. *J Am Vet Med Assoc.* (2008) 233:249–56. doi: 10.2460/javma.233.2.249

114. Leopold A. *A Sand County Almanac*. New York, NY: Oxford University Press (1949).

Validation of a Real-Time PCR for the Detection of *Mycobacterium tuberculosis* Complex Members in Bovine Tissue Samples

Victor Lorente-Leal[1,2], Emmanouil Liandris[1], Elena Castellanos[3], Javier Bezos[1,2], Lucas Domínguez[1,2], Lucía de Juan[1,2] and Beatriz Romero[1*]

[1] VISAVET Health Surveillance Center, Complutense University of Madrid, Madrid, Spain, [2] Animal Health Department, Veterinary Faculty, Complutense University of Madrid, Madrid, Spain, [3] Exosome Diagnostics Inc., Waltham, MA, United States

Correspondence:
Beatriz Romero
bromerom@visavet.ucm.es

Although the post-mortem diagnosis of bovine tuberculosis is mainly achieved through microbiological culture, the development of other techniques to detect *Mycobacterium tuberculosis* complex (MTBC) members directly from tissue samples has been pursued. The present study describes the development, optimization and validation of a Real-Time PCR based on the *mpb70* gene to detect MTBC members in clinical tissue samples from cattle. Specific primers and a hybridization probe were used to amplify MTBC-specific sequences in order to avoid cross-reaction with non-MTBC species. An Internal Amplification Control (IAC) was included in order to assess the presence of PCR inhibitors in the samples. The PCR was optimized to achieve maximum efficiency, and the limit of detection, limit of quantification and dynamic range of the reaction were determined. The specificity of the reaction was tested against 34 mycobacterial and non-mycobacterial species. The diagnostic sensitivity, specificity and positive and negative predictive values (PPV and NPV) of the method were assessed on 200 bovine tissue samples in relation to bacteriological culture. The dynamic range of the reaction spanned from 5 ng/reaction (10^6 genome equivalents) to 50 fg/reaction (10 genome equivalents). The efficiency of the reaction was 102.6% and the achieved R^2 was 0.999. The limit of detection with 95% confidence was 10 genome equivalents/reaction. No cross-reactions with non-MTBC species were observed. The diagnostic sensitivity and specificity values of the *mpb70* specific Real-Time PCR respect to culture were 94.59% (95% CI: 86.73–98.51%) and 96.03% (95% CI: 90.98–98.70%), respectively, with a PPV of 93.33% (95% CI: 85.55–97.07%) and a NPV of 96.80% (95% CI: 92.10–98.74%). The concordance of the Real-Time PCR based on *mpb70* is comparable to that of culture (K = 0.904) showing a great potential for the detection of members of the MTBC in animal tissues.

Keywords: real-time PCR, *Mycobacterium tuberculosis* complex, tuberculosis, detection, bovine tissue

INTRODUCTION

Bovine tuberculosis (bTB) is a chronic infectious disease caused by members of the *Mycobacterium tuberculosis* complex (MTBC), which affects certain species of mammals including cattle (1). Within this group of bacteria, *M. bovis* followed by *M. caprae* are the most frequent species in bovines. Due to its zoonotic potential and to the economic importance of cattle in the EU, this disease is subject to well-established national eradication campaigns in Member States. According to the legislation in force, i.e., 64/432/ECC, the intradermal tuberculin test is the official test in order to classify TB free herds, areas or countries, and microbiological culture is the method of confirmation of MTBC infections in bovine tissues.

The reported recovery rates for culture in general oscillate between 30 and 95% (2–5) while in a recent study using a Bayesian approach, the diagnostic sensitivity and specificity of culture was 78.1 and 99.1%, respectively (6). This variation between studies can be explained by different factors associated with the technique and the samples, which can affect the performance of the method. Firstly, the choice of tissue samples at the abattoir is a key for culture. Abnormal lymph nodes and parenchymatous organs with bTB-compatible lesions must always be included when present. If pathological lesions are not detected then, specific lymph nodes (retropharyngeal, bronchial, mediastinal, supramammary, mandibular, and mesenteric) should be taken for examination and culture. Secondly, the preservation of samples until culture by refrigeration or freezing, together with the step of chemical decontamination, is mandatory in order to decrease the risk of contamination with other microorganisms. Inadequate storage and sample treatment influence the viability of MTBC and can promote the growth of contaminating microorganisms (2). Thirdly, the type of culture media chosen to grow mycobacteria may influence the recovery rate of microbiological culture. MTBC growth can be detected either by colony formation in agar and egg-based solid media (such as Middlebrook 7H10/7H11, Stonebrink or Löwenstein-Jensen with sodium pyruvate), or fluorescence or pressure differences in liquid media (BACTEC 460 TB and MGIT 960 and VersaTREK system). In studies comparing both culture systems, the recovery rates for liquid media are higher than those reported for solid media with values of 80 to 95% and 65 to 82%, respectively (3, 5). The highest recovery rates within liquid systems are recorded for the BACTEC 460 TB system, which is no longer commercially available. In addition, there is a suspected decrease in selectivity of the MGIT 960, which in turn makes liquid media more prone to overgrowth by rapidly growing microorganisms (4, 5). Members of the MTBC are grouped within the slow growing mycobacteria due to their slow replication cycle. As a result, culture detection of MTBC is extremely slow; around 28 days for liquid media and 43 days for solid media for a positive result (2, 3).

In order to overcome the problems associated with the recovery of MTBC by culture, detection of mycobacterial DNA from animal tissue samples using PCR is being considered as an alternative or complementary test to microbiological culture. Since the early 90's, many conventional PCRs have been developed and used for the direct detection of members of the MTBC in bovine samples (7). In those studies including fresh bovine tissue samples from animals with visible and non-visible lesions (VL and NVL), the reported sensitivity and specificity values of PCR with respect to culture showed great variability, ranging from 63 to 97%, and 50 to 97%, respectively (8–10). After the introduction of Real-Time PCR for the detection of MTBC species, sensitivity values increased with respect to conventional PCR. In those studies implementing Real-Time PCR in which bovine tissue samples with VL and NVL were analyzed, diagnostic sensitivity and specificity by Real-Time PCR ranged between 74 to 100% and 97 to 100%, respectively (6, 11–14). The variability in the values between studies depends not only on the type of PCR (conventional, nested or Real-Time PCR), but also on the PCR target (single- or multiple copy) and reagents, the type and number of samples included in the studies, and the DNA isolation methods. The largest study to date assessing the diagnostic performance of Real-Time PCR for the detection of MTBC using a Bayesian approach reported a diagnostic sensitivity of 87.7% and a specificity of 97% (6).

In this study, we describe the development and validation of a Real-Time PCR based on the *mpb70* gene, which encodes for a major antigenic protein conserved in all MTBC species. In addition, we assess its diagnostic performance in fresh bovine tissue samples obtained within the Spanish national eradication campaign.

MATERIALS AND METHODS

Real-Time PCR

PCR Design and Optimization

The *mpb70* gene was the target of this PCR since it encodes for a majorly expressed antigenic protein in *M. bovis*, which is conserved in all members of the MTBC. An *in silico* specificity analysis was carried out, in order to rule out any sequence homologies between other bacterial species, with the Basic Local Alignment Tool (BLAST) from the NCBI, using the *mpb70* CDS from *M. bovis* AF2122/97 (NC_002945.4). The *mpb70* sequence was then used to obtain *mpb70* homologs from the available MTBC genomic sequences deposited in the genbank (NCBI): *M. tuberculosis* H37Rv (NC_000962.3), *M. africanum* strain 25 (CP010334.1), *M. caprae* Allgeau (CP016401.1), *M. microti* strain 12 (CP010333.1), *M. mungi* strain BM22813 (LXTB01000090.1), *M. orygis* strain 112400015 (APKD01000057.1) and *M. canetti* CIPT 140010059 (NC_015848.1).

Oligonucleotides targeting the *mpb70* gene, specific for members of the MTBC, were designed to target a 133bp conserved amplicon with Oligo primer analysis software 6.0 (Molecular Insights, West Cascade, CO, USA): *mpb70*-forward: 5′-CTCAATCCGCAAGTAAACC-3′, *mpb70*-reverse: 5′-TCAGCAGTGACGAATTGG-3′ (15), and *mpb70*-probe: 5′- FAM-CTCAACAGCGGTCAGTACACGGT-BHQ1-3′. The amplicon sequences were obtained and aligned against the available MTBC sequences, as well as with the closest similarities obtained in the *in silico* specificity analysis (e.g., *M. kansasii*, *M. indicus pranii*, or *M. marinum*).

The Real-Time PCRs were carried out using the QuantiFast® Pathogen PCR + IC Kit (QIAGEN, Hilden, Germany). This kit includes an Internal Amplification Control (IAC), as well as specific reagents and primers/probes required for its amplification. It employs MAX™NHS Ester as a reporter dye. Different primer/probe concentrations and extension temperatures were tested in order to achieve maximum replication efficiency.

M. tuberculosis H37Rv DNA was used for the generation of the standard curve and positive controls. Ultra-pure distilled water was used as negative controls. This strain was grown in Löwenstein-Jensen slants in the BSL3 facilities at VISAVET Health Surveillance Center. A loop full of colonies was collected and heat inactivated (100°C) in 200 µl of ultra-pure distilled water during 15 min.

The efficiency and dynamic range of the reaction were assessed in triplicates using a standard curve prepared from a stock of 10 ng/µl of *M. tuberculosis* H37Rv genomic DNA, 10-fold serially diluted to a range of 1 ng/µl to 0.1 fg/µl. DNA concentration and quality of the DNA solution were measured in ten replicates using a nano-drop spectrophotometer (ThermoFisher, Waltham, MA, USA). The dynamic range of the reaction was established as the range of standard curve concentrations at which the coefficient of linearity was >0.997 and the cycle separation between the 10-fold dilutions was close or equal to 3.32 cycles. The limit of quantification was established as the lowest concentration point of the dynamic range of the reaction.

The optimized setup with a final 25 µl volume per reaction, including the Internal Amplification Control (IAC) was: 5 µl of 5x Quantifast Pathogen Master Mix, 2.5 µl of 10x IAC assay, 2.5 µl of 10x Internal Control DNA, 2 µl of 10 pmol/µl *mpb70*-Forward primer, 2 µl of 10 pmol/µl *mpb70*-Reverse primer, 0.75 µl of 10 pmol/µl *mpb70*-probe, 5.25 µl of ultrapure sterile distilled water (Sigma-Aldrich, St. Louis, MO, USA), and 5 µl of DNA sample. Primers and probe were obtained from Eurofins Genomics (Ebersberg, Germany).

All PCR reactions were carried out in a CFX96 Touch™ Real-Time PCR Detection System (Bio-Rad, Hercules, CA, USA) according to the following optimized cycling conditions; 95°C for 5 min followed by 45 2-step cycles of 95°C for 15 s and 60°C for 30 s, with data acquisition at this step.

Analytical Specificity and Sensitivity

The inclusivity of the PCR was tested against seven species of the *M. tuberculosis* complex: *M. tuberculosis*, *M. africanum*, *M. bovis*, *M. bovis* BCG, *M. caprae*, *M. microti*, and *M. pinnipedii*. Selectivity was assessed using a panel of 69 strains from 24 Non-Tuberculous Mycobacteria (NTM) species and 10 non-mycobacterial species (OM: Other Microorganisms); *M. avium* subsp. *hominissuis* ($n = 7$), *M. avium* subsp. *avium* ($n = 3$), *M. avium* group X ($n = 10$), *M. chitae*, *M. colombiense*, *M. europeum*, *M. flavescens*, *M. fortuitum* ($n = 3$), *M. gordonae*, *M. hibernae*, *M. intracellulare*, *M. kansasii* ($n = 9$), *M. marinum* ($n = 2$), *M. neoaurum*, *M. nonchromogenicum* ($n = 4$), *M. parascrofulaceum*, *M. peregrinum* ($n = 2$), *M. phlei* ($n = 2$), *M. scrofulaceum*, *M. seoulense*, *M. shimodei*, *M. smegmatis* ($n = 2$), *M. terrae*, *M. thermoresistible*,

M. vaccae, *Brucella mellitensis*, *Brucella abortus*, *Salmonella enterica* Sv. Typhimurium, *Serratia maucencens*, *Rhodococcus equi*, *Enterococcus hirae*, *Lysteria monocytogenes*, *Nocardia* sp., *Streptomyces* sp., and *Corynebacterium pseudotuberculosis*. DNA for these bacteria was obtained from reference strains and clinical isolates from the VISAVET Health Surveillance Center (Complutense University of Madrid).

The analytical sensitivity or limit of detection (LOD) and intra-assay repeatability were estimated using a new standard curve that was prepared from a 10-fold serially diluted stock of *M. tuberculosis* H37Rv genomic DNA ranging from 1 ng/µl to 10 fg/µl, and one 1:5 dilution thereof to a concentration of 2 fg/µl (10 fg/reaction or 2 genomic equivalents). The reaction was carried out using 20 replicates per concentration and the LOD was established as the concentration in which at least 95% of the replicates were positive. Inter-assay repeatability was assessed in 20 replicates of 10 fg/µl *M. tuberculosis* DNA in a period of 6 months.

M. tuberculosis H37Rv genomic equivalents were obtained from the amount of DNA used for each point of the standard curve using the equation previously described (16): [ng of DNA × $6.023 × 10^{23}$ molecules/mol]/[bp length of genome × 10^9 ng/g × 660 g/mol]. The genome size recorded at the NCBI Genome entry of *M. tuberculosis* H37Rv (NC_000962.3) was used as a reference (i.e., 4.41 Mb). Genomic equivalents for each sample were obtained by extrapolating the Ct values with the quantities from the standard curve.

Selection, Preparation and Culture of Clinical Samples

Two-hundred fresh tissue samples from cattle were randomly selected from samples processed as part of the Spanish national eradication campaign against bTB during the period 2013–2017, based on the Royal Decree 727/2011. Processing took place within the BSL3 facilities of VISAVET Health Surveillance Center. Simple randomization was carried out by assigning a random value to each sample and by sorting them by increasing order. The first 200 samples of this list were included in the study. The selected tissue samples originated from 11 out of the 17 autonomic regions of Spain. Almost half ($n = 99$) of the samples were obtained from Madrid, followed by Castile-La Mancha ($n = 34$), Aragon ($n = 18$), Extremadura ($n = 13$), Valencia ($n = 12$), Murcia ($n = 8$), La Rioja ($n = 6$), Andalusia ($n = 3$), Canary Islands ($n = 3$), Balearic Islands ($n = 3$), and Castile and Leon ($n = 1$).

From the total amount of samples, 118 came from cattle that were positive to the single intradermal tuberculin (SIT) test (bovine PPD ≥ 4 mm), whereas 63 were from SIT-negative animals (bovine PPD ≤ 2 mm) and 4 had inconclusive results (2 mm > bovine PPD < 4 mm) according to the Royal Decree 727/2011. Following the regulation in force, in regions with high prevalence of bTB, SIT inconclusive results were considered as positive. Fifteen animals showed bTB-compatible lesions during routine abattoir inspection of carcasses and were also sent for sample collection and processing. Lymph nodes (retropharyngeal, mandibular, mediastinal, bronchial, prescapular, mesenteric, hepatic, and/or supramammary) and/or organs were then collected for processing, culture and direct PCR.

Once in the laboratory, all tissue samples were visually inspected for lesions and sliced. A total of 78 samples had VL, whereas 122 had NVL. Approximately 2–2.5 g of tissue sample from the same animal were pooled and homogenized in 12 ml sterile distilled water in a Masticator (IUL, Barcelona, Spain) at max speed for up to 5 min. One ml of the homogenized sample was collected for DNA isolation, whereas the remainder of the homogenate was decontaminated with an equal volume of 0.75% (w/v) hexadecyl pyridinium chloride solution in agitation during 30 min (17). Samples were centrifuged during 30 min at 1,300–1,500 g. Pellets were collected with swabs and cultured in Löwenstein-Jensen with sodium pyruvate and Coletsos media (Difco, Spain) at 37°C for a maximum of 3 months. Culture was considered positive when isolates were identified as MTBC by conventional PCR (18) and /or DVR-spoligotyping (19).

Tissue DNA Extraction

DNA from tissues was obtained using the DNeasy Blood & Tissue Kit (QIAGEN) with a few modifications. Briefly, one ml of the homogenized tissue sample was added in a tube containing 100 mg of 0.5 mm and 50 mg of 0.1 mm glass beads and centrifuged for 5 min at 9,000 g. The supernatant was removed from the samples and 200 μl of sterile distilled water and 180 μl of ATL Buffer were added. Samples were then lysed in a Fastprep® FP120 homogenizer (MP Biomedicals, Santa Ana, CA, USA) using 3 cycles of 40 s at a speed of 6.5 m/sec. After an overnight chemical treatment with 20 μl of proteinase K at 56°C, the mechanical lysis step was repeated. Samples were then centrifuged briefly at maximum speed and 300 μl of supernatant were transferred to a new 1.5 ml Eppendorf tube and mixed with 400 μl of a mixture of AL buffer and 96% ethanol (equal volumes). The lysate was transferred to a spin column and was processed according to the manufacturer's instructions. DNA elution was carried out using 200 μl of AE buffer.

Diagnostic Performance

The diagnostic performance of the Real-Time PCR targeting the *mpb70* gene was assessed on 200 randomly selected tissue-extracted DNA samples. The exogenous heterologous IAC supplied with the kit was used to assess the presence or absence of inhibition phenomena. According to the manufacturer, the IAC should show Ct values of 30 ± 3. As a result, complete inhibition was defined when no IAC was amplified and partial inhibition was defined as a Ct > 33 for the IAC. If inhibition was detected, samples were diluted 5-fold and PCR was repeated. Results were compared against microbiological culture, and diagnostic sensitivity and specificity, Positive and Negative Predictive Values (PPV/NPVs) as well as Positive and Negative Likelihood Ratios (PLR and NLRs) were calculated using MedCalc 18.2.1 (MedCalc, Ostend, Belgium). Agreement between culture and Real-Time PCR results was assessed using Cohen's Unweighted Kappa in WinEpi 2.0 (20).

Samples with culture-negative and PCR-positive results were further analyzed by DVR-spoligotyping (detection of spacers) and sequencing of the 16S rRNA gene. Sequencing of a 1,030 bp fragment of the 16S rRNA gene (18) was carried out externally by STABvida (Lisbon, Portugal). The obtained sequences were analyzed using the Bioedit software version 7.1.3.0 (21). Samples that gave a positive result to either of the above two techniques were considered as true positives and were used to re-calculate the diagnostic performance of the Real-Time PCR. On the other hand, for samples with a culture-positive and PCR-negative results DNA extraction and PCR were repeated.

RESULTS

In silico Analysis

Sequence similarity between *mpb70* homologs in members of the MTBC is 99.7–99.8% (data not shown). Even though some non-MTBC species -such as *M. kansasii*, *M. marinum* or *M. gilvum*- have homologous *mpt70/mpb70* sequences (22), sequence similarity with these species is limited (data not shown). Alignments of the *mpb70* amplicons with MTBC species showed 100% identity, with exception of *M. canetti* that had a T/C substitution at position 360 (*M. bovis* AF2122/97 numbering from *mpb70* CDS start). Although this substitution falls within the length of the reverse primer, it did not affect the ability of the primer to anneal to its target in *M. canetti*. *M. indicus pranii*, *M. kansasii* and *M. marinum,* had a considerably lower identity, indicating that specificity issues would be unlikely (data not shown).

Optimization and Analytical Sensitivity and Specificity

For optimization of the PCR reaction and repeatability studies, two 10-fold diluted standard curves were prepared from a 10ng/μl stock of *M. tuberculosis* H37Rv (DNA stock concentrations with Standard Deviations or SDs of 0.35 and 0.97, respectively).

The lowest concentration of DNA detected in the standard curve by the Real-Time PCR was 10 fg/μl (50 fg/reaction or $\sim$ 10 genomic equivalents) with all three replicates showing an amplification curve. The dynamic range of the reaction spanned from 1 ng/μl (5 ng/reaction or approx. 10^6 genome equivalents) to 10 fg/μl (50 fg/reaction or $\sim$ 10 genome equivalents), with an R^2 of 0.999. The upper and lower Ct values of the dynamic range were 20.06 and 36.33, respectively. The quantification limit was set to 10 genome equivalents/ reaction. Replication efficiency was 102.60% with a slope of −3.27.

All 20 replicates with a concentration of 50 fg/reaction were positive for this PCR, whereas only 14/20 of the 10 fg/reaction aliquots were positive. The Ct values of both dilutions were, respectively, 37.07 (SD 0.98) and 38.92 (SD 1.28). Therefore, the limit of detection for this Real-Time PCR with a 95% confidence was 10 fg/μl (50 fg/reaction or 10 genomic equivalents) and the cut-off was set to a Ct < 40.

The Real-Time PCR reacted positively only against members of the MTBC and no cross-reactions were detected against any of the NTMs or non-mycobacterial species tested.

Diagnostic Performance Compared to Microbiological Culture

Two hundred DNA samples obtained from bovine tissues were analyzed using this PCR and microbiological culture. A total of 69 samples were MTBC positive for culture, whereas 131 were negative (**Table 1**). Ten out of the 131 culture-negative samples showed growth of non-tuberculous mycobacteria ($n = 4$) or other microorganisms ($n = 6$) (NTM/OM). The Real-Time PCR detected 71 positive samples, with a minimum and maximum Ct values of 24.39 and 39.35, respectively and a median Ct value of 33.48. Sixty-one out of 69 positive culture samples were also positive for the Real-Time PCR targeting *mpb70*, resulting in a sensitivity relative to culture of 88.41% (95% CI: 74.3 to 94.86%). Ten of the 131 culture-negative samples were positive for the Real-Time PCR, and the specificity value was 92.37% (95% CI: 86.41 to 96.28%). Of the 10 cultures showing growth of NTM/OM, one reacted positively to the direct Real-Time PCR.

The exogenous heterologous IAC used in this PCR detected complete inhibition in only 4 out of 200 samples (2%) and partial inhibition (IAC Ct > 33) in 15 out of 200 samples (7.5%). After dilution, all these samples were PCR negative. One of the completely inhibited samples and 3 of the partially inhibited samples were positive to culture.

PPVs and NPVs were 85.92% (95% CI: 76.97 to 91.76%) and 93.80% (95% CI: 88.72 to 96.67%), respectively. The positive and negative likelihood ratios were, respectively, 11.58 (95% CI: 6.34–21.14) and 0.13 (95% CI: 0.07–0.24). There was a very good correlation between culture and PCR results (Cohen's Unweighted Kappa = 0.802).

Samples with discording results between the two methods used were further analyzed. DNA isolation was repeated for the 8 culture-positive PCR-negative samples. Of these, half ($n = 4$) gave a positive result. For samples with culture-negative and PCR-positive results ($n = 10$), spoligotyping and 16S RNA sequencing were applied and the presence of MTBC DNA was confirmed in 5 of them. Of these, one presented growth by an actinomycete and 4 were negative to culture. These samples, in addition to all culture-positives, were considered to be true positives. As a result, the corrected relative sensitivity and specificity of PCR was calculated to be 94.59% (95% CI: 86.73% to 98.51%) and 96.03% (95% CI: 90.98–98.70%), respectively (**Table 1**). PPVs and NPVs were, then, 93.33% (95% CI: 85.55–97.07%) and 96.80 % (95% CI: 92.10–98.74%). PLRs and NLRs increased to 23.84 (95% CI: 10.08–56.37) and 0.06 (95% CI: 0.02–0.15), respectively. Correlation between culture and PCR increased to 0.904.

Among samples with VL ($n = 78$), 65 and 61 were positive to PCR and culture, respectively (**Table 2**). Three out of 7 culture-negative and PCR-positive samples were shown to contain MTBC DNA by sequencing or spoligotyping. Although 3 culture-positive samples were negative for this PCR, they became positive after the extraction protocol was repeated. Regarding NVL samples (n=122), a total of 6 samples were positive to PCR whereas 116 were found to be negative. In contrast, 8 NVL samples were culture-positive and 114 samples were culture-negative. Of these culture-negative samples, 3 were positive for the Real-Time PCR, of which 2 were confirmed as true positives by sequencing or spoligotyping. On the other hand, 5 culture-positive samples were negative for the *mpb70*-specific PCR. However, one of them was positive after the repetition of the extraction protocol. After confirmation of the true positives, Cohen's Unweighted Kappa between culture and PCR for VL and NVL samples was, respectively, 0.804 and 0.685.

Intra and Inter-Assay Variation

The intra-assay repeatability at a concentration of 10 fg/μl showed an average Ct value of 37.07 with a standard deviation of 0.98 and a coefficient of variation of 2.63%. Inter-assay repeatability using 20 replicates from a stock of 10 fg/μl in a 6 month period showed an average Ct value of 36.70 with a SD of 1.40 and a CV of 3.82%.

DISCUSSION

The purpose of this study was the design, optimization, and validation of the *mpb70* Real-Time PCR for the detection of members of the *M. tuberculosis* complex directly from animal tissue samples. In addition, this study compared the diagnostic performance of this PCR and bacteriological culture using a large number of bovine tissue samples ($n = 200$) collected in the framework of the Spanish bTB eradication program.

The Real-Time PCR targeting the *mpb70* gene showed 100% of inclusivity and selectivity. Moreover, it shows good replication efficiency (102.6%), and an analytical sensitivity of at least 10 genome equivalents with 95% confidence. Furthermore, very little variation was seen at the LOD both within and between assays (CV=2.63 and 3.82%, respectively). In addition, the linear range of the reaction spans from 5 ng/reaction (approximately 10^6 genomic equivalents) to 50 fg/reaction (~ 10 genomic equivalents). Although this PCR was developed for the detection of MTBC, the single-copy nature of the target and the wide linear range of the reaction make this PCR a suitable candidate for absolute quantification studies of MTBC in tissues. In fact, 59 out of the 71 *mpb70* PCR-positive samples showed a Ct value within the dynamic range of the reaction (data not shown). Although the quantification was not possible due to the absence of the standard curve in all runs, the range of concentrations was estimated to be between 2.29×10^5 and 63 genomic equivalents, with an average Ct value of 33.33 (~ 415 genome equivalents).

Overall, there was a good correlation between microbiological culture and PCR results in this study. Furthermore, diagnostic sensitivity and specificity values were very good when compared to microbiological culture (88.41 and 92.37%, respectively). Eight samples were negative to the direct Real-Time PCR but positive to microbiological culture. After repetition of the DNA extraction protocol, half of them became positive to the PCR. This implies that the DNA extraction protocol is very important and directly affects the sensitivity of the PCR. Several factors influence the DNA yield and quality obtained through DNA extraction protocols.

TABLE 1 | Comparison of results obtained by analyzing 200 randomly selected cattle samples by microbiological culture and Real-Time PCR.

		Culture/True positives*				Diagnostic performance	
		Result	+	−	Total	Sensitivity	Specificity
Raw results	PCR	+	61	10	71	88.41% [95% CI: 78.43–94.86%]	92.37% [95% CI: 86.41–96.28%]
		−	8	121	129		
		Total	69	131	200		
Corrected results	PCR	+	70	5	75	94.59% [95% CI: 86.73% to 98.51%]	96.03% [95% CI: 90.98–98.70%]
		−	4	121	125		
		Total	74	126	200		

*Corrected results consider as true positives: (1) those samples that were culture positive, (2) samples that were culture-negative but PCR-positive, and for which MTBC presence was demonstrated by 16S sequencing and/or spoligotyping, and (3) culture-positive and PCR-negative samples that became positive after the DNA extraction was repeated.

TABLE 2 | Comparison of results obtained by analyzing 200 randomly selected veterinary samples by microbiological culture and Real-Time PCR, according to the presence or absence of anatomic lesions.

		Culture (True positives)		
		+	−	Total
VL	PCR +	58 (64)	7 (4)	65 (68)
	PCR −	3 (0)	10	10
	Total	61 (64)	17 (14)	78
NVL	PCR +	3 (6)	3 (1)	6 (7)
	PCR −	5 (4)	111	116 (115)
	Total	8 (10)	114 (112)	122

Culture negative and PCR-positive samples were considered true positives (in brackets) after the confirmation of the presence of MTBC DNA by 16S rRNA gene sequencing and/or spoligotyping.

Firstly, the amount and type of processed tissue could determine the bacterial load in the sample. The extraction protocol used in this study uses a volume of sample that is 1/10 the amount of sample used for microbiological culture, which could produce a loss of sensitivity due to the decreasing amount of bacteria available for extraction. In addition, the presence or absence of lesions can affect the amount of bacteria in the sample which in turn could determine the quantity of available DNA. In this study, the four remaining culture-positive and PCR-negative samples had NVLs, of which 3 were positive to the SIT test. This suggests that the animal may have been at early stages of infection and, therefore, have low bacterial loads. On the other hand, the recovered samples after the second extraction ($n = 4$) had mostly VLs ($n = 3$).

Secondly, the type of disruption technique used can have an important effect in the DNA extraction process. Even though the protocol in this study has been optimized to obtain a high amount of DNA through two mechanical and one overnight chemical lysis steps, improvements in the extraction protocol may reduce the number of discording results. Park et al. showed that increasing the incubation time before mechanical lysis with

ATL buffer up to 3 h increased the DNA yield in *M. avium* subsp. *paratuberculosis* when compared to no pre-treatment (23). On the other hand, an 8-h pre-treatment was detrimental to the amount of extracted DNA, achieving the same amount of DNA as the no pretreatment controls. The effect of reduction in the pre-treatment incubation time should be assessed in the future. Another improvement could include the use of a homogenizer instead of a masticator in the tissue homogenization step, which could release a larger amount of bacteria from tissue samples for extraction.

Furthermore, several factors associated with the extraction protocol may introduce inhibitors in the sample, such as organic compounds or excess host DNA. In order to detect the inhibition of the PCR, the reaction mix includes an exogenous heterologous IAC, with a randomly generated DNA supplied by the manufacturer. By using the IAC, 4 and 15 samples were found to be completely or partially inhibited, respectively. Of these, 1 inhibited and 3 partially inhibited samples were culture-positive, and they remained PCR-negative after a 1:5 dilution. After repeating the extraction protocol on these samples, the inhibited and one partially-inhibited sample became positive, indicating that their dilution may have caused the further dilution of the target DNA and, therefore, may have resulted in the loss of sensitivity in the PCR. Furthermore, this could imply that the inhibitor was not present in the sample and was introduced as a result of the DNA extraction procedure, or that the extraction protocol failed to remove it in the first place. Other reported PCRs also include IACs, but only a few include information regarding the presence or absence of inhibition (11–13). Although no cases of inhibition were detected in these publications, they used endogenous or exogenous homologous IACs, which may present some disadvantages with respect to exogenous heterologous IACs. For instance, the amount of endogenous IAC template (i.e., bovine β-actin gene) varies depending on the type of sample or extraction method used, which means that readouts vary between samples and there is no indication of the level of inhibition present in the sample. In addition, they can overcome inhibitory effects in the sample as they are usually in higher concentrations than the target. Exogenous homologous IAC (i.e., *M. bovis* DNA), on the other hand, are recognized by the target's primers and can, therefore, give rise to competition events that can hinder the amplification of the target DNA in low-concentrated samples, such as those close to the LOD. Exogenous heterologous IACs, such as the ones used in this study, use a consistent amount of control template, different to the target of interest, with a set amplification cycle. As a result, it allows the detection of complete or partial inhibition phenomena and minimizes competition, since the primers and the control target sequence are completely different to those of the target of interest.

Ten samples were negative to culture but positive to the Real-Time PCR. The use of spoligotyping and/or 16S rRNA sequencing on these discording samples showed the presence of MTBC DNA in 5 of them. The inability of culture to detect MTBC in these samples may be due to sample processing issues in which bacterial integrity is hampered and growth is impeded. In addition, very advanced granulomatous lesions may contain lower numbers of viable bacteria than early granulomas (24). Nevertheless, MTBC DNA can still be present in non-viable bacteria in enough quantity to be detected by PCR after purification. Although no histopathological evaluation was done on these samples, 7 of the culture-negative and PCR-positive samples were obtained from animals with VLs whereas 3 were obtained from animals with NVLs. Finally, growth of NTM/OM could be another reason for these discrepancies. In fact, 1 of the 10 tissue samples that showed growth of NTM/OM during culture was positive to this PCR, indicating that the growth of MTBC in culture could have been hampered by the growth of other NTM/OM. The detection of MTBC DNA in this sample by 16S rRNA sequencing and spoligotyping supported the analytical specificity of the *mpb70* oligonucleotides, indicating that the presence of other microorganisms in the sample will not interfere with this PCR.

When the presence of MTBC DNA was confirmed in the discording samples, these were considered as true positives. Therefore, 70 positive samples were correctly identified by PCR, increasing the diagnostic sensitivity and specificity values with respect to culture (from 88.41 to 94.59% and from 92.37 to 96.03%, respectively). PPVs and NPVs were 93.33 and 96.80%, respectively. Furthermore, the PLR was 23.84 indicating a high probability of correctly identifying a bTB-positive tissue sample. In addition, the NLR was very low (0.06), indicating a low probability of a negative result being positive.

The most commonly used genetic target for PCR detection of MTBC species is the IS*6110* transposon (25). Other targets used in the detection of MTBC members in veterinary samples through PCR include the 16S-23S rRNA Internally Transcribed Spacer or ITS (14), *hupB* (26), TbD1 (11), *rv2807* (12), and *devR* (16). The high sequence similarity between the different MTBC species and the single-copy nature of the *mpb70* gene make it also a suitable target for both detection and quantification through Real-Time PCR. Since the early 1990's, the *mpb70* gene has been used extensively for the detection of MTBC species through conventional PCR (18, 27–29). Additionally, it has been used as a target for Real-Time PCR quantification of MTBC members in infected cell culture extracts (15). However, in this study hybridization probes were added to increase specificity.

Although the diagnostic specificity of this PCR was similar (96.03 vs. 97%) to that seen for the Real-Time PCR used by Courcoul et al. targeting the IS*6110* element (6), diagnostic sensitivity was higher in this study (94.59% vs. 87.7%). When compared against a Real-Time PCR detecting the IS*6110* element based on melting curve analysis and hybridization probes (30), the *mpb70*-targeting PCR showed a better correlation with culture results and increased diagnostic sensitivity. A semi-nested Real-Time PCR targeting the IS*6110* showed very similar diagnostic sensitivity, specificity and predictive values to those obtained in this study; 100% diagnostic sensitivity, 97.7% diagnostic specificity, 96.3% PPV and 100% NPV (13). Even though the LOD is lower for this semi-nested Real-Time PCR (1.5fg vs. 50fg), the requirement of two PCR steps increases the risk of cross-contamination. In addition, a Real-Time PCR targeting the 16S-23S ITS showed a moderate diagnostic sensitivity of 73.87% (14).

It is important to consider that the diagnostic performance of this PCR in this study does not give information about the infection status of all animals included in this study, as it only compares culture and PCR on tissue samples. Based on the results of this study and previous publications, direct PCR has some advantages compared to culture for the detection of MTBC species in animal tissue samples. In the first place, PCR takes a few hours to complete in comparison to the weeks required for microbiological culture. Secondly, analytical specificity can be extremely high if the appropriate oligonucleotides are designed, limiting cross-reaction with contaminating microorganisms. This removes the requirement for a decontamination step, decreasing the hazardous conditions applied to the sample. Furthermore, it would reduce the risk of exposure to mycobacteria as it decreases the processing time of tissues with suspected MTBC infections before inactivation, the amount of time spent at BSL3 facilities and the bacterial load to which the user is exposed to. In addition, the *mpb70* PCR showed a comparable limit of detection and diagnostic sensitivity to that seen in IS*6110* PCRs. One disadvantage of the IS*6110* target over the *mpb70* is the risk of horizontal transfer of mobile elements between mycobacterial species, as has been recorded for IS*1245* and *M. kansasii* (31). Moreover, the IS*6110* is present in a variable number of copies within the genome of certain MTBC species, which limits its use in quantitative studies, unlike the *mpb70* gene, which is a single-copy gene.

The results obtained in this study open the possibility of using the direct Real-Time PCR as an alternative to microbiological culture in the short term. Although microbiological culture is still needed for bacterial isolation and molecular characterization with epidemiological purposes, PCR could decrease considerably the time needed until results are obtained, improving the decision making capacity during the eradication campaigns.

In conclusion, the Real-Time targeting the *mpb70* gene is a time-effective and efficient method for the detection of MTBC members in veterinary tissue samples, which shows improved diagnostic performance with respect to culture. In addition, it has a low detection limit of 10 genomic equivalents/reaction of MTBC species. Furthermore, being a single copy gene and having a dynamic range of 10^6-10 genomic equivalents/ reaction, it could be used for quantification studies of as little as 10 genomic equivalents.

AUTHOR CONTRIBUTIONS

VL-L and EL performed all experiments in this study and the *in silico* specificity analysis. EC participated in the design of the *mpb70* specific oligonucleotides used in this study. BR, EL, and LdJ designed the study. LD and LdJ are responsible for the obtaining of samples. VL-L wrote the manuscript with the invaluable insights of EC, JB, EL, LD, BR, and LdJ. BR directed and supervised the complete study.

ACKNOWLEDGMENTS

We would like to thank the excellent work performed by laboratory technicians F. Lozano, T. Alende, A. Gutiérrez, N. Moya, C. Viñolo, D. de la Cruz, and L. Jimenez, in culturing and spoligotyping. We would also like to thank the work carried out by Susana Gómez during the design of the primers and probe, and Pilar Pozo with sequencing. In addition, we would like to appreciate valuable statistical insights given by María Luisa de la Cruz and Julio Álvarez. This work was supported by the Área de Ganadería de la Comunidad de Madrid, the Ministerio de Agricultura, Pesca, Alimentación y Medio Ambiente, and the Programa de Tecnologías Avanzadas en Vigilancia Sanitaria (TAVS) de la Comunidad de Madrid (S2013/ABI2747). This work was supported by the Programa de Tecnologías Avanzadas en Vigilancia Sanitaria (TAVS) from the Comunidad de Madrid (ref. S2013/ABI-2747).

REFERENCES

1. Bezos J, Álvarez J, Romero B Juan L, Dominguez L. Bovine tuberculosis: historical perspective. *Res Veterin Sci.* (2014) 97:S3–4 doi: 10.1016/j.rvsc.2014.09.003
2. Corner LAL, Gormley E, Pfeiffer DU. Primary isolation of *Mycobacterium bovis* from bovine tissues: Conditions for maximising the number of positive cultures. *Vet Microbiol.* (2012) 156:162–71. doi: 10.1016/j.vetmic.2011.10.016
3. Hines N, Payeur JB, Hoffman LJ. Comparison of the recovery of *Mycobacterium bovis* isolates using the BACTEC MGIT 960 system, BACTEC 460 system, and Middlebrook 7H10 and 7H11 solid media. *J Vet Diag Invest.* (2006) 18:243–50. doi: 10.1177/104063870601800302
4. Price-Carter GFYM, Bland K, Joyce MA, Khan F, Surrey M, Lisle GW, et al. Comparison of the BBL mycobacteria growth indicator tube, the BACTEC 12B, and solid media for the isolation of *Mycobacterium bovis*. *J Vet Diag Invest.* (2017) 29:508–12. doi: 10.1177/1040638717697763
5. Robbe-Austerman S, Bravo DM, Harris B. Comparison of the MGIT 960, BACTEC 460 TB and solid media for isolation of *Mycobacterium bovis* in United States veterinary specimens. *BMC Vet Res.* (2013) 9:74. doi: 10.1186/1746-6148-9-74
6. Courcoul A, Moyen J-L, Brugère L, Faye S, Hénault S, Gares H, et al. Estimation of sensitivity and specificity of bacteriology, histopathology and PCR for the confirmatory diagnosis of bovine tuberculosis using latent class analysis. *PLoS ONE.* (2014) 9:e90334. doi: 10.1371/journal.pone.0090334
7. Costa P, Botelho A, Couto I, Viveiros M, Inácio J. Standing of nucleic acid testing strategies in veterinary diagnosis laboratories to uncover *Mycobacterium tuberculosis* complex members. *Front Mol Biosci.* (2014) 1:16. doi: 10.3389/fmolb.2014.00016
8. Liébana E, Aranaz A, Mateos A, Vilafranca M, Gomez-Mampaso E, Tercero JC, et al. Simple and rapid detection of *mycobacterium tuberculosis* complex organisms in bovine tissue samples by PCR. *J. Clin. Microbiol.* (1995) 33:33–6.
9. Stewart LD, McNair J, McCallan L, Gordon A, Grant IR. Improved detection of *mycobacterium bovis* infection in bovine lymph node tissue using immunomagnetic separation (IMS)-Based Methods. *PLoS ONE.* (2013)8:e58374. doi: 10.1371/journal.pone.0058374
10. Wards BJ, Collins DM, Lisle GW. Detection of *Mycobacterium bovis* in tissues by polymerase chain reaction. *Vet Microbiol.* (1995) 43:227–40. doi: 10.1016/0378-1135(94)00096-F
11. Araújo CP, Osório ALAR, Jorge KSG, Ramos CAN, Filho AFS, Vidal CES, et al. Detection of *Mycobacterium bovis* in bovine and bubaline tissues using NEsted-PCR for TbD1. *PLoS ONE.* (2014) 9:e91023. doi: 10.1371/journal.pone.0091023
12. Araújo CP, Osório ALAR, Jorge KSG, Ramos CAN, Filho AFS, Vidal CES, et al. Direct detection of *Mycobacterium tuberculosis* complex in bovine and bubaline tissues through nested-PCR. *Brazil J Microbiol.* (2014) 45:633–40.
13. Costa P, Ferreira AS, Amaro A, Albuquerque T, Botelho A, Couto I, et al. Enhanced Detection of tuberculous mycobacteria in animal tissues using a semi-nested probe-based real-time PCR. *PLoS ONE.* (2013) 8:e81337. doi: 10.1371/journal.pone.0081337
14. Parra A, García N, García A, Lacombe A, Moreno F, Freire F, et al. Development of a molecular diagnostic test applied to experimental abattoir surveillance on bovine tuberculosis. *Vet Microbiol.* (2008) 127:315–24. doi: 10.1016/j.vetmic.2007.09.001
15. Beltran-Beck B, Fuente J, Garrido JM, Aranaz A, Sevilla I, et al. Oral vaccination with heat inactivated *mycobacterium bovis* activates the complement system to protect against tuberculosis. *PLoS ONE.* (2014) 9:e98048. doi: 10.1371/journal.pone.0098048
16. Sevilla IA, Molina E, Elguezabal N, Pérez V, Garrido JM, Juste RA. Detection of Mycobacteria, *Mycobacterium avium* Subspecies, and *Mycobacterium tuberculosis* Complex by a Novel Tetraplex Real-Time PCR Assay. *J Clin Microbiol.* (2015) 53:930–40. doi: 10.1128/JCM.03168-14
17. Corner LA, Trajstman AC. An Evaluation of 1-Hexadecylpyridinium Chloride as a decontaminant in the primary isolation of *mycobacterium bovis* from bovine lesions. *Vet Microbiol.* (1988) 18:127–34. doi: 10.1016/0378-1135(88)90058-2
18. Wilton S, Cousins D. Detection and Identification of Multiple Mycobacterial Pathogens by DNA Amplification in a Single Tube. *Genome Res.* (1992) 1:269–73. doi: 10.1101/gr.1.4.269
19. Kamerbeek J, Schouls L, Kolk A, Agterveld MV, Soolingen D, et al. Simultaneous Detection and strain differentiation of *mycobacterium tuberculosis* for diagnosis and epidemiology. *J Clin Microbiol.* (1997) 35:907–14.
20. Blas ID, Ruiz-Zarzuela I, Vallejo A. WinEpi: working in epidemiology. an online epidemiological tool. In: *Proceedings of the 11th International Symposium on Veterinary Epidemiology and Economics.* (Cairns, QLD) (2006).
21. Hall TA. BioeEdit: a user-friendly biological sequence alignment editor and analysis program for Windows 95/98/NT. *Nucl Acids Symposium Series.* (1999) 41:95–8.
22. Veyrier F, Saïd-Salim B, Behr MA. Evolution of the mycobacterial sigk regulon. *J Bacteriol.* (2008) 190:1891–9. doi: 10.1128/JB.01452-07
23. Park KT, Allen AJ, Davis WC. Development of a novel DNA extraction method for identification and quantification of *Mycobacterium avium* subsp. *paratuberculosis* from tissue samples by real-time PCR. *J Microbiol Methods.* (2014) 99:58–65. doi: 10.1016/j.mimet.2014.02.003
24. Menin Á, Fleith R, Reck C, Marlow M, Fernandes P, Pilati C, et al. Asymptomatic cattle naturally infected with *Mycobacterium bovis* present

exacerbated tissue pathology and bacterial dissemination. *PLoS ONE*. (2013) 8:e53884. doi: 10.1371/journal.pone.0053884

25. Thierry D, Cave MD, Eisenach KD, Crawford JT, Bates JH, Gicquel B, et al. IS*6110*, an IS-like element of *Mycobacterium tuberculosis* complex. *Nucl Acids Res*. (1990) 18:188. doi: 10.1093/nar/18.1.188

26. Mishra A, Singhal A, Chauhan DS, Katoch VM, Srivastava K, Thakral SS, et al. Direct Detection and Identification of *Mycobacterium tuberculosis* and *Mycobacterium bovis* in Bovine Samples by a Novel Nested PCR Assay: Correlation with Conventional Techniques. *J Clin Microbiol*. (2005) 43:5670–8. doi: 10.1128/JCM.43.11.5670-5678.2005

27. Cousins DV, Wilton SD, Francis BR. Use of DNA amplification for the rapid identification of *Mycobacterium bovis*. *Vet Microbiol*. (1991) 27:187–95. doi: 10.1016/0378-1135(91)90010-D

28. Santos N, Geraldes M, Afonso A, Almeida V, Correia-Neves M. Diagnosis of Tuberculosis in the Wild Boar (*Sus scrofa*): a comparison of methods applicable to hunter-harvested animals. *PLoS ONE*. (2010) 5:e12663. doi: 10.1371/journal.pone.0012663

29. Pereira-Suárez AL, Estrada-Chávez Y, Zúñiga-Estrada A, LóPez-Rincón G, Hernández DUM, Padilla-Ramírez FJ, et al. Detection of *Mycobacterium tuberculosis* Complex by PCR in Fresh Cheese from Local Markets in Hidalgo, Mexico. *J Food Protect*. (2014) 77:849–52. doi: 10.4315/0362-028X.JFP-13-389

30. Taylor MJ, Hughes MS, Skuce RA, Neill SD. Detection of *Mycobacterium bovis* in bovine clinical specimens using real-time fluorescence and fluorescence resonance energy transfer probe rapid-Cycle PCR. *J Clin Microbiol*. (2001) 39:1272–8. doi: 10.1128/JCM.39.4.1272-1278.2001

31. RabelloMC, Matsumoto CK, Paula de Almeida LG, Menendez MC, Oliveira RS, et al. First Description of natural and experimental conjugation between mycobacteria mediated by a linear plasmid. *PLoS ONE*. (2010) 7:e29884. doi: 10.1371/journal.pone.0029884

8

TB Control in Humans and Animals in South Africa: A Perspective on Problems and Successes

Christina Meiring*, Paul D. van Helden and Wynand J. Goosen

Division of Molecular Biology and Human Genetics, Faculty of Medicine and Health Sciences, DST-NRF Centre of Excellence for Biomedical Tuberculosis Research, South African Medical Research Council Centre for Tuberculosis Research, Stellenbosch University, Cape Town, South Africa

Correspondence:
Christina Meiring
cmeiring@sun.ac.za

Mycobacterium tuberculosis (M. tb) remains one of the most globally serious infectious agents for human morbidity and mortality, but with significant differences in prevalence across the globe. In many countries, the incidence is now low and declining, but control and eradication remain a distant view. Similarly, the prevalence of bovine TB caused by *Mycobacterium bovis (M. bovis)*, varies significantly across regions, although unlike for *M. tuberculosis*, data are sparse. The reduction in incidence and prevalence and control of both human and bovine TB is difficult and costly, yet some countries have managed to do this with some success. This perspective will consider some of the critical control steps we now know to be important for the control of TB from *M. tuberculosis* in humans living in South Africa, where the incidence of TB is the highest currently experienced. Despite the high incidence of human TB, South Africa has been able to reduce this incidence remarkably in the past few years, despite limited resources and high HIV prevalence. We draw from our experience to ascertain whether we may learn useful lessons from control efforts for both diseases in order to suggest effective control measures for bovine TB.

Keywords: tuberculosis, *Mycobacterium bovis*, bovine TB, infectious diseases, zoonotic TB

INTRODUCTION

Mycobacterium bovis (M. bovis), the causative agent of bovine tuberculosis (BTB), has perhaps the broadest host range of the pathogenic mycobacteria (1). Although the most commonly affected species are members of the Bovidae, even humans can be affected.

Considerably more attention is devoted to control of *Mycobacterium tuberculosis* in humans, than *M. bovis* in its multiple hosts (2). Although there are some similarities between TB control in humans and animals, such as the need for diagnosis, there are also very different disease management options, such as antibiotic therapy for humans, in comparison to test and slaughter for domestic cattle. Disease control measures include the need to find and deal with cases and prevent transmission. Although this seems self-evident, achieving these goals is not simple and require critical activities such as those shown below and discussed later.

Steps to TB control:

1. Awareness
2. Risk factor reduction
3. Access
4. Diagnosis
5. Retention
6. Treatment
7. Adherence
8. Follow up

Actions attributable to these steps allowed South Africa to steadily reduce human TB incidence from a peak of 977/100,000 per annum in 2007 to 781 in 2016. This observed reduction in incidence is perhaps remarkable because the reduction alone exceeds by far the incidence rate seen in most countries (3).

The reported occurrence of bovine TB in South African domestic bovine herds is far lower (**Table 1**), although since full testing coverage is not done the actual numbers are likely to be higher. TB and BTB control activities will be discussed below.

AWARENESS AND STIGMA

Ignorance of TB is rife. For this reason, many organizations tasked with human health care such as WHO (World Health Organization), The Union (International Union Against Tuberculosis and Lung Disease), and MSF (Médecins Sans Frontières), start their campaigns with generating awareness. Such campaigns leverage media, to create interest and awareness.

TABLE 1 | *Mycobacterium bovis* cases reported in South Africa from 2000 to 2018 (Department of Agriculture, Forestry and Fisheries: http://www.daff.gov.za/daffweb3/Branches/Agricultural-Production-Health-Food-Safety/Animal-Health/Epidemiology).

Year	Outbreaks	Cases	Dead/Culled
2000	10	174	181
2001	1	33	1
2002	4	123	32
2003	17	394	370
2004	11	1,525	737
2005	14	747	856
2006	4	42	37
2007	6	102	50
2008	4	50	37
2009	18	36	1,236
2010	8	18	7
2011	7	34	29
2012	3	90	0
2013	2	8	29
2014	8	102	66
2015	8	32	28
2016	3	247	0
2017	1	8	0
2018	3	4	3

Estimated cattle herd size 13.5 million in 2003.

Our own academic department has reached out to schools and communities in multiple activities in 2018 alone. Using past and cured patients to propagate the message through their own experiences can be quite effective at community level. Such public activities have the benefit of addressing and reducing stigma that might be attached to TB. There is now improved awareness amongst the South African public concerning human TB. However, there is little awareness of bovine TB. In general, there has not been much media attention, there is no large or even small-scale campaign, no rallying cry, no catch phrases, and essentially it is left to private and state veterinarians and technicians to work with farmers as they see fit. To date, one awareness day has been organized in only one location, and the limitations of this hardly need to be discussed.

RISK FACTOR REDUCTION

Humans and animals share some common risk factors for TB, such as nutrition or malnutrition, age, crowding, and extent of exposure (4). There are many others which are likely to be restricted to humans or animals only, such as substance abuse in humans and environmental contamination in animals. Many risk factors in humans relate to poverty and are very difficult to address. Risk factors for cattle include historical TB on a farm, movement of animals, TB on neighboring property or in wildlife in contact with domestic stock, prevalence of TB in a herd or area and herd size, multiple premises, poor housing, and nutrition (5). It is often possible to mitigate against these risks for livestock.

A cornerstone of bovine TB control is movement restriction of animals. This is a vital activity, which is not generally possible with humans and therefore presents veterinarians with an enormous advantage to prevent ongoing disease transmission. Most countries have a test and slaughter policy in place for bovine TB in domestic stock (6, 7). However, having a policy and program does not necessarily mean that full coverage is achieved and appropriate action is followed. For example, many resource-poor countries such as South Africa do not have the resources for rigorous testing and there is a lack of compensation to affected livestock owners. Movement restriction requires proper monitoring, which is extremely difficult even under optimal circumstances. Although TB does not have a vector, we can argue that a contaminated environment (soil, water) and multiple hosts may act as reservoirs for infection and therefore also need active management.

ACCESS

In order to capitalize on awareness campaigns, it is vital that access to appropriate facilities and experts are available to persons who are ill. In South Africa, there is a large network of state-funded public health clinics (8) and private practitioners which addresses health problems including TB. In the veterinary field, there is a network of state veterinary services as well as private veterinarians who can deal with bovine TB. However, the veterinary service is far smaller than the human health service component and overall they must deal with far larger numbers of potential hosts on a per capita basis than clinicians for the human population. Testing for bovine TB is voluntary, except for dairy herds. However, there are inadequate numbers of state veterinarians to do regular TB testing, including for dairy herds where compulsory testing every 2 years is required. Therefore, private veterinarians have to be hired at considerable cost to the owners. On occasion, state veterinary services will provide TB testing for impecunious owners or commonage herds. Since there is no compensation paid to owners for culled positive animals or herds that need to be slaughtered, there is little or no incentive for testing to be done, in fact, there can be active resistance to testing.

One of the key elements envisaged for successful TB control remains the goal of a point-of-care (PoC) diagnostic test, the value of which is illustrated by scenarios (**Figure 1**): we highlight firstly the South African human TB diagnostic program prior to 2011, which required three sputum samples from a client on different days over a week. This resulted in a loss to follow up of 17–25% (9, 10). Let us also assume that we use the test still used in many resource-poor settings, i.e., acid-fast staining with diagnostic sensitivity of 50–60%. The implication (**Figure 1** scenario A) is that only a small percentage of patients initiated proper therapy, which allowed ongoing disease and transmission events (8). In a different hypothetical scenario (scenario B), using a test of the same sensitivity but PoC based, with immediate initiation of therapy, the proportion of TB cases that could initiate therapy almost doubles. Scenario B will also imply a reduction in infectiousness time and fewer transmission events. In a third hypothetical scenario (scenario C), an Xpert® MTB/RIF test is conducted (PoC) where indicated, therapy can be initiated immediately. Given the test sensitivity of 82–89% (11, 12), it implies that over 80% of TB cases could initiate therapy. Ignoring specificity discussion to illustrate this point, a high sensitivity PoC diagnostic test results in less loss or default.

By far the majority of the human TB diagnostic tests based on GeneXpert, are done at no cost to clients utilizing public clinics, since laboratory-based tests are done by the National Health Laboratory Service (NHLS, funded by the National Department of Health) which has many laboratories scattered in a network across the country (8). In contrast, the Department of Agriculture, Forestry and Fisheries (DAFF) subsidizes laboratory diagnostics at only one laboratory for BTB in suspect animal cases, but does not pay costs in full. Tests require that samples be taken at necropsy, or that fresh blood samples for immunological tests arrive within hours under ideal conditions, the latter being

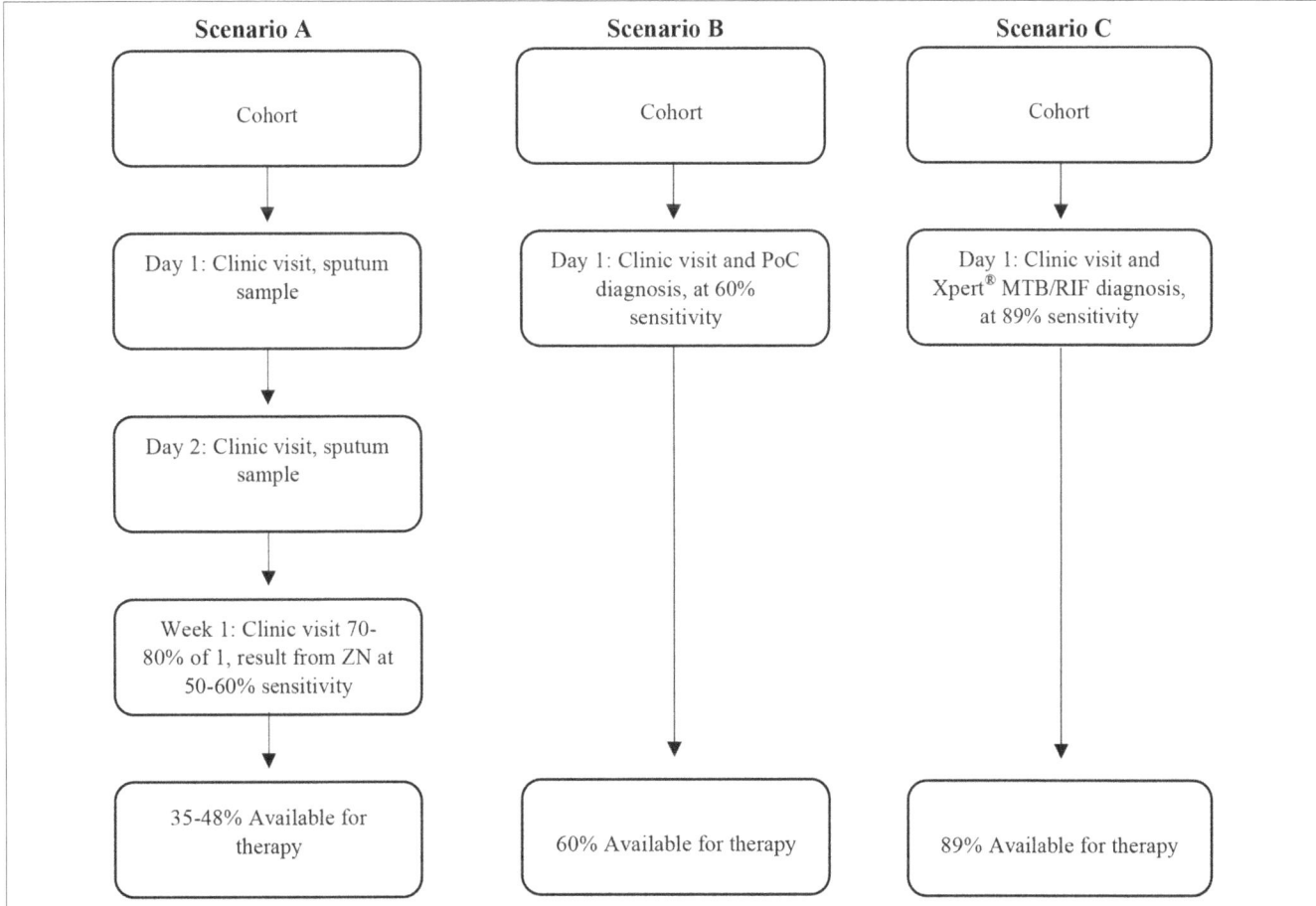

FIGURE 1 | Different scenarios representing different human TB diagnostic approaches which include the sensitivity of the diagnostic tests and corresponding availability of therapy for individuals. Scenario 1 is a previous TB program now obsolete, scenario 2 is hypothetical, illustrating the advantage of point of care test, and scenario 3 is what could be achieved using the GeneXpert system if used for same day diagnosis in the clinic.

largely impossible in a large country with distant rural farms. Owners are not compensated for their animals which will result in a reluctance to test animals. Samples from necropsy are set up for mycobacterial culture followed by speciation (13). Unlike the NHLS, there is only one state lab, Onderstepoort Veterinary Institute (OVI), accredited for testing for bovine TB, largely because there is no financial incentive for other laboratories to be accredited. Such a monopoly is unlikely to be the best way forward.

Clearly, surveillance or suspicion of bovine TB should not lead immediately to slaughter and necropsy. Therefore, non-lethal diagnostics for animals are needed. Only once such diagnostics strongly suggest bovine TB, necropsy, culture, and speciation is done to confirm bovine TB. Bovine TB has been tested for in Bovidae by skin testing and more recently by *in vitro* blood-based interferon gamma (IFN-γ) release assays (IGRA) or other biomarkers (14–19). These tests although useful, are limited owing to the need for blood transport to accredited laboratories under time and temperature constraints, as well as the need for a reasonably well-equipped laboratory. In order to circumvent this logistics problem, serum-based diagnostics are being researched. Serum-based biomarker research in humans shows promise for a diagnostic, but as yet, although sensitivity is high (94%), specificity (73%) is inadequate for implementation (20). However, it may be that such biomarkers discovered for human TB diagnosis, may be applicable to bovine TB.

Bovine TB can also infect many species other than the Bovidae. Therefore, particularly in the case of wildlife, species-specific diagnostic tests may be required. This is necessary to prevent the disease from being maintained in an ecosystem outside of monitored hosts, e.g., cattle or buffaloes and where there may be concerns for endangered species, such as rhinoceroses. Failure to diagnose and treat a TB case has significant downstream cost implications, not least of which is ongoing transmission and disease propagation. Thus, a considerable and ongoing investment in the best diagnostics and control programs to implement these is justified.

RETENTION

Many TB control programs suffer client losses along the care cascade. Such work shows the importance and advantages of the "Holy Grail" of TB researchers, the PoC diagnostic (21). The consequence of losses on the cascade is that successful completion of treatment for TB was estimated to be only 53% of cases (8). In the case of livestock or wildlife, the difficulties involved in accessing animals for repeat testing or dealing with positive responders are familiar to state veterinarians. No similar quantitative care cascade loss studies have been done in veterinary medicine in South Africa and thus information is anecdotal. However, the future cost of missed cases, as for humans, cannot be overemphasized.

TREATMENT

There is perhaps little that can be learnt from current therapeutic management of human TB and extrapolated to animals. The standard treatment for TB in humans is antibiotic therapy (22), which with the exception of animals in captivity is not feasible in animals. Sometimes physical isolation is also practiced, i.e., the TB case is placed in a treatment facility to isolate them from the general populace. For TB in animals, the same basic principle applies: remove the bacterial threat by removing the animal (i.e., physical isolation), usually by slaughter.

ADHERENCE

The basic clinical principle applies: complete the course of treatment. This must apply, whether it is antibiotic treatment in humans, movement control or removal of animals with TB, usually by slaughter. Failure to do so will result in ongoing disease and transmission, and failure to eradicate the problem (22).

FOLLOW-UP

This is an important step and often not done in human TB management in higher incidence areas owing to sheer volume of work and resource limitations. The reason for this activity is that even under ideal conditions and with proper adherence, some individuals will experience recurrent disease. Furthermore, prior to becoming bacillus negative, TB cases can transmit the disease. Ideally, therefore, treated and cured individuals need follow up for at least 2 years (23) and their contacts should be investigated. In the case of free-living humans, particularly in a high incidence society, investigating all contacts is impossible. Likewise for free-ranging wildlife. However, these principles are part of bovine TB control practice in South Africa, i.e., test and remove and subsequent follow up testing and retesting until disease is cleared according to protocol. This practice should always be followed. It is encouraging that even culling of limited infected animals in a free-ranging wildlife system can reduce prevalence rate (7).

Although the steps discussed above are arguably critical for TB control, there are many other factors that are important and will impact on any control measures undertaken. Some of these are discussed further below.

TRANSMISSION

Arguably the most important step in combatting TB is to stop transmission. Close contact is important, but not definitive for transmission. For example, a study in a very high incidence area showed that only a small proportion of human TB cases result from household contact (24, 25). Furthermore, the passive detection of TB cases in high prevalence communities is insufficient to limit disease transmission (8, 26). We still have an inadequate understanding of TB transmission, although we know that aerosol transmission is one of the main sources for humans, and most likely also bovis. In the case of some other animals, it may be ingestion of contaminated meat or biting. Clearly, adequate distance must be maintained to avoid ongoing transmission. Therefore, attention should be given to the potential for a contaminated environment, and there should be space and free airflow such that transmission may be minimized.

INFECTION, LATENCY, AND DISEASE

It is generally stated that (in the absence of immunosuppression), only 10% of infected humans will develop active TB (4, 27). Traditionally and commonly stated: approximately half of those who will develop active disease will do so within 2 years after infection and the other half sometime after that, owing to reactivation of latent infection (LTBI) (28). Controversy characterizes opinions concerning whether a positive diagnostic assay, such as those that are host-based, really prove disease or are indicative of infection but do not necessarily represent disease or the presence of live bacilli. We previously considered four possible states: (1) not exposed, (2) exposed and infected, no response detectable, no sign of disease, (3) infected, bacilli present, no active disease (latent TB), (4) infected, active disease. In clinical medicine, distinguishing between these four states is not necessarily clear. A recent comprehensive review (23), suggests that the burden of disease from latent TB in humans has been vastly overestimated, suggests only three states and that TB has a shorter incubation period than previously thought. If this is correct, it has major implications for public health. Unfortunately, there is little clear-cut data on whether three or four states apply to the multiple animal hosts of *M. bovis,* nor clear-data regarding progression between states.

Therefore, the interpretation of immunological tests for human as well as bovine TB is complex. Possible outcomes of exposure from cattle to *M. bovis* are believed to be in line with that of humans. Briefly, following exposure to bacilli, the innate immune response can either clear the infection or fail to do so. This failure then leads to the need for intervention by the host's adaptive immune response. A successful response leads to the clearance of the infection with no delayed-type hypersensitivity responses (skin test and whole blood gamma interferon release assay negativity), or failure leads to active disease (skin test and IFN-γ release assay positivity) (29). In cattle, failure to detect visible lesions at *post-mortem* examinations does not indicate absence of infection (30). A systematic review of many studies has previously shown that 50% of reactor animals had no visible lesions (31), which was seen in a separate study where only 43% of reactors had visible lesions at slaughter (32). This suggests that as for humans (23) active disease may be significantly underestimated in studies where culture is the gold standard.

Recent modeling suggests that the WHO's (human) TB elimination target cannot be achieved by 2050 using LTBI screening as the sole control strategy (33, 34). The assumptions used include maximum coverage, no imported infections due to travel and migration, and application of an additional 4% annual decrease. This model suggests that a TB incidence of <1/100,000 will only be achieved about 50 years after implementation of LTBI screening and prophylactic treatment (33). These findings are optimistic assumptions, but illustrate the difficulties involved in eliminating TB when LTBI exists. Furthermore, they emphasize that continued surveillance and follow up will be essential. However, if latent TB is far less important than previously assumed, then eradication or good control far sooner than this is possible. Therefore, in veterinary medicine, the approach taken thus far has been wise, i.e., if any test is positive, take action. This should arguably continue to be the case and is probably the reason for the low prevalence of bovine TB in domestic stock in South Africa.

BOVINE TB IN WILDLIFE

Although bovine TB in livestock appears to be of low prevalence in South Africa (**Table 1**), this is not the case in at least three of our large national park systems (35, 36). Thus, far no effective plan has been made to combat it in an open system in South Africa, although some limited culling has been done in one park (7). Such areas pose a risk for spread beyond the park boundaries, but is limited as far as possible by testing, animal movement control, and breeding of disease-free animals, such as TB free herds of African buffalo (37). Insufficient research has been done to show whether or not this disease will impact species to affect the ecosystem and which species are maintenance or end-stage hosts.

ECONOMICS

Stable systems require a healthy society, a healthy economy and a healthy environment. TB, whether in animal or human form impacts on all three of these pillars. The problem with giving inadequate attention to current TB using as the excuse "we can't afford it," will leave us with the situation we currently have. The latest estimates (2014) from WHO are that 1.7 billion humans were latently infected by *M. tuberculosis* (28). We have no idea how many animals are infected by *M. bovis*, as a comparison, but an estimated 147,000 human (zoonotic) cases of bovine TB alone per annum occur (38). This implies many animal cases and neglect now will mean high future costs.

WAY FORWARD

The nature of TB, whether human or animal form, makes eradication in the short term impossible. However, it is clear that transmission must be stopped in order to eradicate the disease. The essential lessons from this are many: one cannot be complacent, one cannot relax vigilance, and care for this disease (39). Active and latent cases must be dealt with before eradication can be considered.

Countries or regions should take the threat of bovine TB seriously. If this is not the case, then perhaps we can learn from one initiative started in South Africa recently to try to improve TB control. A TB Think Tank was established (40) bringing together researchers in the basic sciences, clinical sciences, epidemiology, social sciences, public health, and Health systems experts, and government staff. This body has promoted evidence-based decision-making, and in addition, lobbied successfully for increased funding for TB management (human) in South Africa. By involving national TB control staff and other experts, it is believed that significant impact on TB can be achieved. Similar think tank initiatives could be developed for other settings including bovine TB control to support evidence-based policy development and disease control and lobby for the finances to support such efforts.

AUTHOR CONTRIBUTIONS

All authors listed have made a substantial, direct and intellectual contribution to the work, and approved it for publication.

ACKNOWLEDGMENTS

The authors work was supported by the South African Medical Research Council and National Research Foundation of South Africa.

REFERENCES

1. Good M, Duignan A. Perspectives on the history of bovine TB and the role of tuberculin in bovine TB eradication. *Vet Med Int.* (2011) 2011:410470. doi: 10.4061/2011/410470

2. Olea-Popelka F, Muwonge A, Perera A, Dean AS, Mumford E, Erlacher-Vindel E, et al. Zoonotic tuberculosis in human beings caused by *Mycobacterium bovis*-a call for action. *Lancet Infect Dis.* (2017) 17:e21–5. doi: 10.1016/S1473-3099(16)30139-6

3. WHO (2015). *Global TB Report.*

4. Rieder HL. *Epidemiologic Basis of Tuberculosis Control.* Paris: International Union Against Tuberculosis and Lung Disease (1999). p. 1–162.

5. Skuce RA, AllenAR, McDowell SWJ. Herd-level risk factors for bovine tuberculosis: a literature review. *Vet Med Int.* (2012) 2012:621210. doi: 10.1155/2012/621210

6. De Garine-Wichatitsky M, Caron A, Kock R, Tschopp R, Munyeme M, Hofmeyr M, et al. A review of bovine tuberculosis at the wildlife-livestock-human interface in sub-Saharan Africa. *Epidemiol Infect.* (2013) 141:1342–56. doi: 10.1017/S0950268813000708

7. le Roex N, Cooper D, van Helden PD, Hoal EG, Jolles AE. Disease control in wildlife: evaluating a test and cull programme for bovine tuberculosis in African buffalo. *Transbound Emerg Dis.* (2016) 63:647–57. doi: 10.1111/tbed.12329

8. Naidoo P, Theron G, Rangaka MX, Chihota VN, Vaughan L, Brey ZO, et al. The South African tuberculosis care cascade: estimated losses and methodological challenges. *J Infect Dis.* (2017) 216:S702–13. doi: 10.1093/infdis/jix335

9. Botha E, Den Boon S, Verver S, Dunbar R, Lawrence KA, Bosman M, et al. Initial default from tuberculosis treatment: how often does it happen and what are the reasons? *Int J Tuberc Lung Dis.* (2008) 12:820–3.

10. Claassens MM, Dunbar R, Yang B, Lombard CJ. Scanty smears associated with initial loss to follow-up in South African tuberculosis patients. *Int J Tuberc Lung Dis.* (2017) 21:196–201. doi: 10.5588/ijtld.16.0292

11. Steingart KR, Schiller I, Horne DJ, Pai M, Boehme CC, Dendukuri N. Xpert® MTB/RIF assay for pulmonary tuberculosis and rifampicin resistance in adults. *Cochrane Database Syst Rev.* (2014). CD009593. doi: 10.1002/14651858.CD009593.pub3

12. Theron G, Peter J, van Zyl-Smit R, Mishra H, Streicher E, Murray S, et al. Evaluation of the Xpert MTB/RIF assay for the diagnosis of pulmonary tuberculosis in a high HIV prevalence setting. *Am J Respir Crit Care Med.* (2011) 184:132–40. doi: 10.1164/rccm.201101-0056OC

13. Warren RM, Gey van Pittius NC, Barnard M, Hesseling A, Engelke E, de Kock M, et al. Differentiation of *Mycobacterium tuberculosis* complex by PCR amplification of genomic regions of difference. *Int. J. Tuberc. Lung Dis.* (2006) 10:818–22.

14. Bernitz N, Clarke C, Roos EO, Goosen WJ, Cooper D, van Helden PD, et al. Detection of *Mycobacterium bovis* infection in African buffaloes (*Syncerus caffer*) using QuantiFERON®-TB Gold (QFT) tubes and the Qiagen cattletype® IFN-gamma ELISA. *Vet Immunol Immunopathol.* (2018) 196:48–52. doi: 10.1016/j.vetimm.2017.12.010

15. Goosen WJ, Cooper D, Warren RM, Miller MA, van Helden PD, Parsons SDC. The evaluation of candidate biomarkers of cell-mediated immunity for the diagnosis of Mycobacterium bovis infection in African buffaloes (*Syncerus caffer*). *Vet Immunol Immunopathol.* (2014) 162:198–202. doi: 10.1016/j.vetimm.2014.10.008

16. Goosen WJ, Miller MA, Chegou NN, Cooper D, Warren RM, van Helden PD, et al. Agreement between assays of cell-mediated immunity utilizing *Mycobacterium bovis*-specific antigens for the diagnosis of tuberculosis in African buffaloes (*Syncerus caffer*). *Vet Immunol Immunopathol.* (2014) 160:133–8. doi: 10.1016/j.vetimm.2014.03.015

17. Goosen WJ, Cooper D, Miller MA, van Helden PD, Parsons SDC. IP-10 is a sensitive biomarker of antigen recognition in whole-blood stimulation assays used for the diagnosis of *Mycobacterium bovis* infection in African buffaloes (*Syncerus caffer*). *Clin Vaccine Immunol CVI* (2015) 22:974–8. doi: 10.1128/CVI.00324-15

18. van der Heijden EM, Jenkins AO, Cooper DV, Rutten VPMG, Michel AL. Field application of immunoassays for the detection of Mycobacterium bovis infection in the African buffalo (*Syncerus caffer*). *Vet Immunol Immunopathol.* (2016) 169:68–73. doi: 10.1016/j.vetimm.2015.12.003

19. Waters WR, Thacker TC, Nonnecke BJ, Palmer MV, Schiller I, Oesch B, et al. Evaluation of gamma interferon (IFN-γ)-induced protein 10 responses for detection of cattle infected with *Mycobacterium bovis*: comparisons to IFN-γ responses. *Clin Vaccine Immunol.* (2012) 19:346–51. doi: 10.1128/CVI.05657-11

20. Chegou NN, Sutherland JS, Malherbe S, Crampin AC, Corstjens PL, Geluk A, et al. Diagnostic performance of a seven-marker serum protein biosignature for the diagnosis of active TB disease in African primary healthcare clinic attendees with signs and symptoms suggestive of TB. *Thorax* (2016) 71:785–94. doi: 10.1136/thoraxjnl-2015-207999

21. Uys PW, Warren R, Helden PD, van Murray M, Victor TC. Potential of rapid diagnosis for controlling drug-susceptible and drug-resistant tuberculosis in communities where *Mycobacterium tuberculosis* infections are highly prevalent. *J Clin Microbiol.* (2009) 47:1484–90. doi: 10.1128/JCM.02289-08

22. Rieder HL. *Interventions for Tuberculosis Control and Elimination. Tuberculosis Interventions.* (2002). Available online at: https://www.cabdirect.org/cabdirect/abstract/20023083276 (Accessed June 18, 2018).

23. Behr MA, Edelstein PH, Ramakrishnan L. Revisiting the timetable of tuberculosis. *BMJ* (2018) 362:k2738. doi: 10.1136/bmj.k2738

24. Marais BJ, Hesseling AC, Schaaf HS, Gie RP, van Helden PD, Warren RM. *Mycobacterium tuberculosis* transmission is not related to household genotype in a setting of high endemicity. *J Clin Microbiol.* (2009) 47:1338–43. doi: 10.1128/JCM.02490-08

25. Verver S, Warren RM, Munch Z, Vynnycky E, van Helden PD, et al. Transmission of tuberculosis in a high incidence urban community in South Africa. *Int J Epidemiol.* (2004) 33:351–7. doi: 10.1093/ije/dyh021

26. Claassens M, Schalkwyk C, van Haan L, den Floyd S, Dunbar R, van Helden P, et al. High prevalence of tuberculosis and insufficient case detection in two communities in the Western Cape, South Africa. *PLOS ONE* (2013) 8:e58689. doi: 10.1371/journal.pone.0058689

27. Lin PL, Flynn JL. Understanding latent tuberculosis: a moving target. *J Immunol.* (2010) 185:15–22. doi: 10.4049/jimmunol.0903856

28. Houben RM, Dodd PJ. The global burden of latent tuberculosis infection: a re-estimation using mathematical modelling. *PLOS Med.* (2016) 13:e1002152. doi: 10.1371/journal.pmed.1002152

29. Pollock JM, Neill SD. *Mycobacterium bovis* infection and tuberculosis in cattle. *Vet J.* (2002) 163:115–27. doi: 10.1053/tvjl.2001.0655

30. Clegg TA, Good M, Doyle M, Duignan A, More SJ, Gormley E. The performance of the interferon gamma assay when used as a diagnostic or quality assurance test in *Mycobacterium bovis* infected herds. *Prev Vet Med.* (2017) 140:116–21. doi: 10.1016/j.prevetmed.2017.03.007

31. de la Rua-Domenech R, Goodchild AT, Vordermeier HM, Hewinson RG, Christiansen KH, Clifton-Hadley RS. Ante mortem diagnosis of tuberculosis in cattle: a review of the tuberculin tests, gamma-interferon assay and other ancillary diagnostic techniques. *Res Vet Sci.* (2006) 81:190–210. doi: 10.1016/j.rvsc.2005.11.005

32. O'Hagan MJ, Courcier EA, Drewe JA, Gordon AW, McNair J, Abernethy DA. Risk factors for visible lesions or positive laboratory tests in bovine tuberculosis reactor cattle in Northern Ireland. *Prev Vet Med.* (2015) 120:283–90. doi: 10.1016/j.prevetmed.2015.04.005

33. European Centre for Disease Prevention and Control (2018). *Mathematical Modelling of Programmatic Screening Strategies for Latent Tuberculosis Infection in Countries With Low Tuberculosis Incidence.*

34. WHO (2013). WHO Systematic *Screening for Active Tuberculosis: Principles and Recommendations.* WHO. Available online at: http://www.who.int/tb/tbscreening/en/ (accessed June 20, 2018).

35. Miller MA. *Tuberculosis in South African Wildlife: Why is it Important?* SU Language Centre, editor. Cape Town: Sun Media (2015).

36. Miller M, Michel A, van Helden P, Buss P. Tuberculosis in Rhinoceros: an underrecognized threat? *Transbound Emerg Dis.* (2017) 64:1071–8. doi: 10.1111/tbed.12489

37. Laubscher LL, Hoffman LC. An overview of disease-free buffalo breeding projects with reference to the different systems used in South Africa. *Sustainability* (2012) 4:3124–40. doi: 10.3390/su4113124

38. WHO (2017). *Global Tuberculosis Report.* Geneva.

39. Lienhardt C, Lönnroth K, Menzies D, Balasegaram M, Chakaya J, Cobelens F, et al. Translational research for tuberculosis elimination: priorities, challenges, and actions. *PLOS Med.* (2016) 13:e1001965. doi: 10.1371/journal.pmed.1001965

40. White RG, Charalambous S, Cardenas V, Hippner P, Sumner T, Bozzani F, et al. Evidence-informed policy making at country level: lessons learned from the South African Tuberculosis Think Tank. *Int J Tuberc Lung Dis.* (2018) 22:606–13. doi: 10.5588/ijtld.17.0485

9

Modeling as a Decision Support Tool for Bovine TB Control Programs in Wildlife

Graham C. Smith* and Richard J. Delahay

National Wildlife Management Centre, Animal and Plant Health Agency, York, United Kingdom

*Correspondence:
Graham C. Smith
graham.smith@apha.gov.uk

Computer modeling has a long history of association with epidemiology, and has improved our understanding of the theory of disease dynamics and provided insights into wildlife disease management. A summary of badger bovine TB models and their role in decision making is presented, from a simple initial SEI model, to SEIR (inclusion of a recovered category) and SEI_1I_2 (inclusion of two stages of disease progression) variants, and subsequent spatially-explicit individual-based models used to assess historical badger management strategies. The integration of cattle into TB models allowed comparison of the predicted impacts of different badger management strategies on cattle herd breakdown rates, and provided an economic dimension to the outputs. Estimates of R_0 for bovine TB in cattle and badgers are little higher than unity implying that the disease should be relatively easy to control, which is at odds with practical experience. A cohort of recent models have suggested that combined strategies, involving management of both host species and including vaccination may be most effective. Future models of badger vaccination will need to accommodate the partial protection from infection and likely duration of immunity conferred by the currently available vaccine (BCG). Descriptions of how models could better represent the ecological and epidemiological complexities of the badger-cattle TB system are presented, along with a wider discussion of the utility of modeling for bovine TB management interventions. This includes consideration of the information required to maximize the utility of the next generation of models.

Keywords: badger, model, decision making, bovine tuberculosis, simulation

INTRODUCTION

Mathematical models are both a simplification of reality and a reflection of our current understanding. As a working hypothesis of our supposed reality they can consequently only be shown to be wrong [1]. A good model should only include necessary parameters, although the definition of "necessary" depends on the model's purpose. There are three main types of model: statistical, mathematical and simulation. Statistical models find relationships between parameters and will not be considered here. There is a continuum from mathematical to simulation models, but in general the former are used to investigate how a system works, while the latter, usually mechanistic, can be used to investigate management options.

Bovine tuberculosis (bTB, caused by *Mycobacterium bovis*) is a serious disease of cattle and control can be made more challenging by the involvement of wildlife reservoirs [2]. In the UK and Republic of Ireland, European badgers (*Meles meles*) are implicated in the persistence and spread of infection to cattle (3, 4). In both countries management of the risks of transmission to cattle has focused on culling badgers (5, 6). As badgers are native this imposes certain practical restrictions and attracts controversy. There has also been substantial Government investment in recent years in the development of a badger vaccine (7, 8) with small-scale deployment for research and operational purposes (9, 10).

M. bovis in badgers is a chronic progressive condition, which can lead to debilitating disease and death, although many infected badgers survive for years and prevalence can average about 10–20% or higher (11). Principal sites of infection are the lungs and associated lymph nodes. Badgers may exhibit a range of responses to infection ranging from latency (host infected but bacteria are effectively contained), to generalized disease (12) when they are likely to be most infectious, potentially shedding bacteria in sputum, feces, urine, or pus from wounds or abscesses (13). Once infectious, onward transmission of *M. bovis* occurs by aerosol transmission among animals in close contact, via bite wounding (14), and indirectly through environmental contamination (15, 16). Transmission to cattle is thought to be through contact with bacteria in the environment rather than via direct contact (17, 18).

Mathematical modeling has a long history with the badger-TB system. This has ranged from modeling the dynamics of infection in badger populations, to complex two host badger and cattle systems, and simulating the impact of management to inform disease control policy (see below). Modeling is often referred to as an iterative process. Models can be used to investigate the theoretical aspects of disease ecology and management, data are investigated to determine parameter values, and the models can determine where the data are deficient. If the model output is sensitive to parameter estimates that are uncertain or poorly measured, then this can be used to define new research questions and hence to guide the collection of empirical data to fill gaps and reduce uncertainties. These new data are then incorporated and the process repeated. This iteration rarely occurs in reality since people who generate empirical data and those who write models often work independently. Our research team (the UK National Wildlife Management Centre and its precursors), are therefore relatively unusual in this regard, being responsible for both the longest field study of badgers and bovine TB epidemiology (19), and the evolution of a series of models describing this system. Since reviews of badger/bTB models are already available [e.g., (20, 21)], we provide a historical narrative of the development of these models, the roles they have played in supporting decision-making, and our perspective on the future of modeling in this complex and challenging area of disease management.

HISTORICAL REVIEW

Early badger/bTB models investigated population dynamics in detail since this was the first opportunity to examine data from an ongoing study, resulting in a simple SEI (susceptible, exposed and infectious disease categories) model (22). This work summarized the known information on population dynamics (e.g., fertility and mortality rates). The resultant model suggested

that disease induced mortality was 2.5 times natural mortality and thus exerted a high level of population suppression. The model was used to determine R_0, the expected number of secondary cases produced by one infected case in a completely susceptible population. This is a measure of the transmission potential of a disease and the estimated R_0 lay between 1.9 and 9.7, which reflected the level of parameter uncertainty. This model also explored pseudo-vertical transmission (i.e., mother to offspring transmission via close contact or ingestion of infected milk), the potential presence of asymptomatic carriers of infection, environmental reservoirs and inactive (short-term non-infectious) cases. With hindsight we can see that consideration of these phenomena illustrates the short-fall in empirical evidence on disease progression at the time (23).

The next model was an SEIR (SEI plus a recovered category) model and a parameter search used to refine population and epidemiological values (24). However, the inclusion of a "recovered" class was not itself tested, and has not been implemented in most other models. A further variant was the SEI_1I_2 model which permitted two levels of infectiousness (associated with early and advanced disease) and pseudo-vertical transmission (25). Investigation of six potential model structures suggested that those with two levels of infectiousness had some support.

The construction of an individual-based simulation model permitted the inclusion of territoriality and spatial components (26), which resulted in disease clusters and removed the clear relationship between disease prevalence and population suppression. The use of social groups also meant that the threshold density for disease persistence was now considered as the average minimum social group size that would permit disease maintenance. Although this model also suggested substantial disease-induced population suppression, the effect was reduced by the spatial clustering of disease (26). This was the first model to assess different historical badger management strategies (27): Gassing, Clean Ring, Interim and Live Test strategies (see **Table 1** for definitions). Model outputs suggested that the most efficient strategies were Gassing and the Clean Ring since they may remove foci of infection. The model also explored badger vaccination and concluded that it would take between 10 and 30 years to eradicate bTB with a perfect vaccine, depending on the efficacy of delivery. A later version investigated fertility control (through the use of a theoretical oral contraceptive) and concluded that in isolation this would not eradicate bTB in badgers but that disease control was possible when combined with high levels of culling (30). A simple generic model was used to simulate combined vaccination and fertility control and concluded that the reduced efficacy of vaccination, relative to culling, disappeared when allied with fertility control, and thus a combined approach could be effective (31).

A revision of Smith et al. (25) was the first model to predict limited population suppression (32), which was supported by the field data (33). This model also suggested that culling lactating females only had a limited impact on disease control, which supported the prevailing policy of releasing them.

A return to a simple model investigated the effects of social perturbation [the process of disruption of the social structure of

TABLE 1 | A summary of historical badger control strategies used in England.

Control Strategy	Approach	Estimated Efficacy of control[1]	Area[2]
Gassing	Gassing setts where badgers confirmed with bTB.	90%	Up to 10 km^2
Clean Ring	Cage trap and shoot social groups in an expanding ring where confirmed with bTB	80%	Mean 9 km^2
Interim	Cage trap and shoot badgers on and around confirmed cattle breakdowns	70%	Mean 12 km^2
Live Test	Trial strategy of cage trap and shoot in response to an antibody test.	80%	Mean 1 km^2

[1]from Smith et al. (28), [2]from Krebs et al. (29).

populations subjected to culling: Swinton et al. (34)], which could theoretically increase absolute numbers of infected animals. Both this and a subsequent study (31) also investigated the effect of fertility control, and suggested that lethal control was generally more effective. However, Smith and Cheeseman (31) found that permanent sterility combined with vaccination could be just as effective as lethal control, and would permit disease elimination without risking population extinction. Using updated parameters, a simple mathematical model of badgers and cattle concluded that R_0 was lower than previous estimates, at about 1.1 (35), and was supported by subsequent empirically-derived estimates of 1 to 1.2 (11). These findings suggest that control would require less than a 20% reduction in transmission rates to eliminate disease, although this appears to contrast with field experience.

Simulation models then added cattle, firstly as a simple homogenous set of herds connected to each badger social group (36). This model was used to assess the live test strategy (36), and other historical and prospective strategies (28) including vaccination (37). These studies concluded that the use of a live test required better test sensitivity and that more badgers per group needed testing and that Gassing and the Clean Ring were the most effective historical strategies. The model identified proactive widespread vaccination as the most effective vaccination strategy requiring vaccinating at least 40% of badgers every year to eliminate disease and that combined strategies gave the best initial reduction in cattle herd breakdown rates. Since the models were generating results that could inform policy, there was merit in ensuring the results were robust, so a second independent model was developed using the same input data. Reassuringly, this model gave very similar results (38).

Most of the data came from a field study of bTB epidemiology in badgers (39–42). When the latest models were subjected to sensitivity analysis, the outputs were found to be sensitive to the two infectious classes (particularly the more infectious category, and their mortality rates). This led to more detailed field research, which allowed disease categories and survival rates to be refined (43) and incorporated into subsequent models.

Between 1998 and 2005 a large scale field experiment took place in England, to determine the role of badger culling as a means of controlling bTB in cattle. Results of the Randomised Badger Culling Trial (RBCT) demonstrated that cattle herd breakdown rates were significantly reduced within proactively culled areas, but increased around the edges (4). Subsequent investigations identified significant spatial disruption of badger social group territories after culling (44), which tied in with previous observations of post-cull badger populations, including enhanced movement of surviving animals [reviewed by (45)]. The long-term field data from the Woodchester Park study demonstrated a clear link between badger movement rates and prevalence of bTB in an undisturbed population (46), suggesting that enhanced movements of badgers following culling might have adverse epidemiological outcomes. Thus, the model could now be updated by changing badger behavior (movement probabilities) to generate the pattern of herd breakdowns seen in the field. This approach of pattern-oriented modeling had recently been taking root in ecological models (47, 48). In a subsequent model, badger movement was simulated to match data from field studies (45), and the contact rate amongst badgers increased until the simulated rise in the herd breakdown rate matched that observed during the RBCT (49). The revised model also included a more realistic cattle layer incorporating individual farms and cattle movements, allowing investigation of pre-movement cattle testing, and including farm economics so that a partial cost-benefit analysis could be conducted. Even if most of the badger control costs were borne by the farmer the model concluded that, due to perturbation, the cost-benefit analysis was nearly always negative. Preventing badger immigration, or if perturbation did not occur, an economic benefit was more likely than not (49). If the Government bore the cost of badger culling then even without perturbation, most scenarios indicated an overall economic loss (50).

The Smith et al. (50) model was revised and updated with further field data, and used to investigate different bTB control strategies. In Wales the model was used to inform a decision on what badger management approach to take in an Intensive Action Area (IAA) identified by Government (51–53). The IAA was subjected to badger vaccination, and following 4 years of treatment the model was used to determine the effects of a lack of vaccine in the fifth year (54). This indicated that the fifth year of vaccination would add relatively little to the overall benefit, and no discernable benefit if vaccination was delayed by a year. This suggests that, following 4 years of treatment, herd immunity was raised to a level sufficient to justify a break in vaccination effort. In Northern Ireland, simulations investigated selective badger culling to inform proposals for a trap, live test and cull or vaccinate (TVR) approach (55), which is currently being trialed (56). In England the model was used to assess different culling and vaccination policies and concluded that in order to realize a benefit, badger culling would need to continue for at least 4 years and that low culling efficacy or an early cessation to culling could lead to an increase in the number of herd breakdowns (57).

Other models have investigated different selective or combined badger management strategies (58–60). Supporting previous results, these studies indicated that badger culling may reduce disease prevalence, but alone cannot eradicate bTB, and that combined vaccination strategies may be the most effective. None of the models have found that a single strategy is the most effective, generally agreeing that combined approaches are required, together with strong cattle measures. The deployment of such approaches in the field would provide data to test these predictions. The inability of models to easily eradicate bTB with single approach methods contrasts with the available estimates of R_0, which have suggested that control should be easier to achieve.

Although the principal driver for interest in bTB is to control the disease in cattle, there has been substantially less modeling focused on cattle. However, models of bTB in New Zealand were used to investigate cattle management. These indicated that improved cattle testing (61) and cattle management (62) alone were insufficient to eradicate bTB in the presence of the local wildlife vector (the brushtail possum *Trichosurus vulpecula*). A further model indicated the potential benefits of increased cattle testing, and reduced cattle movement in combination with wildlife vector control (63). These results, combined with output from other models (64–70) were used to inform the eradication strategy (https://ospri.co.nz/our-programmes/tbfree/about-the-tbfree-programme/about-bovine-tb/history-of-tb/).

Other wild mammal species can be infected with *M. bovis* and some may act as maintenance hosts, with potential onward transmission to cattle. In Spain, wild boar *Sus scrofa* and red deer *Cervus elaphus* appear most important as wild reservoirs of infection (71) and in North America white-tailed deer *Odocoileus virginianus* are involved in transmission to cattle (72). A model of bTB in white-tailed deer assessed various vaccination and targeted removal strategies and concluded that vaccination (alone or combined with targeted removal) needed to be undertaken annually to achieve a detectable reduction in prevalence (73), and currently an oral vaccination approach is under investigation (74). However, to date modeling has been applied to a far lesser extent to these situations compared to the badger-cattle bTB system.

The historical evolution of modeling described above clearly indicates where models have been used to inform decision making on bTB control in wildlife. In the badger bTB system, the interplay between field studies and modeling, and the use of models to guide decision making have been particularly prominent. Early models concentrated on increasing our understanding of the system with limited impact on decision making, but derived parameter estimates necessary for later models, which informed further field studies to refine key parameters. Successive models, which have generally included stochasticity, have since played a more explicit role in supporting decision making.

RECOMMENDATIONS

Below we describe a series of recommendations borne out of our experience of data analysis and modeling largely in relation to the badger/bTB system. Our recommendations relate first to themes for future models of bTB in badgers, and second to the presentation of model outputs to decision makers.

Future Models of bTB in Badgers

The following themes could be usefully explored in future models of bTB in badgers, but may also apply to other wildlife disease systems.

1. Recent models suggest that vaccination is a useful tool for controlling bTB in badgers, with the potential to be applied as an exit strategy from culling. Hence, more detailed investigations of vaccination strategies are required. Field and experimental evidence indicate that the current vaccine (BCG) does not provide complete protection from infection (75), but may confer partial protection, or slow down disease progression. To date most models assume that it confers lifetime protection from infection to a given proportion of the vaccinated population. Technically, these models place vaccinated badgers in a different category that has no increased mortality and no ability to infect others. Therefore, these individuals could become infected, and even react to various live tests, but fail to transmit infection, so the models do not actually assume complete protection, but an inability to become infectious. The available empirical data cannot easily distinguish between a proportion of vaccinated animals being very well protected, and all vaccinated animals experiencing slower disease progression. Such partial protection would lead to a reduced efficacy of disease control and requires further investigation in the field and through modeling. Further evidence is also required to determine the duration of protection (whether complete or partial).

2. Intervention duration and frequency have received little attention in models, and could usefully be explored in more detail. Most models assume either continuous or annual application of management, but recent evidence suggests that breaks in treatment may be possible without significant detrimental effects (54). This is important because even short breaks in management of a single year at a time may reduce overall cost and thus improve the economic outcome.

3. Social perturbation in culled badger populations has so far been simulated using a fixed effect, or by pattern-matching model output with field data. Modeling suggests that the presence of perturbation can be pivotal in determining whether a culling strategy is worth pursuing, but perturbation has only been modeled as an on/off effect. Further empirical evidence on the magnitude of perturbation effects encountered under different conditions, and refined model parameterization are vital to more accurately assess likely outcomes of different culling strategies and allow comparison with other approaches.

4. Within-individual level effects have not been explored in badger models. Where animals are tested, or subjected to management interventions (e.g., vaccination) in stochastic models, independence in outcome is assumed. This means that repeated testing (or repeated vaccination), will eventually detect (or sero-convert) every individual. Instead, it may

be that some individuals can never produce a positive test result (or be successfully vaccinated) due to a physiological process/characteristic. This would cause repeated (e.g., annual) management strategies to be less effective, but it is not clear how large such an effect may be.

5. Between-individual effects have not been explored. Most models assume all individuals are the same in terms of their physiological and behavioral responses, although there is clear empirical evidence to the contrary. Social network analyses have revealed individuals occupying different network positions, with associated variation in infection exposure and transmission potential (76). Models that account for individual heterogeneity in transmission rates (within and between species) may be worth investigating with a view to assessing the potential impacts on disease dynamics of removing key individuals in targeted management interventions.

6. Recent interest in selective removal strategies has raised the issue of test performance. In a model the infection status of each individual is perfectly known, whereas test performance determines sensitivity (all infected animals that test negative, regardless of whether latent, infected or infectious). For bTB there is no gold standard test, and thus no way to map an individual onto a simulated categorical state. Thus, test performance is determined globally on the population, and not for each disease state in a model, although empirical evidence suggests some tests have a differential sensitivity according to the stage of disease progression (77, 78). Also, novel probabilistic approaches to describing infection status may help us to incorporate uncertainty in test outcomes and provide a more meaningful way to categorize individuals (79).

7. Theoretical studies have suggested that fertility control may be a useful tool for disease control, particularly in combination with other approaches, but it has yet to be simulated for specific bTB control strategies. Suitable agents are currently available to induce immunocontraception that may last a number of years from a single dose (80) and these are under investigation for badgers, which are unusual in having delayed implantation (http://sciencesearch.defra.gov.uk/Default.aspx?Menu=Menu&Module=More&Location=None&Completed=0&ProjectID=17952).

8. There still appears to be a disconnect between the calculation of R_0 (close to 1.0), and the high level and lengthy duration of control required to achieve disease eradication in stochastic models. The duration of control is not technically a problem, since R_0 indicates the level of control required and tells us nothing about the duration. So this disconnect may be because model simulations are not of sufficient duration, or a result of other issues such as the spatial distribution of animals and disease.

Presenting Model Outputs to Decision Makers

It is clear from our experience that some modeling is more informative to decision makers than others. Below we suggest steps to help improve the relevance of modeling to decision makers.

1. It is important to know whether the purpose of the model is to help inform decision making, or to explore the system under study. In the former, the question to be investigated needs to be clearly articulated, ideally with the involvement of decision makers. The question should be specific, with an example graph or table in mind as the output, which allows both parties to agree on the output metric.

2. What the model does and does not include should be agreed with the decision maker. For example, it should be established whether a wildlife bTB model should include cattle so as to estimate changes in herd breakdown rates, or social perturbation arising from the intervention. The model should include all those components that the decision maker regards as important if they are to trust the output, or demonstrate that such components have very limited effect on the output.

3. Models that are well described and identify their assumptions and limitations, are given more weight by decision makers. Mathematical descriptions of model processes may be required for scientific publication, but flow charts are easier to follow. There are also guidelines to present the description of complex individual based models (81, 82).

4. Model description should include details of verification and validation, and some level of sensitivity and uncertainty analysis. Verification is the process of checking that the model does what is expected, and validation is the process of checking output against real world data (where possible). Sensitivity or uncertainty analysis can be used to demonstrate that a decision should be robust to the parameter uncertainty.

5. Model output is often best described in terms of the potential decision, rather than as a prediction of future trends. Models are simplifications, and are unable to capture the future variability of the real world. However, the performance of two modeled strategies will suffer to the same degree from these issues, and so can provide valuable information on their likely relative benefits and hence inform decision making. For the purposes of comparison it may be useful to determine how often one strategy outperforms another, as this will increase confidence in any selection.

These recommendations have applications beyond the bTB/badger system. Specific themes such as those relating to vaccination efficacy, the potential for management interventions to change host behavior and influence disease dynamics in counter-productive ways, and the performance of diagnostic tests are broadly applicable. This illustrates how the body of work on modeling bTB has contributed to our general understanding of the dynamics and management of disease in wildlife hosts and demonstrated how to model these systems.

AUTHOR CONTRIBUTIONS

All authors listed have made a substantial, direct and intellectual contribution to the work, and approved it for publication.

REFERENCES

1. Lomnicki A. The place of modelling in ecology. *Oikos* (1988) 52:139–42. doi: 10.2307/3565240

2. Palmer MV, Thacker TC, Waters WR, Gortázar C, Corner LAL. *Mycobacterium bovis*: A Model Pathogen at the Interface of Livestock, Wildlife, and Humans. *Vet Med Int.* (2012) 2012:17. doi: 10.1155/2012/236205

3. Griffin JM, Williams DH, Kelly GE, Clegg TA, O'Boyle I, Collins JD, et al. The impact of badger removal on the control of tuberculosis in cattle herds in Ireland. *Prev Vet Med.* (2005) 67:237–66. doi: 10.1016/j.prevetmed.2004.10.009

4. Donnelly CA, Woodroffe R, Cox DR, Bourne FJ, Cheeseman CL, Clifton-Hadley RS, et al. Positive and negative effects of widespread badger culling on tuberculosis in cattle. *Nature* (2006) 439:843–6. doi: 10.1038/nature04454

5. Donnelly CA, Wei G, Johnston WT, Cox DR, Woodroffe R, Bourne FJ, et al. Impacts of widespread badger culling on cattle tuberculosis: concluding analyses from a large-scale field trial. *Int J Infect Dis.* (2007) 11:300–8. doi: 10.1016/j.ijid.2007.04.001

6. Byrne A, White P, McGrath G, O'Keeffe J, Martin S. Risk of tuberculosis cattle herd breakdowns in Ireland: effects of badger culling effort, density and historic large-scale interventions. *Vet Res.* (2014) 45:109. doi: 10.1186/s13567-014-0109-4

7. Lesellier S, Palmer S, Dalley DJ, Davé D, Johnson L, Hewinson RG, et al. The safety and immunogenicity of Bacillus Calmette-Guérin (BCG) vaccine in European badgers (*Meles meles*). *Vet Immunol Immunopathol.* (2006) 112:24–37. doi: 10.1016/j.vetimm.2006.03.009

8. Corner LAL, Murphy D, Costello E, Gormley E. Tuberculosis in European badgers (*Meles meles*) and the control of infection with Bacille Calmette-Guerin vaccination. *J Wildl Dis.* (2009) 45:1042–7. doi: 10.7589/0090-3558-45.4.1042

9. Anon. (2012). More than 1400 badgers vaccinated in Wales. *Vet Rec.* 171:578. doi:10.1136/vr.e8179

10. Aznar I, Frankena K, More SJ, O'Keeffe J, McGrath G, de Jong MCM. Quantification of *Mycobacterium bovis* transmission in a badger vaccine field trial. *Prev Vet Med.* (2018) 149:29–37. doi: 10.1016/j.prevetmed.2017.10.010

11. Delahay RJ, Walker N, Smith GS, Wilkinson D, Clifton-hadley RS, Cheeseman CL, et al. Long-term temporal trends and estimated transmission rates for *Mycobacterium bovis* infection in an undisturbed high-density badger (*Meles meles*) population. *Epidemiol Infect* (2013) 141:1445–56. doi: 10.1017/S0950268813000721

12. Corner LAL, Murphy D, Gormley E. *Mycobacterium bovis* infection in the eurasian badger (*Meles meles*): the disease, pathogenesis, epidemiology and control. *J Comp Pathol.* (2011) 144:1–24. doi: 10.1016/j.jcpa.2010.10.003

13. Clifton-Hadley RS, Wilesmith JW, Stuart FA. *Mycobacterium bovis* in the European badger (*Meles meles*): epidemiological findings in tuberculous badgers from a naturally infected population. *Epidemiol Infect.* (1993) 111:9–19. doi: 10.1017/S0950268800056624

14. Jenkins HE, Cox DR, Delahay RJ. Direction of association between bite wounds and *Mycobacterium bovis* infection in badgers: implications for transmission. *PLoS ONE* (2012) 7:e45584. doi: 10.1371/journal.pone.0045584

15. Courtenay O, Reilly LA, Sweeney FP, Hibberd V, Bryan S, Ul-Hassan A, et al. Is *Mycobacterium bovis* in the environment important for the persistence of bovine tuberculosis? *Biol Lett.* (2006) 2:460–2. doi: 10.1098/rsbl.2006.0468

16. Corner LAL, O'Meara D, Costello E, Lesellier S, Gormley E. The distribution of *Mycobacterium bovis* infection in naturally infected badgers. *Vet J.* (2012) 194:166–72.

17. Drewe JA, O'Connor HM, Weber N, McDonald RA, Delahay RJ. Patterns of direct and indirect contact between cattle and badgers naturally infected with tuberculosis. *Epidemiol Infect.* (2013) 141:1467–75. doi: 10.1017/S0950268813000691

18. Mullen EM, MacWhite T, Maher PK, Kelly DJ, Marples NM, Good M. Foraging Eurasian badgers *Meles meles* and the presence of cattle in pastures. Do badgers avoid cattle? *Appl Anim Behav Sci.* (2013) 144:130–7. doi: 10.1016/j.applanim.2013.01.013

19. McDonald JL, Robertson A, Silk MJ. Wildlife disease ecology from the individual to the population: insights from a long-term study of a naturally-infected European badger population. *J Anim Ecol.* (2018) 87:101–12. doi: 10.1111/1365-2656.12743

20. Smith GC. Models of *Mycobacterium bovis* in wildlife and cattle. *Tuberculosis* (2001) 81:51–64. doi: 10.1054/tube.2000.0264

21. Smith GC. Modelling bovine tuberculosis in wildlife and cattle. In: Smithe LT, editors. *Progress in Tuberculosis Research Nova Science.* New York, NY: Nova Science (2005) p. 249–80.

22. Anderson RM, Trewhella W. Population dynamics of the badger (*Meles meles*) and the epidemiology of bovine tuberculosis (*Mycobacterium bovis*). *Phil Trans R Soc Lond B* (1985) 310:327–81. doi: 10.1098/rstb.1985.0123

23. Cheeseman CL, Little TWA, Mallinson PJ, Rees WA, Wilesmith JW. The progression of bovine tuberculosis infection in a population of *Meles meles* in south-west England. *Acta Zool Fenn.* (1985) 173:197–9.

24. Bentil DE, Murray JD. Modelling bovine tuberculosis in badgers. *J Anim Ecol.* (1993) 62:239–50.

25. Smith GC, Richards MS, Clifton-Hadley RS, Cheeseman CL. Modelling bovine tuberculosis in badgers in England: preliminary results. *Mammalia* (1995) 59:639–50. doi: 10.1515/mamm.1995.59.4.639

26. White PCL, Harris S. Bovine tuberculosis in badger (*Meles meles*) populations in southwest England: the use of a spatial stochastic simulation model to understand the dynamics of the disease. *Phil Trans R Soc Lond B* (1995) 349:391–413.

27. White PCL, Harris S. Bovine tuberculosis in badger (*Meles meles*) populations in southwest England: an assessment of past, present and possible future control strategies using simulation modelling. *Phil Trans R Soc Lond B* (1995) 349:415–32.

28. Smith GC, Cheeseman CL, Clifton-Hadley RS, Wilkinson D. A model of bovine tuberculosis in the badger *Melesmeles*: an evaluation of control strategies. *J Appl Ecol.* (2001) 38:509–19. doi: 10.1046/j.1365-2664.2001.00609.x

29. Krebs JR, Anderson RM, Clutton-Brock T, Morrison I, Young D, Donnelly C. *Bovine Tuberculosis in Cattle and Badgers.* London: MAFF Publications (1997).

30. White PCL, Lewis AJG, Harris S. Fertility control as a means of controlling bovine tuberculosis in badger (*Meles meles*) populations in south-west England: predictions from a spatial stochastic simulation model. *Proc R Soc B* (1997) 264:1737–47. doi: 10.1098/rspb.1997.0241

31. Smith GC, Cheeseman CL. A mathematical model for control of diseases in wildlife populations: culling, vaccine and fertility control. *Ecol Model.* (2002) 150:45–53. doi: 10.1016/S0304-3800(01)00471-9

32. Smith GC, Cheeseman CL, and Clifton-Hadley RS. Modelling the control of bovine tuberculosis in badgers in England: culling and the release of lactating females. *J Appl Ecol.* (1997) 34:1375–86.

33. Wilkinson D, Smith GC, Delahay R, Rogers LM, Cheeseman CL, Clifton-Hadley RS. The effects of bovine tuberculosis (*Mycobacterium bovis*) on mortality in a badger (*Meles meles*) population in England. *J Zool.* (2000) 250:389–95. doi: 10.1111/j.1469-7998.2000.tb00782.x

34. Swinton J, Tuyttens F, Macdonald D, Nokes DJ, Cheeseman CL, Clifton-Hadley R. A comparison of fertility control and lethal control of bovine tuberculosis in badgers: the impact of perturbation induced transmission. *Phil Trans R Soc Lond B* (1997) 352:619–31. doi: 10.1098/rstb.1997.0042

35. Cox DR, Donnelly CA, Bourne FJ, Gettinby G, McInerney JP, Morrison WI, et al. Simple model for tuberculosis in cattle and badgers. *Proc Natl Acad Sci USA.* (2005) 102:17588–93. doi: 10.1073/pnas.0509003102

36. Smith GC, Cheeseman CL, Wilkinson D, Clifton-Hadley RS. A model of bovine tuberculosis in the badger *Meles meles*: the inclusion of cattle and the use of a live test. *J Appl Ecol.* (2001) 38:520–35. doi: 10.1046/j.1365-2664.2001.00610.x

37. Wilkinson D, Smith GC, Delahay RJ, Cheeseman CL. A model of bovine tuberculosis in the badger *Meles meles*: an evaluation of different vaccination strategies. *J Appl Ecol.* (2004) 41:492–501. doi: 10.1111/j.0021-8901.2004.00898.x

38. Shirley MDF, Rushton SP, Smith GC, South AB, Lurz PWW. Investigating the spatial dynamics of bovine tuberculosis in badger populations: evaluating an individual-based simulation model. *Ecol Model.* (2003) 167:139–57. doi: 10.1016/S0304-3800(03)00167-4

39. Cheeseman CL, Wilesmith JW, Ryan J, Mallinson PJ. Badger population dynamics in a high-density area. *Symp Zool Soc Lond.* (1987) 58:279–94.

40. Cheeseman CL, Wilesmith JW, Stuart FA, Mallinson PJ. Dynamics of tuberculosis in a naturally infected Badger population. *Mammal Rev.* (1988) 18:61–72. doi: 10.1111/j.1365-2907.1988.tb00073.x

41. Cheeseman CL, Wilesmith JW, Stuart FA. Tuberculosis: the disease and its epidemiology in the badger, a review. *Epidemiol Infect.* (1989) 103:113–25. doi: 10.1017/S0950268800030417

42. Delahay RJ, Langton S, Smith GC, Clifton-Hadley RS, Cheeseman CL. The spatio-temporal distribution of *Mycobacterium bovis* (bovine tuberculosis) infection in a high density badger population. *J Anim Ecol.* (2000) 69:428–41. doi: 10.1046/j.1365-2656.2000.00406.x

43. Graham J, Smith GC, Delahay RJ, Bailey T, McDonald RA, Hodgson D. Multi-state modelling reveals sex-dependent transmission, progression and severity of tuberculosis in wild badgers. *Epidemiol Infect.* (2013) 141:1429–36. doi: 10.1017/S0950268812003019

44. Woodroffe R, Gilks P, Johnston WT, Le Fevre AM, Cox DR, Donnelly CA, et al. Effects of culling on badger abundance: implications for tuberculosis control. *J Zool.* (2008) 274:28–37. doi: 10.1111/j.1469-7998.2007.00353.x

45. Carter SP, Delahay RJ, Smith GC, Macdonald DW, Riordan P, Etherington TR, et al. Culling-induced social perturbation in Eurasian badgers *Meles meles* and the management of TB in cattle: an analysis of a critical problem in applied ecology. *Proc R Soc B* (2007) 274:2769–77. doi: 10.1098/rspb.2007.0998

46. Vicente J, Delahay RJ, Walker N, Cheeseman CL. Social organization and movement influence the incidence of bovine tuberculosis in an undisturbed high-density badger *Meles meles* population. *J Anim Ecol.* (2007) 76:348–60. doi: 10.1111/j.1365-2656.2006.01199.x

47. Grimm V, Frank K, Jetsch F, Brandl R, Uchmanski J. Pattern-oriented modelling in population ecology. *Sci Tot Environ.* (1996) 183:151–66.

48. Grimm V, Revilla E, Berger U, Jeltsch F, Mooij WM, Railsback SF, et al. Pattern-oriented modeling of agent-based complex systems: lessons from ecology. *Science* (2005) 310:987–91. doi: 10.1126/science.1116681

49. Wilkinson D, Bennett R, McFarlane I, Rushton S, Shirley M, Smith GC. Cost-benefit analysis model of badger (*Meles meles*) culling to reduce cattle herd tuberculosis breakdowns in Britain, with particular reference to badger perturbation. *J Wildl Dis.* (2009) 45:1062–88. doi: 10.7589/0090-3558-45.4.1062

50. Smith GC, Bennet R, Wilkinson D, Cooke R. A cost-benefit analysis of culling badgers to control bovine tuberculosis. *Vet J.* (2007) 173:302–10. doi: 10.1016/j.tvjl.2005.11.017

51. Central Science Laboratory. *Intensive Action Pilot Area - Papers Annex 4.* Welsh Assembly Government (2009). Available online at: https://gov.wales/docs/drah/research/090916annex4en.pdf

52. Central Science Laboratory. *Intensive Action Pilot Area - Papers Annex 5.* Welsh Assembly Government (2009). Available online at: https://gov.wales/docs/drah/research/090916annex5en.pdf

53. Central Science Laboratory. *Intensive Action Pilot Area - Papers Annex 6.* Welsh Assembly Government (2009). Available online at: www.wales.gov.uk/docs/drah/research/090916annex6en.pdf

54. Smith G, Budgey R. *Simulations of the Effect of Badger Vaccination on Bovine Tuberculosis in Badgers and Cattle Within the IAA.* Welsh Government, Welsh Government 10.

55. Smith GC, Delahay RJ, McDonald RA, Budgey R. Model of selective and non-selective management of badgers (*Meles meles*) to control bovine tuberculosis in badgers and cattle. *PLoS ONE* (2016) 11:e0167206. doi: 10.1371/journal.pone.0167206

56. DAERA. *The Test and Vaccinate or Remove (TVR) Wildlife Intervention Research Project: Year 4 Report 2017.* Department of Agriculture, Environment and Rural Affairs, Northern Ireland (2017).

57. Defra. *Comparing Badger (Meles meles) Control Strategies for Reducing Bovine bTB in Cattle in England.* Department for Environment, Food and Rural Affairs London (2010).

58. Hardstaff JL, Bulling MT, Marion G, Hutchings MR, White PCL. Modelling the impact of vaccination on tuberculosis in badgers. *Epidemiol Infection* (2013) 141:1417–27. doi: 10.1017/S0950268813000642

59. Brooks-Pollock E, Wood JLN. Eliminating bovine tuberculosis in cattle and badgers: insight from a dynamic model. *Proc R Soc B* (2015) 282. doi: 10.1098/rspb.2015.0374

60. Abdou M, Frankena K, O'Keeffe J, Byrne AW. Effect of culling and vaccination on bovine tuberculosis infection in a European badger (*Meles meles*) population by spatial simulation modelling. *Prev Vet Med.* (2016) 125:19–30. doi: 10.1016/j.prevetmed.2015.12.012

61. Barlow ND, Kean JM, Hickling G, Livingstone PG, Robson AB. A simulation model for the spread of bovine tuberculosis within New Zealand cattle herds. *Prev Vet Med.* (1997) 32:57–75. doi: 10.1016/S0167-5877(97)00002-0

62. Kao RR, Roberts MG, Ryan TJ. A model of bovine tuberculosis control in domesticated cattle herds. *Proc R Soc B* (1997) 264:1069–76. doi: 10.1098/rspb.1997.0148

63. Barlow ND, Kean JM, Caldwell NP, Ryan TJ. Modelling the regional dynamics and management of bovine tuberculosis in New Zealand cattle herds. *Prev Vet Med.* (1998) 36:25–38. doi: 10.1016/S0167-5877(98)00075-0

64. Barlow ND. A spatially aggregated disease/host model for bovine tb in New Zealand possum populations. *J Appl Ecol.* (1991) 28:777–93.

65. Barlow ND. Control of endemic bovine tb in New Zealand possum populations: results from a simple model. *J Appl Ecol.* (1991) 28:794–809.

66. Barlow ND. Model for controlling bovine tuberculosis in possums. *ASIT Newsletter* (1991) 3:10–11.

67. Barlow ND. A model for the spread of bovine Tb in New Zealand possum populations. *J Appl Ecol.* (1993) 30:156–64.

68. Pfeiffer D, Cochrane T, Stern M, Morris R. A geographical simulation models of bovine tuberculosis in wild possum populations. In: Griffin F, de Lisle G, editors. *Tuberculosis in Wildlife and Domestic Animals.* Dunedin: University of Otago Press (1995). p 165–7.

69. Fulford GR, Roberts MG, Heesterbeek JAP. The metapopulation dynamics of an infectious disease: tuberculosis in possums. *Theor Popul Biol.* (2002) 61:15–29. doi: 10.1006/tpbi.2001.1553

70. Ramsey DSL, Efford MG. Management of bovine tuberculosis in brushtail possums in New Zealand: predictions from a spatially explicit, individual-based model. *J Anim Ecol.* (2010) 47:911–9. doi: 10.1111/j.1365-2664.2010.01839.x

71. Vicente J, Höfle U, Garrido JM, Fernandez-de-Mera IG, Juste R, Barral M, et al. Wild boar and red deer display high prevalences of tuberculosis-like lesions in Spain. *Vet Res.* (2006) 37:107–19. doi: 10.1051/vetres:2005044

72. Schmitt SM, Fitzgerald SD, Cooley TM, Bruning-Fann CS, Sullivan L, Berry D, et al. Bovine tuberculosis in free-ranging white-tailed deer from Michigan. *J Wildl Dis.* (1997) 33:749–58.

73. Cosgrove MK, Campa H, Ramsey DSL, Schmitt SM, O'Brien DJ. Modeling vaccination and targeted removal of white-tailed deer in Michigan for bovine tuberculosis control. *Wildl Soc Bull.* (2012) 36:676–84. doi: 10.1002/wsb.217

74. Dressel D. *Development of Strategies to Orally Deliver Vaccine for Bovine Tuberculosis to White-Tailed Deer of Northeastern Lower Michigan.* Fisheries and Wildlife: Michigan State University (2017).

75. Chambers MA, Rogers F, Delahay RJ, Lesellier S, Ashford R, Dalley D, et al. Bacillus Calmette-Guérin vaccination reduces the severity and progression of tuberculosis in badgers. *Proc R Soc B Biol Sci.* (2011) 278:1913–20. doi: 10.1098/rspb.2010.1953

76. Weber N, Carter SP, Dall SR, Delahay RJ, McDonald JL, Bearhop S, et al. Badger social networks correlate with tuberculosis infection. *Current Biol.* (2013) 23:R915–916. doi: 10.1016/j.cub.2013.09.011

77. Chambers MA, Pressling WA, Cheeseman CL, Clifton-Hadley RS, Hewinson RG. Value of existing serological tests for identifying badgers that shed *Mycobacterium bovis*. *Vet Microbiol.* (2002) 86:183–9. doi: 10.1016/S0378-1135(02)00012-3

78. Chambers MA. Review of the diagnosis of tuberculosis in non-bovid wildlife species using immunological methods – an update of published work since 2009. *Transboun Emerg Dis.* (2013) 60:14–27. doi: 10.1111/tbed.12094

79. Buzdugan SN, Vergne T, Grosbois V, Delahay RJ, Drewe JA. Inference of the infection status of individuals using longitudinal testing data from cryptic populations: towards a probabilistic approach to diagnosis. *Sci Reports* (2017) 7:1111. doi: 10.1038/s41598-017-00806-4

80. Massei G, Cowan D. Fertility control to mitigate human–wildlife conflicts: a review. *Wildl Res.* (2014) 41:1–21. doi: 10.1071/WR13141

81. Grimm V, Berger U, Bastiansen F, Eliassen S, Ginot V, Giske J, et al. A standard protocol for describing individual-based and agent-based models. *Ecol Model.* (2006). 198:115–26. doi: 10.1016/j.ecolmodel.2006.04.023

82. Grimm V, Berger U, DeAngelis DL, Polhill JG, Giske J, Railsback SF. The ODD protocol: a review and first update. *Ecol Model.* (2010) 221:2760–8. doi: 10.1016/j.ecolmodel.2010.08.019

10

Mycobacterium caprae Infection of Red Deer in Western Austria–Optimized use of Pathology Data to Infer Infection Dynamics

Annette Nigsch[1]*, Walter Glawischnig[2], Zoltán Bagó[2] and Norbert Greber[3]

[1] *Department of Animal Sciences, Quantitative Veterinary Epidemiology, Wageningen University, Wageningen, Netherlands,*
[2] *Institute for Veterinary Disease Control, Austrian Agency for Health and Food Safety, Innsbruck and Mödling, Mödling, Austria,* [3] *Department for Veterinary Affairs, Office of the State Government of Vorarlberg, Bregenz, Austria*

*Correspondence:
Annette Nigsch
annettenigsch@gmx.at

Austria is officially bovine tuberculosis (TB) free, but during the last decade the west of the country experienced sporadic TB cases in cattle. Free-ranging red deer are known to be the maintenance host of *Mycobacterium (M.) caprae* in certain areas in Austria, where cattle can become infected on alpine pastures shared with deer. The epidemiology of TB in deer in alpine regions is still poorly understood. To inform decisions on efficient interventions against TB in deer, a method is needed to better capture the infection dynamics on population level. A total of 4,521 free-ranging red deer from Austria's most western Federal state Vorarlberg were TB-tested between 2009 and 2018. *M. caprae* was confirmed in samples from 257 animals. Based on descriptions of TB-like lesions, TB positive animals were categorized with a newly developed lesion score called "Patho Score." Analyses using this Patho Score allowed us to distinguish between endemic, epidemic and sporadic TB situations and revealed different roles of subgroups of infected deer in infection dynamics. Overall, deer in poor condition, deer of older age and stags were the subgroups that were significantly more often TB positive ($p = 0.02$ or smaller for all subgroups). Deer in poor condition ($p < 0.001$) and stags ($p = 0.04$) also showed more often advanced lesions, indicating their role in mycobacterial spread. TB was never detected in fawns, while hinds were the subgroup that showed the fewest advanced lesions. Analysis of outbreaks of TB and lesion development in yearlings provided some evidence for the role of winter feeding as a source for increased infection transmission. Sporadic cases in TB-free areas appear to precede outbreaks in these areas. These currently TB-free areas should receive particular attention in sampling schemes to be able to detect early spreading of the infection. The Patho Score is a quick, easy-to-apply and reproducible tool that provides new insights on the epidemiology of TB in deer at population level and is flexible enough to relate heterogeneous wildlife monitoring data collected following different sampling plans. This lesion score was used for systematic assessment of infection dynamics of mycobacterial infections.

Keywords: tuberculosis, *Mycobacterium caprae*, red deer, Austria, lesion score, infection dynamics

INTRODUCTION

Mycobacterium caprae (*M. caprae*) is part of the *Mycobacterium tuberculosis complex* (MTBC) and is the causal agent of tuberculosis (TB) of cattle and free-ranging red deer (*Cervus elaphus elaphus*) in the border area between western Austria and southern Germany (1–4). In this area, red deer have been identified as TB reservoir that spreads the pathogen through direct or indirect contact to cattle (5). Transmission of TB between wildlife and farmed animals can occur in both directions.

In red deer, TB is a subacute to chronic disease that is associated with emaciation at an advanced stage, but usually does not lead to marked clinical signs (6). TB is commonly diagnosed by presence of lesions in lymph nodes or organs (7). Tonsils are understood to be the main port of entry (8, 9). The medial retropharyngeal lymph nodes drain the tonsils, which is probably the way these lymph nodes become infected (10–12). Accordingly, medial retropharyngeal lymph nodes are often targeted in early detection and monitoring programs (13, 14). As disease progresses within the host, mediastinal and tracheobronchial lymph nodes, lungs, as well as mesenteric lymph nodes can become affected (15). Deer can also show lesions on pleura, in organs within the abdominal cavity, testicles and udder including their regional or subcutaneous lymph nodes (16).

Lesions indicative for TB in red deer range from pinhead-sized to more than 10 cm (in diameter) large granulomas or abscesses. Lesions develop progressively during the subsequent stages of disease and increase in size and number over time. Thin-walled connective tissue capsules containing creamy yellowish-white pus are typical for advanced stages (2, 15–17). These thin-walled abscesses lead in severe cases of generalized TB to high excretion of mycobacteria and thus an increased infectivity of affected animals (6, 18). TB in red deer was reported to be associated with up to 25% of infected animals without macroscopically visible lesions (2, 12). Nugent (19) identified an area in which even 23 (68%) out of 34 culture positive deer had no visible lesions. There are indications that deer that do not die within a year or two of becoming infected can survive for many years (19). Although the detailed pathogenesis of TB in red deer is not fully understood, there is increasing evidence in literature that species-specific stressors, behavioral and environmental factors as well as genetic factors influence susceptibility to mycobacteria (20, 21).

To better understand the development of slowly progressing diseases such as TB on population level, knowledge of the underlying infection dynamics is decisive: when and where did whom spread infection to whom? Especially in the case of wildlife, it is important to exploit all available information to create a valid overall picture and to be able to better target control measures. Another relevant question is the role of subgroups of animals within the deer population for the maintenance and the spread of TB.

This work aims to characterize dynamics of TB transmission within the red deer population to provide evidence for optimized monitoring and control of TB in alpine areas. We also will be investigating whether qualitative and quantitative criteria of TB-like lesions are a suitable indicator to show and measure infection dynamics of TB in deer. On the basis of readily available data, the impact of population structure, time and space will be investigated retrospectively:

- Population structure: do subgroups of animals within the deer population play different roles for the maintenance and the spread of TB?
- Time: did the infection dynamics of TB in red deer in Vorarlberg change between 2009 and 2018?
- Space: are different patterns of infection dynamics observable in the TB zones?

HISTORY OF *Mycobacterium caprae* IN RED DEER IN VORARLBERG, AUSTRIA

Austria is recognized as an officially bovine TB-free (OTF) country since 1999. Anecdotal observations suggest that TB was present in deer in the most western Austrian state of Vorarlberg prior to 1999: animals with spherical abscesses of the mesenteric lymph nodes were seen which were later referred to as "ball deer". But these cases have never been investigated with laboratory diagnostics. The first confirmed TB case in deer in Vorarlberg was recorded in 2006.

In 2008, TB cases in cattle were reported from the neighboring Austrian state Tyrol, which were linked to infected deer. As a consequence, the first systematic deer monitoring was started in Vorarlberg in 2009 with the aim to assess the risk of TB infection spread to its own cattle population. In the first year of this deer monitoring, *M. caprae* was detected in seven out of a total of 71 examined deer. Since then, TB in deer has been under constant observation. The TB cases are concentrated at a hotspot in two valleys (Klostertal and Montafon north of the river Ill, marked in red as "core area" in **Figure 1**). About 25–30 km north of this hotspot, TB is detected sporadically in deer in the border area with Tyrol and Germany.

In the alpine areas of Vorarlberg, agriculture mainly consists of small cattle farms with 5–20 animals in extensive farming. A special management practice is the annual transhumance of cattle on alpine pastures above 1,600 m for up to 100 days during summer. During summer, deer also prefer sub-alpine and alpine areas at altitudes up to 2,500 m, where cooler temperatures predominate, and nutrient-rich forage is available. In certain areas, this traditional grazing leads to intensified contacts between deer and cattle. In 2010 TB was also confirmed in cattle in Vorarlberg. In consequence, control measures targeting deer were started in 2011 with intensive hunting under adapted conditions, i.e. the statuary close season (no hunting allowed) was shortened and limits on culling of antlerless animals were abolished in defined areas. Control measures were continuously extended and intensified in parallel to the developments of TB in deer and cattle in order to meet the required increasing total kill numbers in accordance with the official hunting plan.

In deer, TB prevalence seemed to have reached its plateau in 2013 (22). In the TB zone with the highest prevalence ("core zone"), 16 (25%) out of 62 deer samples examined were TB

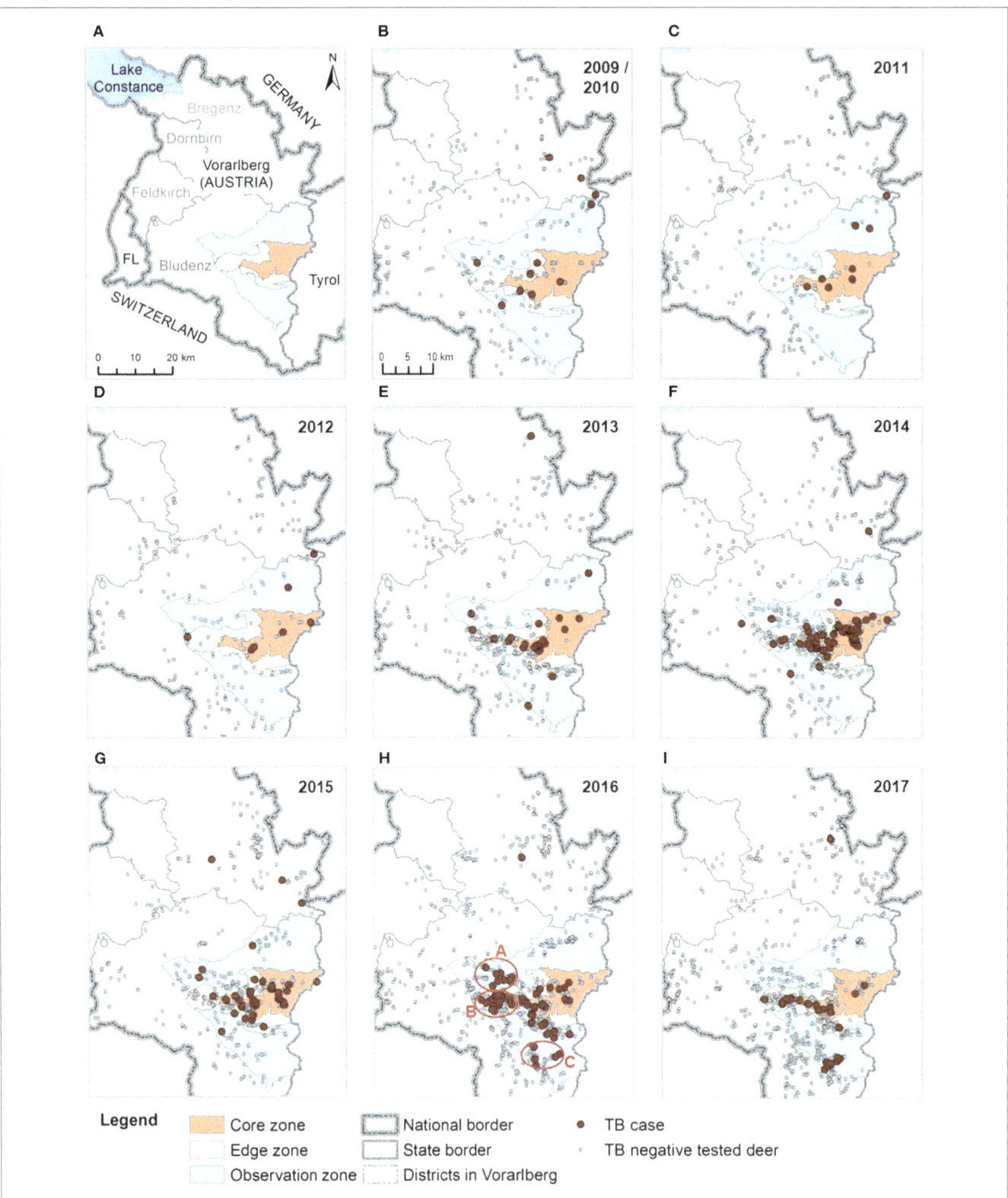

FIGURE 1 | Overview map **(A)** and series of detailed maps of kill locations of TB positive and TB negative deer **(B–I)**, 2009–2017. The core, edge and observation zones form together the TB control area. White areas with kill locations indicate the area outside the TB control area. Cases of the years 2009 and 2010 are shown together in one **(B)**. In 2016 **(H)**, three spots (A–C) with outbreak-like TB are marked in red. FL, Principality of Liechtenstein.

positive in 2013. In the cattle population, TB reached its peak in the winter of 2015/2016 with the detection of *M. caprae* in 30 animals from 13 herds of a total of 9,005 tested cattle from 728 herds (23). In the remaining years between 2013 and 2017, TB was annually confirmed in 4–8 animals from 2 to 7 farms in Vorarlberg (23). The current TB situation does not risk Austria's OTF status yet. The OTF status of a country is based on bovine animals, and a country recognized as OTF will keep this status even though wildlife in the country may be affected, as long as legal conditions are satisfied (Directive 64/432/EEC). However, TB cases in deer require extensive monitoring activities in the cattle population within known deer TB areas. In addition to negative effects on agriculture, hunting and the risk to human health due to this zoonotic agent, annual TB cases led to very high medial and political interest. This interest resulted in part in external pressure for those involved in the control program and reduced their willingness to cooperate in TB control.

Monitoring Tuberculosis in Cattle and Wildlife

All cattle with potential contact to TB-infected deer are annually examined with the comparative intradermal tuberculin skin test between late November and February, and all animals with non-negative skin tests are culled according to legal requirements. Contact animals are traced, and cattle herds are culled if testing indicates a within-herd prevalence of >40%. In addition, all cattle are inspected for TB at the abattoir as part of the national routine TB surveillance. The combination of these measures aims to reduce the risk of undetected TB cases due to imperfect test sensitivity and to ensure that cattle are TB negative in spring before the start of the grazing period. New TB cases diagnosed in cattle in the subsequent testing period led to the conclusion that the main direction of infection is deer-to-cattle, partly followed by spread from cattle-to-cattle within the infected herd. Spoligotyping (24) and mycobacterial interspersed repetitive unit-variable number of tandem repeat typing (25, 26) confirmed for Vorarlberg that all *M. caprae*-positive deer and cattle tested shared the same genotype "Lechtal" (27).

In addition to cattle and red deer, other wildlife species (badgers, foxes, chamois, roe deer) were tested, albeit not systematically. TB could only be detected in a roebuck in 2017, which was hunted in the known TB area (28). Wild boars are rare in Vorarlberg and have not been sampled to date. Based on current evidence, there is no indication of any significant role of other wildlife species in maintenance of TB infection in wildlife populations or for infection transmission to cattle.

Red Deer Management in Vorarlberg

Deer hunting is organized by hunting grounds. Deer hunt is seasonal, with a smaller peak in kills in spring and the main kill season in fall. The fall season accounts for two-thirds of the annual hunting bag. In the winter months between end of December to end of March hunting is generally suspended, with the exception of killing of sick or injured deer. An estimated one third of the deer population is hunter harvested each year, with higher percentages in the TB areas due to control measures in place.

A significant cause for establishment and persistence of TB in deer in Vorarlberg is seen in the marked increase in deer densities in certain regions (29). In the 1970s, a change in deer management practices led to a large increase in deer populations far beyond the natural capacity of deer habitats (30). In parallel, extensive developments in land use, such as growth of settlement areas in alpine valleys, the expansion of infrastructure and increase in tourism have reduced habitat of deer. This meant that deer were forced, against their traditions, to spend the winter at higher altitudes. In order to compensate for limited availability of feed and as strategic intervention to protect avalanche protection forests, winter feeding is nowadays carried out during 140 and 200 days a year (31). Winter feeding not only reduces mortality among weakened animals but will also generate artificially high deer densities around feeding sites. Close contact between animals of different age groups supports direct and indirect transmission of TB (32, 33). Winter feeding of deer is still allowed in Vorarlberg. Since 2017, however, there have been restrictions on choice of feed and more elaborate rules for cleaning and disinfecting feeding sites in spring. Additionally, feeding sites are fenced off with cattle-proof fences during the grazing period (34).

Validated information on deer densities over large-scale administrative areas does not exist for Vorarlberg. However, it is known that densities vary largely across alpine regions with considerable seasonal differences: the highest concentration of deer will be recorded around winter feeding sites on harsh winter days with thick snow cover, with focal concentrations of five up to 300 animals on a small number of hectares. In mild winters, groups of deer at feeding sites will be smaller due to availability of natural feed. In summer, deer are distributed over wider areas and groups of deer grazing together are often small (±10 animals) and will rarely reach group sizes of up to 70–100 animals. Radio telemetry studies showed that the summer habitat of deer in alpine areas can be 1.5–4.5 times larger in size compared to winter habitat (35).

International Aspects of Infection in Wildlife

Sporadic TB cases in deer in the north of Vorarlberg form a shared deer TB area with Tyrol and Germany (5). In addition, neighboring Switzerland and the Principality of Liechtenstein are at risk of introduction of TB by animal trade and cross-border migration of deer (see **Figure 1A**, for an overview map). Radio telemetry studies showed that some deer cross the border after the snowmelt, spend the summer in a neighboring country and return to their winter habitat in their "home" country in autumn. Through these migratory individuals the deer populations of Vorarlberg, Switzerland and Liechtenstein are in seasonal contact (35). Deer are monitored for TB both in deer TB areas of Austria and Germany, as well as in TB-free border areas of Switzerland and Liechtenstein. Efforts are made by the four countries to increase comparability of their currently not yet harmonized monitoring programs in order to obtain a transnational overview of the TB situation in deer, as well as to develop a common control strategy (36).

MATERIALS AND METHODS
Study Population and Deer Monitoring
The study population consisted of all free-ranging red deer examined from February 2009 to March 2018 in the deer monitoring in Vorarlberg. The total of 4,521 sampled animals of all age groups were hunter harvested (99.6%) or found dead (0.4%). According to the deer population structure and in line with requirements of deer monitoring, younger and female deer were examined more frequently, with 1,297 (48.2%) deer ≤ 2 years and 2,170 (55.5%) females. A total of 172 (4.0%) animals were in poor condition.

Deer monitoring is carried out in all parts of Vorarlberg with deer habitats and distinguishes four zones corresponding to TB prevalence: the area with highest prevalence is the 103 km^2 large "core zone", surrounded by the "edge zone" (77 km^2) and the "observation zone" (346 km^2). Core, edge and observation zones form together the 526 km^2 large TB control area (46.95° N to 47.25° in latitude, and from 09.80° to 10.22° W in longitude) in the district of Bludenz. The fourth zone are the remaining deer habitats in Vorarlberg outside the designated TB control area (1,591 km^2) where TB has so far been detected only sporadically in deer, mainly in the north in the district of Bregenz (**Figure 1**). The boundaries of the zones are largely formed by mountain chains and rivers which allow restricted deer movements between zones. Deer abundance is similar in all four zones, with a variation of areas with high and low deer numbers within every zone (37).

Within the 9-year monitoring period, the size of the TB control area and sample size per zone, split by sex and age group, were regularly adjusted depending on case distributions in previous years and published in the annual official deer monitoring program plan (34). Annual sample sizes ranged between 71 and 940 sampled deer. In the hunting season April 2017 to March 2018 all hunter harvested deer except fawns were sampled in core and edge zones ($n = 211$) in accordance with this plan. In the observation zone at least 25% of the hunting bag had to be examined ($n = 215$). Additionally, all deer found dead and sick deer from the whole TB control area had to be investigated. The area outside the TB control area accounted for 401 samples or 20% of the annual hunting bag of deer ≥ 1 year. The sampled deer do not represent a single random sample.

Sampling and Diagnostic Methods
Trained hunters checked the deer at the kill location for external abnormalities. Subsequently, thoracic and abdominal cavities of animals were opened, and internal organs examined visually, and partly palpated. If no tissue abnormalities were observed, the standard sampling consisted of lung with its tributary lymph nodes (tracheobronchal and mediastinal lymph nodes) and larynx with medial retropharyngeal lymph nodes ("head and thorax" samples). As the entire hunting bag was sampled in core and edge zones, requirements for sample materials were relaxed for antlerless deer: the tissues to be sampled could be reduced to the head with medial retropharyngeal lymph nodes ("head-only" samples).

From deer with visible tissue abnormalities, the carcass including all internal organs had to be presented for examination to an official veterinarian. Deer found dead and deer in poor condition were as a rule sampled by veterinarians. In addition to standard sample materials, all parts of the carcass with gross lesions were required to be submitted to the Institute for Veterinary Disease Control, Austrian Agency for Health and Food Safety (AGES), Innsbruck. The reality of the given field conditions is that the sampling process and sampled tissues were quite heterogeneous.

Submitted sample material was pathomorphologically examined and all gross lesions were recorded. Lymph nodes with no visible lesions were dissected into 2–4 mm thick slices to detect even small granulomas. Tissue samples with lesions were cultured for 12 weeks at 37°C and MTBC species differentiation was performed by PCR. The analytical protocol to confirm infection with M. caprae was described by Fink et al. (5) in detail.

Development of the Patho Score
To allow spatial-temporal analysis and comparison of the pathomorphological lesion descriptions in free text, a lesion score ("Patho Score") was developed (**Table 1**). Based on this score, lesions can be subdivided into six categories (score 0–5) depending on their size, number and distribution in the body. The higher the score, the more advanced stage of TB is observed, with score 0 for non-visible lesions. Each examined animal receives a score for the whole package of submitted sample materials. If the sample material is incomplete, Patho Score tends to underestimate disease progress. The interpretation of the score is based on the hypothesis that TB lesions develop progressively and can be grouped and ordered according to their developmental stage.

The criteria for the Patho Score were: a valid, simple and comprehensible measurement tool with good discrimination,

---

TABLE 1 | Patho Score for the categorization of TB-like lesions in deer.

Score	Lesion
0	Non-visible lesion
1	Singular or multiple lesions with <5 mm in Retro 1[a]
2	Singular or multiple lesions with 5–10 mm in Retro 1[a]
3	Singular or multiple lesions with >10 mm in Retro 1[a]
4	Lymph nodes at multiple body sites affected and/or an organ is affected[b]
5	Overall picture: severe progressed TB/generalization[c]

[a] Retro 1, Medial retropharyngeal lymph node with the more advanced lesion. Score 1–3 is based on Retro 1. If both medial retropharyngeal lymph nodes are missing in the sample material, the score for the score levels 1–3 is alternatively based on the lymph node with the most advanced lesion in the submitted sample material.
[b] Retro 1 has score level 3 (>10 mm) and additionally, at least one other lymph node is affected (e.g., Retro 2 with the less advanced lesion, tracheobronchial, mediastinal or mesenteric lymph nodes). By definition, samples with affected organ tissue (lung, pleura, liver, udder, etc.) are categorized at least with score 4, even if the sample material does not contain affected lymph nodes. Reason: According to Cornet's law of localization, the regional lymph node is always affected if the organ is affected (except in chronic organ tuberculosis). Samples consisting only of the head can reach a maximum score of 4.
[c] Example: "Ball deer" with spherical abscessed of the mesenteric lymph nodes, lymphadenitis, lung TB, chronic organ tuberculosis (various organs), severely abnormal lymph nodes.

that is able to take into account heterogeneity of sample material and can be applied retrospectively to historical samples. The development of the score was based on a so-called localization principle:

- In deer monitoring, medial retropharyngeal lymph nodes are the only tissues that must be present in all samples, i.e., both in head-only samples (from antlerless deer hunted in core and edge zone) and also in standard head and thorax samples.
- Three score levels (1–3) are based solely on a medial retropharyngeal lymph node ("Retro 1"). The two higher levels (4–5) are based on the overall picture gained from the examination of the entire sample material.
- The size of the lesion has more influence on the level of the score than the number of lesions.

Development of the Patho Score was carried out in several rounds with evaluations by two raters: the pathologist, who had made the pathomorphological assessment of almost all samples, and an epidemiologist. To test the scoring tool, the two raters independently scored 242 TB positive samples based on available historical free text descriptions. The two test results were compared and samples with discrepancies were discussed. After each round, the definitions of the Patho Score were specified with the aim of obtaining the highest possible inter-rater agreement. With the final version of definitions, agreement was reached in 248 out of 257 samples (observed proportionate agreement of 96.5%). Discrepancies occurred with samples of score 4 or score 5, as the definition of score 5 "overall picture of severe progressed TB" is partly subjective. The categorization will thus in a limited number of samples depend on the rating pathologist.

The scoring of the sample takes on average less than 1 min (including documentation). The definitions of the Patho Score are clear and easy to understand. Training of a pathologist who is specifically experienced with TB is therefore considered not necessary.

As addition to the development of the Patho Score, a second pathologist histologically examined a sub-selection of samples in a blinded experiment to verify the character of the macroscopic lesions and to assess feasibility of standardization of scores. This independent evaluation step revealed that confirmation of the pathogen was a prerequisite for inclusion of a sample in the scoring system, since occasionally (especially with mild lesions) other pathogens can cause comparable lesions (e.g., actinomycotic or mycotic granulomas).

TB positive samples that were examined before October 2017 were scored retrospectively. From October 2017 onwards, all fresh samples were scored by the same pathologist on a continuing basis.

Data Collection and Case Definition

For each sampled animal, data on date of kill event, coordinates and hunting ground of the kill location, age, sex, condition and any further comments by the hunter were recorded in a standardized manner [age groups: males: yearling (1 year), stag III (2–4 years), stag II (5–9 years), stag I (≥10 years), females: yearling (1 year), hind (≥2 years), fawn (from birth till April 1st of following year); condition: good (deer appearing healthy), poor (sick or injured deer with clinical signs)]. Diagnostic results and data on submitted sample materials were recorded by AGES. A central database with all collected data was maintained by the Office of the State Government of Vorarlberg.

Animals were considered a case if *M. caprae* was confirmed by bacterial culture and subsequent species determination. All deer without TB-like lesions or with negative results in bacterial culture were considered negative. In one deer *M. microti* was detected (38), which was classified as (*M. caprae-*) negative in this study. *M. bovis* was never detected.

Inclusion criteria for the analysis were: all deer examined in the deer monitoring with a test result according to the case definition, and presence of a description of the submitted sample material. Excluded were deer that did not meet the minimum requirements for sample material: the sample had to contain at least two of the following lymph nodes or organs: medial retropharyngeal lymph nodes, pulmonary lymph nodes or lung tissue. A total of 4,265 (94.3%) samples met the inclusion criteria (**Figure S1**). Of these, 334 samples (7.8%) had suspicious lesions. *M. caprae* was confirmed in 257 (6.0%) samples, with 7–72 cases per year. Only positive cases were scored with the Patho Score. Since information on sample material was missing for one case, reported results are based on 256 of the 257 confirmed *M. caprae* cases.

Data Analysis

The descriptive analysis of the spatial-temporal development of the Patho Score over a period of nine years and the statistical association between animal-specific risk factors for TB status and Patho Score of advanced TB-like lesions were carried out in STATA (39) using Pearson's chi-squared test, Cochran–Mantel–Haenszel test (MH) and Wald test of homogeneity of stratum-specific odds ratio's (OR). The Patho Score was used as an indicator to systematically show and quantify dynamics of infection. For comparisons of mean Patho Score between subgroups, the arithmetic mean of scores was calculated (reported with the 95% confidence interval (CI)). For the adjusted MH test, the Patho Score was reduced to two levels (low scores: 1–3; and high scores 4–5).

For the MH test, the reference categories were fawns (vs. yearlings and adults >2 years for the variable "age"), males (vs. females for the variable "sex"), good condition (vs. poor condition for the variable "condition"), head-only samples (vs. additional sample tissues for the variable "sample tissue" type) and zone outside the TB control area (vs. observation zone, edge zone and core zone for the variable "zone"). For the binary variable sample tissue "head and thorax," "head, thorax and abdomen," "thorax-only," and "other" samples were subsumed under samples with "additional tissue" (**Table 2**). For the variable zone, the score test for trend of odds was applied; the reported OR

TABLE 2 | Body sites examined and location of TB-like lesions.

Body sites examined	Lesion location						Total (%)	
	Retro[a] (%)		Thorax (%)		Other tissue (%)			
Head-only	115	(98.3)	–	–	4	(3.4)	117	(45.7)
Head and thorax	96	(93.2)	24	(23.3)	1	(1.0)	103	(40.2)
Head, thorax and abdomen	11	(57.9)	11	(57.9)	12	(63.2)	19	(7.4)
Thorax-only	–	–	6	(100)	–	–	6	(2.3)
Other	5	(45.5)	4	(36.4)	3	(27.3)	12[b]	(4.3)
Total	227	(88.7)	45	(17.6)	20	(7.8)	256	(100)

Row percentages of lesion locations may exceed 100% due to lesions at multiple locations in the sample material of an animal. The last column presents column percentages.
[a]*Medial retropharyngeal lymph nodes (present in 248 cases, affected in 227 cases).*
[b]*Only affected sample material was described, but overall information on submitted tissues was missing.*

estimate is an approximation to the OR for a one unit increase in the level of zone).

A causal diagram was used to conceptualize links between the three animal-specific *in vivo* recordable variables age, sex, condition, and the two further explanatory variables sample tissue and zone with the outcomes "TB status" and "Patho Score" and for bias assessment (**Figure 2**). Condition was identified as an intermediate variable on the causal path between both age and sex with TB status and with Patho Score. Age and sex were thus not adjusted for condition to avoid overadjustment. Zone influences age, sex, condition and sample tissue type through zone-specific differences in the sampling within the deer monitoring. The number of sampled tissues is influenced by age, sex and condition according to the deer monitoring program plan, but also influences the chance that an individual of a certain age, sex, or condition becomes a case, or receives a high Patho Score.

The spatial data visualization and analysis was done in ArcGIS (40). Analyses with annual comparisons are based on the official period of the hunting year (April 1st–March 31st), e.g., 2017 includes all deer tested between April 2017 and March 2018. February and March 2009 were counted to the hunting year 2009.

RESULTS

Submitted Sample Material

In a total of 117 (45.7%) out of 256 cases the submitted sample material consisted only of the head or parts of the head including medial retropharyngeal lymph nodes ("head-only," see **Table 2**); 60 (51.3%) of these samples were obtained from hinds and 41 (35.0%) from yearlings. The second largest group were 103 (40.2%) samples consisting of head and thoracic organ tissues ("head and thorax"). See **Table S1** for detailed numbers of deer tested, split by subgroup, TB status and Patho Score.

In 227 (91.5%) out of the 248 samples containing at least one medial retropharyngeal lymph node, this lymph node was affected. Lung or pulmonary lymph nodes were affected in 45 (32.3%) out of 139 samples containing thoracic organ tissues). Other sample tissues with TB-like lesions ("other tissues") comprised parts of the intestine with mesenteric lymph nodes, liver with hepatic lymph nodes, diaphragm with pleura and udder

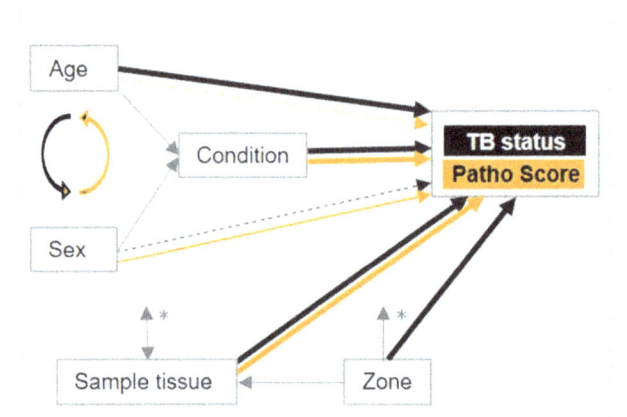

FIGURE 2 | Causal diagram of links between five explanatory variables with the outcomes "TB status" and "Patho Score." Black arrows: links with TB status. Orange arrows: links with Patho Score. For black and orange arrows, thicker arrows indicate stronger evidence for an association with the outcome. Dotted arrows indicate that only one level of the variable appears to be associated with the outcome. Curved arrows indicate interaction between variables. Gray arrows link explanatory variables with each other without any assumptions regarding strength of evidence of an association. *Sample tissue type, age, sex, and condition influence each other in both directions. Zone influences age, sex and condition.

tissue including mammary lymph nodes. Since other tissues were to be presented only in case of visible abnormalities, no valid conclusion can be drawn from these data regarding true frequency of lesions in abdominal organs or other body parts, but they give an overview of the range of lesions and organs affected.

Pathomorphology of Lesions

The pathomorphological abnormalities of TB-like gross lesions corresponded to earlier descriptions on *M. caprae* in red deer in western Austria (4, 5, 16, 41). It could be confirmed that observed lesions predominantly consisted of granulomas and abscesses with creamy pus or caseous cores. With Patho Score 1, lesions were mostly singular, 1–5 mm large granulomas or micro-abscesses in a single lymph node. In 47 (97.9%) of a total of 48 samples with score 1, one or both medial retropharyngeal lymph nodes were affected. Only in one sample, the medial retropharyngeal lymph node itself showed no alterations, but had a 3 mm abscess of creamy-yellowish pus in its immediate vicinity. The exact localization of this lesion could not be identified due to the conduct of the sampling.

Lesions with score 2 were characterized by singular or multiple abscesses with 5–10 mm of diameter, with creamy, purulent-watery or caseous contents, some of which were encapsulated. Score 3 lesions were grossly similar to lesions described for score 2, but with coalescing abscesses that formed singular abscesses with diameters of up to 80 mm. Lesions with score 4 showed a more differentiated picture: in addition to the increasing sizes of typical abscesses in the lymph nodes, numerous miliary granulomas were observed in lymph nodes or the lungs. Lymph nodes were in some cases very small and of firm consistency. Lesions with score 5 corresponded to generalized TB with advanced lesions in multiple lymph nodes and organs with abscesses up to 200 mm in diameter (**Figure S2**).

Cases with head-only samples received a mean score of 2.4 ± 0.2, and cases with additional tissues had a mean score of 3.2 ± 0.2. Within the group of cases with additional tissues mean scores did not differ significantly after adjustment for condition: for animals in poor condition all carcass parts with gross lesions had to be submitted, leading to more sampled tissues with higher numbers of gross lesions. However, among 19 cases with the maximum range of sampled sites (head, thorax and abdomen, **Table 2**), only one case would have received a lower Patho Score if only the standard sample (head and thorax) would have been presented for pathological examination. This was the only case with TB lesions in the mesenteric lymph nodes but without gross lesions in the medial retropharyngeal lymph nodes or thoracic tissues.

Risk Groups for TB Positivity

Figure 3A shows the (crude) apparent prevalences for deer subgroups split by sex, age and condition. **Table 3** list detailed statistical output for this chapter. In the crude analysis the MH chi-squared test showed very strong evidence ($p < 0.001$) for associations between TB status and the explanatory variables sex, age, condition, zone and sample tissue type. In pairwise adjustments against each other, the MH analysis confirmed the strength of association between condition, zone and the sample material and TB status: deer in poor condition had 6.5 times the odds of having TB. For zone, the score test for trend showed an OR of 2.6 for a one unit increase in zone, with the area outside the TB control area as baseline. The crude OR of 0.6 for sample tissue type was confounded by the differing sampling method in the TB zones. In the low prevalence zone outside the TB control area, only 5.1% of submissions were head-only samples. In the observation, edge and core zones, the percentages of head-only samples were 39.0, 66.1, and 62.7%, respectively. After controlling for zone, deer with additional submitted sample tissues had 1.8 times the odds of TB positivity compared to deer with head-only samples.

The Wald test and the comparison with MH adjusted OR for this bivariate analysis suggested sample tissue type and zone as

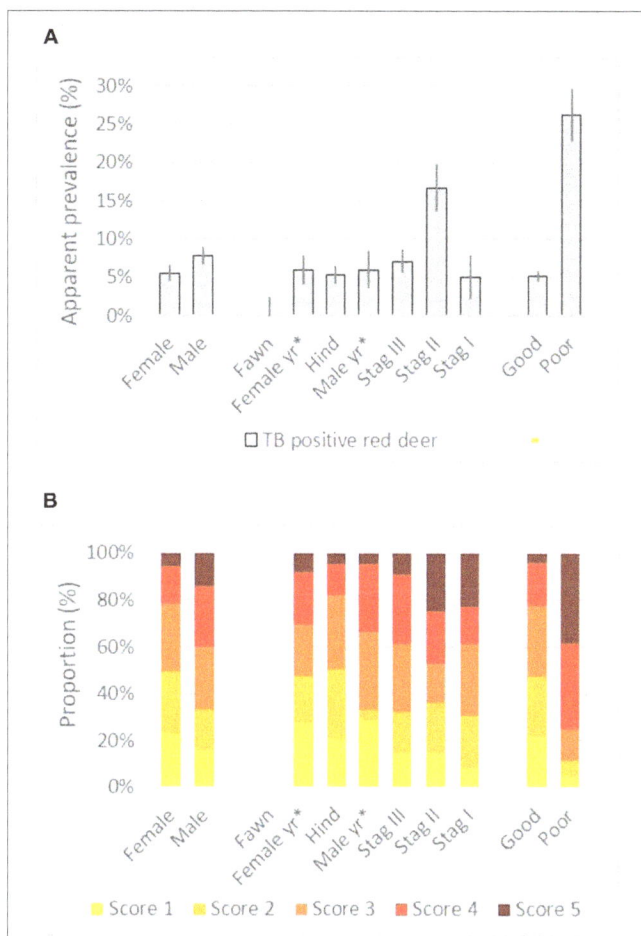

FIGURE 3 | Apparent prevalence with 95% confidence intervals **(A)** and distribution of Patho Scores **(B)**, by sex, sex & age group and condition of TB positive deer ($n = 256$). For better comparability of groups, the Patho Score was normalized in **(B)**. Example how to read the panels: 5.6% of all females were tested TB positive, and of these, 22.3% were categorized with score 1, etc. No sex was recorded for fawns. *yr, yearling, hind: ≥ 2 years, stag III: 2–4 years, stag II: 5–9 years, stag I: ≥ 10 years.

potential confounders for the association between sex and age with TB status. These confounders were thus controlled for in the following analyses. Sex proved to be a weak indicator for TB status: only for the area outside the TB control area, the adjusted MH estimate showed good evidence ($p = 0.01$) for an association between sex and TB status: males had 4.5 times the odds of being TB positive. In the TB control area, age appeared to modify the effect of sex on TB status (and *vice versa*): there was no difference between male and female yearlings ($p = 0.88$). But for adult deer the analysis showed good evidence for an association ($p = 0.02$) between sex and TB status: stags had 1.5 times the odds of being TB positive compared to hinds. The estimated OR was larger for adults with additional sample tissues (OR = 2.2). This association was to a large extent explained by the fact that stags (especially stags II) were more often sick or injured. Out of the 39 cases in adult deer with poor health, 31 (79.5%) were male. After additional adjustment for the intermediate variable condition,

TABLE 3 | Models selected to explain the association between TB status and age, sex, condition of deer, number of submitted sample tissues and TB zone of kill location.

Explanatory variable for TB status	Adjusted for	n (cases)	chi^2	p, MH	OR	95% CI	p, Wald test
Age	Crude MH[a]	4,262[b] (257)	18.50	<0.001	1.55	1.27–1.89	
	Zone, sample tissue	3,982[b] (257)	32.87	<0.001	1.90	1.53–2.39	0.94
Age (males only), in area[c]	Sample tissue	1007[d] (125)	6.63	0.01	2.00	1.17–3.45	0.17
Age (females only), in area[c]	Sample tissue	1,296[d] (118)	3.94	0.05	1.52	1.00–2.30	0.78
Sex	Crude MH[a]	3,912 (257)	7.83	0.005	1.43	1.11–1.85	
Sex, outside area[c]	Age	1,611 (14)	5.97	0.01	4.54	1.19–17.16	0.10
Sex (yearlings only), in area[c]	Sample tissue	746 (56)	0.02	0.88	1.04	0.59–1.85	0.94
Sex (adults only), in area[c]	Sample tissue	1,446 (187)	5.05	0.02	1.53	1.05–2.20	0.02[e]
	Head-only	667 (75)	0.27	0.61	0.85	0.47–1.55	Stratum 1[e]
	Additional tissue	779 (112)	10.04	0.002	2.16	1.33–3.52	Stratum 2[e]
	Sample tissue, condition	1,446 (187)	3.14	0.08	1.41	0.96–2.05	0.12
Condition	Crude MH[a]	4,264 (257)	128.27	<0.001	6.48	4.47–9.41	
	Zone, sample tissue	3,983 (257)	100.46	<0.001	6.62	4.32–10.15	0.12
Sample tissue	Crude MH[a]	3,983 (257)	14.76	<0.001	0.56	0.47–0.79	
	Zone	3,983 (257)	16.84	<0.001	1.76	1.36–2.41	0.31
Zone	Crude MH[a]	4,265 (257)	289.42	<0.001	2.64	2.36–2.95	

For each explanatory variable, the table presents the variables adjusted for, number of independent samples (and cases thereof), (pooled) chi-squared statistic, p-value and estimate of the odds ratio of the Cochran-Mantel-Haenszel (MH) test with 95% confidence interval, and p-value of the Wald test for homogeneity of the odds ratios of the stratified analysis. All tests have one degree of freedom.
[a]Crude MH: MH analysis without adjusting for other variables.
[b]Age in three categories: fawns (reference)—yearlings—adults ≥2 years.
[c]Area: TB control area, consisting of core, edge and observation zones.
[d]Age in two categories: yearlings (reference)—adults ≥2 years, as sex was not recorded for fawns.
[e]Stratum-specific odds ratios need to be reported.

stags had 1.4 times the odds of being TB positive compared to hinds ($p = 0.08$). There was thus only weak statistical support for a controlled direct causal effect of sex *per se* on TB status.

Age *per se* showed to be a good indicator for TB status: After adjusting for zone and sample tissue type, there was even stronger evidence ($p < 0.001$) for an association between age with TB status (adjusted OR = 1.9 vs. crude OR = 1.6). Stratified analysis by sex showed that the odds for TB positivity increased in both sexes with age: stags had 2.0 times the odds of TB positivity compared to male yearlings, and the odds of hinds were 1.5 compared to female yearlings. Out of all subgroups split by sex and age, 5–9 year old stags II showed the highest apparent prevalence of 16.7% (**Figure 3A**). None of the 351 tested fawns was tested TB positive.

Condition was found *per se* to be the most important *in vivo* recordable indicator for TB status. Emaciated, sick or injured deer had after adjusting for zone and sample material around 6.6 times the odds of being tested TB positive compared to deer appearing healthy ($p < 0.001$).

Risk Groups for Advanced Lesions

Figure 3B shows the distribution of the Patho Score for deer subgroups split by sex, age and condition. **Table 4** list detailed statistical output for this chapter. Comparing the crude means of the Patho Score (with levels 1–5), hinds had the lowest mean score (2.5 ± 0.3), followed by yearlings (females: 2.6 ± 0.4; males 2.8 ± 0.5) and stags (stags III: 3.0 ± 0.3; stags II: 3.2 ± 0.4 and stags I: 3.2 ± 0.7). The crude MH analysis showed very strong

evidence ($p < 0.001$) for an association between Patho Score (reduced to two levels high/low) and condition and sample tissue type, and strong evidence ($p = 0.002$) for an association between Patho Score and sex. Deer in poor condition, deer with additional sample tissues and males had 10.5, 3.0, and 2.4 times the odds of having a high Patho Score, respectively. There was no evidence for an association between Patho Score and age or zone in the crude analysis.

Sex appears to be a good indicator for advanced lesions in adult deer: Like with TB status, the Wald test indicated interaction between age and sex in respect to their effect on the Patho Score. Adjusting for sample tissue type showed for yearlings no evidence for an association between sex and Patho Score ($p = 0.83$). For adults however, there was good evidence for an association ($p = 0.04$). Stags had 2.2 times the odds of having advanced lesions compared to hinds.

Age is a weak indicator for score 4–5 lesions: Stratified by sex and adjusted for sample tissue type, there was no statistical support for an association between age and Patho Score with males ($p = 0.77$), although the percentage of advanced lesions increased tendentially with age (except the oldest age group of stags I). Out of all age groups of males, stags II were with 17 (45.9%) of 37 submissions the subgroup with the most lesions with scores 4–5. Females showed an opposing trend: there was some evidence for an association between age and Patho Score ($p = 0.06$). Hinds had 0.4 times the odds, or, in other words, female yearlings had 2.4 times the odds of having a high score compared to hinds. Zone did not confound the association between sex and age with Patho Score; the ORs adjusted for zone did only

TABLE 4 | Models selected to explain the association between Patho Score and age, sex, condition of deer, number of submitted sample tissues and TB zone of kill location.

Explanatory variable for Patho Score	Adjusted for	n	chi^2	p, MH	OR	95% CI	p, Wald test
Sex	Crude MH[a]	256	10.14	0.002	2.44	1.38–4.29	
	Sample tissue	256	2.01	0.16	1.55	0.84–2.87	0.17
Sex (yearlings only)	Sample tissue	57	0.05	0.83	0.87	0.25–3.04	0.65
Sex (adults only)	Sample tissue	199	4.25	0.04	2.15	1.02–4.54	0.14
Age[b]	Crude MH[a]	256	0	0.95	0.98	0.52–1.85	
Age[b] (males only)	Sample tissue	135	0.09	0.77	1.17	0.40–3.40	0.31
Age[b] (females only)	Sample tissue	121	3.51	0.06	0.40	0.15–1.08	0.62
Condition	Crude MH[a]	256	47.15	<0.001	10.53	4.55–24.36	
	Sample tissue	256	35.57	<0.001	9.43	3.92–22.69	0.35
Sample tissue	Crude MH[a]	256	14.84	<0.001	3.02	1.67–5.46	
Zone	Crude MH[a]	256	1.59	0.21	0.83	0.62–1.11	

For each explanatory variable, the table presents the variables adjusted for, number of independent samples (and cases thereof), (pooled) chi-squared statistic, p-value and estimate of the odds ratio of the Cochran-Mantel-Haenszel (MH) test with 95% confidence interval, and p-value of the Wald test for homogeneity of the odds ratios of the stratified analysis. All tests have one degree of freedom.
[a]Crude MH: analysis without adjusting for other variables.
[b]Age in two categories: yearlings (reference)–adults ≥2 years, as TB was never detected in fawns.

marginally differ from the ORs adjusted only for sample tissue type (results not shown).

Condition was again found to be the most important indicator for advanced lesions with scores 4–5. Independent from the levels of age, sex, tissue material or zone, deer in poor condition had 9–10.5 times the odds of showing advanced stages of TB (result shown in **Table 4** are limited to crude analysis and adjustment for sample tissue type). Clinical signs or other abnormalities were recorded for 45 (26.2%) cases; of these 33 (73.3%) received score 4 or 5 (**Figure 3B**). Emaciation was with 12 records the most frequent leading symptom. For another nine deer leg injuries or other injuries were reported. For most cases only non-specific records on the clinical signs were available ("sick," "abnormal behavior"). In general, stags II contributed most to the subgroup of deer in poor condition (19 (42.2%) of 45 cases).

Infection Dynamics in the Years 2009–2017

Geographically, the distribution of TB cases in the core, edge and observation zones remained relatively constant between 2009 and 2012 (**Figures 1B–D**). From 2013 onwards, a redistribution of cases took place: while apparent prevalence decreased in the core zone since 2013, it increased in edge and observation zones in 2013–2016. In the core zone, apparent prevalence was significantly lower (p < 0.03) in 2016 and 2017 with 12.0 (±6.8%) and 10.6% (±8.3%) respectively, compared to 2013–2015 with 21.6–27.6% (±4.7–10.0%) (**Figure 4A**). In the neighboring edge and observation zone apparent prevalence was with 10.1% (±2.2%) in 2016 also significantly higher (p ≤ 0.002) than in 2013 (2.7% ± 2.7%), in 2014 (6.6% ± 3.1%), and also in 2017 (4.8% ± 2.5%). This development was comparable in edge and observation zones and therefore both zones are presented in a joint graph in **Figure 4B**. TB has noticeably spread since 2013, especially in the west and the south of edge and observation zones (**Figures 1E–H**). See **Table S2** for detailed statistics related to apparent prevalences.

Three different patterns of disease occurrence could be identified: endemic disease, epidemics and sporadic cases. These three patterns will be described in more detail.

Endemic Disease

Analyses of the Patho Score showed that all stages of TB occurred together in the core zone. This corresponds to the typical picture of an endemic disease occurrence without much tendency of a change. From 2013 onwards, proportions of all score levels decreased at a fairly similar scale along with a decreasing apparent prevalence (**Figure 4A**) (no p-value reported due to several subgroups with zero individuals). There was still evidence for an active infection cycle in 2016 and 2017, which is revealed by 2% of tested deer with score 1, including yearlings. However, deer with score 5 were missing in sample materials in these last two years with lower apparent prevalences.

Epidemic in a Newly Infected Area

The increase of prevalence was no zone-wide evenly distributed phenomenon but was attributable to three newly infected spots in the edge and observation zones that were confirmed in 2016 (**Figure 1H** shows spots A–C). The 2016 hunting year had both the highest apparent prevalence (10.1% ± 2.2%), and also the highest proportion of higher scores (7% of deer with scores 3–5) recorded so far in these two zones.

Spot B will be described as example for epidemic TB in more detail: This spot was a 23 km^2 large hunting ground located west of the core zone in the edge zone. In 2013, a first case of TB was detected in a female with score 2 (**Figure 5**). In 2014, three animals were positive (all three were females with scores 1 or 3), followed by a case of a yearling with score 1 in 2015. In 2016, five cases were shot right at the beginning of the hunting season in April. This unexpected finding led to an intensified hunting and sampling of deer in this area and resulted in a total of 21 cases out of 93 tested deer. The infection could first be detected in

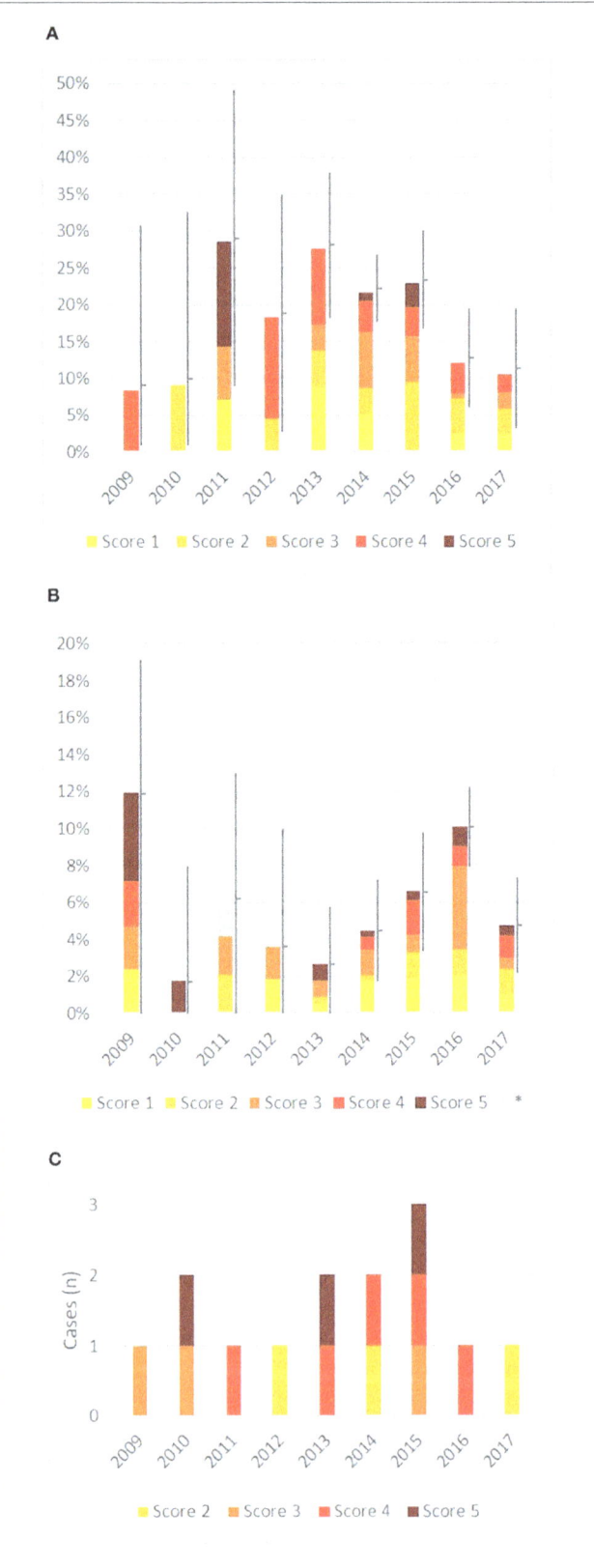

FIGURE 4 | 719 tested deer. **(B)** Edge zone and observation zone (joined) with in total 106 TB positive deer out of 1,733 tested deer. *Data on submitted material was missing for one case marked in grey, therefore no score was assigned. **(C)** Area outside the designated TB control area with in total 14 TB positive deer out of 1,815 tested deer. Colors of cases denote the Patho Score. In **(A,B)**, the bars mark the apparent prevalence with 95% confidence intervals; in **(C)** the number of sporadic cases is shown. Up to 2012, the confidence intervals are large due to lower sample size.

yearlings and females in spring and summer. Only from October 2016 onwards scores 4 and 5 were found (in stags). The first deer with clinical signs was a stage II with score 5 in November.

In two outbreak-like spots in the north-western (spot A) and southern observation zone (spot C), TB was confirmed in 2016 with seven and five cases respectively (**Figure 1H**). In both spots the first cases were also detected in March and April. In spot A, the first case was a stag III with score 1, followed by cases with scores 2 and 3 and 11 month later one case with score 5 (no cases detected in 2017). In spot C, the first case was a female yearling with score 5, followed by cases with scores 1 and 3, and seven more cases in 2017 presenting lesions of all five levels of scores.

Sporadic Cases Outside the Designated TB Control Area

Between February 2009 and March 2018, a total of 14 TB cases were detected outside the designated TB control area, with one to three cases each year (**Figure 4C**). Twelve of these cases were recorded in the district of Bregenz (**Figure 6**). Age and sex distribution among these cases showed with nine males and only one yearling a different pattern compared to the TB control area (**Table S3**). With eight (57.0%) cases with score 4 or 5 lesions, advanced TB stages were frequent, and score 1 lesions were not detected so far. Kill locations were up to 30 km away from each other and in different valleys. On the one hand, cases appeared to be independent in time and space. On the other hand, patterns are visible: all deer were hunted between August and November, and kill locations of eight of the 12 cases lie on an imaginary line (cases numbers 1–5 and 7–9, see **Figure 6**).

DISCUSSION

This study attempts to describe infection dynamics of TB in red deer by using patho-scoring as an additional source of information. The study demonstrates that the infection dynamics of TB are associated with individual animal-specific parameters such as sex, age and condition, and environmental characteristics such as vicinity to other TB areas.

Roles of Subgroups in the Infection Dynamic

Three animal-specific parameters are usually recorded by the hunter before the kill: age, sex, and condition. Older animals and stags were significantly more likely to be TB positive. Stags also had higher Patho Scores than hinds. The subgroups with the lowest apparent prevalence were fawns; and hinds had on average the lowest scores. Effect modification between age and

FIGURE 4 | Development of the Patho Score between 2009 and 2017, stratified by TB zones. **(A)** Core zone with in total 136 TB positive deer out of
(Continued)

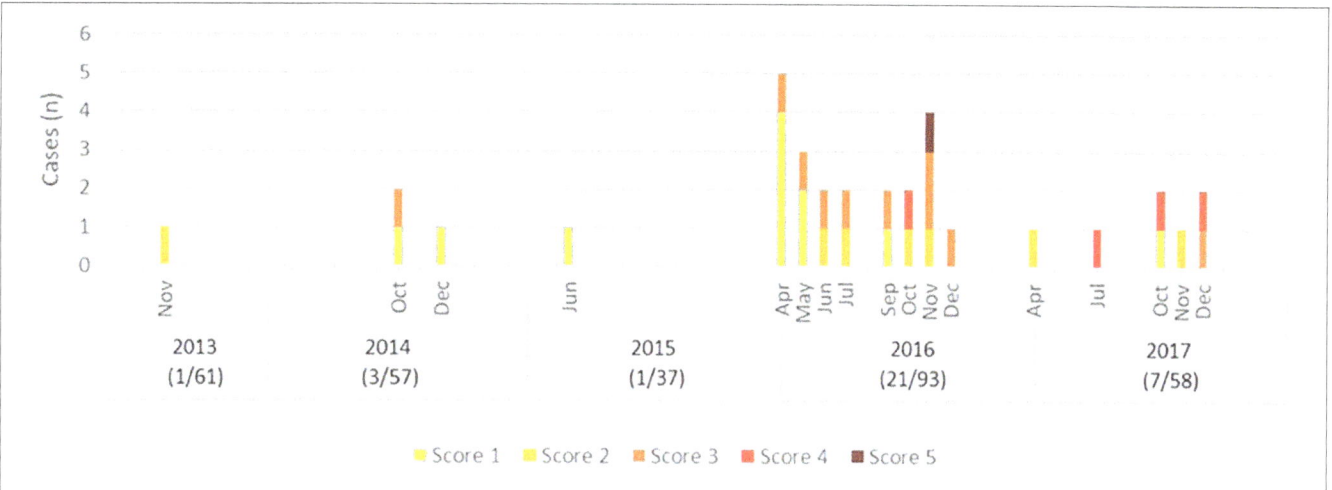

FIGURE 5 | Epidemic curve of TB cases in deer by month of detection for the years 2013–2017, spot B. Colors of cases denote the Patho Score. In Brackets: (number of cases/number of deer tested per year).

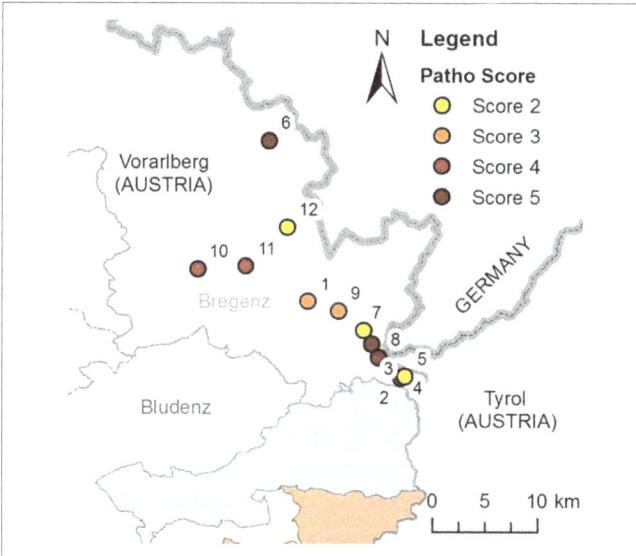

FIGURE 6 | Map of kill locations of 12 TB cases in deer in the area outside the designated TB control area, district of Bregenz. Zones of the TB control area are marked in blue, yellow and red. Case numbers are sorted by kill date: 1: earliest sample from August 2009, 12: latest sample from September 2017). Colors of cases denote the Patho Score (**Table S3** lists the characteristics of cases).

sex on their observed effect on TB status and the developmental stage of lesions could indicate that stags, hinds and yearlings play different roles in the infection dynamics within the infected deer population. These roles for the spread and maintenance of disease of different subgroups should be investigated in more detail to better understand how TB spreads within and between deer populations.

The majority of studies report higher TB prevalence in male deer [reviewed by (42)], including studies from Spain and Michigan (32, 43, 44). In contrast, similar prevalence values were recorded in male and female deer in New Zealand, with a higher

prevalence in young males ≤2 years offset by a lower prevalence in older males > 5 years (19). Lugton et al. (12) observed more gross lesions and more cases of advanced TB in male than female red deer, although this difference was not significant. They interpreted this finding not as a higher susceptibility of males to TB *per se*, but attributed this result to the time the stags were shot, which usually fell into the period during which males were in hard antler. During rutting season, stags experience particular stress from aggression and gathering and maintaining a group of hinds, which may influence the development of lesions (12). The results of this study give some support to this conclusion: after adjusting for the (intermediate variable) condition, there was only weak statistical support for a controlled direct causal effect of sex on TB status. Higher prevalences of TB and advanced lesions in stags were largely attributable to higher proportion of sick or injured deer among males compared to hinds.

TB was not detected in fawns in this study. The observation of no or very low numbers of TB positive fawns has been made on several continents (32, 44, 45) and has been interpreted as indication for the limited importance of dams for the infection of their fawns in free-ranging deer. Conversely, for farmed deer, Griffin et al. (46) described an acute outbreak of TB with a prevalence >90% in young fawns accompanied with a prevalence of 60% in breeding hinds. One feasible explanation would be that the TB status of fawns is indeed directly related to the level of exposure from hinds. In Vorarlberg, hinds were one of the subgroups with the lowest prevalence and also had the lowest Patho Scores. The absence of infection in fawns despite 5% of their mothers being infected could also indicate that direct deer-to-deer transmission is very rare, and fawns are only infected in settings with significant indirect environmental transmission. This might not happen in Vorarlberg until winter feeding begins.

Higher figures of infection in older deer are a common finding in TB literature and are attributed i.a. to long exposure time of this long-lived species and chronicity of TB (12, 44, 47). In Vorarlberg, the group of 5–9 year old stags II had both the highest prevalence of TB positivity and advanced lesions. Over 10 year old stags I were three times less likely to be TB positive compared to stags II, and also less often showed generalized TB (**Figure 3**). The observation that gross lesions are less frequently detected in very old animals was also made by Lugton et al. (12). The authors hypothesized that infected animals may be capable of resolving lesions over time or that susceptible individuals have died, while those remaining have kept the infection under control.

These two different tracks of disease progression could also serve as explanations for the special role of the oldest deer in Vorarlberg: the high numbers of stags II with clinical signs and advanced TB would correspond to the susceptibles that are killed sick or die before they reach the oldest age group. For stags that reach apparently healthy an old age, although they might have been exposed to the pathogen for years, this could indicate some form of natural immunity or clinical latency. An additional explanation could lie in distinct contact patterns. It has been observed that older stags prefer to roam in very small groups of stags or sometimes even become solitary. Such behavior could lead to a limited exposure to the pathogen. To conclude, in case a protective factor could be identified, it would be relevant to investigate whether those "protected" subgroups also show lower infectivity and whether the *in vivo* identification of these animals could be utilized within a selective TB control strategy.

The most important *in vivo* indicator for TB was however the condition. Cases with poor health also had advanced stages of TB (score 4 or the maximum score 5) significantly more often. This relationship was to be expected since the observed clinical signs were likely to be attributable to the disease progress of TB in a considerable number of cases. Research showed that deer with advanced TB can cause massive environmental contamination through the excretion of high numbers of mycobacteria (8, 12, 48). The findings of this study suggest that selective culling that aims at the elimination of potential high shedders should prioritize weak, sick and injured deer, even if no abnormalities indicative for infectious disease are observed. However, to increase the efficiency of a control strategy that includes selective culling, it is advisable to combine findings on risk groups with additional epidemiological information to identify groups of deer with higher exposure or locations with increased risk of environmental contamination, e.g. by targeting groups or areas with earlier detections of deer with scores 4–5.

Patterns of Disease Occurrence

Three different patterns of TB occurrence could be distinguished and characterized: areas with endemic disease, areas with outbreak-like cases, and areas with sporadic cases. This distinction is relevant to assess the infection dynamics in each area and to better inform the selection of targeted prevention and control measures.

Endemic Disease

In the core zone both new infections as well as spreaders with advanced TB were seen, which can lead to further infections. This suggests that an endemic equilibrium has been reached with multiple infection chains occurring in parallel. Surprisingly, only few deer with score 5 were detected in the core zone. In

this zone, deer have been intensively hunted for several years as part of TB control and apparent prevalence is declining. The question remains whether absence of cases with score 5 is causally associated with the decline of the apparent prevalence. To exclude biases due to sampling regime or to confirm other potential reasons these developments need to be further monitored.

Epidemic Disease

Outbreak areas showed the typical picture expected for a point source in a previously disease-free population: the first detected cases presented predominantly early stages of lesions. Over time, more advanced disease stages and cases of generalized disease (score 5) were seen, which eventually were accompanied by clinical signs (**Figure 5**). A characteristic of a point source is that all cases are exposed at one point in time or within a limited period of time and location directly or indirectly to the primary case. Whether the pathogen was introduced by a single "super spreader" or by multiple animals serving as co-primary cases cannot be distinguished from the data. Due to the proximity of outbreak areas to endemically infected areas both scenarios are possible.

In all three outbreaks spots first cases were detected in early spring, pointing toward infection spreading during the winter feeding season. In spring, deer tend to browse still close to the location of their feeding site. It would need to be investigated if through early detection of cases in spring deer belonging to the same winter feeding cohort can be identified. Such a classical approach of tracing back could support targeted hunting of deer at higher risk of infection and thereby prevent that TB establishes permanently in a new area. Whether the three outbreak spots already reached a state of endemic infection or whether control measures were successful in limiting further spread will become clearer within the next 1–2 years. Within one year of detection of the first cases both early and advanced stages of lesions have been found in the three outbreak spots. The case of a yearling killed in April with score 5 indicated that TB can quickly progress to stages where infected individuals may cause massive environmental contamination.

Sporadic Cases

Sporadic cases should receive particular attention: so far, all outbreaks in TB-free areas in Vorarlberg were preceded by sporadic cases. This finding contrasts with the situation in the north of Vorarlberg, where sporadic cases have been recorded for nine years without any indication of spread among the local deer population. Deer abundance and management and size of winter feeding sites are comparable in both the TB control area and the area with sporadic cases, and deer densities are estimated to be high enough to support spread in the resident deer population. The north of Vorarlberg is part of the foothills of the alps with lower mountains and better feed availability for deer. Deer are on average heavier and might thus be in a better physical condition compared to deer in the TB control area. However, it is questionable if this physical advantage is sufficient to prevent the establishment of a new TB spot given that the environmental conditions in the north of Vorarlberg resemble those in the TB areas in nearby southern Germany.

Sporadic cases would be expected in various disease scenarios: they could either indicate that TB became established at a very low level in resident deer and is therefore constantly present—or they could be an indicator for a nearby active TB situation from where cases "spill over" into new areas. For the north of Vorarlberg, the results of the deer monitoring rather support the latter, with regular introductions of infected migratory deer from the TB control area in Vorarlberg or neighboring deer TB areas in Tyrol or Germany. Even in the "TB at a low level" scenario deer with advanced lesions of score 4 or 5 would occasionally spend the winter at feeding sites together with critical numbers of susceptibles. This should eventually lead to the detection of additional cases in resident deer.

Sick deer are likely to isolate themselves from their social group. It could be observed that deer with severe TB were commonly found alone and well away from other deer (12). If sporadic cases seen in the north of Vorarlberg are such isolated deer that have migrated from affected areas, this means that even advanced TB is no obstacle for diseased animals to move over long distances. The pattern of sporadic cases being mostly older stags is consistent with results from a telemetry study in the south of Vorarlberg: this study showed that stags more often migrate over long distances up to 30 km across mountains and have a larger mean home range size of 6,400 hectares, compared to females with 2,600 hectares (35). The kill sites of sporadic cases were in distances between 1 and 13 km from the borders to Tyrol, Germany and the TB control area of Vorarlberg. The origin of migratory deer can therefore not be determined based merely on the distance of the kill site to the closest TB area. Cross-border cooperation is needed to better understand the dynamics of TB in this border area. Comparative genomic analyses could provide insights into the relationship of mycobacteria circulating in the different affected regions.

Lesion Presence as Indicator for Disease Progress

At individual animal-level, environmental factors as well as animal-specific factors are understood to influence progression of TB and other diseases within the infected body (20, 21). This implies that the time period to progress from one stage of lesions to the next might vary considerably between infected individuals.

Latency is an important characteristic of *M. tuberculosis* infection in humans (49, 50) described it also as the most frequent expression of *M. bovis* infection in badgers. In cattle, latent TB infections are not considered to be common (51), and *M. bovis* infection of cattle usually results in a slowly progressive disease (52). For red deer, it is not known how often latent TB infections occur and which role they play in infection dynamics. Studies on *M. caprae* in red deer in Austria (4) and Germany (2) and *M. bovis* in red deer in Spain (44, 53) and New Zealand (8, 12, 19) showed that the pathogen could be detected in 22–68% of deer samples without visible lesions. Gavier-Widen et al. (54) argued that this non-visible lesion presentation in animals was likely to include latent cases or merely early-stage infections that do not yet present macroscopic lesions. However, it is uncertain if animals with non-visible lesions would eventually

develop progressive disease or if these infections can be cured spontaneously (52, 54). Until host immune mechanisms of red deer are not better understood, inferences on the potential time of TB infection based on lesion need to be made with caution. Especially with adult deer, score 1 lesions cannot be put on a level with recent infections without any supporting epidemiological data. However, lack of gross lesions in the total of 351 tested fawns till December in combination with presence of small lesions detected from April onwards in yearlings of the same birth cohort indicate that these score 1 lesions indeed correspond to recent infections that potentially occurred during the winter feeding period.

Being aware of these open questions, results of this work nevertheless support the approach that an analysis of tissue lesions at population-level is still useful to monitor developments in infection dynamics. The Patho Score allows visualization and quantification of these dynamics. The Patho Score presented in this study focuses on lesions in medial retropharyngeal lymph nodes and discriminates particularly between mild to moderate stages of lesions. At the population level these lesions generally indicate recent infections (11, 33). Predominance of lesions in medial retropharyngeal lymph nodes reported in this study was previously described for *M. caprae* in Austrian red deer by Fink et al. (5) and Nigsch (22). This observation corresponds to results of studies from other countries (11, 15, 53) and supports the conclusion that monitoring programs that focus on the examination of lymphoid tissue of the head are capable to detect a significant portion of TB-infected red deer (53) and are also suitable for early detection of TB.

Applications of the Patho Score

Lesion scores are regularly used in experimental TB challenge studies of cattle, deer and other wildlife, where tissue materials can be sampled under standardized situations (21, 55–57). With naturally infected deer, lesion scores were applied to study infection patterns and effects of TB on deer, to assess the role of deer in perpetuating TB among cattle or to develop sampling protocols (17, 19, 53). In this study, the Patho Score was used to identify risk groups for advanced TB stages and to characterize areas with different patterns of disease occurrence. For many analyses, such as detailed analyses of outbreaks or analyses of sporadic cases, the absolute number of TB cases was too low to obtain statistically significant results. These mainly descriptive analyses are thus considered as exploratory. One strength of the Patho Score is certainly that with the descriptive information it generates, it provides a much more differentiated insight into the TB situation compared to prevalence data alone, at no extra costs. This information can then be used for forming hypotheses to be investigated via more rigorous, multivariable statistical methods in a next step, and for guiding early disease management efforts until those hypotheses are validated.

The overarching goal of deer monitoring is to protect cattle against TB infections from deer. For Vorarlberg, no studies are available on the interaction between cattle and deer, but the main route of infection is assumed to be indirect transmission. The Patho Score helps to identify areas with an increased risk of environmental contamination by deer with advanced stages of

TB, or areas where the risk of infection could increase rapidly due to recent outbreaks in deer. Identification of these high-risk areas is an important prerequisite for targeted measures toward disease prevention in cattle.

Future applications of the Patho Score include comparing infection dynamics of TB in different countries or to support comparison of different monitoring systems, e.g., how successful is the monitoring system to detect very small TB lesions.

Limitations

Deer monitoring and sampling are conducted under field conditions: by definition, the hunting bag is not a simple random sample of the local deer population. On the one hand, some age groups are underrepresented in the hunting bag as red deer management favors a specific age pyramid. On the other hand, the hunting law foresees that obviously sick and injured animals must be harvested for welfare purposes. In the TB control area all sick and injured deer had to be examined and were thus likely to be overrepresented in the sample.

In addition, only tissue material with gross lesions was selected for further examinations to confirm TB. Tissue without lesions was considered TB negative. Lesion-based monitoring tends to underestimate the prevalence. These limitations were known to the authors before the development of the Patho Score. Therefore, the challenge was to develop a valid tool under the given conditions, which is capable to take account of the heterogeneity of the available historical longitudinal data.

A critical task was to assess the impact of missing lymph nodes or other organ tissues in individual samples for the correct categorization with the Patho Score. The association between number of sample tissues and Patho Score was significant. Deer represented with thoracic or abdominal tissues in addition to heads received more frequently a high score of 4 or 5. However, submission of more tissues in addition to the standard sample (head and thorax) has only in one case led to a higher score. The reason for this lies in the definitions for score 4 and 5 (**Table 1**): samples with one affected organ (lung, pleura, liver, udder, etc) are categorized at least with score 4, and one severely affected body site is sufficient to receive score 5. Submission of more abnormal tissues will not necessarily increase a high score.

"Head-only" samples could by definition only reach a maximum score of 4. Sample selection in the current deer monitoring might thus underestimate the proportion of high scores and thereby the proportion of potential super-spreaders among identified cases. However, the amount of submitted tissues and severity of clinical lesions were also causally related: for deer with visible organ abnormalities, deer monitoring required that more tissues including all affected body sites were sampled. The potential bias in selection of sample material was accounted for twofold: firstly, by adjusting for the amount of sample material in the statistical analysis, and secondly by the final interpretation of the Patho Score: in this study, scores 4 and 5 were both interpreted to be more relevant for spreading disease, with score 5 being considered as an advanced stage of score 4. Standardization of sample material (if logistically feasible) would have a positive effect on the overall sensitivity of deer monitoring and furthermore would increase validity of the Patho Score.

Even though deer monitoring will underestimate true prevalence, the authors hypothesize that comparative analyses over time and space remain valid, as sampling mode and diagnostic protocol did not change greatly over the 9-year monitoring period. With lesion-based monitoring the role of animals with non-visible lesions for the infection dynamic could not be investigated. Such an investigation would require culturing of key lymph nodes from all deer, including those with non-visible lesions. However, it can be assumed that deer with gross lesions play at least for pathogen spread a more important role. With 4,521 examined samples virtually the whole range of stages of lesions could be explored. For an external evaluation of validity of the Patho Score, it would be of interest to apply this score on data from other regions to estimate the effect of field conditions.

Recommendations

The assessment of TB-like lesions showed various practical approaches on how to gain better insight into the infection dynamics through the targeted selection of animals to be sampled in early spring to early identify new spots of infection. Identified risk groups for TB and advanced lesions should receive particular attention in infection control programs. Special attention require also sporadic cases in TB-free areas: they do not necessarily indicate that the infection already spreads locally but these sporadic cases appear to be a precursor of outbreaks among resident deer populations. In this context, one relevant question for further research would be: what constellation of animal-specific parameters, lesions, season and other measurable conditions would signal a transition of an area with sporadic cases to an outbreak area or to an area with an endemic level of infection presence?

The next step to draw a holistic picture of the infection dynamics would be to include home range size, habitat selection and deer-to-deer interaction within and between deer populations in this alpine setting in more detail to investigate potential seasonality of infections and to better characterize the role of specific subgroups in maintenance and spread of TB. Furthermore, characteristics of the pathogen should be considered in addition to host-specific, environmental and human interaction related parameters. This could be taken into account in the form of genomic analyses of infection chains between animals or between subpopulations of animals. With the ultimate goal to better understand host-pathogen interactions for this important pathogen. For this task it will be very valuable to link data generated by pathology, diagnostics, epidemiology and systems biology research.

CONCLUSION

This is the first study of *M. caprae* in red deer in the Austrian state of Vorarlberg that describes development of TB and its infection dynamics over the last decade. The study proposes the use of TB-like lesions in a so-called Patho Score as a mirror for infection dynamics. With the Patho Score, a new instrument is introduced to complement monitoring of TB in red deer in western Austria and to systematically visualize and quantify infection dynamics at no additional costs. This work shows the breadth of application possibilities of this lesion score. The analysis adds some evidence regarding the critical role of winter feeding sites for spread of TB infections in young deer. The identification of geographic areas with differing patterns of disease occurrence demonstrated that TB does spread in Vorarlberg within several geographically connected subpopulations with separate infection cycles. TB spreads only slowly between valleys but migrating infected deer might introduce the agent into new areas.

To the best knowledge of the authors, this is the first study that uses a lesion score for the systematical description of the infection dynamics of mycobacterial disease. Due to the cross-border TB situation, the possibility to systematically compare TB dynamics based on heterogeneous data is an important added value.

ETHICS STATEMENT

All animal sampling was post-mortem in accordance with the official deer monitoring program plan of the Office of the State Government of Vorarlberg. Wildlife samples came from hunter-harvested individuals that were shot during the legal hunting season, or individuals found dead, independently and prior to our research. According to national legislation (Austrian Tierversuchsgesetz 2012 – TVG 2012, BGBl. I Nr. 114/2012) no permission or consent was required for conducting this type of study.

AUTHOR CONTRIBUTIONS

AN, WG, and NG designed the study. WG and ZB carried out the laboratory work. WG and NG entered and prepared the data for the analysis. AN, WG, and ZB developed the Patho Score. AN performed the analysis. AN, WG, and ZB drafted the preliminary manuscript. All authors participated in the review and the editing of the draft and approved its final version.

ACKNOWLEDGMENTS

In the first place, the authors would like to thank all hunters and official veterinarians from Vorarlberg. Without their support the implementation of the deer monitoring would not have been possible. We would like to acknowledge Hubert Schatz for sharing his expertise in wildlife ecology. We also want to thank Ynte Schukken and Mart de Jong for valuable professional discussions. This study received financial support from the Office of the State Government of Vorarlberg, the Austrian Agency for Health and Food Safety and Wageningen University.

REFERENCES

1. Greber N. *Monitoring tuberculosis* (M. caprae) in red deer and follow-up risk-based tuberculin-testing of cattle (In German: Monitoring auf Tuberkulose beim Rotwild durch M. caprae und nachfolgende risikobasierte Tuberkulintests bei Rindern). In: *Proceedings of the DACh Epidemiology Meeting.* Vienna (2011).

2. Müller M, Hafner-Marx A, Ehrlein J, Ewringmann T, Ebert U, Weber BK, et al. Pathomorphological alterations of tuberculosis in red deer (In German. Pathomorphologische Veränderungen bei der Tuberkulose des Rotwildes). *Amtstierärztlicher Dienst und Lebensmittelkontrolle* (2014) 21:251–8.

3. Prodinger WM, Eigentler A, Allerberger F, Schönbauer M, Glawischnig W. Infection of red deer, cattle, and humans with *Mycobacterium bovis* subsp. *caprae* in western Austria. *J Clin Microbiol.* (2002) 40:2270–2. doi: 10.1128/JCM.40.6.2270-2272.2002

4. Schoepf K, Prodinger WM, Glawischnig W, Hofer E, Revilla-Fernandez S, Hofrichter J, et al. A two-years' survey on the prevalence of tuberculosis caused by *Mycobacterium caprae* in red deer (*Cervus elaphus*) in the Tyrol, Austria. *ISRN Veter Sci.* (2012) 2012:7. doi: 10.5402/2012/245138

5. Fink M, Schleicher C, Gonano M, Prodinger WM, Pacciarini M, Glawischnig W, et al. Red deer as maintenance host for bovine tuberculosis, Alpine region. *Emerg Infect Dis.* (2015) 21:464. doi: 10.3201/eid2103. 141119

6. Clifton-Hadley R, Wilesmith J. Tuberculosis in deer: a review. *Veter Record* (1991) 129:5–12. doi: 10.1136/vr.129.1.5

7. Buchan G, Griffin J. Tuberculosis in domesticated deer (*Cervus elaphus*): a large animal model for human tuberculosis. *J Compar Pathol.* (1990) 103:11–22. doi: 10.1016/S0021-9975(08)80131-4

8. Lugton IW, Wilson PR, Morris RS, Griffin JF, de Lisle GW. Natural infection of red deer with bovine tuberculosis. *NZ Veter J.* (1997) 45:19–26. doi: 10.1080/00480169.1997.35983

9. Mackintosh C, Griffin J. "Epidemiological aspects of deer tuberculosis research," in *Proceedings of a Deer Course for Veterinarians Deer Branch, the Association* (1994). pp. 106–15.

10. Griffin J, Buchan G. Aetiology, pathogenesis and diagnosis of *Mycobacterium bovis* in deer. *Veter Microbiol.* (1994) 40:193–205. doi: 10.1016/0378-1135(94)90055-8

11. Lisle GW, de Havill PF. Mycobacteria isolated from deer in New Zealand from 1970 - 1983. *NZ Veter J.* (1985) 33:138–40. doi: 10.1080/00480169.1985.35198

12. Lugton IW, Wilson PR, Morris RS, Nugent G. Epidemiology and pathogenesis of *Mycobacferium bovis* infection of red deer (*Cervus elaphus*) in New Zealand. *NZ Veter J.* (1998) 46:147–56. doi: 10.1080/00480169.1998.36079

13. Nigsch A, Ryser MP, Henschel A, Schneeberger D, Suter D, Jakob P. *Manual Tuberculosis in Wildlife (In German: Handbuch Tuberkulose beim Wild).* 1st editon. Bern: Federal Food Safety and Veterinary Office (2014). Available online at: https://www.bundespublikationen.admin.ch/cshop_bbl/b2c/start/(carea=002 4817F68691EE1B4B08AD5B235D00F&citem=0024817F68691EE1B4B08AD 5B235D00F2C59E545D7371ED481E9BBBAE8DB3F4D)/.do German, French, Italian.

14. Palmer M, O'Brien DJ, Griffin F, Delahay RJ. Tuberculosis in wild and captive deer. Many Hosts of Mycobacteria: Tuberculosis, Leprosy and Other Mycobacterial Diseases of Man and Animals. Wallingford: CABI (2015).

15. Mackintosh CG, De Lisle GW, Collins DM, Griffin JFT. Mycobacterial diseases of deer. *NZ Veter J.* (2004) 52:163–74. doi: 10.1080/00480169.2004.36424

16. Glawischnig W, Allerberger F, Messner C, Schönbauer M, Prodinger WM. Endemic Tuberculosis in free-ranging red deer (Cervus elaphus hippelaphus) in the Northern limestone Alps (In German: Tuberkulose-Endemie bei freilebendem Rotwild (Cervus elaphus hippelaphus) in den nördlichen Kalkalpen). *Wiener tierärztliche Monatsschrift* (2003) 90:38–44.

17. Johnson LK, Liebana E, Nunez A, Spencer Y, Clifton-Hadley R, Jahans K, et al. Histological observations of bovine tuberculosis in lung and lymph node tissues from British deer. *Veter J.* (2008) 175:409–12. doi: 10.1016/j.tvjl.2007.04.021

18. Vicente J, Barasona JA, Acevedo P, Ruiz-Fons JF, Boadella M, Diez-Delgado I, et al. Temporal trend of tuberculosis in wild ungulates from Mediterranean S pain. *Transbound Emerg Dis.* (2013) 60:92–103. doi: 10.1111/tbed.12167

19. Nugent G. *The Role of Wild Deer in the Epidemiology and Management of Bovine tuberculosis in New Zealand.* Lincoln: Lincoln University (2005).

20. Griffin J, Thomson A. Farmed deer: a large animal model for stress. *Domest Ani Endocrinol.* (1998) 15:445–56. doi: 10.1016/S0739-7240(98)00016-2

21. Mackintosh CG, Qureshi T, Waldrup K, Labes RE, Dodds KG, Griffin JF. Genetic resistance to experimental infection with *Mycobacterium bovis* in red deer (*Cervus elaphus*). *Infect immun.* (2000) 68:1620–5. doi: 10.1128/IAI.68.3.1620-1625.2000

22. Nigsch A. *Tuberculosis in wildlife in the area of Vorarlberg. Expert opinion on the current sitation 2015/2016 (In German: Tuberkulose beim Wild im Raum Vorarlberg. Expertise zur aktuellen Situation 2015/2016).* Federal Food Safety and Veterinary Office (2016). Available online at: https://www.researchgate.net/publication/315628448_Tuberculosis_in_wildlife_in_the_region_of_Vorarlberg_Expertise_on_the_current_situation_20152016_in_German

23. KVG. *Communication Platform Consumer Protection. Tuberculosis (In German: Kommunikationsplattform VerbraucherInnengesundheit. Tuberkulose)* (2018). Available online at: https://www.verbrauchergesundheit.gv.at/tiere/krankheiten/tbc.html

24. Kamerbeek J, Schouls L, Kolk A, van Agterveld M, van Soolingen D, Kuijper S, et al. Simultaneous detection and strain differentiation of *Mycobacterium tuberculosis* for diagnosis and epidemiology. *J Clin Microbiol.* (1997) 35:907–14.

25. Mazars E, Lesjean S, Banuls AL, Gilbert M, Vincent V, Gicquel B, et al. High-resolution minisatellite-based typing as a portable approach to global analysis of *Mycobacterium tuberculosis* molecular epidemiology. *Proc Natl Acad Sci USA.* (2001) 98:1901–6. doi: 10.1073/pnas.98.4.1901

26. Supply P, Allix C, Lesjean S, Cardoso-Oelemann M, Rüsch-Gerdes S, Willery E, et al. Proposal for standardization of optimized mycobacterial interspersed repetitive unit-variable-number tandem repeat typing of *Mycobacterium tuberculosis. J Clin Microbiol.* (2006) 44:4498–510. doi: 10.1128/JCM.01392-06

27. Domogalla J, Prodinger WM, Blum H, Krebs S, Gellert S, Müller M, et al. Region of difference 4 in alpine *Mycobacterium caprae* isolates indicates three variants. *J Clin Microbiol.* (2013) 51:1381–8. doi: 10.1128/JCM.02966-12

28. Greber N. *Red Deer Monitoring 2017 (In German: Bericht Rotwildmonitoring 2017).* Vorarlberger:Jagd (2018).

29. FIWI. *Tuberculosis in Alpine Wildlife. Monitoring, Diagnostics and Potential Control Strategies of Tuberculosis in Wild Animals in the Alpine Provinces of Austria, Germany, Italy and Switzerland.* Report: Work package 3 - "Epidemiology, University of Veterinary Medicine Vienna, Research Institute of Wildlife Ecology, Department of Integrative Biology and Evolution ,Vienna (2013). Available online at: https://www.era-learn.eu/network-information/networks/emida/emida-2009-research-call/tuberculosis-in-alpine-wildlife-monitoring-diagnostics-and-potential-control-strategies-of-tuberculosis-in-wild-animals-in-the-alpine-provinces-of-austria-germany-italy-and-switzerland

30. Reimoser F, Tataruch F, Klansek E. *Regional Planning Concept for Hoofed Game Management in Vorarlberg With Special Consideration of Forest Decline. (in German: Regionalplanungskonzept zur Schalenwildbewirtschaftung in Vorarlberg unter besonderer Berücksichtigung des Waldsterbens).* University of Veterinary Medicine Vienna (1988). Available online at: http://www.vorarlberg.at/pdf/regionalplanungskonzept19.pdf

31. Reimoser F, Spoerk J, Duscher A, Agreiter A. *Evaluation of the Wildlife - Environment - Situation in the State of Vorarlberg With Special Consideration of the Impact of the Hunting Law of Vorarlberg on Forest and Wildlife (Comparison 1988 - 2003). (in German: Evaluierung der Wild - Umwelt - Situation im Bundesland Vorarlberg unter besonderer Beruecksichtigung der Auswirkungen des Vorarlberger Jagdgesetzes auf Wald und Wild (Vergleich 1988 - 2003)).* University of Veterinary Medicine Vienna, University of Natural Ressources and Life Science, Vienna. (2005). Available online at: http://www.vorarlberg.at/pdf/evaluierungderwild_umwelt.pdf

32. O'Brien DJ, Schmitt SM, Fierke JS, Hogle SA, Winterstein SR, Cooley TM, et al. Epidemiology of Mycobacterium bovis in free-ranging white-tailed deer, Michigan, USA, 1995–2000. *Prevent Veter Med.* (2002) 54:47–63. doi: 10.1016/S0167-5877(02)00010-7

33. Palmer M, Waters W, Whipple D. Lesion development in white-tailed deer (*Odocoileus virginianus*) experimentally infected with *Mycobacterium bovis. Veter Pathol.* (2002) 39:334–40. doi: 10.1354/vp.39-3-334

34. Office of the State Government of Vorarlberg. Measures for the Prevention and Control of Tuberculosis 2018. In: *German: Schwerpunktmaßnahmen 2018 zur Tbc-Vorbeugung und -Bekämpfung* (2018). Available online at: https://vorarlberg.at/web/land-vorarlberg/contentdetailseite/-/asset_publisher/qA6AJ38txu0k/content/abschussplanerfuellung?article_id=219568

35. FIWI. *Tagging of Red Deer in the Border Triangle (Vorarlberg, Principality of Liechtenstein and Canton Grisons).* Final report, Part A – Data analysis (In German: Rotwildmarkierung im Dreiländereck, (Vorarlberg, Fürstentum Liechtenstein, Kanton Graubünden)). Forschungsinstitut für Wildtierkunde und Ökologie FIWI. Veterinärmedizinische Universität Wien (2014).

36. Federal Food Safety and Veterinary Office. *Four Alpine Countries Join Forces to Fight Tuberculosis in Wildlife (In German: Vier Alpenländer Gehen Gemeinsam Gegen die Tuberkulose beim Wild vor).* Press release (2018). Available online at: https://www.blv.admin.ch/blv/de/home/dokumentation/nsb-news-list.msg-id-70029.html. German, French, Italian

37. Office of the State Government of Vorarlberg. *Hunting statistics Vorarlberg.* (2018) Available online at: http://vorarlberg.at/vorarlberg/landwirtschaft_forst/landwirtschaft/jagd/weitereinformationen/jagdstatistik.htm

38. Glawischnig W, Hofer E, Weinberger H, Pohl B, Revilla-Fernandez S, Schöpf K. A severe case of red deer Tuberculosis caused by Mycobacterium microti. In: *13th European Wildlife Disease Association Conference.* Larissa (2018).

39. StataCorp. *Stata Statistical Software: Release 14.* College Station, TX: StataCorp LP (2015).

40. ESRI. *ArcGIS Desktop: Release 10.* Redlands, CA: Environmental Systems Research Institute (2011).

41. Glawischnig W. *Tuberculosis in Wildlife (In German: Tuberkulose bei Wildtieren).* Jagd in Tirol (2009).

42. Nugent G, Gortazar C, Knowles G. The epidemiology of *Mycobacterium bovis* in wild deer and feral pigs and their roles in the establishment and spread of bovine tuberculosis in New Zealand wildlife. *NZ Veter J.* (2015) 63(Supp. 1):54–67. doi: 10.1080/00480169.2014.963792

43. Vicente J, Höfle U, Garrido JM, Fernández-de-Mera IG, Acevedo P, Juste R, et al. Risk factors associated with the prevalence of tuberculosis-like lesions in fenced wild boar and red deer in south central Spain. *Veter Res.* (2007) 38:451–64. doi: 10.1051/vetres:2007002

44. Vicente J, Höfle U, Garrido JM, Fernández-De-Mera IG, Juste R, Barral M, et al. Wild boar and red deer display high prevalences of tuberculosis-like lesions in Spain. *Veter Res.* (2006) 37:107–19. doi: 10.1051/vetres:2005044

45. Lugton I. Mucosa-associated lymphoid tissues as sites for uptake, carriage and excretion of tubercle bacilli and other pathogenic mycobacteria. *Immunol. Cell Biol.* (1999) 77:364–72. doi: 10.1046/j.1440-1711.1999.00836.x

46. Griffin J, Chinn D, Rodgers C. Diagnostic strategies and outcomes on three New Zealand deer farms with severe outbreaks of bovine tuberculosis. *Tuberculosis* (2004) 84:293–302. doi: 10.1016/j.tube.2003.11.001

47. Zanella G, Duvauchelle A, Hars J, Moutou F, Boschiroli ML, Durand B. Patterns of lesions of bovine tuberculosis in wild red deer and wild boar. *Veter Rec.* (2008) 163:43–7. doi: 10.1136/vr.163.2.43

48. Griffin J, Mackintosh C. Tuberculosis in deer: perceptions, problems and progress. *Veter J.* (2000) 160:202–19. doi: 10.1053/tvjl.2000.0514

49. Sjögren I, Sutherland I. Studies of tuberculosis in an in relation to infection in cattle. *Tubercle* (1975) 56:113–27. doi: 10.1016/0041-3879(75)90022-7

50. Corner LA, O'Meara D, Costello E, Lesellier S, Gormley E. The distribution of *Mycobacterium bovis* infection in naturally infected badgers. *Veter J.* (2012) 194:166–72. doi: 10.1016/j.tvjl.2012.03.013

51. Liebana E, Johnson L, Gough J, Durr P, Jahans K, Clifton-Hadley R, et al. Pathology of naturally occurring bovine tuberculosis in England and Wales. *Veter J.* (2008) 176:354–60. doi: 10.1016/j.tvjl.2007.07.001

52. Waters WR, Palmer MV. *Mycobacterium bovis* infection of cattle and white-tailed deer: translational research of relevance to human tuberculosis. *ILAR J.* (2015) 56:26–43. doi: 10.1093/ilar/ilv001

53. Martín-Hernando MP, Torres MJ, Aznar J, Negro JJ, Gandía A, Gortázar C. Distribution of lesions in red and fallow deer naturally infected with *Mycobacterium bovis*. *J Compar Pathol.* (2010) 142:43–50. doi: 10.1016/j.jcpa.2009.07.003

54. Gavier-Widén D, Cooke MM, Gallagher J, Chambers MA, Gortázar C. A review of infection of wildlife hosts with Mycobacterium bovis and the diagnostic difficulties of the "no visible lesion" presentation. *NZ Veter J.* (2009) 57:122–31. doi: 10.1080/00480169.2009.36891

55. Ballesteros C, Garrido JM, Vicente J, Romero B, Galindo RC, Minguijón E, et al. First data on Eurasian wild boar response to oral immunization with BCG and challenge with a *Mycobacterium bovis* field strain. *Vaccine* (2009) 27:6662–8. doi: 10.1016/j.vaccine.2009.08.095

56. Vordermeier H, Chambers MA, Cockle PJ, Whelan AO, Simmons J, Hewinson RG. Correlation of ESAT-6 specific IFN-production with pathology in cattle following BCG vaccination against experimental bovine tuberculosis. *Infect Immun.* (2002) 70:3026–32. doi: 10.1128/IAI.70.6.3026-3032.2002

57. Wangoo A, Johnson L, Gough J, Ackbar R, Inglut S, Hicks D, et al. Advanced granulomatous lesions in *Mycobacterium bovis*-infected cattle are associated with increased expression of type I procollagen, $\gamma\Delta$(WC1+) T cells and CD 68+ cells. *J Compar Pathol.* (2005) 133:223–34. doi: 10.1016/j.jcpa.2005.05.001

Development and Evaluation of a Serological Assay for the Diagnosis of Tuberculosis in Alpacas and Llamas

Jose A. Infantes-Lorenzo [1,2], Claire E. Whitehead [3], Inmaculada Moreno [4], Javier Bezos [1], Alvaro Roy [1], Lucas Domínguez [1,5], Mercedes Domínguez [4†] and Francisco J. Salguero [2*†]

[1] VISAVET Health Surveillance Centre, Universidad Complutense de Madrid, Madrid, Spain, [2] Department of Pathology and Infectious Diseases, School of Veterinary Medicine, University of Surrey, Guildford, United Kingdom, [3] Camelid Veterinary Services Ltd, Reading, United Kingdom, [4] Unidad de Inmunología Microbiana, Centro Nacional de Microbiología, Instituto de Salud Carlos III, Madrid, Spain, [5] Departamento de Sanidad Animal, Facultad de Veterinaria, Universidad Complutense de Madrid, Madrid, Spain

*Correspondence:
Francisco J. Salguero
f.salguerobodes@surrey.ac.uk

† These authors have contributed equally to this work

South American camelids are susceptible to tuberculosis, caused mainly by *Mycobacterium bovis* and *M. microti*. Despite the tuberculin skin test being the official test for tuberculosis, it has a very low sensitivity in these species (14–20%). Serological tests present the advantages of being rapid, easy to perform and facilitate analysis of large numbers of samples in a short period of time. Novel antigen discovery and evaluation would provide enhanced detection of specific antibodies against members of *M. tuberculosis* complex. Here, we describe the development and evaluation of an ELISA-type immunoassays to use in the diagnosis of tuberculosis in llamas and alpacas based on P22, a multiprotein complex obtained by affinity chromatography from bovine Purified Protein Derivative (bPPD), that showed high sensitivity and specificity in mice, cattle and goats. This work was performed in two stages. First, a preliminary panel of samples collected from tuberculosis-free ($n = 396$) and *M. bovis*-infected herds ($n = 56$) was assayed, obtaining high specificity (100%) and sensitivity ranging from 63 to 96%. Subsequently, the use of the serological assay was tested using samples from two herds suffering from clinical *M. bovis* ($n = 88$) and *M. microti* ($n = 25$) infection to evaluate the ability of the ELISA to detect infected animals. 11 out of 88 alpacas were positive to the ELISA in a *M. bovis* outbreak and 7 out of 25 in a *M. microti* outbreak. The P22 ELISA potentially provides a sensitive and specific platform for improved tuberculosis surveillance in camelids.

Keywords: South American camelids, diagnosis, ELISA, P22, tuberculosis

INTRODUCTION

To date, tuberculosis (TB) is one of the most important diseases globally, both in animals and humans (1, 2). Animal TB has a broad range of domestic and wild mammal species hosts, including South American Camelids (SAC) that have become increasingly popular as production animals in recent years. Although llamas and alpacas are gaining more importance in fiber production (3, 4), these animals also have companion animal value and may have regular contact with humans and other susceptible animal species. SACs are a potential source of different pathogens that might be transmitted to humans and could pose a risk to human health (5). Among these diseases, alpacas and llamas are very susceptible to TB, caused by bacteria from the *Mycobacterium tuberculosis* complex (MTC), mainly by *M. bovis* and *M. microti* (6, 7).

The diagnosis of tuberculosis in SAC has been mainly based on the tuberculin skin test, both single and comparative intradermal tuberculin test (SIT and SCIT, respectively), but these show poor performance in general in these species (8–10) and low sensitivity between 14 and 20%. A sensitivity of only 14% was found in one llama herd outbreak for animals that presented with visible lesions at post-mortem examination within 3 months of the SCIT test (11). In another report, only one llama tested positive out of five that were subsequently found to have visible lesions from which *M. bovis* was cultured (12). The interferon gamma (IFN-γ) test, based on the stimulation of blood cells with Purified Protein Derivatives (PPDs) and subsequent detection of the IFN-γ released, has been also developed for the diagnosis of TB, but it has been difficult to standardize, is labor-intensive, and in SAC yields a low sensitivity and specificity (63.6 and 89.1%, respectively) (13). In addition, in-house and commercial serological assays for the detection of specific antibodies have been previously investigated with a wide range of results (8, 11–14), but have been tested in a low number of animals.

Serological tests have been able to detect infected animals before the onset of clinical disease (8). In addition, the booster effect on the antibody response caused after injection of tuberculin has been reported as a strategic option to increase the sensitivity of serological assays in some species (15, 16). In general terms, the specificity of the serological assays are moderate to high, ranged from 84.6 to 98%, depending on the study and serological test employed (13, 17, 18). However, they showed low to moderate sensitivity, ranging from 43 to 75%, even using sera samples collected after intradermal PPD injection (7, 13, 17, 18). More details of the serological test evaluated in SAC are provided in **Table 1**. For these reasons, it is necessary to develop and evaluate new assays in order to provide more sensitive and specific options for the serological diagnosis of TB in SACs.

The aim of the present study was to develop and evaluate a novel ELISA type assay for the detection of specific antibodies of MTC in alpacas and llamas based on P22 multiprotein complex (20), which is affinity-purified from the PPD of *M. bovis,* and has been shown to provide greater sensitivity in other host species (15, 16). The P22-based ELISA was tested in serum samples from alpacas naturally infected with *M. bovis* and *M. microti* from Spain and England and uninfected llamas and alpacas from Peru and England.

MATERIALS AND METHODS

This work was performed in two stages: the first one included a preliminary panel of samples collected in TB-free and naturally

M. bovis-infected herds to set the optimal cut-off point and calculate specificity and sensitivity of the ELISA; in a second stage, two farms suffering from clinical TB infection under different epidemiological situations were used to validate the test. Handling of the animals, testing and sampling were performed by accredited veterinarians. These were residual samples collected as part of routine surveillance or during breakdown sampling. All samples used in this study were serum samples. The animals used in this study were not experimental animals. All handling and sampling procedures were performed by veterinarians in accordance with the local legislation (Real Decreto 53/2013 in Spain, Ley de Protección y Bienestar animal N° 30407 in Peru, and the The Veterinary Surgeon Act 1966 in England).

Assessment of Specificity and Sensitivity

The specificity of the serological tests was evaluated in two different TB-free herds of alpacas and llamas located in different regions in Peru (19). The first alpaca herd was located at 4,000 m of altitude in La Libertad (northwest) and the second llama herd was located at approximately 4,200 m of altitude in Puno (southeast). 120 alpacas (104 male and 16 female) and 40 llamas (all female) were tested. Both herds were considered TB-free (based on long history of TB-free infection, absence of compatible lesions and epidemiological investigations). No lesions consistent with TB were observed in any animal in the 5 years prior to the study during slaughterhouse surveillance and no TB outbreak was reported on farms near the herds of the study. In addition, one TB-free herd from southern England was also included. 236 samples were available from adult alpacas at this herd including 93 males and 143 females. The regulatory program for TB surveillance in SAC in England can be found in the Bovine TB Eradication Programme for England (http://apha.defra.gov.uk).

The sensitivity was evaluated using serum samples from animals (n = 56) from a herd located in central Spain where an *M. bovis* outbreak was detected. The herd was a mix of alpacas of Suri and Huacaya breed. No previous history of TBs was reported before this outbreak. In December 2011, field veterinarians detected clinical signs (anorexia, cachexia, respiratory distress) and/or sudden deaths in three alpacas. Compatible TB-like lesions were observed in the post-mortem examination of one of these alpacas and *M. bovis* infection was subsequently confirmed by bacterial culture (18). A total of 67 animals were slaughtered and subjected to post-mortem examination within 4 weeks after the ante-mortem tests. Animals with positive *M. bovis* cultures and/or presence of visible TB-like lesions compatible with TB (n = 56) were included in the study to assess sensitivity. Serum samples for detection of specific antibodies were collected prior to PPD inoculation and 15 days after.

Testing the ELISA Under Field Conditions in Two TB Outbreaks

The analysis was carried out in two herds with natural *M. bovis* or *M. microti* infection confirmed by the presence of lesions compatible with TB and/or microbiological culture. Herd A consisted of 88 animals of Huacaya breed in England. This farm was selected due to a TB outbreak commencing in November

TABLE 1 | Details of different serodiagnostic tests in llamas and alpacas.

Assay test	Specie	Number of animals ($n_{Se} + n_{Sp}$)	Antigens	Sensitivity (%)	Specificity (%)	References
Enzyme linked immunosorbent assay (ELISA)	Alpaca	65	MPB83	43.1	–	(18)
	Llama and alpaca	160	MPB83	–	96.3	(19)
	Alpacas	52 + 306	MPB70 and MPB83	69.2	97.4	(13)
	Alpacas	52 + 257	M. bovis antigens[a]	66.7	96.9	(13)
VetTB STAT-PAK	Llama	14	MPB83, ESAT-6 and CFP-10	64.3	–	(11)
	Llama and alpaca	8 + 79	MPB83, ESAT-6 and CFP-10	62.5	89.9	(8)
	Llama and alpaca	52 + 279	MPB83, ESAT-6 and CFP-10	73.1	94.6	(17)
	Alpacas	52 + 306	MPB83, ESAT-6 and CFP-10	67.3	97.4	(13)
Dual-path platform (DPP)	Llama and alpaca	52 + 279	MPB70 and MPB83	75	97.5	(17)
	Alpacas	52 + 306	MPB70 and MPB83	57.7	96.7	(13)
Multiantigen print immunoassay (MAPIA)	Llama	14	M. bovis antigens[b]	100	–	(11)
	Llama and alpaca	8 + 79	M. bovis antigens[c]	87.5	97.5	(8)

nSe, number of TB positive animals used for evaluation of Se; nSp, number of negative animals used for evaluation of Sp.

[a] bPPD, ESAT6, CFP10, Rv3616c, MPB83, MPB70, and an MPB70 peptide.

[b] ESAT-6, CFP-10, MPB64, MPB59, MPB70, MPB83, the 16-kDa protein, the 38-kDa protein, two fusion proteins comprising CFP10/ESAT-6 and the 16-kDa protein/MPB83, and two native antigens, bPPD and M. bovis culture filtrate.

[c] Purified recombinant proteins (ESAT-6, CFP10, MPB70, MPB83, Mtb8, Mtb48, Acr1, and the 38 kDa protein), two native antigens, MPB83 protein and M. bovis culture filtrate (MBCF), and four protein fusions (CFP10/ESAT-6, Acr1/MPB83, F10, and F6).

2016. Two initial clinical cases were disclosed at necropsy with compatible TB lesions and M. bovis was isolated. Subsequently, a whole herd SCIT was performed and one alpaca was culled on the basis of a positive test. This alpaca was found to have lesions at necropsy. Serological testing took place 14 days later using Enferplex and cervid-DPP tests: two animals tested positive on the Enferplex test, were culled but found to have no visible lesions. All animals were skin-tested again 3 months later (using bovine tuberculin only) and also bled for further serological analysis (Enferplex only) 10 days following the skin test. Three animals were found positive on serology and were culled. At necropsy examination, two of these animals had no visible lesions while the third alpaca was found to have atypical lesions, comprising multiple small caseous lesions in a prescapular lymph node.

The herd B outbreak of TB was detected a herd of approximately 80 animals located in England in July 2017. The owner had performed surveillance serological testing (Enferplex) in May and identified a single animal that tested positive. At a retest 1 month later, the animal remained positive and was culled voluntarily on the basis of suspicion of disease. He was found to have lesions in the liver as well as bronchial and hepatic lymph nodes but no lesions in the lungs. At whole herd skin testing (SCIT), three further animals were disclosed and culled, although no visible lesions were found. At serological testing performed after the skin test, six animals were identified as positive on Enferplex and culled. Five of these animals had atypical lesions identified at post-mortem examination while the sixth had typical lesions in the lungs. A seventh alpaca was culled as a dangerous contact and also displayed atypical lesions at necropsy. 25 samples were available for analysis from 22 Suri alpacas (3 males and 19 females), one Huacaya male alpaca and two male llamas. M microti was never successfully cultured from these cases although PCR testing of lesion material was positive for M microti.

Development of an Indirect and a Competitive ELISA

An in-house indirect ELISA that detects antibodies against a protein complex named P22, purified by affinity chromatography from bovine PPD [CZ Veterinaria (Porriño, Spain)] was developed. The indirect ELISA was performed as described previously with minor modifications (15). Briefly, plates were coated with P22 (10 μg/ml) and then blocked with 5% skimmed milk powder solution in phosphate buffered saline (PBS). After three washes with PBS plus 0.05%Tween 20 (PBST), sera were added in duplicate at 1:100 dilutions in skimmed milk and incubated for 60 min at 37°C. The optimal dilution of test serum was determined before by evaluating the reactivity of serum diluted from 1:10 to 1:640. 100 µl of detection antibody (Anti-llama IgG-HRP conjugate at 1:4,000 were added and the plates were incubated for 30 min at room temperature (RT). As before, the secondary antibody was titrated from 1:1,000 to 1:8,000 to choose the optimal dilution. The reaction was developed by adding 100 µl of o-phenylenediamine dihydrochloride substrate (FAST OPD, Sigma–Aldrich, St Louise, USA) incubated for 15 min in darkness and RT conditions. After that, the reaction was stopped with 50 µl of H_2SO_4 (3 N). The optical density (OD) was measured at 492 nm with an ELISA reader.

Negative control serum was obtained from TB-free llama previously described as *M. bovis* culture negative from TB-free areas and was included in every plate in quadruplicate. Positive controls were obtained from llamas previously described as *M. bovis*-infected confirmed by the presence of TB compatible lesions and *M. bovis* positive culture.

In order to reduce the cross-reactivity with non-tuberculous mycobacteria (NTM), a competitive ELISA was included. In this case the serum samples were diluted in skimmed milk supplemented with avian PPD [CZ Veterinaria (Porriño, Spain)] at 150 µg/ml. Only samples that yielded positive results to the indirect ELISA were analyzed by the competitive ELISA.

Data Treatment

Sample results were expressed as an ELISA percentage (E%), calculated by the following formula: [sample E% = (mean sample OD/(2 × mean of negative control OD)) × 100]. Specificity was calculated in the TB-free population using the formula [Sp = true negatives/(true negatives + false positives) × 100]. Sensitivity was calculated in the TB-infected population by the formula [Se = true positives/(true positives + false negatives) × 100]. The cut-off value was calculated using a ROC analysis and was defined as the value at which the highest sum of Se plus Sp was obtained (21). Confidence intervals for Se and Sp were calculated using the 95% Wilson's confident interval (Epitools, Ausvet Pty Ltd., Canberra, Australia).

RESULTS

The ROC analysis evidenced the diagnostic value the P22 ELISA in SAC (**Figure 1**). The cut-off value was defined as the ratio of the mean sample OD to the double of the mean OD of the negative control. The P22 ELISA with a cut-off value set at 100 E% showed the best balance between sensitivity and specificity. Modifying the cut-off value (>100E%<) resulted in either a decreased specificity or a constant sensitivity and a cut-off value of 100 was, therefore, chosen for the P22 ELISA.

The data including sensitivity, specificity, positive predictive value, negative predictive value and area under the curve (AUC), using confidence intervals of 95% (95% CI) for the ELISA with a chosen cut-off value of 100, are summarized in **Table 2**. Once the optimal cut-off was calculated, the specificity and sensitivity was studied in greater depth.

Determination of Test Specificity

Specificity of the P22 ELISA in llama and alpaca herds is shown in **Table 3**. The 396 animals from TB-free herds were negative to the indirect ELISA. Thus, overall the specificity of P22 indirect

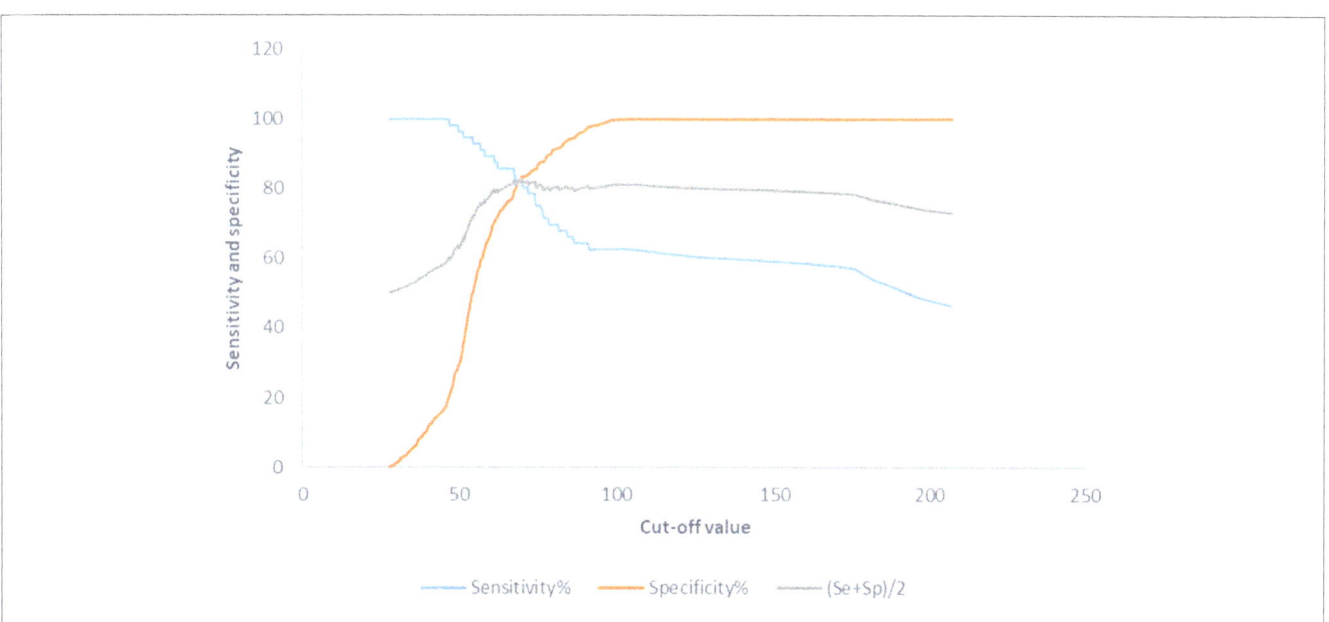

FIGURE 1 | Diagnostic value graphics for the tuberculosis indirect ELISA in SACs when using the P22 as an antigen. Sensitivity (Se), specificity (Sp) and their semi-sum are the percentages on the Y-axis and the cut-off value on the X-axis.

TABLE 2 | Sensitivity (Se), specificity (Sp), positive predictive value (PPV), negative predictive value (NPV) and area under the curve (AUC) with 95% confidence intervals (CI₉₅) in the chosen cut-off value of 100 for P22 indirect ELISA in llamas and alpacas.

Se		Sp		PPV		NPV		AUC
%	CI₉₅	%	CI₉₅	%	CI₉₅	%	CI₉₅	
62.5	49.4–74	100	99–100	100	90.1–100	95	92.4–96.7	0.91

TABLE 3 | Specificity and 95% Wilson's confident interval of the ELISA using serum samples from llama and alpacas taken before and 5 days after the SCIT test.

Country	Specie	Total	Pre-SCIT N^a	Pre-SCIT Sp^b	Post-SCIT N^a	Post-SCIT Sp^b
Peru	Alpaca	120	0	100 (96.9–100)	0	100 (96.9–100)
Peru	Llama	40	0	100 (91.2–100)	0	100 (91.2–100)
UK	Alpaca	236	0	100 (98.4–100)	–	–
	Total	396	0	100 (99–100)	0	100 (97.7–100)

^{a} Number of positive animals.
^{b} 95% Confidence interval for specificity.

ELISA was 100% (95% CI 99–100) in llamas and alpacas. In the absence of any positive animal, the competitive ELISA was not carried out.

Determination of Test Sensitivity

The sensitivity achieved with P22 indirect ELISA in the samples from Spain was 62.5% (35/56) (95% CI 49.4–74) before PPD inoculation, and 96.4% (54/56) (95% CI 87.9–99) 15 days after PPD inoculation (**Table 4**). The competitive ELISA showed similar sensitivity.

Study of Two TB Outbreaks in England

M. bovis Outbreak

In herd A, of the 88 animal analyzed, 11 were positive to indirect ELISA (**Figure 2**). However, three animals had E% over 150 and the remaining eight animals had values between 100 and 150%. The competitive ELISA showed similar results. The same three animals had over E% 150 again and only seven were between 100 and 150%, one less than using the indirect ELISA. This animal was negative in competitive ELISA and positive in indirect ELISA maybe due to cross reaction by NTM. Considering that four animals had visible lesions at necropsy, three were positive to both the indirect and competitive ELISA.

M. microti Outbreak

In herd B, 25 serum samples were analyzed. Seven animals were positive in both indirect and competitive ELISA. Only one animal showed an E% value close to the cut-off point. The other six animals that had an E% over 300 (**Figure 2**), had visible lesions at post-mortem examination. Two animals with visible lesions at necropsy were negative to the ELISAs.

TABLE 4 | Sensitivity and 95% Wilson's confident interval of indirect (Ei) and competitive ELISA (Ec) in TB-infected animals based on post-mortem examination (culture positive and/or presence of visible TB lesions).

N of animals	Pre-SCIT Ei	Pre-SCIT Ec	15 days after SCIT Ei	15 days after SCIT Ec
56	62.5 (49.4–74)	60.7 (47.6–72.4)	96.4 (87.9–99)	96.4 (87.9–99)

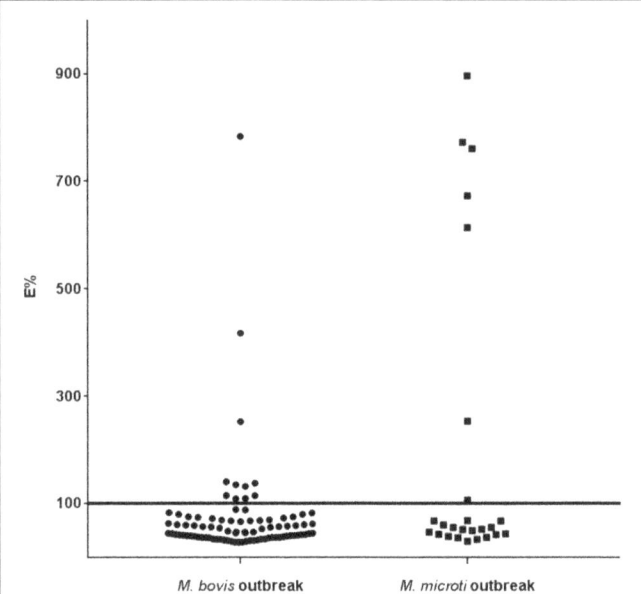

FIGURE 2 | Histogram of the ELISA E% value of individual llama or alpaca tested by indirect ELISA using P22 as antigen in *M. bovis* and *M. microti* outbreaks. The horizontal line represents the chosen cut-off value.

DISCUSSION

Since alpacas became an important animal in Europe and more tools for the diagnosis of TB in alpacas are needed, our results suggest that the indirect P22 ELISAs described here can provide better sensitivity and specificity than other TB antibody detection tests currently used in alpacas and could be used to detect both *M. bovis* and *M. microti* infection in SAC. As the indirect ELISA showed a specificity of 100%, and the purpose for the competitive ELISA was to remove antibodies against proteins shared between *M. tuberculosis complex* and non-tuberculous mycobacteria, the competitive ELISA is not useful in this case to improve the specificity of the diagnosis. Therefore, we focused on the indirect ELISA and propose this ELISA as a new tool for the diagnosis of TB in SACs.

Several serological tests for detection of antibodies against TB described previously showed specificity range from 84 to 98% (13, 17, 19). The P22 ELISA achieved an excellent specificity of 100%, higher than all serological test described up to date for diagnosis of TB in camelids. In addition, no effect of the injection of PPD was observed. The number of animal included in this study was large enough to have a reliable specificity data, including with samples 5 days after PPD injection. However, further studies with samples taken 15 days after the skin test are necessary to confirm this finding because 5 days post-PPD may be insufficient to observe optimal antibody boost.

Regarding sensitivity, our ELISA yielded a moderate average sensitivity of 62.5%, similar to those reported by other serological assays in SACs, which are between 43 and 74% (13, 17, 18). These results are similar to those obtained for TB in bovine using a P22-based ELISA test (15). Using samples obtained 15 days after skin test, the sensitivity of P22 ELISA increased to 96%. This result was higher than reported by all previous serological assays using samples 15 days post-skin test, which sensitivity was between 77 and 89% (18). This boosting effect has been reported in TB in goats, bovines and alpacas (16, 18, 22). Casal et al. (22) demonstrated that sensitivity was significantly higher in cattle using samples collected 15 days post-skin test (ranging from 66.7 to 85.2%). Our results obtained using samples 15 days after injection of PPD were promising and suggested that the P22 ELISA could be a useful TB diagnostic tool in SACs. Taking a blood sample at 15 days post-PPD injection would require an additional veterinary visit, with an associate cost. For this reason, it may not be suitable as a routine method. Despite the costly strategy, the increase of the sensitivity to almost 100%could justify its use in certain situations. The booster effect, including the P22 ELISA, has also been described as a useful approach in cases of explosive TB outbreaks in other species as goats (16).

Humoral response occurs primarily in advances stage of infection and its detection has been considered less effective in early stages of TB infection (23, 24). However, although the skin test is the official diagnostic test for TB in alpacas, SIT test showed poor performances in terms of sensitivity and our results showed a higher sensitivity than SIT. Similar results were obtained previously (11, 13, 18). The combination of the skin test and a serological assay could be an approach to maximize the detection of infected animal instead of IFN-γ because of low sensitivity and difficulties to perform (18). Therefore, implementation of serology in parallel with the skin test could reach sensitivity of 100% (18). Since serology represents a rapid and inexpensive assay, a previous study recommended testing the same samples using several serological assays for a better diagnosis of infected animals (13). In this sense, our P22 ELISA may serve as a preferred technique for the diagnosis of TB,

together with other serological assays or skin test. In addition, previous published batches of P22 showed similar qualitative and quantitative composition (20) and, consequently make P22 a stable and reliable product.

TB in SACs is mainly caused by M. bovis and M. microti, and has been reported in several European countries including Spain, the Netherlands, Switzerland, Ireland and the UK (7, 9, 14, 25). The present study has demonstrated the potential of the ELISA in serodiagnosis of TB due to M. bovis and also M. microti. The high OD observed in six M. microti and three M. bovis infected animals suggest a new promising sensitive serological test. Moreover, out of four animals in M. bovis outbreak and eight animals in M. microti outbreak with visible lesions, three and six animals, respectively were positive to the ELISA, showing a good ability to detect animals in advance stages of diseases, which are considered to be the major excretors of bacterias (26, 27). In addition, the low rates of positive results found in the herd A also confirm the high specificity of the assays. Eight and one animals in herds A and B, respectively had an E% close to the cut-off. However, the specificity of the ELISA was 100% and, for this reason, the cross-reaction with other proteins in P22 shared with environmental mycobacteria was discarded. The level of antibodies in these animals was low and consequently the OD in the ELISA was also low.

In conclusion, the new multiprotein complex named P22 could be an alternative antigen for the detection of specific M. tuberculosis complex antibodies in SAC. Moreover, the P22-based indirect ELISA can be used as a cost effective, rapid and reliable tool for the large-scale screening and therefore, support the detection and management of tuberculosis in llamas and alpacas.

AUTHOR CONTRIBUTIONS

CW, JB, AR, and LD obtained the serum samples from the animals. JI-L, CW, IM, MD, and FS performed the laboratory techniques. JI-L, CW, MD, and FS wrote the manuscript that was edited, discussed and reviewed and accepted by all authors.

ACKNOWLEDGMENTS

Authors would like to thank Ana Belén Martinez and Soledad Crespo for their technical assistance and María Luisa de la Cruz for her support in statistical analysis.

REFERENCES

1. Schiller I, Waters WR, Vordermeier HM, Jemmi T, Welsh M, Keck N, et al. Bovine tuberculosis in Europe from the perspective of an officially tuberculosis free country: trade, surveillance and diagnostics. Vet Microbiol. (2011) 151:153–9. doi: doi: 10.1016/j.vetmic.2011.02.039

2. Pesciaroli M, Alvarez J, Boniotti MB, Cagiola M, Di Marco V, Marianelli C, et al. Tuberculosis in domestic animal species. Res Vet Sci. (2014) 97:S78–85. doi: 10.1016/j.rvsc.2014.05.015

3. Barlow AM, Mitchell KA, Visram KH. Bovine tuberculosis in llama (Lama glama) in the UK. Vet Rec. (1999) 145:639–40.

4. D'Alterio GL, Knowles TG, Eknaes EI, Loevland IE, Foster AP. Postal survey of the population of South American camelids in the United Kingdom in 2000/01. Vet Rec. (2006) 158:86–90. doi: 10.1136/vr.158.3.86

5. Halsby K, Twomey DF, Featherstone C, Foster A, Walsh A, Hewitt K, et al. Zoonotic diseases in South American camelids in England and Wales. Epidemiol Infect. (2017) 145:1037–43. doi: 10.1017/S0950268816003101

6. Twomey DF, Crawshaw TR, Anscombe JE, Farrant L, Evans LJ, McElligott WS, et al. TB in llamas caused by Mycobacterium bovis. Vet Rec. (2007) 160:170. doi: 10.1136/vr.160.5.170

7. Zanolari P, Robert N, Lyashchenko KP, Pfyffer GE, Greenwald R, Esfandiari J, et al. Tuberculosis caused by Mycobacterium microti

in South American camelids. *J Vet Intern Med.* (2009) 23:1266–72. doi: 10.1111/j.1939-1676.2009.0377.x

8. Lyashchenko KP, Greenwald R, Esfandiari J, Meylan M, Burri IH, Zanolari P. Antibody responses in New World camelids with tuberculosis caused by *Mycobacterium microti*. *Vet Microbiol.* (2007) 125:265–73. doi: 10.1016/j.vetmic.2007.05.026

9. Ryan E, Dwyer P, Connolly D, Fagan J, Costello E, More S. Tuberculosis in alpaca (Lama pacos) on a farm in Ireland. 1. A clinical report. *Ir Vet J.* (2008) 61:527–31. doi: 10.1186/2046-0481-61-8-527

10. Garcia-Bocanegra I, Barranco I, Rodriguez-Gomez IM, Perez B, Gomez-Laguna J, Rodriguez S, et al. Tuberculosis in alpacas (*Lama pacos*) caused by *Mycobacterium bovis*. *J Clin Microbiol.* (2010) 48:1960–4. doi: 10.1128/JCM.02518-09

11. Dean GS, Crawshaw TR, de la Rua-Domenech R, Farrant L, Greenwald R, Higgins RJ, et al. Use of serological techniques for diagnosis of *Mycobacterium bovis* infection in a llama herd. *Vet Rec.* (2009) 165:323–4. doi: 10.1136/vr.165.11.323

12. Twomey DF, Collins R, Cranwell MP, Crawshaw TR, Higgins RJ, Dean GS, et al. Controlling tuberculosis in a llama (*Lama glama*) herd using clinical signs, tuberculin skin testing and serology. *Vet J.* (2012) 192:246–8. doi: 10.1016/j.tvjl.2011.05.014

13. Rhodes S, Holder T, Clifford D, Dexter I, Brewer J, Smith N, et al. Evaluation of gamma interferon and antibody tuberculosis tests in alpacas. *Clin Vaccine Immunol.* (2012) 19:1677–83. doi: 10.1128/CVI.00405-12

14. Alvarez J, Bezos J, Juan L, Vordermeier M, Rodriguez S, Fernandez-de-Mera IG, et al. Diagnosis of tuberculosis in camelids: old problems, current solutions and future challenges. *Transbound Emerg Dis.* (2012) 59:1–10. doi: 10.1111/j.1865-1682.2011.01233.x

15. Casal C, Infantes JA, Risalde MA, Diez-Guerrier A, Dominguez M, Moreno I, et al. Antibody detection tests improve the sensitivity of tuberculosis diagnosis in cattle. *Res Vet Sci.* (2017) 112:214–21. doi: 10.1016/j.rvsc.2017.05.012

16. Bezos J, Roy A, Infantes-Lorenzo JA, Gonzalez I, Venteo A, Romero B, et al. The use of serological tests in combination with the intradermal tuberculin test maximizes the detection of tuberculosis infected goats. *Vet Immunol Immunopathol.* (2018) 199:43–52. doi: 10.1016/j.vetimm.2018.03.006

17. Lyashchenko KP, Greenwald R, Esfandiari J, Rhodes S, Dean G, de la Rua-Domenech R, et al. Diagnostic value of animal-side antibody assays for rapid detection of *Mycobacterium bovis* or *Mycobacterium microti* infection in South American camelids. *Clin Vaccine Immunol.* (2011) 18:2143–47. doi: 10.1128/CVI.05386-11

18. Bezos J, Casal C, Alvarez J, Diez-Guerrier A, Rodriguez-Bertos A, Romero B, et al. Evaluation of the performance of cellular and serological diagnostic tests for the diagnosis of tuberculosis in an alpaca (*Vicugna pacos*) herd naturally infected with Mycobacterium bovis. *Prev Vet Med.* (2013) 111:304–13. doi: 10.1016/j.prevetmed.2013.05.013

19. Bezos J, Romero B, Delgado A, Alvarez J, Casal C, Venteo A, et al. Evaluation of the specificity of intradermal tuberculin and serological tests for diagnosis of tuberculosis in alpaca (*Vicugna pacos*) and llama (*Lama glama*) herds under field conditions in Peru. *Vet Rec.* (2014) 174:532. doi: 10.1136/vr.102463

20. Infantes-Lorenzo JA, Moreno I, Risalde MLA, Roy A, Villar M, Romero B, et al. Proteomic characterisation of bovine and avian purified protein derivatives and identification of specific antigens for serodiagnosis of bovine tuberculosis. *Clin Proteomics* (2017) 14:36. doi: 10.1186/s12014-017-9171-z

21. Aurtenetxe O, Barral M, Vicente J, de la Fuente J, Gortazar C, Juste RA. Development and validation of an enzyme-linked immunosorbent assay for antibodies against *Mycobacterium bovis* in European wild boar. *BMC Vet Res.* (2008) 4:43. doi: 10.1186/1746-6148-4-43

22. Casal C, Diez-Guerrier A, Alvarez J, Rodriguez-Campos S, Mateos A, Linscott R, et al. Strategic use of serology for the diagnosis of bovine tuberculosis after intradermal skin testing. *Vet Microbiol.* (2014) 170:342–51. doi: 10.1016/j.vetmic.2014.02.036

23. Pollock JM, Neill SD. *Mycobacterium bovis* infection and tuberculosis in cattle. *Vet J.* (2002) 163:115–27. doi: 10.1053/tvjl.2001.0655

24. Welsh MD, Cunningham RT, Corbett DM, Girvin RM, McNair J, Skuce RA, et al. Influence of pathological progression on the balance between cellular and humoral immune responses in bovine tuberculosis. *Immunology* (2005) 114:101–11. doi: 10.1111/j.1365-2567.2004.02003.x

25. Twomey DF, Crawshaw TR, Anscombe JE, Barnett JE, Farrant L, Evans LJ, et al. Assessment of antemortem tests used in the control of an outbreak of tuberculosis in llamas (*Lama glama*). *Vet Rec.* (2010) 167:475–80. doi: 10.1136/vr.c4192

26. Waters WR, Maggioli MF, McGill JL, Lyashchenko KP, Palmer MV. Relevance of bovine tuberculosis research to the understanding of human disease: historical perspectives, approaches, and immunologic mechanisms. *Vet Immunol Immunopathol.* (2014) 159:113–32. doi: 10.1016/j.vetimm.2014.02.009

27. Santos N, Almeida V, Gortazar C, Correia-Neves M. Patterns of *Mycobacterium tuberculosis*-complex excretion and characterization of super-shedders in naturally-infected wild boar and red deer. *Vet Res.* (2015) 46:129. doi: 10.1186/s13567-015-0270-4

Impact of Genetic Selection for Increased Cattle Resistance to Bovine Tuberculosis on Disease Transmission Dynamics

Kethusegile Raphaka [1,2], Enrique Sánchez-Molano [1], Smaragda Tsairidou [1], Osvaldo Anacleto [1,3], Elizabeth Janet Glass [1], John Arthur Woolliams [1], Andrea Doeschl-Wilson [1†] and Georgios Banos [1,4*†]

[1] The Roslin Institute and Royal (Dick) School of Veterinary Studies, University of Edinburgh, Edinburgh, United Kingdom, [2] Department of Agricultural Research, Gaborone, Botswana, [3] Instituto de Ciências Matemáticas e de Computação, Universidade de São Paulo, São Carlos, Brazil, [4] Scotland's Rural College, Edinburgh, United Kingdom

*Correspondence:
Georgios Banos
Georgios.Banos@roslin.ed.ac.uk

[†] These authors have contributed equally to this work

Bovine tuberculosis (bTB) poses a challenge to animal health and welfare worldwide. Presence of genetic variation in host resistance to *Mycobacterium bovis* infection makes the trait amenable to improvement with genetic selection. Genetic evaluations for resistance to infection in dairy cattle are currently available in the United Kingdom (UK), enabling genetic selection of more resistant animals. However, the extent to which genetic selection could contribute to bTB eradication is unknown. The objective of this study was to quantify the impact of genetic selection for bTB resistance on cattle-to-cattle disease transmission dynamics and prevalence by developing a stochastic genetic epidemiological model. The model was used to implement genetic selection in a simulated cattle population. The model considered various levels of selection intensity over 20 generations assuming genetic heterogeneity in host resistance to infection. Our model attempted to represent the dairy cattle population structure and current bTB control strategies in the UK, and was informed by genetic and epidemiological parameters inferred from data collected from UK bTB infected dairy herds. The risk of a bTB breakdown was modeled as the percentage of herds where initially infected cows (index cases) generated secondary cases by infecting herd-mates. The model predicted that this risk would be reduced by half after 4, 6, 9, and 15 generations for selection intensities corresponding to genetic selection of the 10, 25, 50, and 70% most resistant sires, respectively. In herds undergoing bTB breakdowns, genetic selection reduced the severity of breakdowns over generations by reducing both the percentage of secondary cases and the duration over which new secondary cases were detected. Selection of the 10, 25, 50, and 70% most resistant sires reduced the percentage of secondary cases to <1% in 4, 5, 7, and 11 generations, respectively. Similarly, the proportion of long breakdowns (breakdowns in which secondary cases were detected for more than 365 days) was reduced by half in 2, 2, 3, and 4 generations, respectively. Collectively, results suggest that genetic selection could be a viable tool that can complement existing management and surveillance methods to control and ultimately eradicate bTB.

Keywords: bovine tuberculosis, resistance, susceptibility, epidemiological model, genetic selection, prevalence

INTRODUCTION

Bovine tuberculosis (bTB) is an infectious zoonotic disease of cattle caused by *Mycobacterium bovis* (*M. bovis*) that is endemic in many parts of the world (1). Notably, bTB continues to be a challenge in the United Kingdom (UK) despite a national eradication programme being in place for over five decades (2). In the UK, bTB control is mainly based on the culling of cattle that react positively to the single intradermal comparative cervical tuberculin test, commonly known as the skin test. When at least one positive reactor to the skin test is detected in a herd during routine testing, a "breakdown" status is declared, and animal movement restrictions are imposed on that herd. The herd is then systematically tested every 2 months and animals reacting positively to the skin test are sent to slaughter. When all animals test negative to two consecutive tests the breakdown officially ends and the herd re-enters routine surveillance (3).

In addition to herds being subjected to compulsory regular testing, other control measures are applied in relation to bio-security (2, 4). However, so far, the existing control strategies have proven insufficient to eradicate the disease. This may be partially attributed to the low sensitivity of the skin test, potentially leading to undetected infected animals that contribute to the recurrence of breakdowns (5). Another contributing factor is the existence of wildlife reservoirs of *M. bovis* (for example, the Eurasian badger in the UK) (6). The problem persists and there is no clear evidence for a decline (7), despite the UK government spending over £175 million annually in the control of the disease (8). While Scotland was declared officially bTB free (OTF) in 2009, the governments of England and Wales have set a goal to become OTF by 2038 (4, 9). Thus, genetic selection for increased resistance of cattle to bTB may provide a potential complementary strategy (10) to achieve this goal.

Quantitative genetic studies have shown that there is genetic variation in cattle resistance to bTB (11–15). Therefore, it would be feasible to reduce disease prevalence and breakdown severity through selectively breeding for enhanced host resistance to the disease. In the UK, genetic evaluations of individual dairy cattle for resistance to bTB have been available since 2016. Availability of genetic evaluations enables the bovine industry to select sires based on their inherent capacity to produce more resistant progeny (16). However, before embarking on intense selection for enhanced resistance to bTB, it is important to understand the impact of such a selection process on disease risk and prevalence (17).

Genetic epidemiological models have been used to evaluate the role of genetic selection in populations undergoing an epidemic (17–19). Such models have been applied to a variety of diseases in farm animals including sea lice infection in the Atlantic salmon (20), bacterial (21, 22), and nematode (23) infestations in sheep, and Marek's disease in chickens (24). These studies estimated the impact of host genetic variation and genetic selection for increased host resistance on disease prevalence and spread. Several epidemiological models specific to bTB in cattle have been proposed (5, 25–31). None of them, however, has accounted for genetic variation in host resistance or considered genetic selection as a potential control option. In

the present study, we propose an epidemiological model which, unlike previous models for bTB, incorporates genetic variation of disease resistance in the host, and models genetic selection.

Disease progression in previous epidemiological bTB models has been typically assumed to follow transition from the state of susceptible (*S*) to exposed (*E*), to test-sensitive (diagnosable; *T*), and finally to Infectious (*I*; *SETI* model). Typically, a susceptible animal becomes infectious only after going through the exposed and test-sensitive states (5, 27, 28, 30, 31). Pathogen transmission in the *SETI* model is such that infected animals that are test-sensitive and react positively to the skin test are removed before they become infectious. If this is the case, identification of infected animals through frequent comprehensive testing and immediate removal of test-positive animals as being currently carried out in the UK should substantially reduce bTB prevalence. However, given the current gap of knowledge about the relationship between *M. bovis* excretion and skin test response, and considering the persistence and general increase in bTB incidence over the past decade in the UK (7), other models of disease transmission dynamics need to be explored.

In the present study we considered a *SEIT* model where an animal becomes infectious (*I*) before infection can be detected by the skin test (*T*). This model implies that infected cattle may become infectious before they can be diagnosed and removed. Compared to the *SETI* model, *SEIT* represents the "worst case" scenario in terms of bTB transmission. The model follows the suggestion that all tuberculous cattle with lesions, particularly in the respiratory tract, should be considered as potential excretors of *M. bovis*, thus constituting sources of infection for other animals both within and across herds (32, 33).

The aim of the present study was to determine the impact of genetic selection for enhanced host resistance to bTB on cattle-to-cattle transmission dynamics and bTB prevalence using a *SEIT* epidemiological model.

MATERIAL AND METHODS

The impact of selection for increased resistance to bTB on the risk and severity of bTB breakdowns were investigated using a simulated, genetically heterogeneous cattle population. The proposed genetic epidemiological model was designed to simulate *M. bovis* infection dynamics in closed herds within the current UK bTB testing policy, firstly in the absence of selection and secondly following genetic selection for enhanced host resistance (reduced susceptibility) over 20 generations, with different selection intensities.

Simulated Populations

Non-overlapping generations of a dairy cattle population ($N = 20,000$) were generated comprising 50% males and 50% females. A founder generation was created, where sires and dams were randomly chosen and mated to create the base population. This base population was generated assuming a sire-to-offspring ratio of 1:50, thus being consistent with the national policy in reporting genetic evaluations for bTB in the UK (R. Mrode, personal communication, 2017). Large half-sib families were thus created, reflecting a realistic dairy cattle population structure where, with the extensive use of artificial insemination, sires tend to have large numbers of progeny (daughters). Given that genetic selection of the best sires is the key component of selective breeding programmes in dairy cattle, selection was carried out based on estimated breeding values of sires generated as outlined below. This is also consistent with the current industry practice to only consider sire bTB genetic evaluations in selection.

Incorporating Genetic Variation in Host Susceptibility

Cattle susceptibility to bTB was modeled as a polygenic trait consistent with an infinitesimal model assuming presence of many loci each with a small additive effect on the trait (15, 34). More specifically, genetic variation for susceptibility was assumed to follow a normal distribution in the log scale, since previous studies suggested that disease traits are usually skewed (20, 35–37) and a log transformation is commonly used to achieve data normality (38). Considering that genetic evaluation methods may not capture all the additive genetic variance (σ_a^2) associated with a trait, therefore, both the true genetic value of an individual (TBV) for susceptibility and the corresponding estimated breeding value (EBV) were simulated drawing from normal distributions $N(0, \sigma_a^2)$ and $N(0, r^2\sigma_a^2)$, respectively, where r was the accuracy of the estimate. Thus, in the founder population, TBVs and EBVs were simulated from a multivariate normal distribution $MVN(0, \mathbf{G})$, where $\mathbf{G}$ corresponded to the genetic variance-covariance matrix. The covariance between TBVs and EBVs was derived as $cov_{TBV,EBV} = \text{r}*\sqrt{\sigma_a^2}*\sqrt{\sigma_a^2 r^2}$. An additional term, the prediction error (PE) for each animal was computed as the difference between TBV and EBV.

In further generations, TBVs of the offspring of two selected animals were equal to the average TBV of the parents plus an individual Mendelian sampling (MS) term reflecting the random sampling and combination of parental alleles. This latter term followed a normal distribution $N(0, 0.5(1 - \overline{F})\sigma_a^2)$, where $\overline{F}$ corresponded to the average inbreeding coefficient of the parents. In a similar way, the TBVs of the offspring were decomposed into EBV and PE, both being computed as the average of the respective parental values plus the corresponding MS terms, which were now drawn from normal distributions $N(0, 0.5(1 - \overline{F})\sigma_{EBV}^2)$ and $N(0, 0.5(1 - \overline{F})\sigma_{PE}^2)$, respectively. Therefore, simulated TBVs, EBVs, and PEs were computed for each offspring as:

$$EBV_{offspring} = \overline{EBV}_{parents} + MS_{EBV}$$

$$PE_{offspring} = \overline{PE}_{parents} + MS_{PE}$$

$$TBV_{offspring} = EBV_{offspring} + PE_{offspring}$$

In all generations, environmental effects were generated from a normal distribution $N(0, \sigma_e^2)$, where σ_e^2 corresponded to the environmental variance and was kept constant through all generations. Finally, the individual phenotypic value for underlying susceptibility to bTB i.e., g_i of each individual animal i was computed as the sum of the animal's TBV plus the corresponding environmental effect E, i.e., $g_i = TBV_i + E_i$.

Distribution of Animals Into Individual Herds

Currently, genetic evaluations for bTB in the UK assess the resistance of sires based on disease incidence of their daughters as described in Banos et al. (39). Therefore, breakdowns were simulated here based only on female offspring produced in each generation; the latter corresponds to 2–4 years in dairy cattle. A pool of selected sires was created, and female offspring were randomly allocated into 100 herds comprising 100 individuals each. Every selected sire contributed at least one daughter into one herd. Breakdowns were then simulated within each herd as outlined below.

The Epidemic Within Herd Transmission Model

A stochastic within-herd bTB transmission model was developed to simulate bTB spread in each herd and provide estimates of severity and duration of bTB breakdowns (**Supplementary Figure 1**). In particular, a compartmental *SEIT* model was assumed in which susceptible cows progress between the four infection states: (1) Susceptible state (S), where the animal is not infected but susceptible to infection; (2) Exposed state (E), where the animal is infected but not infectious and is undetectable by the skin test; (3) Infectious state (I), where the animal is able to infect others but is still undetectable by the skin test; (4) Test-sensitive state (T), where the infectious animal is now detectable by the skin test. Furthermore, the model incorporated the current UK policy of a 60 days routine skin test performed on all animals following the onset of a breakdown. At the specific test-days, infected animals at detectable state T may be diagnosed as reactors assuming a test sensitivity of Ω. Cows that reacted positively to the skin test were removed from the herd, in line with the UK official test-and-cull procedure (**Supplementary Figure 1**).

Infection (transition from state S to E) was modeled as a Poisson distribution process with time dependent average infection rate $\lambda(t) = \alpha + \beta(I(t) + T(t))$, where $I(t)$ and $T(t)$ were the number of animals in the herd at the I and T states at time t, respectively, and the parameters α and β represented transmission coefficients for external sources of infection (aggregate of all potential sources of external infection including wildlife, infected move-in cattle and infected cattle from contiguous farms) and for within-herd cattle-to-cattle transmission, respectively (**Supplementary Figure 1**) (30, 31). A density dependent mode of transmission was assumed as herd size is known to be correlated to bTB incidence and persistence (40–42). Progression of infected cows from E to I state and from I to T state occurred at average rates σ and γ, respectively (**Supplementary Figure 1**).

Individual variation in susceptibility was incorporated into the model through each individual's log-normally distributed susceptibility phenotype calculated as outlined above. The individual infection rate of individual i at time t was then defined as $\lambda_i(t) = e^{g_i}(\alpha + \beta(I(t) + T(t)))$, where g_i refers to the normally distributed susceptibility value specified by the genetic model above. In contrast to the population averages for α, β

σ, and γ, which were kept constant over successive generations, the average susceptibility g changed over generations because of genetic selection.

To generate a sufficient number of herds experiencing breakdowns in the first generation, the epidemic in each herd was started by two randomly chosen infectious individuals in state I, termed "index cases." Two individuals were chosen here instead of one to ensure that breakdowns did not die out within the first 60 days of duration. This editing step allowed us to generate enough data to test the various genetic selection practices described below.

Disease progression within each herd was then simulated as a series of random independent events representing the transition of an animal between two successive states in the compartmental $SEIT$ model. The time to the next event (inter-event time), the corresponding event type (for example, transition from S to E), and the corresponding individual experiencing the transition were determined using Gillespie's direct algorithm adapted to heterogeneous populations as outlined in Lipschutz-Powell et al. (35).

Possible events in our model were the infection of a susceptible animal (transition from S to E), an exposed animal becoming infectious (transition from E to I), an infectious animal becoming test-sensitive (transition from I to T) and a test-sensitive animal being removed from the herd after testing positive to the skin test (transition from T to R). However, the latter event was modeled separately at time intervals of 60 days according to the official skin test schedule. For the other events the inter-event time was sampled from an exponential distribution with rate equal to the sum of all process rates calculated as $R_{total} = \sum_{i=1}^{N_S} e^{g_i} (\alpha + \beta (I + T)) + \sigma N_E + \gamma N_I$, where Nx is the total number of animals in each x state within the herd. In other words, the time to the next event was estimated as $-\ln(y)/R_{total}$, where $y \sim U(0, 1)$. The specific event type e that occurs at that particular time was sampled by drawing a random variable from a distinct distribution with probability $\frac{p(e)=R_e}{R_{total}}$. R_e is the rate of occurrence of the specific event. The individual in the particular event was then chosen randomly, and in the case of infection (S to E) it was weighted by the individual's susceptibility phenotype.

In line with the current bTB control strategy, the epidemic in each herd was simulated until the end of a bTB breakdown, defined by two consecutive negative skin tests for all herd members (3). During the epidemic, the number of individuals in each disease state together with the corresponding times was recorded, and based on these, the total number of reactors and the duration of each epidemic (i.e., the time from beginning to end of a breakdown) were derived.

Model Parameterization and Validation

Input parameters for the epidemiological bTB model illustrated in **Supplementary Figure 1** were based on real field data used for national genetic evaluations for bTB in the UK. These data consisted of 1,210,652 cow records from 10,589 herds where breakdowns had been declared between the years 2000 and 2014. The mean number of animals per herd in the dataset was 114, and the recorded number of infected animals referred to reactors diagnosed by the skin test. Based on the latest bTB epidemiological study in the UK (31) the value of the external rate of infection α in the simulation (**Supplementary Figure 1**) was set to 5×10^{-7} days^{-1}. Furthermore, a skin test sensitivity (Ω) of 0.60 was used as in Banos et al. (39), which is the value considered in the current official UK genetic evaluation for bTB resistance. To determine the remaining parameter values of the $SEIT$ model (β, σ, γ, as well as genetic and environmental variances for underlying susceptibility), multiple parameter combinations were tested and the corresponding model output was compared to the following characteristics derived from analyzing the field data: mean percentage of skin-test reactors per breakdown (8.5%), mean duration of breakdown from official onset to end (366 days), and genetic variance (0.0032) and heritability (0.10) of the observed bTB phenotype indicating presence (reactor) or absence (non-reactor) of bTB. We derived these estimates from the analysis of the above-mentioned field data using the model described in Banos et al. (39).

The bTB susceptibility phenotype g in the $SEIT$ model (**Supplementary Figure 1**) corresponds to the underlying scale of the binary presence or absence of the disease trait in the data analyses (39) (observed scale). To make the model results concordant with the observed scale, a range of different genetic and environmental variance estimates for the underlying scale in the base population were explored and the corresponding heritability and genetic variance estimates on the observed scale were calculated. The final genetic and environmental variances chosen for the simulated data on the observed scale and used to generate the base population were those that were closest to the real field data estimates on the observed scale.

In order to study the impact of variation in epidemiological parameters on disease epidemic and genetic selection, two additional simulation scenarios were run, one assuming a 10-fold increase in the rate of external infection ($\alpha = 5 \times 10^{-6}$ days^{-1}) and another considering a lower sensitivity of the skin test ($\Omega = 0.30$); the latter is similar to the lower credible interval obtained in the meta-analysis of skin-test sensitivity by Nuñez-Garcia et al. (43).

Genetic Selection Process and Impact

Firstly, epidemics were simulated for 20 generations without any genetic selection (100% of sires used for breeding) in order to establish the baseline of bTB transmission dynamics. Subsequently, truncation selection of genetically resistant sires was simulated for 20 generations. Sires were selected for breeding based on their underlying susceptibility EBVs. Different levels of selection intensity were explored by selecting the 10, 25, 50, and 70% most resistant (least susceptible) sires. These reflect different potential selection strategies against the disease. Selected sires were randomly mated with cows. Dams were randomly selected in each generation. Population size and sex ratios were kept constant across generations. The female offspring of these sires then formed the next generation of individuals for which bTB epidemics were simulated.

The impact of genetic selection on bTB prevalence was assessed in each generation by estimating the mean underlying susceptibility to *M. bovis* infection in the population as well as the risk and severity of breakdowns. A breakdown was assumed to have occurred when at least one secondary case was produced from the index cases within a herd. Otherwise, in the absence of a secondary case a "no breakdown" was declared and duration equal to 0 days was assigned. Therefore, the risk of a breakdown (probability of a breakdown occurring) was defined as the proportion of simulated epidemics that resulted in at least one secondary case (infected cow other than the index cases that seeded the epidemic). The severity of a breakdown was then assessed by estimating the percentage of secondary cases and the duration of their occurrence within the breakdown (duration of secondary cases). Breakdowns were categorized as mild, moderate, and severe based on mean percentage of secondary cases being less or equal to 3% (only 1 secondary case), 3–10%, and above 10% (10% equating 50% of breakdowns in the distribution) respectively. Breakdowns were also categorized as short, medium and long depending on whether the duration of secondary cases was less than or equal to 180 days, between 180 and 365 days, and above 365 days, respectively.

Finally, to assess the impact of the *SEIT* model assumption that animals become first infectious and then test-sensitive, the same simulations were run separately assuming a *SETI* epidemiological model. In the latter, infected animals were test-sensitive, hence detectable, before they became infectious. The same parameters were used as for the *SEIT* model.

In all cases, each selection scenario reflecting one of the four selection intensities described above was replicated 50 times. Results were averaged across all herds and replicates for each generation.

RESULTS

Parameter Values and Model Fit to Real Data

Parameter values were identified to ensure that simulated and real bTB breakdowns shared similar characteristics with respect to the distributions of mean percentage of reactors per breakdown, total duration of breakdown, genetic and phenotypic variance and heritability of susceptibility on the observed scale (**Figure 1**; **Table 1**). The distributions of both the mean percentage of reactors per breakdown and the total duration of breakdown were more long-tailed in real data compared to simulated data (**Figure 1**), probably because real data were affected by more extreme and unpredictable environmental conditions than those modeled in the simulation. Significant correlations ($p < 0.001$) were found between mean percentage of infected individuals per breakdown and mean duration of breakdown in both datasets; however, the correlation was smaller in real data (0.43) than in simulated data (0.85), for the same reason as stated above.

The rate of progression from the E to I state, σ, corresponded to an exposed state duration ($1/\sigma$) of 25 days (**Table 1**). The rate of progression γ from I to T state suggested that, once a cow becomes infectious, she is expected to respond to the skin test within ($1/\gamma$) 2 days.

Impact of Genetic Selection on Underlying Susceptibility

Genetic selection resulted in a reduction in the mean underlying susceptibility to bTB and the corresponding genetic variance (**Supplementary Figure 2**). The initial underlying susceptibility phenotype in the base population was simulated with a mean of zero, hence the decrease in susceptibility due to selection is depicted by negative values in **Supplementary Figure 2B**. Greater reduction was observed for higher selection intensities. As expected, no change in genetic variance and mean susceptibility was observed over generations in absence of selection.

Impact of Genetic Selection on Epidemic Profiles

Figure 2 shows the *SEIT* profiles (proportions of individuals in different states of the *SEIT* model) over successive generations for different selection intensities. The proportion of infected animals, including those in the exposed, infectious and test-sensitive states, was high before selection and significantly reduced after implementation of selection. As expected, there was no significant reduction in the number of infected individuals and duration of the epidemic over generations when no selection was performed (**Figure 2A**). Selection noticeably affected both the epidemic risk (illustrated here by the decreasing number of epidemic profiles over successive generations in **Figures 2B–E**) and severity (illustrated here by the number of infected (*E*, *T*, and *I*) individuals and epidemic duration). As expected, the higher the selection intensity, the stronger was the impact on the epidemic profile (**Figures 2B–E**).

Impact of Genetic Selection on Risk of a Breakdown to Occur

Figure 3 shows a decrease in the probability of a breakdown occurring with increasing selection intensity. Prior to selection, the mean probability of occurrence of a breakdown was 81.8%. When higher selection intensities were applied corresponding to selection of the 10 and 25% most resistant sires, this probability was halved after 4 and 6 generations, respectively. A similar result was achieved for lower selection intensities (50 and 70% most resistant sires) after 9 and 15 generations, respectively.

Impact of Genetic Selection on Percentage of Secondary Cases and Duration of Their Occurrence Within Breakdowns

Genetic selection led to a decline in the percentage of secondary cases per breakdown (**Figure 4A**). To reduce the percentage of secondary cases per breakdown to <1%, 4, 5, 7, and 11 generations of selection were required when 10, 25, 50, and 70% most resistant sires were selected, respectively. The corresponding duration of secondary case occurrence within a breakdown in these generations was reduced by more than half to 114.9, 125.5, 139.9, and 141.8 days for the four selection intensities, respectively, compared to 326.1 days before selection was introduced (**Figure 4B**). Furthermore, selection for 12 and 17 generations was required to eliminate the epidemics (occurrence of secondary cases less than or equal to 0.1%) when 10 and

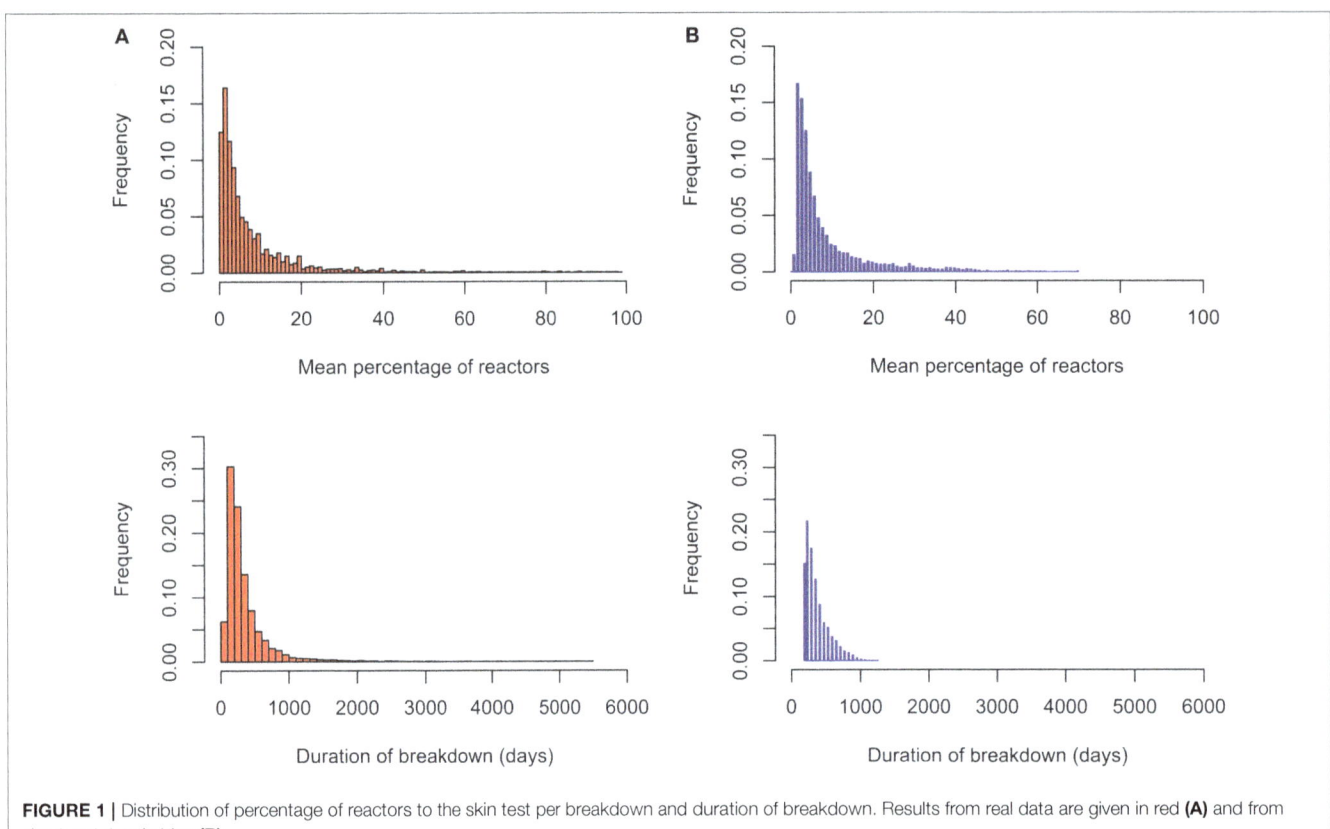

FIGURE 1 | Distribution of percentage of reactors to the skin test per breakdown and duration of breakdown. Results from real data are given in red **(A)** and from simulated data in blue **(B)**.

25% most resistant sires were selected, respectively. However, elimination of bTB was not possible with lower selection intensities (greater proportion of sires selected) during the simulated selection period of 20 generations. In the absence of selection, the percentage of secondary cases and time for induction of secondary cases fluctuated around the initial mean (**Figures 4A,B**).

The effects of genetic selection when breakdowns were categorized according to severity are illustrated in **Figure 5** and **Supplementary Figure 3**. Prior to selection, the proportion of mild, moderate and severe breakdowns was 0.46, 0.32, and 0.22, respectively. During selection, the overall severity of breakdowns decreased across generations (**Figure 5**). When high selection intensities were applied (selection of the 10 or 25% most resistant sires), almost all breakdowns became mild by generation 10 (**Figure 5A**). However, it was only when selection of the 10% most resistant sires was implemented that breakdowns became short at the end of selection (**Supplementary Figure 3A**). Proportion of long breakdowns was reduced by more than 50% after 2, 2, 3, and 4 generations for selection of 10, 25, 50, and 70% most resistant sires, respectively (**Supplementary Figure 3B**). In the absence of selection, severity of breakdowns remained constant, with slight fluctuations across generations (**Figure 5**; **Supplementary Figure 3**).

The above results collectively demonstrate how genetic selection has the potential to reduce the probability of a breakdown occurring and the severity of the breakdowns that do eventually occur.

Impact of Variation in Epidemiological Parameters

Scenarios with a 10-fold increase in the external rate of infection ($\alpha = 5 \times 10^{-6}$ days^{-1} instead of 5×10^{-7} days^{-1}) are shown in **Supplementary Data Sheet 1**. All other parameters being the same, this increase led to a small non-significant tendency toward more severe breakdowns in early generations but did not influence the impact of genetic selection on disease epidemic, probability of breakdown occurrence and severity of breakdowns.

The reduction of the skin test sensitivity to 0.30 from 0.60 led to an increase in the severity of breakdowns in terms of number of secondary cases and duration but did not affect the probability of a breakdown to occur (**Supplementary Data Sheet 2**). Importantly, the impact of genetic selection on the disease transmission dynamics was similarly demonstrable in the case of reduced sensitivity of the skin test.

Comparison Between SEIT and SETI Models

The impact of genetic selection on the risk and severity of breakdowns under the two models were very similar (**Supplementary Figure 4**). For the same parameter values, slightly more secondary cases per breakdown were generated

TABLE 1 | Epidemiological and genetic parameters of bovine tuberculosis in simulated and real (field) data.

	Simulated data	Real data
PERCENTAGE OF REACTORS TO THE SKIN-TEST (%)		
Average	8.7	8.5
Range (min–max)	0.0–70	0.08–98.0
3rd Quartile	10.0	9.5
Standard deviation	9.5	12.4
DURATION OF BREAKDOWN (NO. DAYS)		
Average	365.9	365.7
Range (min–max)	180.0–1,260	60.0–5,457
3rd Quartile	420.0	409.0
Standard deviation	174.7	395.1
EPIDEMIOLOGICAL PARAMETERS		
Rate of external infection (α) [days^{-1}]	5×10^{-7}	
Transmission coefficient (β)	0.012	
Rate from exposed to infectious state (σ) [days^{-1}]	0.04	
Rate from infectious to test-sensitive state (γ) [days^{-1}]	0.5	
Rate of detection (Ω)	0.60	
GENETIC PARAMETERS OF SUSCEPTIBILITY		
Underlying scale		
Genetic variance	0.3	
Environmental variance	0.3	
Accuracy of selection	0.63	
Observed scale		
Genetic variance	0.0034	0.0032
Phenotypic variance	0.032	0.031
Heritability	0.106	0.103

with the *SEIT* (6.8%) compared to the *SETI* (5.8%) model in the base population (unselected population). The same number of generations was required in either model to reduce the probability (risk) of a breakdown to occur by half. Similarly, the difference in time required to achieve a certain percentage of reduction (e.g., 50%) in secondary cases or time for induction of secondary cases between the two models was always less than one generation (**Supplementary Figure 4**).

DISCUSSION

Considerable advances in infectious disease control may be achieved by selective breeding programmes that include disease resistance of animals in the breeding goal (44). In this context, a breeding programme that exploits existing genetic variation in host susceptibility to bTB could form an important part of the national bTB eradication strategy (11–13, 15, 39). However, quantitative genetics theory alone cannot predict how genetic gain in disease resistance translates

into reduction of bTB breakdown risk and severity. The novelty of the present study lies in (i) the development of a genetic epidemiological model that combines for the first time quantitative genetics and epidemiological dynamics of bTB, and (ii) the ability of this model to assess the consequences of genetic selection for enhanced host resistance on bTB prevalence and dynamics.

Our choice of model parameter values was informed by previous literature estimates (5, 27–31, 45) and bTB field data in order to represent UK field conditions. Similarities between model and field or experimental data are essential for drawing reliable conclusions from model predictions (46). In the present study, real data were somewhat more variable than simulated data as manifested by a wider range and greater standard deviation. Otherwise, the simulated model outputs, including mean values and genetic parameters, were similar to results obtained from field data analysis. The distributions of percentage of reactors to the skin test in both real and simulated data were characteristically skewed to the right and correlated with breakdown duration. Skewness in the distribution of disease traits may be attributed to between animal genetic variation (20) and also environmental effects (47). In the real data, other factors such as differences in herd size, management, badger prevalence and climatic conditions are likely to contribute to the diversity observed in epidemic characteristics (42, 48, 49). Many of these factors are recorded in practice, and can be captured by statistical models and accounted for in the genetic evaluation. Other, non-systematic sources of variation would constitute noise in the statistical models. Increasing model complexity by including various systematic or non-systematic effects into the simulation model may increase variability in the model predictions, but would not affect selection response.

Although the bTB model in the present study differs from previous epidemiological bTB models that did not incorporate genetic variation in the host, the estimated population average transmission coefficient β was within the range of transmission coefficients (0.006–0.014 days^{-1}) previously reported (5, 27, 29, 31, 50). The duration of the exposed state (*E*) in our model was 25 days, thus slightly higher than the 20 days estimated by O'Hare et al. (31) using UK data and a *SETI* model. In our study, an animal that became infectious was expected to become detectable within 2 days. This short time interval may be sufficient for some additional infected animals to infect others prior to their own diagnosis and subsequent removal from the herd. This may partly explain the persistence of bTB in the UK despite the on-going regime of skin testing and slaughtering of positive reactors. The 2 days between the *I* and *T* states in the present study is comparable to the 1.8 days estimated by Conlan et al. (5), where early infectiousness was assumed (considering animals in both *E* and *T* states in the *SETI* model to be infectious). In their model the *E* state was referred to as the occult state to denote that, although infectious, animals were not detectable by the skin test (5). These estimates would imply that, once animals are infectious a relatively short time is required before they can be detected by the skin test.

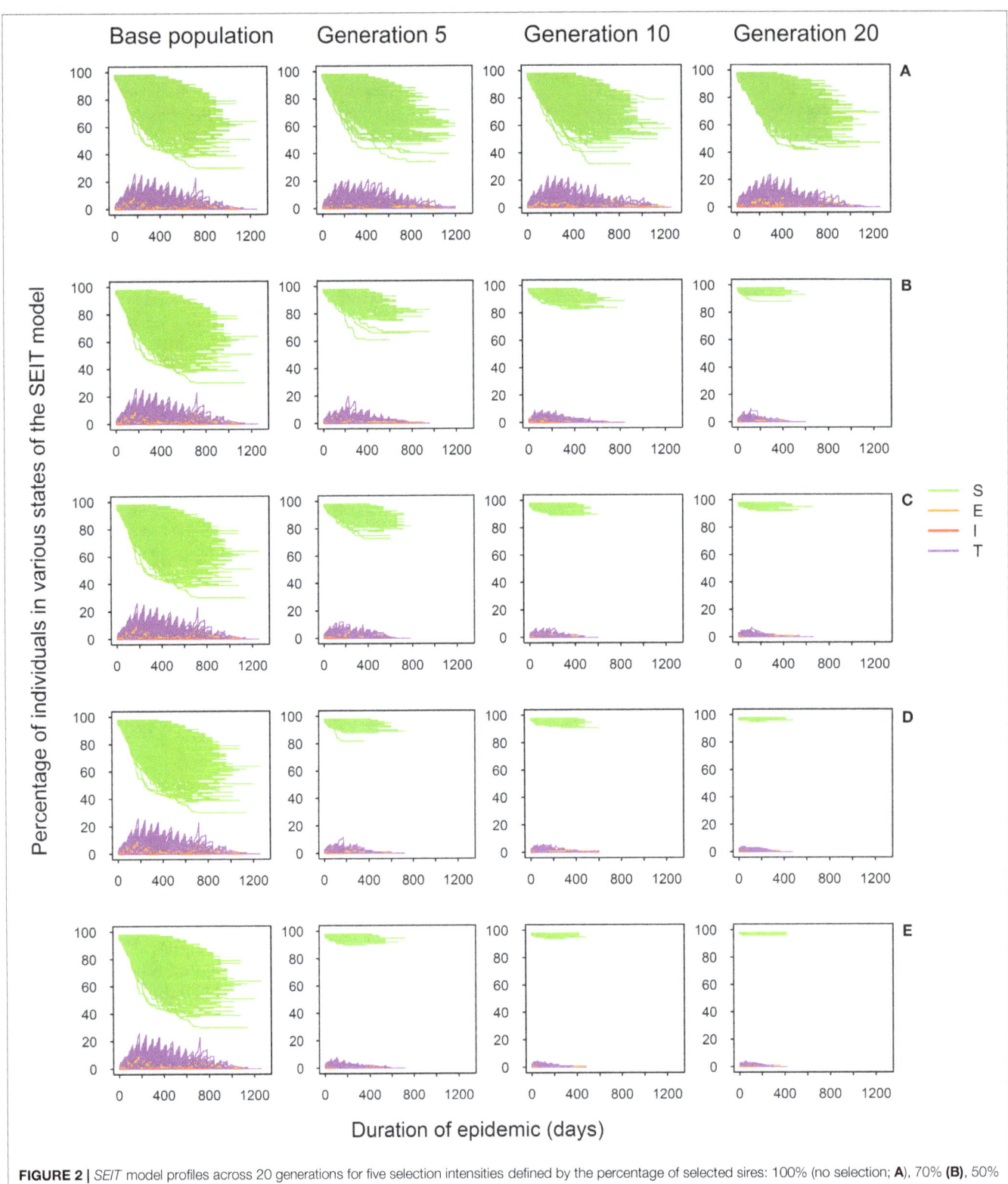

FIGURE 2 | *SEIT* model profiles across 20 generations for five selection intensities defined by the percentage of selected sires: 100% (no selection; **A**), 70% **(B)**, 50% **(C)**, 25% **(D)**, and 10% **(E)**; proportion of susceptible (*S*), exposed (*E*), infectious (*I*), and test-sensitive (*T*) individuals during the course of the epidemic.

Several important implications arise from our results as far as interpretation of bTB transmission and evaluation of control strategies are concerned, particularly with regards to the implementation of genetic selection for increased host disease resistance. Although the potential of the latter as a complementary strategy for disease control has been recognized

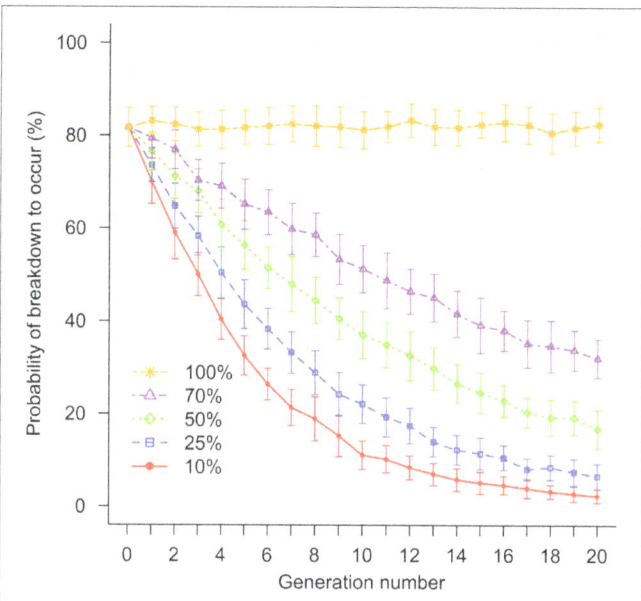

FIGURE 3 | Impact of genetic selection on risk of breakdown (probability of a breakdown to occur). Selection intensities correspond to selection of the 10, 25, 50, 70, and 100% (no selection) most resistant sires.

(10), its utility in terms of reducing disease risk, prevalence, and severity has not been previously assessed.

Susceptibility on the underlying scale affects the probability of an individual to become infected. Therefore, as animals become more resistant, the expectation is for them to become less likely to be infected. Our results demonstrate how reduction in individual infection probability as a result of genetic selection for host resistance to bTB relates to the probability of breakdowns to happen in the first place. Equally important, even when a breakdown was to occur, it would be less severe in terms of number of infected individuals and duration compared to a no selection scenario. Thus, our results are in agreement with previous studies that demonstrated that selection can reduce both the risk and severity of epidemics for other diseases in livestock and fish (17, 20, 21, 51, 52). This is expected to lead to a reduction, not only in frequency of future breakdowns but also in economic losses, as prolonged breakdowns consume substantial resources. Furthermore, as selection reduces the number of reactors during a bTB breakdown, it is also expected to reduce the risk of recurrence (53, 54). Recurrence has been found to be high in the UK, where 23% (38%) of breakdowns recur within 12 (24) months despite the on-going testing regime (55).

We explored the amount of genetic progress in bTB resistance when sires were selected at different levels of selection intensity. Simulating different selection intensities provides insights into future options for breeders. In all cases, our model predicted that most benefits would emerge within the first 5–10 generations of selection. The lowest selection intensity considered here, corresponding to selection of the 70% genetically most resistant sires, reflects a conservative approach that may be taken by breeders regarding novel traits in the breeding programme (G. Banos, unpublished data available upon request). Our results

suggest that with such low selection intensity, genetic selection alone would not eradicate bTB by the time England and Wales are set to achieve OTF status (year 2038, which would correspond to 4–5 generations in conventional breeding programmes or about 2–2.5 generations in genomic breeding programmes). Thus, it would be tempting to consider medium to high selection intensities in the breeding programme. However, care must be taken when higher selection intensities are opted for because of possible antagonistic genetic correlations between bTB and other important dairy traits (56) in the breeding goal. Antagonism would imply that genetically improving one trait compromises the other and may be dealt with using an optimized selection index of multiple traits.

Selection could be applied complementarily to other interventions including existing measures in order to expedite the eradication process. In the context of the genetic-epidemiological model described here, this would include continued efforts to reduce the external source of infection, referring to wildlife-to-cattle, and neighboring and incoming cattle-to-local cattle transmission. Furthermore, improvement of sensitivity of major bTB diagnostic tools such as the skin test and abattoir inspection could translate into an increased removal rate of infected cattle and, hence, reduce the average herd infectivity; further research would be needed to quantify such possible benefits. Other options not included in our model such as selecting for increased resistance in dams in addition to sires, genetic selection to reduce infectivity in addition to susceptibility (57), and genomic selection could also be explored. The latter has a potential to considerably shorten the generation interval and expedite genetic gains (58, 59).

Given the global importance of bTB, a large number of epidemiological models for bTB transmission have been published in the scientific literature (5, 25, 30, 31, 45, 50, 60). The models differ widely in their scope and purpose, although the majority of models focus on estimating transmission parameters and transmission routes from epidemiological data, or explore the impact of different surveillance or control options on bTB prevalence. To the best of our knowledge, this is the first model that incorporates genetic disease control strategies.

To model within-herd transmission dynamics, the epidemiological bTB model in the present study adopted a similar compartmental approach as in recently published stochastic epidemiological bTB models that have been fitted to UK bTB data (5, 30, 31). However, to assess the impact of genetic selection on bTB prevalence and dynamics, we adopted the *SEIT* transmission model, while a more optimistic *SETI* model in terms of transmission has been previously used in the majority of epidemiological studies. Information about the suitability of *SEIT* or *SETI* models for bovine tuberculosis is non-existent. In other diseases, both *SETI* and *SEIT* models have proven to be biologically reasonable. Diseases in humans such as HIV or hepatitis C show epidemiological processes concordant with the *SEIT* model, with window periods between infection and detection when the infected individuals are also infectious (61). Furthermore, in case of human tuberculosis, the window period for the Mantoux test (a skin test based in the presence of immune response against tuberculin) is

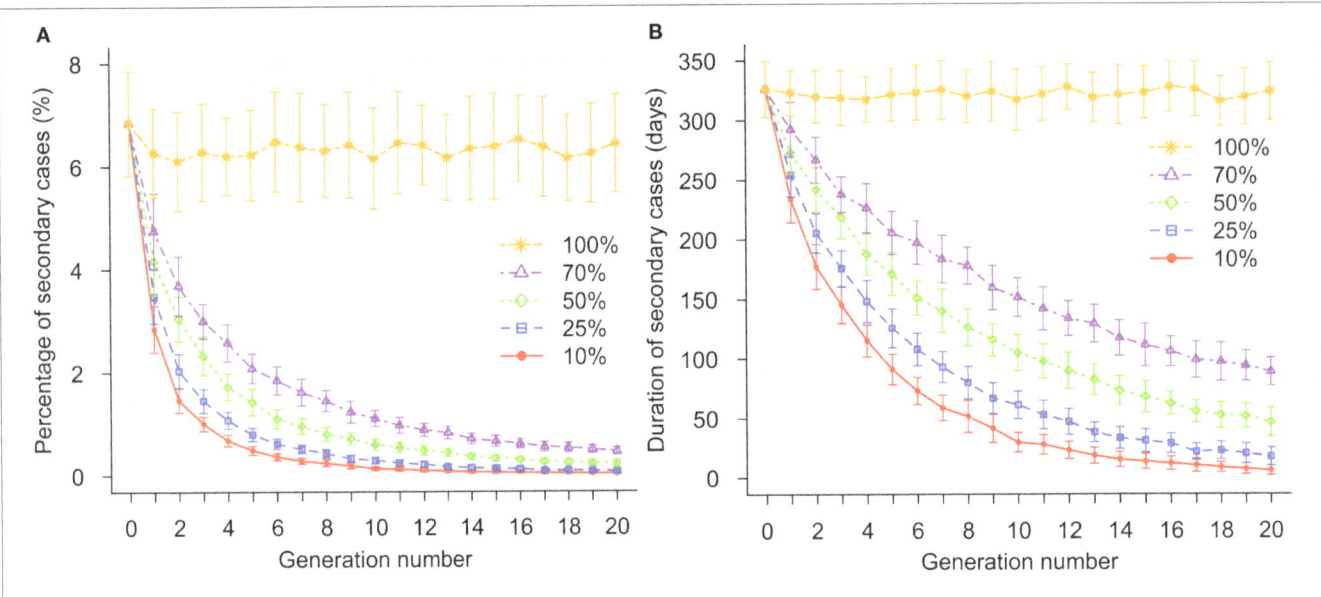

FIGURE 4 | Impact of genetic selection on percentage of secondary cases **(A)** and duration of secondary case occurrence **(B)** within a breakdown. Selection intensities correspond to selection of the 10, 25, 50, 70, and 100% (no selection) most resistant sires.

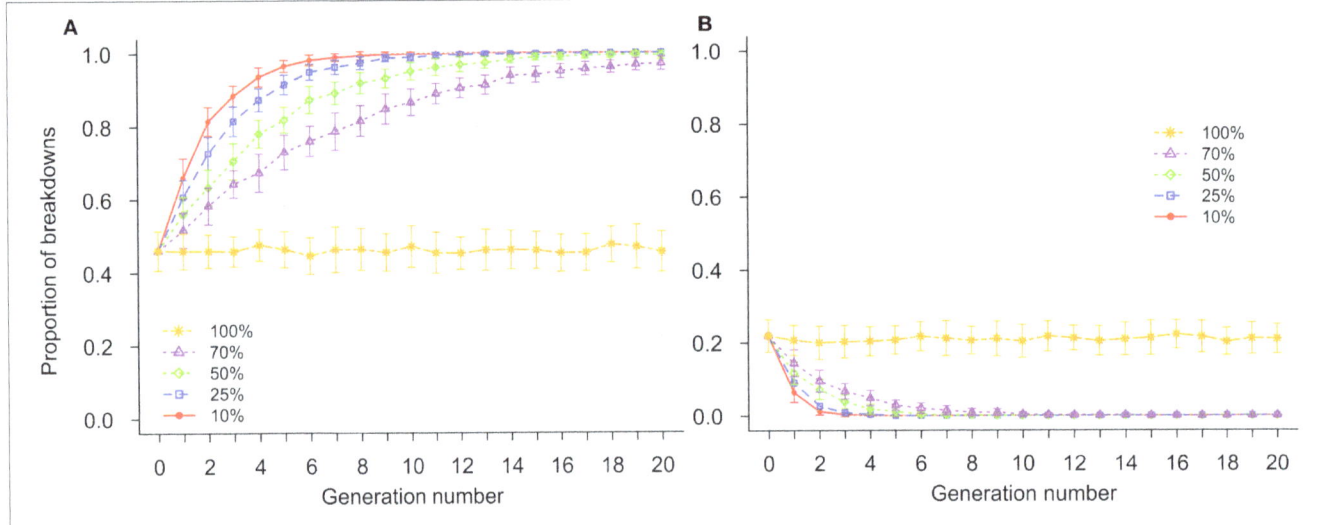

FIGURE 5 | Impact of genetic selection on the percentage of secondary case(s) occurrence within a breakdown; mild (≤3% secondary cases - **A**) and severe (>10% secondary cases - **B**); selection intensities correspond to selection of the 10, 25, 50, 70, and 100% (no selection) most resistant sires.

between 2 and 6 weeks (62), with an incubation period for the disease of 2–12 weeks, thus potentially allowing enough time for individuals to become infectious before the window period closes. This is particularly true when the individual has a slow immune response that delays detection. While the onset of infectiousness in relation to reactivity to the skin test is currently not known, inference based approaches have demonstrated an equally good model fit to empirical data if cattle were assumed to become infectious without epidemiological latency, i.e., before entering the detectable state (5). Results from the present study demonstrated that the *SEIT* model indeed represented the "worst" case scenario resulting in more secondary cases per

breakdown than the *SETI* model. The number of secondary cases increased in the *SEIT* model because animals became infectious and could infect others before being detected and removed. However, despite the difference between the models in terms of bTB transmission, the present study showed that the impact of genetic selection tended not to differ much between the two models. The similarity between the models may be partly attributed to the relatively short time interval of 2 days estimated between the *I* and *T* states. Differences between the model predictions might have been more pronounced if this time interval was longer and the contribution of the external force of infection (α) higher.

Some important assumptions warrant further discussion. In the present study, the external source of infection (α) was kept constant across generations. However, selection is expected to reduce external infection because as animals become more resistant and the number of infectious cows declines, cattle-to-cattle and cattle-to-wildlife-to-cattle transmissions are expected to reduce over time. Therefore, keeping the external source of infection constant in the simulations depicts a somewhat conservative approach regarding the favorable impact of genetic selection. Similarly, the accuracy of selection was kept constant in the simulations, but may also decline as bTB outbreaks decrease across generations and genetically resistant cows become harder to identify. Lower accuracies could slow down response to selection. However, continuous bTB field data collection combined with optimized bTB genetic evaluation methods would counter the effect of reduction in disease prevalence and maintain accuracy of selection over generations. A common concern about genetic control strategies is the impact of selection for host resistance on potential pathogen evolution, which may slow down the predicted genetic gain in host resistance. However, in the case of bTB, the relatively low genetic variability of *M. bovis strains* within cattle populations (63), combined with the evidence from quantitative genetics studies incorporated in the model that host resistance is controlled by many genes, implies that this risk can be considered as negligible (64).

Even though the model aimed to mimic the overall population structure of UK dairy herds, demographic characteristics were not explicitly included in the present study. Not including specific demographic characteristics would particularly affect the estimates of breakdown risk, which are conditional on the introduction of infected cows in each herd. It should be noted that whilst these estimates are useful means to quantify and compare selection response, they differ from the absolute risk of a bTB breakdown, which also depends on the probability of index cases to occur in the first place and on various additional factors not considered in the model, such as cattle movement across herds of different sizes, or different management characteristics and exposure to wildlife (40, 42, 49).

Furthermore, the parameters used in the present study were obtained from literature estimates and statistical comparison of simulated with real disease data. Whilst this approach is very common for epidemiological prediction models (20, 21, 23, 25, 27), it cannot be guaranteed that alternative sets of parameter values would not provide a better model fit to the data. To test this, more sophisticated statistical inference techniques (30, 31, 37) would be required. Thus, future modeling studies may build on our work, including explicit descriptions of additional risk factors associated with bTB prevalence combined with statistical inference techniques for parameter estimation.

Apart from genetic variation in cattle resistance to bTB, no other sources of genetic or individual variation in the model parameters were included in the model. This is in line with standard animal breeding approaches, which focus primarily on selection for disease resistance. Although it is possible that cows may also vary genetically in the duration of the exposed or infectious state, or even in their skin test sensitivity, including genetic variation in the corresponding epidemiological model parameters may affect epidemiological characteristics within each generation (19, 22), but will not affect the predicted responses to selection for disease resistance. Also, within the context of the above assumptions, changing the values of some key epidemiological parameters did not seem to affect the impact of genetic selection on disease transmission dynamics manifested by probability of breakdown occurrence and severity of breakdowns. However, these parameters would largely determine the dynamics of a bTB epidemic, especially when genetic selection is not taken into account. Specifically, our analyses revealed that a decreased sensitivity of the skin test would lead to more severe breakdowns, affecting both the number of secondary cases and the duration of breakdowns. Therefore, the development of diagnostics with high sensitivity that would allow early and accurate detection of infected individual is strongly encouraged.

In the present study, the purpose of some simplifications was to allow a clear demonstration of the predicted effects of genetic selection for enhanced host resistance against the disease on the evolution and dynamics of epidemics. We maintain that the predicted impact of selection is still relevant when such simplifications are lifted. For example, we assumed that all herds in the simulation had the same size, which was similar to the average herd size in the UK dairy cattle population. In reality, herd size varies implying possibly different individual profiles of epidemics in larger vs. smaller herds. However, at population level, the overall epidemic profile will reflect that of the average-sized herd. Furthermore, sire distribution across herds is independent of herd size meaning the overall accuracy of genetic evaluation and selection would not be very close to what was simulated here.

The genetic-epidemiological model developed in the present study provides the first quantitative estimates of the impact of selection for increased resistance on bTB prevalence. In all cases, selection for increased resistance translates into noticeable epidemiological benefits. Strong selection intensities on bTB resistance would particularly benefit high risk geographic areas where the disease is highly prevalent and highly resistant sires are required. The prospects of assimilating bTB resistance into the national selection programme are convincing despite the moderate heritability of the trait. For example, while heritability of clinical mastitis in dairy cattle is low and unfavorably correlated with milk production traits, mastitis is nonetheless included in selective breeding programmes in several countries (65, 66).

CONCLUSIONS

We developed a genetic epidemiological model to investigate the impact of genetic selection for enhanced bTB resistance on disease prevalence and dynamics. Results demonstrated that genetic selection could substantially reduce bTB prevalence and severity of breakdowns over generations of selection. Our study also highlights the importance of considering genetic selection as an additional control tool that can complement existing strategies. Considering genetic selection is pertinent, especially with the view of accelerating the control and eradication of bTB to achieve the national goal of OTF status by 2038 as planned in England and Wales. Future work could consider additional genetic selection strategies such as selection for resistant dams and selection for reduced individual animal infectivity.

AVAILABILITY OF DATA

Data generated from the present study will be made available on request to qualified researchers.

AUTHOR CONTRIBUTIONS

KR, AD-W, EG, JW, and GB designed the study. KR and ES-M performed the analysis. KR, ES-M, ST, OA, AD-W, and GB interpreted the results. KR prepared the manuscript. KR, ES-M, ST, OA, EG, JW, AD-W, and GB revised the manuscript and improved its content.

ACKNOWLEDGMENTS

Field data used in the present study for comparisons were availed by Edinburgh Genetic Evaluation Services (EGENES) within the Scotland's Rural College.

SUPPLEMENTARY MATERIAL

Supplementary Data Sheet 1 | Simulated scenario with increased rate of external infection ($\alpha = 5 \times 10^{-6}$ instead of 5×10^{-7}), all other parameters remaining constant. Figures shown are: *SEIT* model profiles across 20 generations for five selection intensities defined by the percentage of selected sires: 100% (no selection; **A**), 70% **(B)**, 50% **(C)**, 25% **(D)**, and 10% **(E)**; proportion of susceptible (*S*), exposed (*E*), infectious (*I*), and test-sensitive (*T*) individuals during the course of the epidemic. Impact of genetic selection on risk of breakdown (probability of a breakdown to occur). Selection intensities correspond to selection of the 10, 25, 50, 70 and 100% (no selection) most resistant sires. Impact of genetic selection on percentage of secondary case(s) occurrence within a breakdown; mild ($\leq$3% secondary cases—**A**) and severe (>10% secondary cases—**B**); selection intensities correspond to selection of the 10, 25, 50, 70, and 100% (no selection) most resistant sires. Impact of genetic selection on the

duration of secondary case(s) within a breakdown; short ($\leq$180 days - **A**) and long (>365 days - **B**); selection intensities correspond to selection of the 10, 25, 50, 70, and 100% (no selection) most resistant sires.

Supplementary Data Sheet 2 | Simulated scenario with decreased sensitivity of the skin test (0.30 instead of 0.60), all other parameters remaining constant. Figures shown are: *SEIT* model profiles across 20 generations for five selection intensities defined by the percentage of selected sires: 100% (no selection; **A**), 70% **(B)**, 50% **(C)**, 25% **(D)**, and 10% **(E)**; proportion of susceptible (*S*), exposed (*E*), infectious (*I*), and test-sensitive (*T*) individuals during the course of the epidemic. Impact of genetic selection on risk of breakdown (probability of a breakdown to occur). Selection intensities correspond to selection of the 10, 25, 50, 70, and 100% (no selection) most resistant sires. Impact of genetic selection on percentage of secondary cases **(A)** and duration of secondary case occurrence **(B)** within a breakdown. Selection intensities correspond to selection of the 10, 25, 50, 70, and 100% (no selection) most resistant sires. Impact of genetic selection on the percentage of secondary case(s) occurrence within a breakdown; mild ($\leq$3% secondary cases - **A**) and severe (>10% secondary cases **B**); selection intensities correspond to selection of the 10, 25, 50, 70, and 100% (no selection) most resistant sires. Impact of genetic selection on the duration of secondary case(s) within a breakdown; short ($\leq$180 days - **A**) and long (>365 days - **B**); selection intensities correspond to selection of the 10, 25, 50, 70, and 100% (no selection) most resistant sires.

Supplementary Figure 1 | Scheme of the compartmental genetic-epidemiological bTB model. The compartments depict the transition between different animal disease states [Susceptible, Exposed (latent), Infectious and Test-sensitive (detectable)] in the adopted *SEIT* model with assumed heterogeneity in underlying host susceptibility to bTB. Once cows in the Test-sensitive state are diagnosed, they are removed from the herd (Removed compartment). The transition between the compartments depends on the background infection (B), the population average values for the epidemiological parameters: transmission coefficient, β; rate of infection from external sources, α; force of infection from herd-mates, λ; progression rate from Exposed to Infectious state, σ; progression rate from Infectious to Test-sensitive state, γ; skin test sensitivity, Ω; and the distribution of the underlying susceptibility of cattle to bTB (g). Genetic selection affects the g and, thus the individual and average rates of progression from Susceptible to the subsequent states.

Supplementary Figure 2 | Impact of genetic selection on the host underlying susceptibility to bovine tuberculosis. Changes in genetic variation **(A)** and mean susceptibility on the underlying scale **(B)**; selection intensities correspond to selection of the 10, 25, 50, 70, and 100% (no selection) most resistant of sires.

Supplementary Figure 3 | Impact of genetic selection on the duration of breakdown; short ($\leq$180 days - **A**) and long (>365 days - **B**); selection intensities correspond to selection of the 10, 25, 50, 70, and 100% (no selection) most resistant sires.

Supplementary Figure 4 | Impact of genetic selection on average risk of breakdown, and percentage and duration of secondary case(s) occurrence within breakdown in the *SEIT* **(A)** and *SETI* **(B)** models. Selection intensities correspond to selection of the 10, 25, 50, 70, and 100% (no selection) most resistant sires. The dashed horizontal lines represent reduction by 50%.

REFERENCES

1. Fitzgerald S, Kaneene J. Wildlife reservoirs of bovine tuberculosis worldwide: hosts, pathology, surveillance, and control. *Vet Pathol.* (2013) 50:488–99. doi: 10.1177/0300985812467472
2. Department for Environment Food and Rural Affairs (DEFRA). *Bovine TB Eradication Programme for England.* (2011). Available online at: https://assets.publishing.service.gov.uk/government/uploads/system/uploads/attachment_data/file/69443/pb13601-bovinetb-eradication-programme-110719.pdf (Accessed July 9, 2018).
3. Department for Environment Food and Rural Affairs (DEFRA). *Bovine TB: Get Your Cows Tested in England.* (2015). Available online at: https://www.gov.uk/guidance/bovine-tb-getting-your-cattle-tested-in-england (Accessed May 3, 2017).
4. Department for Environment Food and Rural Affairs (DEFRA). *The Strategy for Achieving Officially Bovine Tuberculosis Free Status for England.* (2014). Available online at: https://www.gov.uk/government/uploads/system/uploads/attachment_data/file/300447/pb14088-bovine-tb-strategy-140328.pdf (Accessed May 25, 2017).
5. Conlan AJ, McKinley TJ, Karolemeas K, Pollock EB, Goodchild AV, Mitchell AP, et al. Estimating the hidden burden of bovine tuberculosis in Great Britain. *PLoS Comput Biol.* (2012) 8:e1002730. doi: 10.1371/journal.pcbi.1002730
6. Gallagher J, Clifton-Hadley R. Tuberculosis in badgers; a review of the disease and its significance for other animals. *Res Vet Sci.* (2000) 69:203–17. doi: 10.1053/rvsc.2000.0422
7. Lawes J, Harris K, Brouwer A, Broughan J, Smith N, Upton P. Bovine TB surveillance in Great Britain in 2014. *Vet Rec.* (2016) 178:310–5. doi: 10.1136/vr.i1616

8. Abernethy DA, Upton P, Higgins IM, McGrath G, Goodchild AV, Rolfe SJ, et al. Bovine tuberculosis trends in the UK and the Republic of Ireland, 1995-2010. *Vet Rec.* (2013) 172:312. doi: 10.1136/vr.100969

9. Department for Environment Food and Rural Affairs (DEFRA). *Quarterly Publication of National Statistics on the Incidence and Prevalence of Tuberculosis (TB) in Cattle in Great Britain – to End December 2016.* (2017). Available online at: https://assets.publishing.service.gov.uk/government/uploads/system/uploads/attachment_data/file/69443/pb13601-bovinetb-eradication-programme-110719.pdf (Accessed May 25, 2017).

10. Allen AR, Minozzi G, Glass EJ, Skuce RA, McDowell SW, Woolliams JA, et al. Bovine tuberculosis: the genetic basis of host susceptibility. *Proc Biol Sci.* (2010) 277:2737–45. doi: 10.1098/rspb.2010.0830

11. Bermingham ML, More SJ, Good M, Cromie AR, Higgins IM, Brotherstone S, et al. Genetics of tuberculosis in Irish Holstein-Friesian dairy herds. *J Dairy Sci.* (2009) 92:3447–56. doi: 10.3168/jds.2008-1848

12. Brotherstone S, White I, Coffey M, Downs S, Mitchell A, Clifton-Hadley R, et al. Evidence of genetic resistance of cattle to infection with *Mycobacterium bovis. J Dairy Sci.* (2010) 93:1234–42. doi: 10.3168/jds.2009-2609

13. Richardson IW, Bradley DG, Higgins IM, More SJ, McClure J, Berry DP. Variance components for susceptibility to *Mycobacterium bovis* infection in dairy and beef cattle. *Gen Sel Evol.* (2014) 46:77. doi: 10.1186/s12711-014-0077-1

14. Tsairidou S, Woolliams JA, Allen AR, Skuce RA, McBride SH, Wright DM, et al. Genomic prediction for tuberculosis resistance in dairy cattle. *PLoS ONE* (2014) 9:e96728. doi: 10.1371/journal.pone.0096728

15. Raphaka K, Matika O, Sánchez-Molano E, Mrode R, Coffey MP, Riggio V, et al. Genomic regions underlying susceptibility to bovine tuberculosis in Holstein-Friesian cattle. *BMC Genet.* (2017) 18:27. doi: 10.1186/s12863-017-0493-7

16. Agriculture and Horticulture Development Board (AHDB). (2016). *TB Advantage.* Available online at: http://dairy.ahdb.org.uk/technical-information/breeding-genetics/tb-advantage/ (Accessed May 21, 2017).

17. MacKenzie K, Bishop SC. Utilizing stochastic genetic epidemiological models to quantify the impact of selection for resistance to infectious diseases in domestic livestock. *J Anim Sci.* (2001) 79:2057–65. doi: 10.2527/2001.7982057x

18. Springbett A, MacKenzie K, Woolliams J, Bishop S. The contribution of genetic diversity to the spread of infectious diseases in livestock populations. *Genetics* (2003) 165:1465–74.

19. Nath M, Woolliams J, Bishop S. Assessment of the dynamics of microparasite infections in genetically homogeneous and heterogeneous populations using a stochastic epidemic model. *J Anim Sci.* (2008) 86:1747–57. doi: 10.2527/jas.2007-0615

20. Gharbi K, Matthews L, Bron J, Roberts R, Tinch A, Stear M. The control of sea lice in Atlantic salmon by selective breeding. *J R Soc Interface* (2015) 12:20150574. doi: 10.1098/rsif.2015.0574

21. Nieuwhof GJ, Conington J, Bishop SC. A genetic epidemiological model to describe resistance to an endemic bacterial disease in livestock: application to footrot in sheep. *Gen Sel Evol.* (2009) 41:19. doi: 10.1186/1297-9686-41-19

22. Doeschl-Wilson AB, Davidson R, Conington J, Roughsedge T, Hutchings MR, Villanueva B. Implications of host genetic variation on the risk and prevalence of infectious diseases transmitted through the environment. *Genetics* (2011) 188:683–93. doi: 10.1534/genetics.110.125625

23. Bishop SC, Stear MJ. Modeling of host genetics and resistance to infectious diseases: understanding and controlling nematode infections. *Vet Parasitol.* (2003) 115:147–66. doi: 10.1016/S0304-4017(03)00204-8

24. Nath M. Development of a genetic epidemiological model for Marek's disease in poultry. In: *Proceedings of the 8th World Congress on Genetics Applied to Livestock Production* (Belo Horizonte) (2006).

25. Barlow N, Kean J, Hickling G, Livingstone P, Robson A. A simulation model for the spread of bovine tuberculosis within New Zealand cattle herds. *Prev Vet Med.* (1997) 32:57–75. doi: 10.1016/S0167-5877(97)00002-0

26. Kao R, Roberts M, Ryan T. A model of bovine tuberculosis control in domesticated cattle herds. *Proc Biol Sci.* (1997) 264:1069–76. doi: 10.1098/rspb.1997.0148

27. Fischer E, Van Roermund H, Hemerik L, Van Asseldonk M, De Jong M. Evaluation of surveillance strategies for bovine tuberculosis (*Mycobacterium bovis*) using an individual based epidemiological model. *Prev Vet Med.* (2005) 67:283–301. doi: 10.1016/j.prevetmed.2004.12.002

28. Biek R, O'Hare A, Wright D, Mallon T, McCormick C, Orton RJ, et al. Whole genome sequencing reveals local transmission patterns of *Mycobacterium bovis* in sympatric cattle and badger populations. *PLoS Pathog.* (2012) 8:e1003008. doi: 10.1371/journal.ppat.1003008

29. Bekara MA, Courcoul A, Benet JJ, Durand B. Modeling tuberculosis dynamics, detection and control in cattle herds. *PLoS ONE* (2014) 9:e108584. doi: 10.1371/journal.pone.0108584

30. Brooks-Pollock E, Roberts GO, Keeling MJ. A dynamic model of bovine tuberculosis spread and control in Great Britain. *Nature* (2014) 511:228–31. doi: 10.1038/nature13529

31. O'Hare A, Orton RJ, Bessell PR, Kao RR. Estimating epidemiological parameters for bovine tuberculosis in British cattle using a Bayesian partial-likelihood approach. *Proc Biol Sci.* (2014) 281:20140248. doi: 10.1098/rspb.2014.0248

32. McIlroy S, Neill S, McCracken R. Pulmonary lesions and *Mycobacterium bovis* excretion from the respiratory tract of tuberculin reacting cattle. *Vet Rec.* (1986) 118:718–21. doi: 10.1136/vr.118.26.718

33. Neill S, Hanna J, O'brien J, McCracken R. Excretion of *Mycobacterium bovis* by experimentally infected cattle. *Vet. Rec.* (1988) 123:340–3. doi: 10.1136/vr.123.13.340

34. Bermingham ML, Bishop SC, Woolliams JA, Pong-Wong R, Allen AR, McBride SH, et al. Genome-wide association study identifies novel loci associated with resistance to bovine tuberculosis. *Heredity* (2014) 112:543–51. doi: 10.1038/hdy.2013.137

35. Lipschutz-Powell D, Woolliams JA, Bijma P, Doeschl-Wilson AB. Indirect genetic effects and the spread of infectious disease: are we capturing the full heritable variation underlying disease prevalence? *PLoS ONE* (2012) 7:e39551. doi: 10.1371/journal.pone.0039551

36. Lipschutz-Powell D, Woolliams JA, Doeschl-Wilson AB. A unifying theory for genetic epidemiological analysis of binary disease data. *Genet Sel Evol.* (2014) 46:1–12. doi: 10.1186/1297-9686-46-15

37. Anacleto O, Garcia-Cortés LA, Lipschutz-Powell D, Woolliams JA, Doeschl-Wilson AB. A novel statistical model to estimate host genetic effects affecting disease transmission. *Genetics* (2015) 201:871–84. doi: 10.1534/genetics.115.179853

38. Green M, Green L, Schukken Y, Bradley A, Peeler E, Barkema H, et al. Somatic cell count distributions during lactation predict clinical mastitis. *J Dairy Sci.* (2004) 87:1256–64. doi: 10.3168/jds.S0022-0302(04)73276-2

39. Banos G, Winters M, Mrode R, Mitchell A, Bishop SC, Woolliams JA, et al. Genetic evaluation for bovine tuberculosis resistance in dairy cattle. *J Dairy Sci.* (2017) 100:1272–81. doi: 10.3168/jds.2016-11897

40. Reilly L, Courtenay O. Husbandry practices, badger sett density and habitat composition as risk factors for transient and persistent bovine tuberculosis on UK cattle farms. *Prev Vet Med.* (2007) 80:129–42. doi: 10.1016/j.prevetmed.2007.02.002

41. Brooks-Pollock E, Keeling M. Herd size and bovine tuberculosis persistence in cattle farms in Great Britain. *Prev Vet Med.* (2009) 92:360–5. doi: 10.1016/j.prevetmed.2009.08.022

42. Humblet M-F, Boschiroli ML, Saegerman C. Classification of worldwide bovine tuberculosis risk factors in cattle: a stratified approach. *Vet Res.* (2009) 40:1–24. doi: 10.1051/vetres/2009033

43. Nuñez-Garcia J, Downs SH, Parry JE, Abernethy DA, Broughan JM, Cameron AR, et al. Meta-analyses of the sensitivity and specificity of ante-mortem and post-mortem diagnostic tests for bovine tuberculosis in the UK and Ireland. *Prev Vet Med.* (2018) 153:94–107. doi: 10.1016/j.prevetmed.2017.02.017

44. Berry DP, Bermingham ML, Good M, More SJ. Genetics of animal health and disease in cattle. *Ir Vet J.* (2011) 64:5. doi: 10.1186/2046-0481-64-5

45. Barlow N. Non-linear transmission and simple models for bovine tuberculosis. *J Anim Ecol.* (2000) 69:703–13. doi: 10.1046/j.1365-2656.2000.00428.x

46. Brooks-Pollock E, de Jong M, Keeling MJ, Klinkenberg D, Wood JL. Eight challenges in modelling infectious livestock diseases. *Epidemics* (2015) 10:1–5. doi: 10.1016/j.epidem.2014.08.005

47. Stear M, Boag B, Cattadori I, Murphy L. Genetic variation in resistance to mixed, predominantly *Teladorsagia circumcincta* nematode infections of sheep: from heritabilities to gene identification. *Parasite Immunol.* (2009) 31:274–82. doi: 10.1111/j.1365-3024.2009.01105.x

48. Karolemeas K, McKinley T, Clifton-Hadley R, Goodchild A, Mitchell A, Johnston W, et al. Predicting prolonged bovine tuberculosis breakdowns in Great Britain as an aid to control. *Prev Vet Med.* (2010) 97:183–90. doi: 10.1016/j.prevetmed.2010.09.007

49. Skuce RA, Allen AR, McDowell SW. Herd-level risk factors for bovine tuberculosis: a literature review. *Vet Med Int.* (2012) 2012:621210. doi: 10.1155/2012/621210

50. Perez AM, Ward MP, Charmandarián A, Ritacco V. Simulation model of within-herd transmission of bovine tuberculosis in Argentine dairy herds. *Prev Vet Med.* (2002) 54:361–72. doi: 10.1016/S0167-5877(02)00043-0

51. MacKenzie K, Bishop S. A discrete-time epidemiological model to quantify selection for disease resistance. *Anim Sci.* (1999) 69:543–51. doi: 10.1017/S1357729800051390

52. Lipschutz-Powell D, Woolliams JA, Bijma P, Pong-Wong R, Bermingham ML, Doeschl-Wilson AB. Bias, accuracy, and impact of indirect genetic effects in infectious diseases. *Front Genet.* (2012) 3:215. doi: 10.3389/fgene.2012.00215

53. Olea-Popelka F, White P, Collins J, O'Keeffe J, Kelton D, Martin, S. Breakdown severity during a bovine tuberculosis episode as a predictor of future herd breakdowns in Ireland. *Prev Vet Med.* (2004) 63:163–72. doi: 10.1016/j.prevetmed.2004.03.001

54. Wolfe DM, Berke O, Kelton DF, White PW, More SJ, O'Keeffe J, et al. From explanation to prediction: a model for recurrent bovine tuberculosis in Irish cattle herds. *Prev Vet Med.* (2010) 94:170–7. doi: 10.1016/j.prevetmed.2010.02.010

55. Karolemeas K, McKinley TJ, Clifton-Hadley RS, Goodchild AV, Mitchell A, Johnston WT, et al. Recurrence of bovine tuberculosis breakdowns in Great Britain: risk factors and prediction. *Prev Vet Med.* (2011) 102:22–9. doi: 10.1016/j.prevetmed.2011.06.004

56. Bermingham ML, More SJ, Good M, Cromie AR, Higgins IM, Berry DP. Genetic correlations between measures of *Mycobacterium bovis* infection and economically important traits in Irish Holstein-Friesian dairy cows. *J Dairy Sci.* (2010) 93:5413–22. doi: 10.3168/jds.2009-2925

57. Tsairidou S, Anacleto O, Raphaka K, Sanchez-Molano E, Banos G, Woolliams JA, et al. Enhancing genetic disease control by selecting for lower host infectivity. In: *11th World Congress on Genetics Applied to Livestock Production* (Auckland) (2018).

58. Schaeffer L. Strategy for applying genome-wide selection in dairy cattle. *J Anim Breed Genet.* (2006) 123:218–23. doi: 10.1111/j.1439-0388.2006.00595.x

59. Hayes BJ, Bowman PJ, Chamberlain A, Goddard M. Invited review: genomic selection in dairy cattle: progress and challenges. *J Dairy Sci.* (2009) 92:433–43. doi: 10.3168/jds.2008-1646

60. Anderson RM, Trewhella W. Population dynamics of the badger (*Meles meles*) and the epidemiology of bovine tuberculosis (*Mycobacterium bovis*). *Philos Trans R Soc Lond B Biol Sci.* (1985) 310:327–81. doi: 10.1098/rstb.1985.0123

61. Pilcher CD, Christopoulos KA, Golden M. Public health rationale for rapid nucleic acid or p24 antigen tests for HIV. *J Infect Dis.* (2010) 201(Suppl. 1):S7–15. doi: 10.1086/650393

62. Nayak S, Acharjya B. Mantoux test and its interpretation. *Indian Dermatol Online J.* (2012) 3:2. doi: 10.4103/2229-5178.93479

63. Patane JS, Martins J Jr, Castelao AB, Nishibe C, Montera L, Bigi F, et al. Patterns and processes of *Mycobacterium bovis* evolution revealed by phylogenomic analyses. *Genome Biol. Evol.* (2017) 9:521–35. doi: 10.1093/gbe/evx022

64. Kemper KE, Goddard ME, Bishop SC. Adaptation of gastrointestinal nematode parasites to host genotype: single locus simulation models. *Genet Sel Evol.* (2013) 45:14. doi: 10.1186/1297-9686-45-14

65. Philipsson J, Lindhé B. Experiences of including reproduction and health traits in Scandinavian dairy cattle breeding programmes. *Livestock Prod Sci.* (2003) 83:99–112. doi: 10.1016/S0301-6226(03)00047-2

66. Bell MJ, Pryce J, Wilson P. A comparison of the economic value for enteric methane emissions with other biological traits associated with dairy cows. *Am Res J Agric.* (2016) 2:1–17. doi: 10.21694/2379-1047.16002

Wild Animal Tuberculosis: Stakeholder Value Systems and Management of Disease

Eamonn Gormley* and Leigh A. L. Corner

School of Veterinary Medicine, University College Dublin, Dublin, Ireland

*Correspondence:
Eamonn Gormley
egormley@ucd.ie

When human health is put at risk from the transmission of animal diseases, the options for intervention often require input from stakeholders whose differing values systems contribute to decisions on disease management. Animal tuberculosis (TB), caused principally by *Mycobacterium bovis* is an archetypical zoonotic pathogen in that it can be transmitted from animals to humans and *vice versa*. Although elimination of zoonotic transmission of TB to humans is frequently promoted as the *raison d'être* for TB management in livestock, in many countries the control strategies are more likely based on minimizing the impact of sustained infection on the agricultural industry. Where wild animals are implicated in the epidemiology of the disease, the options for control and eradication can require involvement of additional stakeholder groups. Conflict can arise when different monetary and/or societal values are assigned to the affected animals. This may impose practical and ethical dilemmas for decision makers where one or more species of wild animal is seen by some stakeholders to have a greater value than the affected livestock. Here we assess the role of stakeholder values in influencing TB eradication strategies in a number of countries including Ireland, the UK, the USA, Spain, France, Australia, New Zealand and South Africa. What it reveals is that the level of stakeholder involvement increases with the complexity of the epidemiology, and that similar groups of stakeholders may agree to a set of control and eradication measures in one region only to disagree with applying the same measures in another. The level of consensus depends on the considerations of the reservoir status of the infected host, the societal values assigned to each species, the type of interventions proposed, ethical issues raised by culling of sentient wild animals, and the economic cost benefit effectiveness of dealing with the problem in one or more species over a long time frame. While there is a societal benefit from controlling TB, the means to achieve this requires identification and long-term engagement with all key stakeholders in order to reach agreement on ethical frameworks that prioritize and justify control options, particularly where culling of wild animals is concerned.

Keywords: tuberculosis, *Mycobacterium bovis*, animals, wildlife, stakeholders, value systems

INTRODUCTION

With increased global interest in the emergence of new infectious diseases, the role of animals in the transmission of infection to humans has become a focus of attention (1). The reasons for the spread of infections are complex and multifactorial and can involve changes in human populations and densities, modifications in animal husbandry practices, and changes to the ecological environment leading to human intrusion into wildlife habitats that hitherto remained undisturbed (2, 3). It is the increased risk of transmission to humans that is most often the foundation for efforts to understand the epidemiology of animal disease and the implementation of preventative measures to minimize transmission (4, 5). A case in point is tuberculosis (TB) in animals and the danger it has historically posed to humans. Commonly referred to as "bovine tuberculosis" despite the causative organisms, most frequently *Mycobacterium bovis*, being capable of infecting a wide range of mammalian species, the perceived risk is reflective of the historical close association between livestock and humans (6, 7). During the early part of the twentieth century, in the period preceding the pasteurization of milk, transmission of infection *via* contaminated milk was a serious public health problem in the industrialized world, leading to many thousands of cases of human TB with high mortality rates (8, 9). The discipline of epidemiology (as we understand it today) was then largely non-existent. To the extent that attempts to address the disease in all its forms (cattle and human TB) were driven by competing stakeholder interests (e.g., dairy industry, public health agencies, government), more often than not it resulted in stasis and a complete failure to reduce disease incidence (10). Many countries in Europe eventually achieved eradication of TB from cattle through the roll out of government-regulated compulsory national screening programmes in cattle, and have since maintained this status through monitoring of animals for typical TB lesions at the slaughter house (11). For some of those countries that failed to achieve eradication, despite intensive testing, there was an awareness that the epidemiology of the disease was complicated by other possible sources of infection, notably wildlife (12). This militated against any quick-fix solutions to solve the problems. Instead it lead to decades of research to unravel what has turned out in many circumstances to be extremely complex epidemiology.

There have been few systematic studies worldwide to assess the extent of wildlife TB and it is often the case that studies are only initiated when there is spillover of TB into livestock, or where there is a high value placed on the species by particular stakeholders. Wild animal populations infected with TB are currently found in North and South America, Europe, Africa and Australasia (12). However, the finding of TB in wild animals in any particular environment does not constitute proof that they are a significant source of infection for livestock, companion animals or humans (13). Indeed it reveals little in terms of whether the affected species is a self-sustaining maintenance host or a dead-end spillover host. This distinction is critical for the development of strategies to control the disease in livestock as it can impact on the perspectives and level of engagement among a range of stakeholders. Depending on the reservoir status stakeholders may assign different value systems to the wildlife species and this can directly influence the type of management systems put in place. When TB is found in a free-ranging wildlife population the prevention of spread to other animals, especially livestock is often the immediate priority followed by the prevention of geographic spread. The identification of maintenance hosts is therefore of paramount importance in understanding the epidemiology because the disease can persist

indefinitely in the absence of specific management and control programs. If it is established that wild animals are important in the epidemiological cycle and act as a source of risk to livestock, the decision making process as to the preferred actions will primarily depend on the considerations of the reservoir status of the infected host and the broader societal values assigned to each species by stakeholders. With spillover hosts, there may be a broad consensus reached among a limited number of stakeholders that an aggressive response to dealing with the reservoir host is the most effective strategy for stamping out the disease. However, if disease becomes established in a maintenance host, this will attract the attention of a broader range of stakeholders and there will be more complex ethical issues raised from culling of sentient wild animals and the economic cost benefit effectiveness of dealing with the problem in one or more species over a long time frame.

How to deal with the disease problems in cattle, arising from infected wildlife, has in the past often proven to be a quandary for stakeholders, in that government and industry supported measures (e.g., wildlife disease surveillance, culling) were not, at least in the beginning, underpinned by strong scientific evidence (14, 15). Rather, they were often pragmatic choices based on basic, simplistic epidemiological principles that aimed to deliver cost-effective beneficial results to the livestock industry in the short to medium term while awaiting the relatively slow pace of research to decipher the epidemiology and translate the results into policy decisions (14, 16). As a result, the primary driver for disease management in livestock has most often been based on economics and the impact of sustained infection on the agricultural industry (17, 18). In countries where wildlife have been considered as a potential source of infection the programmes evolved as the initial poor epidemiological understanding became clear, both from experience and also resulting from focused research both within the targeted species, and from assessing the risk of spread to other species (16, 19). However, as is often the case with scientific investigations into complex problems there can be an absence of certainty, and this has lead to conflict between the demands of different stakeholders (20).

STAKEHOLDER VALUE SYSTEMS AND WILDLIFE

"Wildlife stakeholder" broadly describes any person or group with an interest in wildlife. The levels of interest and the weighted values that each stakeholder assigns to particular wildlife can be highly variable, and defining the moral and ethical viewpoints of stakeholders that influences their level of engagement can be difficult. This is because there is likely to be a complex interplay between the values that each stakeholder places on wildlife and how it is linked to their moral perspectives on animal rights, animal-human health, conservation and biodiversity (21). Value systems for wildlife have been broadly classified into a number of groups according to their (a) economic importance, (b) nutritional value, (c) ecological role, and (d) socio-cultural significance (22). Quantifying the values with a high degree of certainty can be problematic as it mostly relies on data collected from surveys assessing preferences of stakeholders (23).

Stated preference methodologies, such as choice experiments allow for a structured method of data generation that helps to identify the factors influencing alternative choice scenarios (24). This approach is based on the assumption that individuals will select the choice that they expect will give them the highest benefit (utility), when presented with a set of alternatives. Its advantage over simple stated preference methods is that it allows for the valuation of attributes that characterize a particular scenario, rather than just valuing the scenario itself. Within each scenario there can be a scale of positive and negative values. For example, within the large game reserves in Africa, wildlife conservation activities can have a net positive value because of the significant beneficial impact on the local economy, also through the enhancement of local ecosystems from maintenance of biodiversity, and the cultural significance of wildlife for local communities. Negative values can accrue, for example, if there is crop or other habitat destruction because of over-abundance of particular species (e.g., large herbivores). As another example in the context of TB, choice experiment studies carried out in the UK have shown that badger management policies attract very high values: the surveys revealed that the public places high values on government policies that avoid culling of badgers (25).

Where wildlife start to encroach and compete with human interests negative value perceptions can increase among an expanded range of stakeholders. The divergence of values can lead to conflicts between those who place higher values on human activities (e.g., farming) and livelihoods and those who value the protection and welfare of wild animals. How these differences are reconciled can depend on the environmental and animal ethics perspectives of the stakeholders (26). These perspectives range from a contractarian viewpoint where there is a hypothetical social agreement to manage wildlife wisely for human benefit, to an animal rights focused viewpoint where there is no societal obligation to manage or interfere in any way with the well-being of wildlife. For many stakeholders with a general or transient interest in wildlife the ethical perspectives are likely to represent a blend of different viewpoints combining multiple value systems e.g., utilitarian and animals rights based values, such that respect for wildlife is acknowledged while at the same time adopting a value system allowing for the sacrifice of the interests of some animals for the greater benefit of others. The recognition that wild animals are a source of zoonotic diseases, particularly animal TB, can quickly change the number of stakeholders involved and increase the range of ethical perspectives: it can quickly shift the balance from high values associated with the natural rights of wild animals to much lower values as the threat of TB intensifies. The threat from infected wildlife can, on the one hand, be viewed as a serious agricultural problem with potential significance for broader human activities and health. A contrary perspective can assign higher net values to the affected wildlife species because of the belief that the disease impact is mostly restricted to the livestock industry or that the threat is overstated. Where there is a lack of objective data to support a particular perspective, this can lead to disagreements between those stakeholders who primarily value animal welfare and rights, and those who value the perceived greater benefits to society. Added difficulties arise from trying to define measures of benefit, for example, how can society assess and compare the pain and suffering experienced by slaughter of cattle and culling of wildlife? How are ethical views influenced by the presence of disease in one or both species? Do TB control programmes strike the correct balance between protecting the livestock industry and valuing the benefits of wildlife existing in their natural habitats? If TB was restricted to wildlife, how many stakeholders would be concerned for their fate? From studying the evolution and operation of TB control programmes in different parts of the world, we argue that the presence of TB in wild animals can lead to a change in ethical frameworks, and also involve a wider range and higher level of stakeholder engagement in the strategies employed to deal with the problem. The values of the interested parties appear to be based on an *ad hoc* blend of economic considerations, livelihood activities, knowledge, ethical perspectives, social acceptance, ecological concerns, cultural significance, and political will. This results in significant challenges for the selection of control policies where one or more species of wild animal is seen by some stakeholders to have a greater value than the affected livestock. It can also lead to demands for exceptionally high quality scientific evidence to justify particular interventions. Not all species are of equal significance in the epidemiology of disease, not all are considered equal when subjected to disease management, nor are they always equal in the eyes of stakeholders.

To try and get a better understanding of how policy decisions to manage TB in wildlife are influenced by stakeholders, we have looked at a number of established TB control programmes worldwide where there is strong evidence of epidemiological involvement of wildlife in the transmission of infection. We highlight the influence of stakeholder values on the management of the disease where the contexts differed. The approaches to disease control range from relatively uncomplicated management systems in Australia where there was strong consensus between stakeholders because of the negative value pest status of the wild animals to the highly complex epidemiology of disease in South Africa where multiple species of high positive conservation value are affected and a diverse range of stakeholder groups are involved in the debate on how to control and manage the disease.

WILDLIFE TB IN AUSTRALIA

Australia has been uniquely successful in eradication of TB from cattle against the background of a significant wildlife reservoir of infection in an area of one state, the Northern Territory (NT). Eradication was achieved following agreement of key stakeholders to the program, which included addressing the problem of wildlife reservoirs of infection (27). The last known cases of TB in Australia were detected in 2002: two cases in buffalo herds in the NT and a secondary case in a cattle herd in Queensland (28). Studies had revealed that *M. bovis* infection in animals was limited to two maintenance hosts: domestic cattle and feral water buffalo (*Bubalus bubalis*), with infection recorded in only one other wild animal host, feral pigs (*Sus scrofa*) (29, 30). There were only two reports of infection in other domestic grazing animal species: in goats co-grazing with infected cattle (31) and in fallow deer (*Dama dama*) (32). Also, as well as being a maintenance host for TB, feral water buffalo and feral pigs were classified as invasive pest animal species that were causing a major negative impact on the environment of the coastal wetlands of the NT.

The Australian history of bovine TB control mirrors that of other developed countries, with an evolution from a voluntary program in the early twentieth century to a national program commencing in 1970 (33). The initial focus was on removal of diseased dairy cattle to minimize the threat to the human population. Reduction in prevalence was rapid and by the 1960s only a few pockets of infection remained among the southern states where dairy herds were dominant. However, the threat of trade restrictions for meat and dairy products imposed by trading partners in Europe and US lead to the launch of the national Brucellosis and Tuberculosis Eradication Campaign (BTEC), which ran from 1970–1997. The cattle industry was a key stakeholder in this campaign which included herd test and slaughter, compensation payments, tracing of animal movements, all backed up by a dedicated laboratory service. Aerial mustering and ground shooting was used in the large farms in northern Australia with whole herd culling of infected herds during the final stages. It was notable that domesticated water buffalo herds in this region were managed similar to local cattle herds and were subject to a test and slaughter strategy.

Feral water buffalo were only found in the NT having been introduced there in the mid-1800s. In the 1960s the prevalence of TB in slaughtered bulls was 16%. In 1970 at the commencement of the BTEC program, the disease was endemic in buffalo across most of their range (34) with the prevalence of lesions in abattoir slaughtered animals ranging up to 8.2% (35). The buffalo population peaked in the 1980s at around 350,000 head with the majority being unmusterable feral stock. With agreement between some of the stakeholders, that is, state and federal governments, pastoralists and conservationists, a decision was made to eradicate the wild buffalo herds by culling. The culling operations were effective and buffalo were eradicated from the coastal plains of the NT, except for a few domesticated buffalo herds and, at the request of the indigenous Aboriginal land owners, up to 60,000 animals were allowed to remain in the northeast corner of the state, where no TB was ever recorded in cattle or buffalo.

There was strong social, political, and cattle industry support for eradication of feral buffalo with the principal justification being the risk of transmission to cattle, even though there was only limited interaction between buffalo and cattle and no evidence of significant cross-species transmission (13). There was minimal objection to the eradication program from the small commercial buffalo capturing industry. The scientific evidence of damage to the coast flood plains caused by buffalo, leading to saltwater intrusion into the freshwater flood plains, resulting in the loss of habitat for native animals, and birds, was well documented (36). The coastal plains included the Kakadu National Park, a World Heritage site.

When the focus of the Australian national TB eradication program was extended to the pastoral grazing areas of northern Australia there was trepidation among stakeholders as feral pigs were considered as a possible reservoir of M. bovis infection.

These suids were widespread and numerous in the region, and though the prevalence of confirmed M. bovis infection in some studies was high at 19.2% (30) it was subsequently considered from the distribution of TB lesions that they constituted a spillover host with a minimal risk of onwards transmission from pigs to other animal species. It is likely the feral pigs became infected by scavenging on carcasses of tuberculous cattle and water buffalo (13). No direct intervention was taken against the feral pig population and it was later shown that after eradication of TB from cattle and the eradication of buffalo, TB prevalence in feral pigs declined significantly (29). Unlike in New Zealand, infection with M. bovis was never reported in the common brushtail possum (Trichosurus vulpecula). Elsewhere, the absence of infection among native wildlife allowed the focus of the TB campaign to remain on cattle and buffalo. Following the end of BTEC, all subsequent buffalo herds were derived from populations where infection had never been present. Since 2011, infection with M. bovis has been classified as an exotic disease of cattle in Australia (37).

NEW ZEALAND AND TB IN WILDLIFE

The New Zealand history of bovine TB control parallels that of Australia, starting with voluntary testing of dairy cattle herds in 1941 and moving to stringent and compulsory test and slaughter programmes in 1961 (14, 16). When progress stalled, the discovery of the disease in wildlife was recognized as a possible constraint to eradication (38). Epidemiological studies in New Zealand identified 14 species infected with M. bovis, but only three, domestic cattle, domestic deer and brushtail possums, were identified as maintenance hosts, though wild ferrets (Mustela furo) were considered as possibly a maintenance host in very limited areas (16, 39). Although not considered as maintenance hosts, feral pigs and wild deer, along with the ferret, have proved invaluable as sentinel hosts for surveillance of TB in possum populations (40). The current testing program for cattle and deer is based on the risks associated with transmission of infection from possums (14). The brushtail possum is a small arboreal marsupial, first introduced into New Zealand from Australia in 1837 to establish a commercial fur trade (41). They were officially classified as a pest species in 1948. The possum population reached a peak of around 50–70 million in the 1980s. The original public perception of possums as harmless changed when it was shown that they might pose a great threat to survival of native fauna, including the iconic kiwi (42). Although first shown to be infected in the mid–1960s, the findings in the 1970s revealed that possums were a maintenance reservoir host for M. bovis, and strongly implicated in the transmission of infection to cattle. Studies also showed that possums were highly susceptible to infection resulting in a rapidly disseminated and fatal disease (41, 43). Although generally avoiding cattle, terminally ill possums display abnormal behavior patterns which could bring them into contact with inquisitive cattle (44, 45).

The early government-led initiatives to control TB in cattle subsequently evolved into a public-private partnership between the government and the livestock industries with a remit to conduct wide scale possum control (16). The objective of the national program was to eradicate *M. bovis* from New Zealand and this received general societal and industry stakeholder support (46, 47). The broad geographic distribution of tuberculous possum populations and the large number of other species affected initially made the prospects of eradication unlikely even though there was support for the TB eradication program, especially the focus on possum culling (48). In recent years a choice experiment survey of the NZ public was carried out to assess the non-monetary benefits to native forest biodiversity arising from TB-related possum control (48). This revealed strong public stakeholder support for the benefits of possum control, particularly the values placed on the observable effects of improved forest canopies and the positive impact on native bird, insect and plant species. The main criticism of possum control has subsequently been aimed at the methods used to cull possums, especially the use of sodium fluoroacetate (1080) by aerial application (49, 50).

The early possum control measures helped to significantly lower the incidence of disease in cattle herds, but relied on basic assumptions of the epidemiology, rather than any hard scientific evidence (41, 51). Where large scale possum control measures were successful, the TB levels in the sentinel species also declined, demonstrating that targeting resources at one key maintenance reservoir had a direct beneficial effect on other species (52). Currently the population of possums is estimated to be in the order of 30 million. As a result of the possum culling, also controls on the movement of cattle and deer, and TB testing, the number of infected herds in NZ has dropped from ~1,700 deer and cattle herds at the peak in 1995 to 41 herds in 2015 (14, 16).

BADGER TB IN IRELAND AND THE UK

In recent times the most controversial wild animal TB control strategies in Ireland and the UK have revolved around the European badger (*Meles meles*) with deep polarization of opinion among many of the stakeholders, particularly in the UK (53). The role of badgers in the epidemiology of TB in cattle in the UK and Ireland has been subject to intensive investigations since *M. bovis* infection was first identified in badgers in England in 1971 and subsequently in Ireland in 1974 (54, 55). Over the preceding 10 years substantial progress had been made in reducing the incidence of TB in cattle in both countries due to mandatory herd screening programmes (9, 56, 57). When progress stalled, and badgers were found to be infected, local badger culling operations resulted in an apparent decline of disease in cattle (57, 58). Over the next two decades evidence accumulated through large scale culling studies that strongly implicated badgers in the TB transmission cycle (59–63). The advent of DNA genotyping of *M. bovis* isolates also revealed that prevalent genotypes were common in both cattle and badgers sharing the same environment, providing evidence of cross-species transmission (64, 65). Tuberculosis in badgers is a chronic slowly progressive disease (66) and infected badgers satisfy the criteria to be a maintenance reservoir host for *M. bovis* in Ireland and the UK (13). They are highly susceptible to infection

and the predominant location of lesions suggest that infection among badgers occurs principally *via* the respiratory route with transmission from infected bite wounds being of secondary importance (67, 68). The social structure of badgers facilitates close interactions that lead to an increased risk of transmission. Pseudovertical transmission from dam to cub is likely to be a key factor in maintenance of infection within local populations (66).

In the Republic of Ireland the national TB eradication plan commenced in the late 1950's, and the strategy has succeeded in decreasing TB incidence in cattle and maintaining it at a relatively low level (69). This has been achieved using a program of sustained cattle testing and targeted badger culling (70). Prior to the implementation of a national badger culling strategy in the Republic of Ireland, two separate badger culling studies (East Offaly Project and the Four Area Study) confirmed the role of badgers in the epidemiology of TB in cattle. Both trials showed a significant drop in cattle TB prevalence in areas where badgers were proactively culled in comparison to the control areas (60, 63). A separate study conducted in County Laois between 1989 and 2005 also provided evidence that badger culling had a positive impact on the risk of future TB breakdowns in cattle and a positive protective effect on herds neighboring the index herd (71). Badger culling was incorporated into the national TB eradication strategy in 2004. As a compromise with stakeholders who had reservations about the strategy, there was a limit imposed on which individual setts could be culled in the relation to the index herd and the proportion of the badger population subjected to culling. Since then, the Irish culling program has focused on areas with high incidence of infection in cattle; areas in which studies have shown the highest infection prevalence in badgers (72). Culling is only conducted following an exhaustive epidemiological investigation to rule out other causes of herd breakdowns (e.g., residual infection, contiguous herd spread, purchase of undiagnosed infected animals), and where badgers are considered as a likely source of infection. Analysis of data generated from culling studies has shown a beneficial long-term decrease in cattle TB (71) and also TB in the badgers of the re-emergent population (73). The culling of badgers in Ireland at national level is considered as an interim strategy to minimize transmission to cattle pending the development of a suitable and effective vaccine. Most stakeholders have accepted culling of badgers, albeit with reservations (72). These reservations are mainly framed around the evidence base that implicates badgers in the epidemiology of TB in cattle, that there is an effective control programme in place for infected herds, and whether culling of badgers is an acceptable measure when the benefits to cattle are difficult to quantify against a background of other control measures focused on cattle.

In the UK there are a large number of stakeholders with diametrically opposing views involved in the debates on the TB control strategy. Culling of badgers to control TB in cattle has proved extremely controversial since it commenced in 1973. Concerns over badger welfare arose from the Ministry of Agriculture, Fisheries and Food (MAFF) policy of gassing setts with hydrogen cyanide, leading to a number of commissioned reports over the following decades, with no clear resolution as to how the scientific evidence should inform policy. The

Zuckermann review in 1980 recommended sampling of badgers in the vicinity of affected farms and culling at setts if badgers tested positive (74). In 1986 the Dunnet report questioned the efficacy and the cost sustainability of this "clean ring" strategy (75). The Krebs report concluded that though the evidence was indirect, badgers were a significant source of infection in cattle and recommended an experimental trial to quantify the impact of badger culling on cattle TB (76). The Randomized Badger Culling Trial (RBCT) was carried out between 1998–2006 with the objectives to generate scientific evidence for the role of badgers in cattle TB, and to help formulate appropriate policy measures. However, it ended up highly divisive and the legacy of the trial continues today. Cassidy (77) argues that the design, scale and complexity of the trial, including ongoing disruption by anti-cull protesters made it extremely difficult to generate a strong evidence base that might have otherwise been gathered in more conventional small case controlled studies. The trial area consisted of 10 sets of "triplets" areas, each containing a proactive-culling area, a reactive-culling area with culling only in response to a cattle TB cattle breakdown and a survey-only area where no culling was conducted. The trial results showed that the incidence of bovine TB in cattle dropped by 19% in the proactive-culling area. However, the proactive culling was also associated with a 29% increase in cattle TB in the area outside the culling zone (62, 78). The increase in cattle TB outside of the culling area was attributed to the "perturbation" effect, where the social behavior of badgers was altered by the culling activities, leading to increased interactions and transmission rates to cattle in the area outside of the badgers normal territories (78, 79). Reactive culling was abandoned early in the trial as it was believed to increase, rather than decrease, the incidence of TB in cattle in these areas.

Since its completion, the conclusions of the RBCT have been disputed and the data re-interpreted many times. In its final report, the government appointed Independent Science Group (ISG), which oversaw the trial, concluded that "badger culling can make no meaningful contribution to cattle TB control in Britain" (78). This viewpoint was somewhat contradicted by the (also-) government commissioned follow-up King review which found that badger culling "could make a significant contribution to the control of cattle TB in those areas of England where there is a high and persistent incidence of TB in cattle, provided removal takes places alongside an effective programme of cattle controls" (80). Cassidy (77) points out that the ISG took a broad perspective to their remit and combined analysis and policy issues to reach their conclusions, whereas the King review restricted the focus to the scientific evidence, without taking account of policy considerations and animal welfare concerns. The situation has not been helped by the perceived inability of successive governments to formulate a long-term policy that balances the pros and cons of the moral arguments used by stakeholders. Changes in the UK government over the years has lead to major policy shifts on badger control measures, further emphasizing the inability of government stakeholders to implement evidence based policies while taking account of the viewpoints of interested parties (53, 77). The Labor government of 2006–2010 accepted the findings of the ISG and resisted pressure from the Nation Farmers Union (NFU) and

the British Veterinary Association (BVA) to endorse culling. The Conservative—Liberal Democrats coalition government (2010–2015) changed policy and agreed to introduce culling on a limited scale. While the majority of politicians and many stakeholder groups recognized the role that badgers played in the epidemiology of TB in cattle, there was less agreement on the strength of the RBCT scientific evidence and also the economics and ethics of large scale culling. Pilot culls commenced in Somerset and Gloucestershire in 2013 attracting major opposition from a large cross section of community groups and organizations. When it was reported that the trials failed to meet the pre-determined limits of humaneness and efficacy, this served only to galvanize opposition that demanded a cessation of culling. The effectiveness of the culling operations was also questioned and despite all of the confounders associated with the design (e.g., failure to achieve reduction of targeted population, differences in levels of implementation), it appeared that badger culling was associated with a reduction in cattle TB incidence (81). As cattle TB rates continued to climb in the UK, the Conservative government in 2015, although fully attuned to the unpopularity of culling, expanded the culling areas to placate the demands of the farming industry. Elsewhere, contrasting policies operated in other parts of the UK experiencing problems with cattle TB. The Assembly in Wales has resisted a badger culling policy but instead has increased the range of cattle control measures and focused on vaccination of badgers (82). In Northern Ireland the local Assembly agreed to a badger Test, Vaccinate and Release (TVR) trial to gauge the effectiveness of this approach on cattle TB rates. The strategy involves capturing live badgers in an area with a high level of cattle TB, testing the badgers for TB, vaccinating those that test negative to the disease and removing those that test positive (83). A survey of farmers attitudes to TB control strategies in Northern Ireland revealed a willingness to allow vaccination and culling of badgers on their land with an overall preference for vaccination, and less concern about public opposition (84).

The multi-dimensional aspects and complexity of the evolution of cattle TB policy in the UK raises many questions on the ethics and value systems of stakeholders in the context of culling of badgers. The role of the media is of key importance in framing the viewpoints of many of the principal actors (85). Where there is difficulty in understanding the complexity of the scientific evidence, the press can influence perspectives by over-simplifying the arguments for or against a particular strategy e.g., culling or vaccination, and this can help to fuel the controversies. This can lead to poorly thought out policy decisions, which may reinforce perceptions of mismanagement. Surveys of farmers in new endemic TB areas in the UK have revealed a fatalistic attitude to the problem, where many believed that bad luck played a role in herds contracting TB, but also mediated by perceptions of the political aspects of the disease and the lack of trust in government (86, 87). Similar perceptions were found in Northern Ireland where interviews with focus groups (cattle and beef farmers, private and state veterinarians) revealed differences in perceptions and knowledge of the disease among the different actors (88). It was concluded that a "one-size-fits-all" approach to control policy would be unlikely to succeed without recognizing the heterogeneities of many aspects of disease transmission and the multiple framings of the disease by different stakeholders.

McCulloch and Reiss have described the history and evolution of government policy toward control of TB in badgers in the UK (53). They argue that the debate can be distilled into two questions related to quantifying the role that badgers play in the epidemiology and whether the current control options are effective, practical (in controlling transmission) and socially acceptable? They conclude that policy should not be based exclusively on scientific evidence, economics or public opinion. Rather, they propose that the ethical issues need to be addressed by independent experts according to moral frameworks that question what is right, and what is justifiable, and taking into account the impact of policy on the morally affected stakeholders. McCulloch and Reiss separately analyse these frameworks from a utilitarian perspective (89). This approach strives to achieve a balance between the competing interests of stakeholders in order to achieve the greatest utility benefit for all. But it raises the question as to who are the greatest beneficiaries and how can one measure and quantify the utility benefit? In this context there is a generally perceived human benefit from farming arising mainly from production of high quality food leading to good public health. But there is also a strong societal benefit and positive value from maintaining undisturbed badger populations in their native habitats (25). Because of TB there are conflicting viewpoints on these utility benefits among stakeholders. McCulloch and Reiss argue that according to utilitarian theory, *"the slaughter of a cow or the culling of a badger with a life of net positive value will result in a loss of utility. All else being equal, the killing of a cow or badger that could be expected to continue with a life of net positive value is, therefore,* prima facie *morally wrong, simply because it reduces total utility"* They suggest that killing of badgers can be morally justifiable if it results in greater overall utility, e.g., the replacement of the (badger) utility by cattle, or an increase in human utility through improved farming economic benefits accruing from culling of badgers. They then pose the question as to how much culling of badgers is acceptable to justify the increased utility value of cattle? The contention from the ethics of utilitarianism is that the correct policy is one which produces overall highest utility. But this relies on an understanding of the consequences of the policy such that the impact of different policies can be objectively compared and measured. Their analysis concluded that non-culling approaches including badger vaccination policy options resulted in higher overall utility, and was superior to the badger culling option. In the absence of agreement among stakeholders, vaccination of badgers offers a utilitarian solution, and is now considered as a strategy that can address many of the negative issues associated with culling (90).

WILDLIFE TB IN SPAIN AND FRANCE

In continental western Europe, Spain is considered to have a complex epidemiology of TB involving multiple mycobacterium species, animal species and several maintenance hosts including cattle, deer and wild boar (91). Domestic goats, sheep and free-ranging domestic pigs are also implicated in the transmission cycle and often share common pasture land with cattle (92–94). Infections with *Mycobacterium caprae* is common in goats and has been known to spill over to cattle (92). Badgers have also been shown to be infected with *M. bovis* though the impact on livestock is unclear and may differ according to the region (95). For example, badger numbers are more abundant in the cooler Atlantic influenced regions in the north of the country where molecular typing of *M. bovis* strains has shown that they are common to badgers and cattle (96). In the southern mediterranean region of Spain wild boar are believed to be maintenance reservoirs of infection (97). These animals are well-adapted to the seasonal variability in food and water sources, and their mobility and scavenging on infected carrion (e.g., deer) likely influences the pathogenesis of disease which is frequently associated with head, pulmonary and disseminated TB lesions (97). Wild boar are considered as a significant risk factor for TB breakdowns in cattle (98), likely resulting from indirect contact (99).

High densities of wild boar are often maintained by artificial feeding to support a vibrant hunting industry, typically in fenced game estates many of which also house deer, cattle, sheep and pigs in free ranging systems (100). During the hot season experienced in southern regions of Spain, wild boar and other wild species congregate at high densities at watering holes increasing contact rates and the probability of both transmission within and across species (101). Surveys of *M. bovis* prevalence in Doñana National Park (DNP) in southern Spain have revealed prevalences of 52% in wild boar, 27% in red deer and 18.0 % in fallow deer (102). In areas where cattle are absent, prevalences have reached 92% in wild boar (102). The congregation of boar at feeding sites is associated with the high risk of tuberculosis in deer (103). The DNP is also one of the last refuges of the critically endangered Iberian lynx (*Lynx pardinus*), which along with foxes (*Vulpes vulpes*) are considered as spill over hosts (104, 105). In comparison, the prevalence of TB in wild boar in the Atlantic influenced habitats of Northern Spain is significantly lower when compared with the mediterranean habitats (96). This is likely due to lower densities in the northern regions, lower levels of artificial management, less congregation at water holes; all of these factors impacting on infection transmission rates.

As in many other European countries TB eradication in Spain was initially driven by the high prevalence of disease in cattle. When research revealed a multi-host epidemiology of disease, this brought additional stakeholders, including government, hunting lobbies, agricultural industry, and conservationists into the discussion on how best to manage the problem. Culling of wild boar has been shown to be an effective and strategic measure to reduce prevalence, and with the added likely benefit of a decrease in transmission to other species (106). However, culling of animals has also caused conflict among stakeholders while policy makers have attempted to balance the competing interests of hunters, producers, and conservationists. The principal reason is because the hunting estates require managed high densities of animals to maximize commercial returns and hunting groups are resistant to widescale culling (107).

Research has continued in Spain to monitor changes in the occurrence of TB and to unravel the complexities of the epidemiology with a long term view to measure the impact of interventions that may reduce transmission rates among all affected species (108). A questionnaire survey was carried out among key stakeholders (veterinarians, livestock owners and farmers) in south central Spain to gauge their opinions on specific intervention strategies chosen by a panel of experts that included veterinarians engaged in research into wildlife and disease management in the study area (20). Although banning of supplementary feeding of wildlife on cattle farms was ranked by the experts as the most effective control option, this opinion was not shared by hunters and farmers as a practical measure. Overall, hunters and farmers showed the highest levels of agreement for the top-ranked interventions (ban on supplementary feeding, restricting access to waterholes, increased frequency of cattle testing, removal of discarded offal from hunting land) while hunters and veterinarians agreed least. This study highlighted the diverse attitudes of different stakeholders to a range of intervention strategies and probably reflected differences in opinion on the broader epidemiological picture. The opinions of farmers and hunters were more aligned because of their converged interests in the same parcels of land required for their activities, whereas the perspectives of veterinarians were primarily guided by principles of disease management while trying to balance the interests of all stakeholders including policy makers (20).

France was declared officially TB free in 2000, but since then sporadic outbreaks of TB in cattle have continued in a number of regions in the south-west and east of the country (109, 110). TB was also first identified in wild red deer in the northern Normandy region of France in 2001. By 2006, prevalence rates remained high in deer (24%) and wild boar (42%) despite culling of these animals to reduce densities (111). TB infection was subsequently diagnosed in badgers in the areas most affected by TB in cattle (112). Arising from increased concerns over broader wildlife involvement in cattle TB outbreaks (TB in wildlife occuring in areas with cattle TB), the French General Directorate for Food (DGAL) and institutions involved in animal health and wildlife management established a national surveillance system "Sylvatub" in 2011 (113). This serves to co-ordinate the activities to detect and monitor TB in wildlife, and involves a wide range of national and local stakeholders including hunting and wildlife agencies, cattle breeders, pest controllers, trapper associations, veterinary associations and public administrators. The objective is to develop a broad national understanding of the risks associated with TB in wildlife allowing for the design and implementation of control strategies. An evaluation of stakeholder perceptions of the Sylvatub has revealed overall satisfaction with the system, the utility of helping farmers being the primary motivating factor (114). The improved understanding of TB epidemiology was also cited as a motivating factor for participation. Disincentives to participation included practical difficulties, regulatory hurdles, time-consuming activities, economic and material constraints.

The results of this evaluation appear to feed into the same stakeholder narrative in other countries experiencing wildlife TB problems, in spite of a low impact on TB rates in cattle.

TB IN WILDLIFE IN USA

The success of TB control in a wildlife species can crucially depend on the support or otherwise of individual or groups of stakeholders. In the USA white-tailed deer (*Odocoileus virginianus*) are the principal wildlife maintenance hosts implicated in transmission of TB to livestock in Michigan and Minnesota (115). Although there have been significant differences between the two states in the prevalence of TB in deer and the size of areas containing infected deer, the responses to the disease have been contrasted by temporal, social, economic, and logistical factors.

The US National Bovine TB Eradication Program was launched in 1917 following years of often fractious debate on the merits of different control options based around meat inspection and the recently developed tuberculin skin test (8, 15). Pasteurization of milk for human consumption had commenced almost a decade earlier in Chicago and New York, and other major cities, to reduce the risks associated with zoonotic TB and other diseases. Stringent application of the test and slaughter control measures lead to rapid success in controlling the disease and by 1940 prevalence was reduced to <0.5% in every state (116). Prevalence in livestock was recorded as 0.003% in 1994. Between 2001 and 2011, 92 US cattle herds were diagnosed as TB infected and several constraints to eradication were identified including changed management practices, importation of infected animals and the emergence of the disease in cervid species, particularly wild white-tailed deer in Michigan and Minnesota (116).

The disease was first reported in wild deer in Michigan in 1975 and was considered an isolated event (117). In 1994 it was detected again in a hunter shot deer close to the original case, providing for early but inconclusive evidence of a possible wildlife reservoir. It was the impetus for the state to initiate a TB control programme targeted at wildlife and farmed deer. In 1995 after the first year of systematic wildlife surveillance, 4.9% of deer sampled were culture positive for *M. bovis* in the core outbreak area (~1,500 km^2) (118). With the disease eradication plan underway, addressing both the deer and the cattle populations, there was resistance mounted by some of the large number of stakeholders, with no universal acceptance for the proposed control measures (119). While there was overall support among deer hunters, livestock producers and agricultural business for the eradication of TB, there were differences in the knowledge and perceptions of the threats of TB, leading to a lack of support for eradication measures (120). As a major stakeholder, the hunting industry did not consider that the extent of the disease problem warranted reduction of deer numbers in the infected areas, and they were opposed to the banning of supplemental feeding and baiting which had helped to increase deer densities. From an epidemiological perspective, this provided opportunities for contact between infected and susceptible animals either by direct contact or contamination of food (121, 122). Agricultural producers relying on crop production for sale of feed to the hunters also considered the measures as a threat to their business. Among livestock producers, including those with most to lose from the TB outbreaks, only 57% supported further reductions in deer numbers. These differences in values among the key stakeholders and problems with compliance constrained the ongoing control efforts and TB in cattle and wildlife (123, 124) and TB breakdowns in cattle continued, preventing the state from regaining its former TB free status. Between 1994 and 2010 there were however only 50 cattle farms positive for TB, and of those within the TB core area the most likely source of infection for the herd was wildlife. The majority of TB infections in other wildlife including coyotes (*Canis latrans*), racoons (*Procyon lotor*), red fox (*Vulpes vulpes*), bobcat (*Felis rufus*) and black bear (*Ursus americanus*) have been found in the northern portion of the Michigan's Lower Peninsula which contains the core area and probably amounts to them being spillover hosts (125). The full state of Michigan has still not regained its TB free status from the USDA (123).

When TB was detected in white-tailed deer and cattle in Minnesota in 2005 there was a rapid and aggressive response (119). The control of TB was framed by implementation of a strong management programme by the Minnesota Department of Natural Resources. The outbreak was confined to a small area of <425 km^2. By 2011 only 12 beef cattle herds and 27 white-tailed deer had been diagnosed with TB. The result of studies to investigate the factors associated with deer-cattle transmission had implicated deer visits and damage to stored cattle feed as a major risk factor (123). The decision was made to eradicate infection from both the cattle and deer populations by culling both species and this inevitably placed an economic burden on both the cattle industry and recreational deer hunters. A new deer management unit was created that allowed for additional hunting opportunities. Private landowners were issued with shooting permits to remove an unlimited number of deer on their lands, with the proviso that samples were submitted for TB-testing and the carcasses used for venison, thus avoiding wastage. A recreational feeding ban for deer and elk was put in place in 2006 in the TB endemic areas and monitored by enforcement officers. The plan was highly successful in reducing the prevalence of TB and by 2011, there were no recorded cases of TB in deer or cattle in Minnesota (119). As a result the state re-gained its TB free status from the USDA (119).

Although the key stakeholder groups in Michigan and Minnesota were similar and likely motivated by the same concerns, the outcomes of the TB eradication programmes in each state were markedly different. There are a number of factors that may have contributed to the divergent outcomes. The control efforts in Minnesota benefited from the issues revealed from the interventions of the Michigan campaign. With the disease emerging much later in Minnesota there was political pressure to quickly stamp out the disease before it became endemic. Thus, control measures were implemented much earlier after discovery of the outbreak in Minnesota, whereas the disease was present for at least 20 years before control measures were applied in

Michigan. Although there was some resistance to deer culling from hunters in Minnesota there was also the realization that TB eradication in the short term was beneficial to the industry in the long term. The demands for strong action from the cattle industry also made it easier for politicians to implement aggressive actions.

Carstensen et al. describe a combination factors that may have contributed to the different levels of stakeholder acceptance in both states and the more aggressive response in Minnesota (119). They highlight that the core area of the TB outbreak in Minnesota was 29% of that in Michigan. Also, the terrain topography and the substantially higher proportion of publicly owned land in Minnesota facilitated access for shooting of deer. Use of helicopters for aerial shooting to remove deer was controversial, though strong engagement with all stakeholders through public meetings helped to alleviate concerns. While baiting and feeding of deer were illegal in the core outbreak areas of both Michigan and Minnesota, baiting was illegal in Minnesota more than a decade prior to the finding of TB in cattle or free-ranging deer. The land ownership in Michigan's core area comprised 90% private land, including hunting areas, making it difficult to enforce compliance with the law. The number of farms in the affected area of Minnesota was twice that of Michigan's core area, helping to increase the political clout of the cattle industry in Minnesota. A buy out program was available to cattle producers in Minnesota's TB outbreak area to help reduce the cattle population at risk. A high proportion of eligible farms accepted the buy-out, and ~6,200 cattle were removed from the TB affected area. A similar buy out was not facilitated in Michigan. What these factors illustrate is how differences in the value systems of the same stakeholders in each state affected the outcome of the disease eradication measures. From a value systems perspective the utility value of the deer in Michigan was given a higher overall nominal score because of the powerful hunting lobby, whereas, in Minnesota the concerns of the agricultural lobby trumped the hunting industry allowing the state officials to implement a much more forceful control plan.

WILDLIFE TB IN AFRICA

The number of wild animal species involved in the highly complex epidemiology of TB in South Africa poses particular challenges for identifying and engaging with stakeholders in order to seek broad consensus on control strategies (126). The African continent is home to a vast and diverse range of indigenous wild mammals, many, if not most, of which it can be assumed are susceptible to infection with TB (127). Given the lack of any reliable hard data, it is not known with certainty if the disease was originally introduced by human activities or if it always had a presence in wildlife at some level, with the open and expansive landscape facilitating interactions and new incidents of infection across multiple species (128). The advent of molecular typing of strains isolated from cattle has revealed the presence of three geographically distinct *M. bovis* clonal complexes in Africa, the African Af1 complex dominant in sub-Saharan West-central Africa (Mali, Cameroon, Chad and Nigeria), African Af2 found in East Africa (Uganda, Burundi, Tanzania and Ethiopia) and

European Eu1 complex in South Africa (129–131). The presence of the Eu1 strain is associated with the arrival of the Dutch and British colonial settlers in South Africa with TB infected cattle, and represented a significant event in the emergence and spread of TB among native animals.

TB was first identified in cattle in South Africa in the late nineteenth century, and in indigenous kudu (*Tragelaphus strepsiceros*) in 1928 (127). In the following decades the disease was diagnosed in an increasing number of wildlife species including duiker (*Sylvicapra grimmia*), and springbok (*Antidorcas marsupilias*). More recently research has focused on the Hluhluwe-iMfolozi Park (960 km^2) and Kruger National Park (19,485 km^2) where it is believed that TB was transmitted to the African buffalo (*Syncerus caffer*) from domestic cattle in the 1950s (132). Among the many wildlife species affected the buffalo is considered to be the principal maintenance reservoir of infection, although kudu also appear to maintain the infection (132–134). By 1995, the disease had spread northwards from the southern part of the Kruger and since then has affected many different animal species including lion (*Panthera leo*), cheetah (*Acinonyx jubatus*), kudu, leopard (*Panthera pardus*), chacma baboon (*Papio ursinus*) (135–137), black rhinoceros (*Diceros bicornis*) (138, 139) and white rhinoceros (*Ceratotherium simum*) (140). There was also evidence of spillover to neighboring livestock (141). Molecular strain typing has shown that the infection had spread by clonal expansion of the Eu1 strain type and spread to game farms and reserves in Mpumalanga, Limpopo, KwaZulu-Natal, Free State and North West Provinces, affecting at least 16 different animal species (142).

In South Africa a voluntary test and slaughter scheme for cattle was initiated in 1969, and by 1991 had reduced the disease prevalence to 0.04%. However, primarily due to financial and resource reasons this level of success was not sustained, and the disease levels increased thereafter (132).

There is only limited basic epidemiology known for most African wild mammal species other than buffalo (143). As the disease became established in maintenance hosts it was inevitable that the infection transmitted to predator species, including lions, hyena (*Crocuta crocuta*), leopard and cheetah, and a range of scavengers and omnivores (142). These, as with other predators, are probably spillover hosts where the infection is unlikely to be sustained in the absence of external sources of infection. The pattern of generalized TB in the prey species (including buffalo and antelope species) increases the likelihood of transmission following ingestion of infected organs and tissues.

In South Africa, all aspects of wildlife have provided lucrative business opportunities with increased global interest in ecotourism, trade in wild animals and conservation (132). The number of wildlife has increased considerably in South Africa in recent years, both in national parks and private game reserves. Iconic African wildlife species are exported worldwide to zoos for conservation and can attract very high purchase fees (139). In the absence of any reliable ante-mortem diagnostic tests for TB this poses great challenges to controlling spread of infection when animals are translocated to reserves within Africa or exported worldwide. There are many recorded examples of tuberculosis in rhinoceros housed in zoos going back over 100 years yet in that time there have been relatively few advances in development of sensitive diagnostic tests other than relying on observation and clinical symptoms (139). The finding in the Kruger National Park of an infected free-ranging black rhinoceros (138) and in the white rhinoceros (140), species recognized as critically endangered and near threatened by the International Union for Conservation of Nature, has serious implications for the conservation measures for rhinoceroses, and movement out of the Park for breeding and conservation reasons.

With the expanding range of African animals infected with TB, it is difficult for programme managers to deal with the problem given the enormous costs involved, notwithstanding the paucity of epidemiological information available for single species let alone unraveling the complexities of the infection in multi-species hosts (132, 144). The deficiency in the epidemiology of the multi-host system prevents any single proposed programme from claiming precedence. In South Africa control of animal diseases is regulated by the Department of Agriculture, Forestry and Fisheries (DAFF) though there are many local, national and international stakeholders involved, including ecologists, veterinarians, conservationists, animal rehabilitation centers, ecotourism companies, game capture operations, national and provincial parks, hunting companies, the cattle industry, wildlife ranching etc. Given the diverse range of the interest groups, there is likely to be as many conflicting opinions on how to manage the problems. For example, although TB is endemic in many buffalo populations, it does not appear to be detrimental to their population structure, nor are TB test positive buffalo more likely to be subjected to predation by lions (145). This may lead to opposing viewpoints from those groups who believe the presence of TB has minimal ecological impact and, for example, veterinarians motivated to eradicate disease. Spillover of disease to high value predators does raise concerns from many additional stakeholders. It is unlikely that TB can now be eradicated from the community of affected species by current available methods and policies are likely to be framed around management of the disease to minimize spread. Test and slaughter programmes, if available, may serve to decrease local prevalence but are unlikely to achieve eradication. Resources may be focused on species of highest monetary or conservation value, thus providing short to mid range economic benefit but achieving little in the context of eradication of the disease from free-living animals. Vaccination may provide a potential solution in the future, however it would need to be cost-effective, and any chance of success will also require many additional studies to improve epidemiological knowledge and understand how control measures directed at one or more species affects the dynamics of disease in multi-host systems (146).

VACCINATION OF WILDLIFE AGAINST TB

Where culling of animals is not considered a feasible option (for whatever reason) as a disease management tool, vaccination of wild animals against TB is often promoted as an alternative strategy, primarily because it provides for a non-destructive approach to controlling disease and addresses animal welfare concerns, as well as conservation concerns arising from deliberate killing of wild animals (147, 148). The purpose of vaccination is to reduce the incidence of infection leading to lower levels of intra-species spread of infection, as well as transmission to other wild species and livestock (149). By reaching and maintaining a threshold level of coverage the vaccine will also confer protection to the non-vaccinated proportion of the population through the generation of herd immunity. Over time, and with an effective vaccine, the disease will eventually disappear from the vaccinated population. The BCG vaccine, used extensively in humans, has been shown to work in a variety of animal species (147, 150, 151), and more recently an alternative heat inactivated *M. bovis* (HIMB) vaccine candidate has shown some promise in a range of species (152–154). These vaccines can be delivered by injection or oral bait. BCG is a live vaccine and a single dose can provide a long duration of protection against natural exposure to infection (155).

In deciding on the appropriate control strategies to employ, the desired outcome needs to be carefully considered in order to avoid further conflict among stakeholders. For example, vaccination of badgers may address conservation concerns arising from culling a protected species, with the added benefit of protecting cattle from badger—cattle transmission. However, the time frames to achieve eradication will be much longer when compared with culling (156). Studies of UK farmers' perceptions of vaccination as a means to control TB have also revealed cautious attitudes to this strategy (157). It has been noted that the media paid more attention to vaccination when the controversies over culling escalated (85), and wildlife groups have heavily promoted the vaccine strategy. While there is good field data to show that the vaccine can protect badgers in their natural environment, the scientific evidence of a direct link between badger vaccination and time scales for a positive impact in reducing TB breakdowns in cattle is lacking. This serves to reduce farmers' confidence in vaccination, which in part reflects their lack of trust in the ability of government to control the disease (86). There is also a viewpoint among farmers of over-population of badgers that is consistent with a preference for culling of badgers above vaccination (158). If farmers believe that there is little that can be done to control the disease, a vaccination strategy is also unlikely to alleviate such concerns. Elsewhere, BCG vaccination may be of use in countries without established control or eradication programmes where testing and slaughter of reactor cattle is not practiced or considered acceptable for economic, social or religious reasons.

DISCUSSION

The eradication of TB from animals has faced many challenges since studies commenced in cattle, when in the early 1890s Koch's old tuberculin was found to be useful as a diagnostic tool for TB (159). Along with pasteurization of milk and slaughter of infected animals, these measures would eventually herald a new age where the impact of zoonotic TB was effectively controlled. From today's perspective it seems extraordinary to consider

that stakeholders did not universally welcome these approaches as a potential panacea to reduce the burden of infection in humans. To understand this we must take account of some of the value systems that underpinned opposition to the policy at the time. In the US, which launched its TB eradication program in 1917, when TB was causing greater morbidity and mortality among cattle than all other diseases, there was often complacency and resistance to mass tuberculin testing of animals (8, 15). The TB problem was seen as wholly intractable and any broad scale measures would result in unacceptable economic losses. At that time there was also considerable resistance, particularly in the UK, from the dairy industry to any government imposed interventions that would increase production costs and where the benefits were largely unproven (10). During this period it was primarily veterinarians who supported the campaign of compulsory inspection, animal slaughter, pasteurization, and any other measures that might help to eradicate the disease (10). However, there were also many in the profession whose livelihoods depended on the custom of farmers and were opposed to some of the proposed measures. Given the high burden of disease in cattle there was also the view among interested parties that mass screening and slaughter of infected animals would decimate the dairy industry (10). The historical record highlights the different perspectives of stakeholders in dealing with a serious zoonotic disease, which in the end only succeeded in stalling progress to reduce the incidence of zoonotic TB. The emergence of the discipline of epidemiology in the past fifty years has increased our understanding of many of the risk factors associated with TB in cattle and wildlife, but it has also generated and molded the viewpoints of many different stakeholders. There is now better knowledge of wildlife sources of TB infection that are implicated in the transmission cycle of disease to cattle. It might be logical to conclude therefore, that the improved scientific knowledge base should lead to more rational and manageable control options. However, where these affected wildlife species have a high societal value, it has created a new set of stakeholders with often conflicting perspectives that is redolent of the antagonism among interested parties in the early twentieth century. Zoonotic TB may no longer be the potent driver for disease control that it was in previous decades. Instead, the rationale for TB eradication is now driven mainly by economic, trade, animal rights and conservation concerns (18, 132, 160). Each of these drivers brings elements of different moral frameworks and ethical perspectives, which sometimes clash because of the difficulties and uncertainties associated with control of the disease.

The examples of TB management in the different countries portray a range of single and multi-host wild animal systems implicated in the transmission cycle of TB that involves livestock. In most cases epidemiological investigations have helped reveal the reservoir status (maintenance or spillover) of many of the species involved, and this has informed the type of control measure applied (14, 161). How policy makers decide on the appropriate intervention strategies to address each concern is extremely difficult, but it must, by necessity, take account of the stakeholder perspectives in the local environment where the disease is proving problematic to eradicate (46). In New Zealand, for example, the economic impact of TB transmission from possums to cattle has been reduced significantly in recent years. Nevertheless, there is broad acceptance for continued culling of possums given their perceived status as an environmental pest species. Although there has been disquiet about the widespread use of sodium fluoroacetate (1080) in the environment (49), studies have shown high societal value placed on the conservation co-benefits as a result of culling (48). Adopting the rationale of McCulloch and Reiss (89), there is measurable net utility benefit to New Zealand biodiversity, ecology and agriculture arising from culling of possums, which validates the utilitarian approach to solve the problem.

In contrast, the culling of badgers in the UK is not short of controversy and reflects the polarized perspectives and viewpoints of the principal stakeholders. These would include the dairy and beef cattle industries and associated beneficiaries on one hand, and conservationists, animal rights groups and environmentalists on the other (53). The broad middle ground of opinion may be influenced by arguments from either side. All would agree that eradication of TB is a desirable goal though they might disagree on where the control programme should be focused. The issue at hand is how TB control is best achieved and what strategies are likely to be most effective (162). Despite being a protected species in the Republic of Ireland and the UK, the culling of badgers in order to reduce densities as a means of minimizing transmission to cattle has been central to the wildlife disease control programmes (72). This is justified by the positive outcomes achieved in New Zealand following culling of possums (14). Nevertheless, in the UK this has not detracted from the determination of opponents of the current policy to resist expansion of culling areas and to advocate for complete cessation of culling (53). It appears that there is a broad range of complex evidential and ethical perspectives at play among the principal actors. Arising from the RBCT, there are continued debates as to whether reactive or pro-active culling is the most effective strategy (163, 164). It is argued by some that the scientific evidence is not sufficiently strong to warrant culling policies (165). Others adopt a moral framework based on animal health and welfare (i.e., the moral harm from culling wild animals is inconsistent with empathy, compassion or benevolence) concluding that it is fundamentally unethical and inhumane to indiscriminately kill a protected wild species that is an integral part of the natural countryside (166). The impact of culling badgers on other animals also comes into play: opportunistic analysis associated with the RBCT has shown that population counts of hedgehogs doubled over a 5-year period from the start of cull, demonstrating potential ecological consequences of badger culling and the direct impact it has on other animal species (167). These viewpoints reflect the different moral and ethical frameworks underpinning the diverse range of opinions. According to Cassidy, the societal values and cultural framing of the badger in the UK as being "good" or "bad" is at the root of the polarized opinions on how to deal with the TB problem (168). In her essay she traces the conflict as far back as the sixteenth century when badgers were listed in the Tudor Vermin Act among animals believed to interfere with human activity, and attracted a bounty per head killed. The notion

of badgers being a positive cultural iconic wildlife species was promulgated in early twentieth century literature, particularly through the influence of stories such as "The Wind in the Willows" (169), notwithstanding the social attitudes that lead to ambivalence over cruel practices such as badger baiting, which took place widely over many decades until recently.

The current arguments for and against culling of badgers in the UK broadly align with the opposing framings of the badger and the societal values assigned to the badger by either side of the debate (53, 168). On the one hand they play a defining role in the perceptions of a healthy natural countryside, while on the other they pose a serious economic threat to the cattle industry by virtue of their TB status. The approach of McCulloch and Reiss is of relevance here in that by comparing the consequential outcomes of different control strategies e.g., culling vs. vaccination, it does allow for a measurable impact of different policies (89). They propose that policy decisions affecting sentient animals be subject to a mandatory Animal Welfare Impact Assessment (AWIA) based on the arguments that (a) sentient animals are owed moral considerations, (b) there is public concern about how policy impacts on the welfare of animals, and (c) international treaties pay full regard to animal welfare (170). The desired endpoint is an overall policy that defines the greatest level of benefit (who benefits and by how much?) while accounting for the different moral frameworks that fuel the disputes. It is of interest to note that the level of acrimony between opposing sides appears to be much greater in England compared with Wales, Northern Ireland and the Republic of Ireland. Although there are no comparable sociological studies, it has been suggested that the controversies in England reflect in some part the traditional different attitudes to the countryside between urbanized and rural societies (168). Ireland has historically been a largely agrarian society with few large urban centers (compared to UK), and this may have informed attitudes to the badgers and to their place in the countryside. This makes it relatively less problematic to generate policies with clearly identifiable beneficiaries.

Some stakeholders have questioned the cost-benefit of continued costly surveillance of TB given that milk pasteurization is highly effective at killing *M. bovis*, and the risk of infection from infected meat is negligible (160). While the case may have merit from the viewpoint of agricultural economics, it does represent a narrow perspective on public spending on an animal health issue. Engaging the opinions of other stakeholders, as we have asserted, serves to broaden the arguments for continued surveillance. Many countries have successfully eradicated TB and there is a societal benefit to having disease-free cattle. In other parts of the developing world, pasteurization of milk or meat inspection is not routine and *M. bovis* in unpasteurized milk poses a zoonotic risk to consumers (171, 172). If developed countries are not seen to lead the way in progressing toward eradication this might dis-incentivize others to follow similar pathways.

We have shown here that the level of engagement and ethical perspectives of stakeholders can change when wildlife disease management becomes part of an eradication programme (46). One of the major problems for policy makers is identifying the main beneficiaries of any programme, simply because there are so many worthy candidates. In recent years, and driven by the need to better understand the disease, there have been many studies reporting new TB diagnostic tests for a variety of high value animal species (173–182). Knowledge of the extent of the disease in these animals is the first step in addressing the problem, which may prove to be very costly. The control of animal TB needs also to be considered in the context of the OIE "One health" strategy to control zoonotic diseases (183). This will require increased cooperation and communication between an expanded range of stakeholders engaged in human and animal health, the industry sector, conservation, ecologists, educators, farmers, and interested public etc. Reaching agreement on a common and standardized value system for animals may be extremely challenging, but it could represent a first step in devising solutions for TB that are realistic and achievable.

AUTHOR CONTRIBUTIONS

EG and LC contributed equally to this review including critical analysis of published data and preparation of the manuscript. The opinions expressed in this paper are solely those of the authors.

ACKNOWLEDGMENTS

We would like to acknowledge funding and support provided by the Department of Agriculture, Food & the Marine Food (DAFM) for all of the badger studies in Ireland. We are very grateful for constructive discussions with Paul Livingstone (NZ), Ana Balseiro (Spain), Sven Parsons (SA), Dan O'Brien (USA) and Lin Marie De Klerk (SA), and for valuable insights into animal TB in their respective countries.

REFERENCES

1. Jones KE, Patel NG, Levy MA, Storeygard A, Balk D, Gittleman JL, et al. Global trends in emerging infectious diseases. *Nature* (2008) 451:990–3. doi: 10.1038/nature06536

2. McMahon BJ, Morand S, Gray JS. Ecosystem change and zoonoses in the Anthropocene. *Zoonoses Public Health* (2018) 65:755–65. doi: 10.1111/zph.12489

3. Jones BA, Grace D, Kock R, Alonso S, Rushton J, Said MY, et al. Zoonosis emergence linked to agricultural intensification and environmental change. *Proc Natl Acad Sci USA.* (2013) 110:8399–404. doi: 10.1073/pnas.1208 059110

4. Kaneene JB, Miller R, Steele JH, Thoen CO. Preventing and controlling zoonotic tuberculosis: a One Health approach. *Vet Ital.* (2014) 50:7–22. doi: 10.12834/VetIt.1302.08

5. O'Reilly LM, Daborn CJ. The epidemiology of *Mycobacterium bovis* infections in animals and man. *Tuber Lung Dis.* (1995) 76(Suppl. 1):1–46. doi: 10.1016/0962-8479(95)90591-X

6. Grange JM, Collins CH. Bovine tubercle bacilli and disease in animals and man. *Epidemiol Infect.* (1987) 99:221–34. doi: 10.1017/S0950268800 067686

7. Katale BZ, Mbugi EV, Kendal S, Fyumagwa RD, Kibiki GS, Godfrey-Faussett P, et al. Bovine tuberculosis at the human-livestock-wildlife interface: is it a public health problem in Tanzania? A review. *Onderstepoort J Vet Res.* (2012) 79:463. doi: 10.4102/ojvr.v7 9i2.463

8. Olmstead AL, Rhodes PW. An impossible undertaking: the eradication of bovine tuberculosis in the United States. *J Econ Hist.* (2004) 64:734–72. doi: 10.1017/S0022050704002955

9. Reynolds D. A review of tuberculosis science and policy in Great Britain. *Vet Microbiol.* (2006) 112:119–26. doi: 10.1016/j.vetmic.2005. 11.042

10. Atkins PJ. Lobbying and resistance with regard to policy on bovine tuberculosis in Britain 1900-1939: an inside/outside model. In: Condrau F, Worboys M, editors. *Tuberculosis Then and Now: Perspectives on the history of an Infectious Disease.* Montreal, QC: McGill-Queen's University Press (2010). 248 p.

11. Reviriego Gordejo FJ, Vermeersch JP. Towards eradication of bovine tuberculosis in the European Union. *Vet Microbiol.* (2006) 112:101–9. doi: 10.1016/j.vetmic.2005.11.034

12. Palmer MV, Thacker TC, Waters WR, Gortazar C, Corner LA. *Mycobacterium bovis*: a model pathogen at the interface of livestock, wildlife, and humans. *Vet Med Int.* (2012) 2012:236205. doi: 10.1155/2012/ 236205

13. Corner LA. The role of wild animal populations in the epidemiology of tuberculosis in domestic animals: how to assess the risk. *Vet Microbiol.* (2006) 112:303–12. doi: 10.1016/j.vetmic.2005.11.015

14. Livingstone PG, Hancox N, Nugent G, Mackereth G, Hutchings SA. Development of the New Zealand strategy for local eradication of tuberculosis from wildlife and livestock. *N Z Vet J.* (2015) 63(Suppl. 1):98–107. doi: 10.1080/00480169.2015.1013581

15. Palmer MV, Waters WR. Bovine tuberculosis and the establishment of an eradication program in the United States: role of veterinarians. *Vet Med Int.* (2011) 2011:816345. doi: 10.4061/2011/816345

16. Livingstone PG, Hancox N, Nugent G, de Lisle GW. Toward eradication: the effect of *Mycobacterium bovis* infection in wildlife on the evolution and future direction of bovine tuberculosis management in New Zealand. *N Z Vet J.* (2015) 63(Suppl. 1):4–18. doi: 10.1080/00480169.2014. 971082

17. Bernues A, Manrique E, Maza MT. Economic evaluation of bovine brucellosis and tuberculosis eradication programmes in a mountain area of Spain. *Prev Vet Med.* (1997) 30:137–49. doi: 10.1016/S0167-5877(96) 01103-8

18. Gordon SV. Bovine TB: stopping disease control would block all live exports. *Nature* (2008) 456:700. doi: 10.1038/456700b

19. Palmer MV. *Mycobacterium bovis*: characteristics of wildlife reservoir hosts. *Transbound Emerg Dis.* (2013) 60(Suppl. 1):1–13. doi: 10.1111/tbed. 12115

20. Cowie CE, Gortazar C, White PC, Hutchings MR, Vicente J. Stakeholder opinions on the practicality of management interventions to control bovine tuberculosis. *Vet J.* (2015) 204:179–85. doi: 10.1016/j.tvjl.2015. 02.022

21. Ryser-Degiorgis MP, Pewsner M, Angst C. Joining the dots - understanding the complex interplay between the values we place on wildlife, biodiversity conservation, human and animal health: a review. *Schweiz Arch Tierheilkd.* (2015) 157:243–53. doi: 10.17236/sat00018

22. Chardonnet P, des Clers B, Fischer J, Gerhold R, Jori F, Lamarque F. The value of wildlife. *Rev Sci Tech.* (2002) 21:15–51. doi: 10.20506/rst.21.1.1323

23. Hanneman WM. Valuing the environment through contingent valuation. *J Econ Perspect.* (1994) 8:19–43. doi: 10.1257/jep.8.4.19

24. Hanley N, Wright R, Adamowicz W. Using choice experiments to value the environment. . *Environ Resour Econ.* (1998) 11:413–28. doi: 10.1023/A:1008287310583

25. Bennet RM, Willis KG. Public values for badgers, bovine TB reduction and management strategies. *J Environ Plann Manag.* (2008) 51:511–23. doi: 10.1080/09640560802116996

26. Gamborg C, Palmer C, Sandoe P. Ethics of wildlife management and conservation: what should we try to protect? *Nat Educ Knowl.* (2012) 3:8.

27. Radunz B. Surveillance and risk management during the latter stages of eradication: experiences from Australia. *Vet Microbiol.* (2006) 112:283–90. doi: 10.1016/j.vetmic.2005.11.042

28. More SJ, Radunz B, Glanville RJ. Lessons learned during the successful eradication of bovine tuberculosis from Australia. *Vet Rec.* (2015) 177:224–32. doi: 10.1136/vr.103163

29. McInerney J, Small KJ, Caley P. Prevalence of *Mycobacterium bovis* infection in feral pigs in the Northern Territory. *Aust Vet J.* (1995) 72:448–51. doi: 10.1111/j.1751-0813.1995.tb03486.x

30. Corner LA, Barrett RH, Lepper AW, Lewis V, Pearson CW. A survey of mycobacteriosis of feral pigs in the Northern Territory. *Aust Vet J.* (1981) 57:537–42. doi: 10.1111/j.1751-0813.1981.tb00428.x

31. Cousins DV, Francis BR, Casey R, Mayberry C. *Mycobacterium bovis* infection in a goat. *Aust Vet J.* (1993) 70:262–3. doi: 10.1111/j.1751-0813.1993.tb08045.x

32. Robinson RC, Phillips PH, Stevens G, Storm PA. An outbreak of *Mycobacterium bovis* infection in fallow deer (*Dama dama*). *Aust Vet J.* (1989) 66:195–7. doi: 10.1111/j.1751-0813.1989.tb09806.x

33. Cousins DV, Roberts JL. Australia's campaign to eradicate bovine tuberculosis: the battle for freedom and beyond. *Tuberculosis* (2001) 81:5–15. doi: 10.1054/tube.2000.0261

34. McCool CJ, Newton-Tabrett DA. The route of infection in tuberculosis in feral buffalo. *Aust Vet J.* (1979) 55:401–2. doi: 10.1111/j.1751-0813.1979.tb15912.x

35. Hein WR, Tomasovic AA. An abattoir survey of tuberculosis in feral buffaloes. *Aust Vet J.* (1981) 57:543–7. doi: 10.1111/j.1751-0813.1981.tb00429.x

36. Cobb SM. Saltwater intrusion and mangrove encroachment of coastal wetlands in the alligator rivers region, Northern Territory, Australia. In: *Supervising Scientist for the Alligator Rivers R, Australia*. Supervising S, editor. Darwin, NT: Supervising Scientist (2007).

37. Turner A. Endemic disease control and regulation in Australia 1901-2010. *Aust Vet J.* (2011) 89:413–21. doi: 10.1111/j.1751-0813.2011.00811.x

38. Davidson RM. The role of the Opossum in spreading tuberculosis. *N Z J Agric.* (1976) 133:21–5.

39. Byrom AE, Caley P, Paterson BM, Nugent G. Feral ferrets (*Mustela furo*) as hosts and sentinels of tuberculosis in New Zealand. *N Z Vet J.* (2015) 63(Suppl. 1):42–53. doi: 10.1080/00480169.2014.981314

40. Nugent G, Gortazar C, Knowles G. The epidemiology of *Mycobacterium bovis* in wild deer and feral pigs and their roles in the establishment and spread of bovine tuberculosis in New Zealand wildlife. *N Z Vet J.* (2015) 63(Suppl. 1):54–67. doi: 10.1080/00480169.2014.963792

41. Nugent G, Buddle BM, Knowles G. Epidemiology and control of *Mycobacterium bovis* infection in brushtail possums (*Trichosurus vulpecula*), the primary wildlife host of bovine tuberculosis in New Zealand. *N Z Vet J.* (2015) 63(Suppl. 1):28–41. doi: 10.1080/00480169.2014.963791

42. Nugent G. Possum feeding patterns: dietary tactics of a reluctant folivore. In: Montague TL, editor. *The Brushtail Possum: Biology, Impact and Management of an Introduced Marsupial*. Lincoln: Manaaki Whenua Press (2000). p. 10–23.

43. Jackson R, Cooke MM, Coleman JD, Morris RS. Naturally occurring tuberculosis caused by *Mycobacterium bovis* in brushtail possums (*Trichosurus vulpecula*): I. An epidemiological analysis of lesion distribution. *N Z Vet J.* (1995):306–14. doi: 10.1080/00480169./1995.35911

44. Paterson BM, Morris RS, Weston J, Cowan PE. Foraging and denning patterns of brushtail possums, and their possible relationship to contact with cattle and the transmission of bovine tuberculosis. *N Z Vet J.* (1995) 43:281–8. doi: 10.1080/00480169./1995.35907

45. Paterson BM, Morris RS. Interactions between beef cattle and simulated tuberculous possums on pasture. *N Z Vet J.* (1995) 43:289–93. doi: 10.1080/00480169./1995.35908

46. Livingstone P, Hancox N. Managing bovine tuberculosis: successes and issues. In: Chambers M, Gordon S, Olea-Popelka F, and Barrow P, editors. *Bovine Tuberculosis*. CABI (2018). p. 225–47. doi: 10.1079/9781786391520.0225

47. Russell JC. A comparison of attitudes towards introduced wildlife in New Zealand in 1994 and 2012. *J R Soc N Z.* (2014) 44:136–51. doi: 10.1080/03036758.2014.944192

48. Tait P, Saunders C, Nugent G, Rutherford P. Valuing conservation benefits of disease control in wildlife: a choice experiment approach to bovine tuberculosis management in New Zealand's native forests. *J Environ Manag.* (2017) 189:142–9. doi: 10.1016/j.jenvman.2016.12.045

49. Green W, Rohan M. Opposition to aerial 1080 poisoning for control of invasive mammals in New Zealand: risk perceptions and agency responses. *J R Soc N Z.* (2012) 42:185–213. doi: 10.1080/03036758.2011.556130

50. Morgan D, Warburton B, Nugent G. Aerial prefeeding followed by ground based toxic baiting for more efficient and acceptable poisoning of invasive small mammalian pests. *PLoS ONE* (2015) 10:e0134032. doi: 10.1371/journal.pone.0134032

51. Caley P, Hickling GJ, Cowan PE, Pfeiffer DU. Effects of sustained control of brushtail possums on levels of *Mycobacterium bovis* infection in cattle and brushtail possum populations from Hokotaka, New Zealand. *N Z Vet J.* (1999) 47:133–42. doi: 10.1080/00480169.1999.36130

52. Nugent G, Whitford J, Yockney IJ, Cross ML. Reduced spillover transmission of *Mycobacterium bovis* to feral pigs (*Sus scofa*) following population control of brushtail possums (*Trichosurus vulpecula*). *Epidemiol Infect.* (2012) 140:1036–47. doi: 10.1017/S0950268811001579

53. McCulloch SP, Reiss MJ. Bovine tuberculosis and badger control in Britain: science, policy and politics. *J Agric Environ Ethics* (2017) 30:469–84. doi: 10.1007/s10806-017-9686-3

54. Muirhead RJ, Gallagher J, Burns KJ. Tuberculosis in wild badgers in Gloucestershire: epidemiology. *Vet Rec.* (1974) 95:552–5. doi: 10.1136/vr.95.24.552

55. Noonan NL, Sheane WD, Harper LR, J. RP. Wildlife as a possible reservoir of bovine tuberculosis. *Irish Vet J.* (1975) 29:1.

56. Abernethy DA, Denny GO, Menzies FD, McGuckian P, Honhold N, Roberts AR. The Northern Ireland programme for the control and eradication of *Mycobacterium bovis*. *Vet Microbiol.* (2006) 112:231–7. doi: 10.1016/j.vetmic.2005.11.023

57. More SJ, Good M. The tuberculosis eradication programme in Ireland: a review of scientific and policy advances since 1988. *Vet Microbiol.* (2006) 112:239–51. doi: 10.1016/j.vetmic.2005.11.022

58. Clifton-Hadley RS, Wilesmith JW, Richards MS, Upton P, Johnston S. The occurrence of *Mycobacterium bovis* infection in cattle in and around an area subject to extensive badger (*Meles meles*) control. *Epidemiol Infect.* (1995) 114:179–93. doi: 10.1017/S0950268800052031

59. O'Mairtin D, Williams DH, Griffin JM, L.A. D, Eves JA. The effect of a badger removal programme on the incidence of tuberculosis in an Irish cattle population. *Prev Vet Med.* (1998) 34:47–56.

60. Griffin JM, Williams DH, Kelly GE, Clegg TA, O'Boyle I, Collins JD, et al. The impact of badger removal on the control of tuberculosis in cattle herds in Ireland. *Prev Vet Med.* (2005) 67:237–66. doi: 10.1016/j.prevetmed.2004.10.009

61. Donnelly CA, Wei G, Johnston WT, Cox DR, Woodroffe R, Bourne FJ, et al. Impacts of widespread badger culling on cattle tuberculosis: concluding analyses from a large-scale field trial. *Int J Infect Dis.* (2007) 11:300–8. doi: 10.1016/j.ijid.2007.04.001

62. Donnelly CA, Woodroffe R, Cox DR, Bourne FJ, Cheeseman CL, Clifton-Hadley RS, et al. Positive and negative effects of widespread badger culling on tuberculosis in cattle. *Nature* (2006) 439:843–6. doi: 10.1038/nature04454

63. Eves JA. Impact of badger removal on bovine tuberculosis in east Co Offaly. *Irish Vet J.* (1999) 52:199–203.

64. Costello E, O'Grady D, Flynn O, O'Brien R, Rogers M, Quigley F, et al. Study of restriction fragment length polymorphism analysis and spoligotyping for epidemiological investigation of *Mycobacterium bovis* infection. *J Clin Microbiol.* (1999) 37:3217–22.

65. Biek R, O'Hare A, Wright D, Mallon T, McCormick C, Orton RJ, et al. Whole genome sequencing reveals local transmission patterns of *Mycobacterium bovis* in sympatric cattle and badger populations. *PLoS Pathog.* (2012) 8:e1003008. doi: 10.1371/journal.ppat.1003008

66. Corner LA, Murphy D, Gormley E. *Mycobacterium bovis* infection in the Eurasian badger (*Meles meles*): the disease, pathogenesis, epidemiology and control. *J Comp Pathol.* (2011) 144:1–24. doi: 10.1016/j.jcpa.2010.10.003

67. Corner LA, Costello E, Lesellier S, O'Meara D, Sleeman DP, Gormley E. Experimental tuberculosis in the European badger (*Meles meles*) after endobronchial inoculation of *Mycobacterium bovis*: I. Pathology

and bacteriology. *Res Vet Sci.* (2007) 83:53–62. doi: 10.1016/j.rvsc.2006.10.016

68. Corner LA, O'Meara D, Costello E, Lesellier S, Gormley E. The distribution of *Mycobacterium bovis* infection in naturally infected badgers. *Vet J.* (2012) 194:166–72. doi: 10.1016/j.tvjl.2012.03.013

69. More SJ, Houtsma E, Doyle L, McGrath G, Clegg TA, de la Rua-Domenech R, et al. Further description of bovine tuberculosis trends in the United Kingdom and the Republic of Ireland, 2003–2015. *Vet Rec.* (2018) 183:717. doi: 10.1136/vr.104718

70. More SJ, Good M. Understanding and managing bTB risk: perspectives from Ireland. *Vet Microbiol.* (2015) 176:209–18. doi: 10.1016/j.vetmic.2015.01.026

71. Olea-Popelka FJ, Fitzgerald P, White P, McGrath G, Collins JD, O'Keeffe J, et al. Targeted badger removal and the subsequent risk of bovine tuberculosis in cattle herds in county Laois, Ireland. *Prev Vet Med.* (2009) 88:178–84. doi: 10.1016/j.prevetmed.2008.09.008

72. Sheridan M, Good M, More SJ, Gormley E. The impact of an integrated wildlife and bovine tuberculosis eradication program in Ireland. In: Thoen CO, Steele JH, Kaneene JB, editors. *Zoonotic Tuberculosis: Mycobacterium bovis and Other Pathogenic Mycobacteria, 3rd Edn.* Wiley Blackwell (2014), p. 323–40. doi: 10.1002/9781118474310.ch28

73. Corner LA, Clegg TA, More SJ, Williams DH, O'Boyle I, Costello E, et al. The effect of varying levels of population control on the prevalence of tuberculosis in badgers in Ireland. *Res Vet Sci.* (2008) 85:238–49. doi: 10.1016/j.rvsc.2007.11.010

74. Zuckermann OM. *Badgers, Cattle and Tuberculosis.* London: HM Stationary Office (1980).

75. Dunnet GM, Jones DM, McInerney JP. *Badgers and Bovine Tuberculosis: Review of Policy.* London: HM Stationary Office (1986).

76. Krebs J, Anderson R, Clutton-Brock T, Morrison I, Young D, Donnelly C. *Bovine Tuberculosis in Cattle and Badgers - Report by the Independent Scientific Review Group.* Ministry of Agriculture, Fisheries and Food (1997).

77. Cassidy A. 'Big science' in the field: experimenting with badgers and bovine TB, 1995–2015. *Hist Philos Life Sci.* (2015) 37:305–25. doi: 10.1007/s40656-015-0072-z

78. Bourne FJ, Donnelly CA, Cox DR, Gettinby G, McInerney JP, Morrison WI, et al. *Bovine TB: The Scientific Evidence—Final Report of the Independent Scientific Group on Cattle TB.* London: Independent Scientific Group on Cattle TB (2007).

79. Woodroffe R, Donnelly CA, Cox DR, Bourne FJ, Cheeseman CL, Delahay RJ, et al. Effects of culling on badger *Meles meles* spatial organization: Implications for the control of bovine tuberculosis. *J Appl Ecol.* (2006) 43:1–10. doi: 10.1111/j.1365-2664.2005.01144.x

80. King D, Roper TJ, Young D, Woolhouse MEJ, Collins DA, Wood P. *Bovine Tuberculosis in Cattle and Badgers: A Report by the Chief Scientific Adviser.* London (2007).

81. Brunton LA, Donnelly CA, O'Connor H, Prosser A, Ashfield S, Ashton A, et al. Assessing the effects of the first 2 years of industry-led badger culling in England on the incidence of bovine tuberculosis in cattle in 2013-2015. *Ecol Evol.* (2017) 7:7213–30. doi: 10.1002/ece3.3254

82. Anon. Different TB pictures require different approaches to control, says Wales' CVO. *Vet Rec.* (2017) 181:551. doi: 10.1136/vr.j5430

83. DAERA. *TVR Wildlife Intervention Research Project - Year 4 Report (2017)* (2018).

84. O'Hagan MJ, Matthews DI, Laird C, McDowell SW. Farmers' beliefs about bovine tuberculosis control in Northern Ireland. *Vet J.* (2016) 212:22–6. doi: 10.1016/j.tvjl.2015.10.038

85. Naylor R, Manley W, Maye D, Enticott G, Ilbery BW, Hamilton-Webb A. The framing of public knowledge controversies in the media: a comparative analysis of the portrayal of badger vaccination in the English National, Regional and Farming Press. *Soc Rural.* (2017) 57:3–22. doi: 10.1111/soru.12105

86. Enticott G, Maye D, Fisher R, Ilbery B, Kirwan J. Badger Vaccination: dimensions of trust and confidence in the governance of animal disease. *Environ Plann A* (2014) 46:2881–97. doi: 10.1068/a130298p

87. Enticott G, Maye D, Carmody P, Naylor R, Ward K, Hinchliffe S, et al. Farming on the edge: farmer attitudes to bovine tuberculosis in newly endemic areas. *Vet Rec.* (2015) 177:439. doi: 10.1136/vr.103187

88. Robinson PA. Framing bovine tuberculosis: a 'political ecology of health' approach to circulation of knowledge(s) about animal disease control. *Geogr J.* (2017) 183:285–94. doi: 10.1111/geoj.12217

89. McCulloch SP, Reiss MJ. Bovine tuberculosis and badger culling in england: a utilitarian analysis of policy options. *J Agric Environ Ethics* (2017) 30:511–33. doi: 10.1007/s10806-017-9680-9

90. Gormley E, Corner LA. Control strategies for wildlife tuberculosis in Ireland. *Transbound Emerg Dis.* (2013) 60(Suppl. 1):128–35. doi: 10.1111/tbed.12095

91. Gortazar C, Delahay RJ, Mcdonald RA, Boadella M, Wilson GJ, Gavier-Widen D, et al. The status of tuberculosis in European wild mammals. *Mammal Rev.* (2012) 42:193–206. doi: 10.1111/j.1365-2907.2011.00191.x

92. Rodriguez S, Bezos J, Romero B, de Juan L, Alvarez J, Castellanos E, et al. *Mycobacterium caprae* infection in livestock and wildlife, Spain. *Emerg Infect Dis.* (2011) 17:532–5. doi: 10.3201/eid1703.100618

93. Munoz-Mendoza M, Romero B, Del Cerro A, Gortazar C, Garcia-Marin JF, Menendez S, et al. Sheep as a potential source of bovine TB: epidemiology, pathology and evaluation of diagnostic techniques. *Transbound Emerg Dis.* (2016) 63:635–46. doi: 10.1111/tbed.12325

94. Di Marco V, Mazzone P, Capuccio MT, Boniotti MB, Aronica V, Russo M, et al. Epidemiological significance of the domestic black pig (*Sus scrofa*) in maintenance of bovine tuberculosis in Sicily. *J Clin Microbiol.* (2012) 50:1209–18. doi: 10.1128/JCM.06544-11

95. Balseiro A, Gonzalez-Quiros P, Rodriguez O, Francisca Copano M, Merediz I, de Juan L, et al. Spatial relationships between Eurasian badgers (*Meles meles*) and cattle infected with *Mycobacterium bovis* in Northern Spain. *Vet J.* (2013) 197:739–45. doi: 10.1016/j.tvjl.2013.03.017

96. Munoz-Mendoza M, Marreros N, Boadella M, Gortazar C, Menendez S, de Juan L, et al. Wild boar tuberculosis in Iberian Atlantic Spain: a different picture from Mediterranean habitats. *BMC Vet Res.* (2013) 9:176. doi: 10.1186/1746-6148-9-176

97. Martin-Hernando MP, Hofle U, Vicente J, Ruiz-Fons F, Vidal D, Barral M, et al. Lesions associated with *Mycobacterium tuberculosis* complex infection in the European wild boar. *Tuberculosis* (2007) 87:360–7. doi: 10.1016/j.tube.2007.02.003

98. Hardstaff JL, Marion G, Hutchings MR, White PC. Evaluating the tuberculosis hazard posed to cattle from wildlife across Europe. *Res Vet Sci.* (2014) 97(Suppl.):S86–93. doi: 10.1016/j.rvsc.2013.12.002

99. Kukielka E, Barasona JA, Cowie CE, Drewe JA, Gortazar C, Cotarelo I, et al. Spatial and temporal interactions between livestock and wildlife in South Central Spain assessed by camera traps. *Prev Vet Med.* (2013) 112:213–21. doi: 10.1016/j.prevetmed.2013.08.008

100. Vicente J, Barasona JA, Acevedo P, Ruiz-Fons JF, Boadella M, Diez-Delgado I, et al. Temporal trend of tuberculosis in wild ungulates from Mediterranean Spain. *Transbound Emerg Dis.* (2013) 60(Suppl 1.):92–103. doi: 10.1111/tbed.12167

101. Barasona JA, Vicente J, Diez-Delgado I, Aznar J, Gortazar C, Torres MJ. Environmental presence of *Mycobacterium tuberculosis* complex in aggregation points at the wildlife/livestock interface. *Transbound Emerg Dis.* (2017) 64:1148–58. doi: 10.1111/tbed.12480

102. Gortazar C, Torres MJ, Vicente J, Acevedo P, Reglero M, de la Fuente J, et al. Bovine tuberculosis in Doñana Biosphere Reserve: the role of wild ungulates as disease reservoirs in the last Iberian lynx strongholds. *PLoS ONE* (2008) 3:e2776. doi: 10.1371/journal.pone.0002776

103. Vicente J, Hofle U, Garrido JM, Fernandez-de-Mera IG, Acevedo P, Juste R, et al. Risk factors associated with the prevalence of tuberculosis-like lesions in fenced wild boar and red deer in south central Spain. *Vet Res.* (2007) 38:451–64. doi: 10.1051/vetres:2007002

104. Perez J, Calzada J, Leon-Vizcaino L, Cubero MJ, Velarde J, Mozos E. Tuberculosis in an Iberian lynx (*Lynx pardina*). *Vet Rec.* (2001) 148:414–5. doi: 10.1136/vr.148.13.414

105. Millan J, Jimenez MA, Viota M, Candela MG, Pena L, Leon-Vizcaino L. Disseminated bovine tuberculosis in a wild red fox (*Vulpes vulpes*) in southern Spain. *J Wildl Dis.* (2008) 44:701–6. doi: 10.7589/0090-3558-44.3.701

106. Boadella M, Vicente J, Ruiz-Fons F, de la Fuente J, Gortazar C. Effects of culling Eurasian wild boar on the prevalence of *Mycobacterium bovis* and Aujeszky's disease virus. *Prev Vet Med.* (2012) 107:214–21. doi: 10.1016/j.prevetmed.2012.06.001

107. Gortazar C, Acevedo P, Ruiz-Fons F, Vicente J. Disease risks and overabundance of game species. *Eur J Wildl Res.* (2006) 52:81–7. doi: 10.1007/s10344-005-0022-2

108. Cowie CE, Marreos N, Gortazar C, Jaroso R, White PC, Balseiro A. Shared risk factors for multiple livestock diseases: a case study of bovine tuberculosis and brucellosis. *Res Vet Sci.* (2014) 97:491–7. doi: 10.1016/j.rvsc.2014.09.002

109. Cavalerie L, Courcoul A, Boschiroli ML, Réveillaud E, Gay P. Tuberculose bovine en France en 2014: une situation stable. *Bull Epidémiol Santé Anim.* (2014) 71:4–11.

110. Bouchez-Zacria M, Courcoul A, Durand B. The Distribution of bovine tuberculosis in cattle farms is linked to cattle trade and badger-mediated contact networks in South-Western France, 2007-2015. *Front Vet Sci.* (2018) 5:173. doi: 10.3389/fvets.2018.00173

111. Zanella G, Durand B, Hars J, Moutou F, Garin-Bastuji B, Duvauchelle A, et al. *Mycobacterium bovis* in wildlife in France. *J Wildl Dis.* (2008) 44:99–108. doi: 10.7589/0090-3558-44.1.99

112. Payne A, Boschiroli ML, Gueneau E, Moyen JL, Rambaud T, Dufour B, et al. Bovine tuberculosis in "Eurasian" badgers (*Meles meles*) in France. *Eur J Wildl Res.* (2013) 59:331–9. doi: 10.1007/s10344-012-0678-3

113. Reveillaud E, Desvaux S, Boschiroli ML, Hars J, Faure E, Fediaevsky A, et al. Infection of wildlife by *Mycobacterium bovis* in France assessment through a national surveillance system, Sylvatub. *Front Vet Sci.* (2018) 5:262. doi: 10.3389/fvets.2018.00262

114. Riviere J, Le Strat Y, Hendrikx P, Dufour B. Perceptions and acceptability of some stakeholders about the bovine tuberculosis surveillance system for wildlife (Sylvatub) in France. *PLoS ONE* (2018) 13:e0194447. doi: 10.1371/journal.pone.0194447

115. Miller RS, Sweeney SJ. *Mycobacterium bovis* (bovine tuberculosis) infection in North American wildlife: current status and opportunities for mitigation of risks of further infection in wildlife populations. *Epidemiol Infect.* (2013) 141:1357–70. doi: 10.1017/S0950268813000976

116. Naugle AL, Schoenbaum M, Hench CW, Henderson OL, Shere J. Bovine tuberculosis eradication in the United States: a century of progress. In: Thoen CO, Steele JH, Kaneene JB, editors. *Zoonotic Tuberculosis: Mycobacterium Bovis and Other Pathogenic Mycobacteria, 3rd Ed.* Wiley Blackwell (2014). p. 235–51. doi: 10.1002/9781118474310.ch21

117. Schmitt SM, Fitzgerald SD, Cooley TM, Bruning-Fann CS, Sullivan L, Berry D, et al. Bovine tuberculosis in free-ranging white-tailed deer from Michigan. *J Wildl Dis.* (1997) 33:749–58. doi: 10.7589/0090-3558-33.4.749

118. O'Brien DJ, Schmitt SM, Fitzgerald SD, Berry DE, Hickling GJ. Managing the wildlife reservoir of *Mycobacterium bovis*: the Michigan, USA, experience. *Vet Microbiol.* (2006) 112:313–23. doi: 10.1016/j.vetmic.2005.11.014

119. Carstensen M, O'Brien DJ, Schmitt SM. Public acceptance as a determinant of management strategies for bovine tuberculosis in free-ranging U.S. wildlife. *Vet Microbiol.* (2011) 151:200–4. doi: 10.1016/j.vetmic.2011.02.046

120. Dorn ML, Mertig AG. Bovine tuberculosis in Michigan: stakeholder attitudes and implications for eradication efforts. *Wildl Soc Bull.* (2010) 33:539–52. doi: 10.2193/0091-7648(2005)33[539:BTIMSA]2.0.CO;2

121. Palmer MV, Waters WR, Whipple DL. Shared feed as a means of deer-to-deer transmission of *Mycobacterium bovis*. *J Wildl Dis.* (2004) 40:87–91. doi: 10.7589/0090-3558-40.1.87

122. Rudolph BA, Riley SJ, Hickling GJ, Frawley BJ, Garner MS, Winterstein SR. Regulating hunter baiting for white-tailed deer in Michigan: Biological and social considerations. *Wildl Soc Bull.* (2006) 34:314–21. doi: 10.2193/0091-7648(2006)34[314:RHBFWD]2.0.CO;2

123. Gilsdorf MJ, Kaneene JB. The importance of *M. bovis* infection in cervids on the eradication of bovine tuberculosis in the United States. In: Thoen CO, Steele JH, Kaneene JB, editors. *Zoonotic Tuberculosis: Mycobacterium bovis and Other Pathogenic Mycobacteria, 3rd Edn.* Wiley Blackwell (2014). p. 263–75. doi: 10.1002/9781118474310.ch23

124. VerCauteren KC, Lavelle MJ, Campa H. Persistent spillback of bovine tuberculosis from white-tailed deer to cattle in michigan, USA: status, strategies, and needs. *Front Vet Sci.* (2018) 5:301. doi: 10.3389/fvets.2018.00301

125. Bruning-Fann CS, Schmitt SM, Fitzgerald SD, Fierke JS, Friedrich PD, Kaneene JB, et al. Bovine tuberculosis in free-ranging carnivores from Michigan. *J Wildl Dis.* (2001) 37:58–64. doi: 10.7589/0090-3558-37.1.58

126. Michel AL, Muller B, van Helden PD. *Mycobacterium bovis* at the animal-human interface: a problem, or not? *Vet Microbiol.* (2010) 140:371–81. doi: 10.1016/j.vetmic.2009.08.029

127. Renwick AR, White PC, Bengis RG. Bovine tuberculosis in southern African wildlife: a multi-species host-pathogen system. *Epidemiol Infect.* (2007) 135:529–40. doi: 10.1017/S0950268806007205

128. De Garine-Wichatitsky M, Caron A, Kock R, Tschopp R, Munyeme M, Hofmeyr M, et al. A review of bovine tuberculosis at the wildlife-livestock-human interface in sub-Saharan Africa. *Epidemiol Infect.* (2013) 141:1342–56. doi: 10.1017/S0950268813000708

129. Smith NH, Berg S, Dale J, Allen A, Rodriguez S, Romero B, et al. European 1: a globally important clonal complex of *Mycobacterium bovis*. *Infect Genet Evol.* (2011) 11:1340–51. doi: 10.1016/j.meegid.2011.04.027

130. Muller B, Hilty M, Berg S, Garcia-Pelayo MC, Dale J, Boschiroli ML, et al. African 1, an epidemiologically important clonal complex of *Mycobacterium bovis* dominant in Mali, Nigeria, Cameroon, and Chad. *J Bacteriol.* (2009) 191:1951–60. doi: 10.1128/JB.01590-08

131. Berg S, Garcia-Pelayo MC, Muller B, Hailu E, Asiimwe B, Kremer K, et al. African 2, a clonal complex of *Mycobacterium bovis* epidemiologically important in East Africa. *J Bacteriol.* (2011) 193:670–8. doi: 10.1128/JB.00750-10

132. Michel AL, Bengis RG, Keet DF, Hofmeyr M, Klerk LM, Cross PC, et al. Wildlife tuberculosis in South African conservation areas: implications and challenges. *Vet Microbiol.* (2006) 112:91–100. doi: 10.1016/j.vetmic.2005.11.035

133. Michel AL, Bengis RG. The African buffalo: a villain for inter-species spread of infectious diseases in southern Africa. *Onderstepoort J Vet Res.* (2012) 79:453. doi: 10.4102/ojvr.v79i2.453

134. Gey van Pittius NC, Perrett KD, Michel AL, Keet DF, Hlokwe T, Streicher EM, et al. Infection of African buffalo (*Syncerus caffer*) by oryx bacillus, a rare member of the antelope clade of the *Mycobacterium tuberculosis* complex. *J Wildl Dis.* (2012) 48:849–57. doi: 10.7589/2010-07-178

135. Keet DF, Kriek NP, Penrith ML, Michel A, Huchzermeyer H. Tuberculosis in buffaloes (*Syncerus caffer*) in the Kruger National Park: spread of the disease to other species. *Onderstepoort J Vet Res.* (1996) 63:239–44.

136. Keet DF, Kriek NP, Bengis RG, Grobler DG, Michel A. The rise and fall of tuberculosis in free-ranging chacma baboon troop in the Kruger National Park. *Onderstepoort J Vet Res.* (2000) 67:115–22.

137. Viljoen IM, van Helden PD, Millar RP. *Mycobacterium bovis* infection in the lion (*Panthera leo*): current knowledge, conundrums and research challenges. *Vet Microbiol.* (2015) 177:252–60. doi: 10.1016/j.vetmic.2015.03.028

138. Miller MA, Buss PE, van Helden PD, Parsons SD. *Mycobacterium bovis* in a free-ranging black rhinoceros, Kruger National Park, South Africa, 2016. *Emerg Infect Dis.* (2017) 23:557–8. doi: 10.3201/eid2303.161622

139. Miller M, Michel A, van Helden P, Buss P. Tuberculosis in Rhinoceros: An Underrecognized Threat? *Transbound Emerg Dis.* (2017) 64:1071–8. doi: 10.1111/tbed.12489

140. Miller MA, Buss P, Parsons SDC, Roos E, Chileshe J, Goosen WJ, et al. Conservation of white rhinoceroses threatened by bovine tuberculosis, South Africa, 2016-2017. *Emerg Infect Dis.* (2018) 24:2373–5. doi: 10.3201/eid2412.180293

141. Musoke J, Hlokwe T, Marcotty T, du Plessis BJ, Michel AL. Spillover of *Mycobacterium bovis* from wildlife to livestock, South Africa. *Emerg Infect Dis.* (2015) 21:448–51. doi: 10.3201/eid2103.131690

142. Hlokwe TM, van Helden P, Michel AL. Evidence of increasing intra and inter-species transmission of *Mycobacterium bovis* in South Africa: are we losing the battle? *Prev Vet Med.* (2014) 115:10–7. doi: 10.1016/j.prevetmed.2014.03.011

143. De Vos V, Bengis RG, Kriek NP, Michel A, Keet DF, Raath JP, et al. The epidemiology of tuberculosis in free-ranging African buffalo (*Syncerus caffer*) in the Kruger National Park, South Africa. *Onderstepoort J Vet Res.* (2001) 68:119–30.

144. Dippenaar A, Parsons SDC, Miller MA, Hlokwe T, Gey van Pittius NC, Adroub SA, et al. Progenitor strain introduction of *Mycobacterium bovis* at the wildlife-livestock interface can lead to clonal expansion of the disease in a single ecosystem. *Infect Genet Evol.* (2017) 51:235–8. doi: 10.1016/j.meegid.2017.04.012

145. Cross PC, Heisey DM, Bowers JA, Hay CT, Wolhuter J, Buss P, et al. Disease, predation and demography: assessing the impacts of bovine tuberculosis on African buffalo by monitoring at individual and population levels. *J Appl Ecol.* (2009) 46:467–75. doi: 10.1111/j.1365-2664.2008.01589.x

146. Caron A, Cornelis D, Foggin C, Hofmeyr M, de Garine-Wichatitsky M. African buffalo movement and zoonotic disease risk across transfrontier conservation areas, Southern Africa. *Emerg Infect Dis.* (2016) 22:277–80. doi: 10.3201/eid2202.140864

147. Buddle BM, Parlane NA, Wedlock DN, Heiser A. Overview of vaccination trials for control of tuberculosis in cattle, wildlife and humans. *Transbound Emerg Dis.* (2013) 60(Suppl. 1):136–46. doi: 10.1111/tbed.12092

148. Buddle BM, Vordermeier HM, Chambers MA, de Klerk-Lorist LM. Efficacy and safety of BCG vaccine for control of tuberculosis in domestic livestock and wildlife. *Front Vet Sci.* (2018) 5:259. doi: 10.3389/fvets.2018.00259

149. Gormley E, Corner LA. Control of tuberculosis in badgers by vaccination: where next? *Vet J.* (2011) 189:239–41. doi: 10.1016/j.tvjl.2011.03.007

150. Palmer MV, Thacker TC, Waters WR. Vaccination of white-tailed deer (*Odocoileus virginianus*) with *Mycobacterium bovis* bacillus Calmette Guerin. *Vaccine* (2007) 25:6589–97. doi: 10.1016/j.vaccine.2007.06.056

151. Gormley E, Ni Bhuachalla D, O'Keeffe J, Murphy D, Aldwell FE, Fitzsimons T, et al. Oral vaccination of free-living badgers (*Meles meles*) with Bacille Calmette Guerin (BCG) vaccine confers protection against tuberculosis. *PLoS ONE* (2017) 12:e0168851. doi: 10.1371/journal.pone.0168851

152. Balseiro A, Altuzarra R, Vidal E, Moll X, Espada Y, Sevilla IA, et al. Assessment of BCG and inactivated *Mycobacterium bovis* vaccines in an experimental tuberculosis infection model in sheep. *PLoS ONE* (2017) 12:e0180546. doi: 10.1371/journal.pone.0180546

153. Garrido JM, Sevilla IA, Beltran-Beck B, Minguijon E, Ballesteros C, Galindo RC, et al. Protection against tuberculosis in Eurasian wild boar vaccinated with heat-inactivated *Mycobacterium bovis*. *PLoS ONE* (2011) 6:e24905. doi: 10.1371/journal.pone.0024905

154. Beltran-Beck B, Romero B, Sevilla IA, Barasona JA, Garrido JM, Gonzalez-Barrio D, et al. Assessment of an oral *Mycobacterium bovis* BCG vaccine and an inactivated *M. bovis* preparation for wild boar in terms of adverse reactions, vaccine strain survival, and uptake by nontarget species. *Clin Vaccine Immunol.* (2014) 21:12–20. doi: 10.1128/CVI.00488-13

155. Tompkins DM, Buddle BM, Whitford J, Cross ML, Yates GF, Lambeth MR, et al. Sustained protection against tuberculosis conferred to a wildlife host by single dose oral vaccination. *Vaccine* (2013) 31:893–9. doi: 10.1016/j.vaccine.2012.12.003

156. Brooks-Pollock E, Wood JL. Eliminating bovine tuberculosis in cattle and badgers: insight from a dynamic model. *Proc Biol Sci.* (2015) 282:20150374. doi: 10.1098/rspb.2015.0374

157. Enticott G, Maye D, Ilbery B, Fisher R, Kirwan J. Farmers' confidence in vaccinating badgers against bovine tuberculosis. *Vet Rec.* (2012) 170:204. doi: 10.1136/vr.100079

158. Maye D, Enticott G, Naylor R, Ilbery BW, Kirwan JR. Animal disease and narratives of nature: farmers' reactions to the neoliberal governance of bovine Tuberculosis. *J Rural Stud.* (2014) 36:401–10. doi: 10.1016/j.jrurstud.2014.07.001

159. Good M, Bakker D, Duignan A, Collins DM. The history of *in vivo* tuberculin testing in bovines: tuberculosis, a "One Health" Issue. *Front Vet Sci.* (2018) 5:59. doi: 10.3389/fvets.2018.00059

160. Torgerson PR, Torgerson DJ. Public health and bovine tuberculosis: what's all the fuss about? *Trends Microbiol.* (2010) 18:67–72. doi: 10.1016/j.tim.2009.11.002

161. Kriek N. Tuberculosis in animals in South Africa. In: Thoen CO, Steele JH, Kaneene JB, editors. *Zoonotic Tuberculosis: Mycobacterium bovis and other pathogenic mycobacteria, 3rd Edn.* Wiley Blackwell (2014). p. 99–108. doi: 10.1002/9781118474310.ch9

162. Godfray HC, Donnelly CA, Kao RR, Macdonald DW, McDonald RA, Petrokofsky G, et al. A restatement of the natural science evidence base relevant to the control of bovine tuberculosis in Great Britain. *Proc Biol Sci.* (2013) 280:20131634. doi: 10.1098/rspb.2013.1634

163. Vial F, Donnelly CA. Localized reactive badger culling increases risk of bovine tuberculosis in nearby cattle herds. *Biol Lett.* (2012) 8:50–3. doi: 10.1098/rsbl.2011.0554

164. Karolemeas K, Donnelly CA, Conlan AJ, Mitchell AP, Clifton-Hadley RS, Upton P, et al. The effect of badger culling on breakdown prolongation and recurrence of bovine tuberculosis in cattle herds in Great Britain. *PLoS ONE* (2012) 7:e51342. doi: 10.1371/journal.pone.0051342

165. Jenkins HE, Woodroffe R, Donnelly CA. The duration of the effects of repeated widespread badger culling on cattle tuberculosis following the cessation of culling. *PLoS ONE* (2010) 5:e9090. doi: 10.1371/journal.pone.0009090

166. McCulloch SP, Reiss MJ. Bovine Tuberculosis policy in England: would a virtuous government Cull Mr Badger? *J Agric Environ Ethics* (2017) 30:551–63. doi: 10.1007/s10806-017-9687-2

167. Trewby ID, Young R, McDonald RA, Wilson GJ, Davison J, Walker N, et al. Impacts of removing badgers on localised counts of hedgehogs. *PLoS ONE* (2014) 9:e95477. doi: 10.1371/journal.pone.0095477

168. Cassidy A. Vermin, victims and disease: UK framings of badgers in and beyond the bovine TB controversy. *Soc Rural.* (2012) 52:192–214. doi: 10.1111/j.1467-9523.2012.00562.x

169. Grahame K. *The Wind in the Willows*: London: Methuen (1908).

170. McCulloch SP, Reiss MJ. The development of an Animal Welfare Impact Assessment (AWIA) tool and its application to bovine tuberculosis and badger control in England. *J Agric Environ Ethics* (2017) 30:485–510. doi: 10.1007/s10806-017-9684-5

171. Zarden CF, Marassi CD, Figueiredo EE, Lilenbaum W. *Mycobacterium bovis* detection from milk of negative skin test cows. *Vet Rec.* (2013) 172:130. doi: 10.1136/vr.101054

172. Ereqat S, Nasereddin A, Levine H, Azmi K, Al-Jawabreh A, Greenblatt CL, et al. First-time detection of *Mycobacterium bovis* in livestock tissues and milk in the West Bank, Palestinian Territories. *PLoS Negl Trop Dis.* (2013) 7:e2417. doi: 10.1371/journal.pntd.0002417

173. Bruns AC, Tanner M, Williams MC, Botha L, O'Brien A, Fosgate GT, et al. Diagnosis and Implications of *Mycobacterium Bovis* Infection in Banded Mongooses (*Mungos Mungo*) in the Kruger National Park, South Africa. *J Wildl Dis.* (2017) 53:19–29. doi: 10.7589/2015-11-318

174. Angkawanish T, Morar D, van Kooten P, Bontekoning I, Schreuder J, Maas M, et al. The elephant interferon gamma assay: a contribution to diagnosis of tuberculosis in elephants. *Transbound Emerg Dis.* (2013) 60(Suppl. 1):53–9. doi: 10.1111/tbed.12098

175. Morar D, Schreuder J, Meny M, van Kooten PJ, Tijhaar E, Michel AL, et al. Towards establishing a rhinoceros-specific interferon-gamma (IFN-gamma) assay for diagnosis of tuberculosis. *Transbound Emerg Dis.* (2013) 60 Suppl 1:60–6. doi: 10.1111/tbed.12132

176. Miller M, Buss P, Hofmeyr J, Olea-Popelka F, Parsons S, van Helden P. Antemortem diagnosis of *Mycobacterium bovis* infection in free-ranging African lions (*Panthera leo*) and implications for transmission. *J Wildl Dis.* (2015) 51:493–7. doi: 10.7589/2014-07-170

177. Olivier TT, Viljoen IM, Hofmeyr J, Hausler GA, Goosen WJ, Tordiffe ASW, et al. Development of a gene expression assay for the diagnosis of *Mycobacterium bovis* infection in african lions (*Panthera leo*). *Transbound Emerg Dis.* (2017) 64:774–81. doi: 10.1111/tbed.12436

178. Parsons SD, Gous TA, Warren RM, de Villiers C, Seier JV, van Helden PD. Detection of *Mycobacterium tuberculosis* infection in chacma baboons (*Papio ursinus*) using the QuantiFERON-TB gold (in-tube) assay. *J Med Primatol.* (2009) 38:411–7. doi: 10.1111/j.1600-0684.2009.00367.x

179. Parsons SD, Menezes AM, Cooper D, Walzl G, Warren RM, van Helden PD. Development of a diagnostic gene expression assay for tuberculosis and its use under field conditions in African buffaloes (*Syncerus caffer*). *Vet Immunol Immunopathol.* (2012) 148:337–42. doi: 10.1016/j.vetimm.2012.04.025

180. Parsons SDC, Morar-Leather D, Buss P, Hofmeyr J, McFadyen R, Rutten V, et al. The kinetics of the humoral and interferon-gamma immune responses to experimental *Mycobacterium bovis* infection in the white rhinoceros (*Ceratotherium simum*). *Front Immunol.* (2017) 8:1831. doi: 10.3389/fimmu.2017.01831

181. Roos EO, Olea-Popelka F, Buss P, de Klerk-Lorist LM, Cooper D, Warren RM, et al. IP-10: a potential biomarker for detection of *Mycobacterium bovis*

infection in warthogs (*Phacochoerus africanus*). *Vet Immunol Immunopathol.* (2018) 201:43–8. doi: 10.1016/j.vetimm.2018.05.007

182. Roos EO, Olea-Popelka F, Buss P, Hausler GA, Warren R, van Helden PD, et al. Measuring antigen-specific responses in *Mycobacterium bovis*-infected warthogs (*Phacochoerus africanus*) using the intradermal tuberculin test. *BMC Vet Res.* (2018) 14:360. doi: 10.1186/s12917-018-1685-8

183. Olea-Popelka F, Fujiwara PI. Building a Multi-Institutional and Interdisciplinary Team to develop a zoonotic tuberculosis roadmap. *Front Public Health* (2018) 6:167. doi: 10.3389/fpubh.2018.00167

Evaluation of Three Commercial Interferon-γ Assays in a Bovine Tuberculosis Free Population

Giovanni Ghielmetti[1]*, Patricia Landolt[1], Ute Friedel[1], Marina Morach[2], Sonja Hartnack[3], Roger Stephan[1] and Sarah Schmitt[1]

[1] Section of Veterinary Bacteriology, Institute for Food Safety and Hygiene, University of Zurich, Zurich, Switzerland, [2] Institute for Food Safety and Hygiene, University of Zurich, Zurich, Switzerland, [3] Section of Epidemiology, University of Zurich, Zurich, Switzerland

*Correspondence:
Giovanni Ghielmetti
giovanni.ghielmetti@vetbakt.uzh.ch

The interferon-γ assay has been used worldwide as an ancillary test for the diagnosis of bovine tuberculosis (bTB). This study aimed to describe, based on the bTB-free status in Switzerland, the difference of applying a more stringent cutoff point of 0.05 compared with 0.1 for bTB surveillance. Moreover, the effect of time between blood collection and stimulation, culture results, optical density values, and the influence of testing different breeds were evaluated. Blood samples from a total of 118 healthy cows older than 6 months were tested with three commercial interferon-gamma assays. To confirm the bTB-free status of the tested animals and to investigate potential cross-reactions with nontuberculous mycobacteria, pulmonary and abdominal lymph nodes in addition to ileal mucosa from each cattle were used for the detection of viable *Mycobacteria* spp. by specific culture. Significant differences regarding the proportion of false-positive results between the two Bovigam tests and between Bovigam 2G and ID Screen were found. Samples analyzed with Bovigam 2G were 2.5 [95% confidence interval (CI) 1.6–3.9] times more likely to yield a false-positive test result than samples analyzed with Bovigam TB. Similarly, the odds ratio (OR) for testing samples false-positive with ID Screen compared with Bovigam TB was 1.9 (95% CI 1.21–2.9). The OR for testing false-positive with ID Screen compared with Bovigam 2G was less to equally likely with an OR of 0.75 (95% CI 0.5–1.1). When using a cutoff of 0.05 instead of 0.1, the OR for a false-positive test result was 2.2 (95% CI 1.6–3.1). Samples tested after 6 h compared with a delayed stimulation time of 22–24 h were more likely to yield a false-positive test result with an OR of 3.9 (95% CI 2.7–5.6). In conclusion, applying a more stringent cutoff of 0.05 with the Bovigam 2G kit generates a questionable high number of false-positive results of one of three tested animals. Furthermore, specific breeds might show an increased risk to result false-positive in the Bovigam 2G and the ID Screen assays.

Keywords: cattle, bovine tuberculosis, diagnosis, interferon-gamma assay, *Mycobacterium bovis*, *Mycobacterium avium* subsp *paratuberculosis*, *Mycobacterium avium* subsp *hominissuis*, *Mycobacterium persicum*

INTRODUCTION

Bovine tuberculosis (bTB) is a chronic zoonotic disease caused by *Mycobacterium bovis* and *Mycobacterium caprae* (1). Cattle (*Bos Taurus*) are considered to be the main reservoir of bTB, and eradication programs worldwide focus primarily on this domestic species (2). Although such programs were able to significantly reduce the prevalence of the disease and some industrialized countries are considered to have official bTB-free status, specific geographical areas are still faced with this burden. Despite remarkable public and private efforts, the causes of this failure are multiple, including the varying clinical signs, intrinsic features of these bacteria such as the broad host spectrum and environmental resilience, the transmission modalities, and the absence of accurate *antemortem* diagnostic test applicable in the field (3–5).

The standard method for *antemortem* bTB detection and international trade of cattle is the tuberculin test, which involves the intradermal injection of bovine tuberculin purified protein derivative (PPDB) in the cervical area or the caudal fold of the tail (6). Skinfold thickness at the injection site is measured before and 72 h after PPDB is injected to calculate any increase. In addition, cutaneous reactions such as induration and swelling are evaluated. A more specific variant of the single intradermal test [single intradermal cervical comparative test (SICCT)] involves the additional injection of avian tuberculin (PPDA) into different sites, theoretically enabling distinction between animals infected with bTB and those responding to PPDA as a result of exposure to mycobacteria other than *Mycobacterium tuberculosis* complex (MTBC) (6). There are numerous known weaknesses associated with tuberculin skin testing, e.g., variations in specificity (Sp) and sensitivity (Se) related to different PPD products or even from batch-to-batch, the subjective injection and measurement ability of the test performer, and the necessity of restraining the animals twice (7, 8).

To overcome some of the mentioned drawbacks, a whole-blood cellular assay using a sandwich enzyme immunoassay (EIA) for the bovine cytokine interferon-gamma (IFN-γ) has been developed and used as a standalone or ancillary test to the intradermal tuberculin test for diagnostic purposes (9, 10). There are numerous advantages of the IFN-γ assay over the skin tests, including that the animals are captured only once, inconclusive tests can be readily repeated, quantification of the lymphocytes reaction to various stimulants is based on optical densities (ODs), and stimulation controls are included. Moreover, the IFN-γ assay may detect bTB-infected animals up to 60–120 days earlier than the single cervical tuberculin test (11–13).

The first IFN-γ assay (Bovigam TB, Thermo Fisher Scientific, Reinach, Switzerland) is now Office International des Epizooties-certified as an ancillary assay to the tuberculin test and may be authorized to maximize detection of infected cattle (Council Directive 64/432/ECC), including bTB-freedom certification for animals or products movement purposes and prevalence estimation (14). Switzerland was faced with bTB with two distinct outbreaks in 2013–2014 (15). At the time of writing, these events represent the last detection of *M. bovis* and *M. caprae* in domestic or wild animals in Switzerland. Although the first

event was caused by the reemergence of an undetected *M. bovis* strain that circulated in the Swiss cattle population over at least 15 years, the second outbreak originated from cattle infected during summer pasturing in an Austrian endemic area (16, 17). Consequent test and cull measures based primarily on SICCT and comprehensive epidemiological contact-tracing investigation enabled the preservation of the official bTB-free status. Under these circumstances, the IFN-γ assay was used in the late stage of the epidemiological investigations as an ancillary test for non-negative SICCT animals.

In addition to the ongoing slaughterhouse surveillance through *postmortem* meat inspection, a nationwide monitoring program (LyMON) for early detection of bTB was started in 2013 (18). Meat inspectors were encouraged to submit altered bovine lymph nodes to the bTB reference laboratory for macroscopic inspection and culture for mycobacteria. Over an 8-year period, lymph nodes originated from 793 cows were sliced into thin sections (1–2 mm) and investigated for the presence of lesions compatible with bTB. Suspicious samples ($n = 121$) were homogenized and tested for the presence of MTBC DNA by real-time polymerase chain reaction (PCR) and cultured in mycobacterial selective media (15). Moreover, in 2014, a red deer monitoring program involving two bordering Swiss Cantons and the Principality of Liechtenstein was implemented (19). Over a 7-year period, retropharyngeal and mediastinal lymph nodes of 1,382 randomly and risk-based selected red deer, such as emaciated individuals or animals killed by motor vehicles, and 33 other wild animals (roe deer, fallow deer, fox, chamois, and Alpine ibex) were investigated macroscopically by trained personnel. Of these, a total of 412 wild animals were additionally tested for the presence of MTBC DNA by real-time PCR and cultured in mycobacterial selective media (15). No further bTB cases were detected after the two mentioned outbreaks in cattle, and although *M. caprae* is still endemic in the Austrian border region, none of the investigated red deer and other wild animals resulted positive.

Although the described surveillance measures testified that the Swiss population is currently free of bTB, punctual reintroductions through illegal imports or wildlife movements are possible. Therefore, in accordance with the European Food Safety Authority's scientific opinion, EIA cutoff thresholds should be evaluated in each country based on the local epidemiological conditions to ameliorate the accuracy of the IFN-γ assay (20). Hence, these modifications of the laboratory evaluation criteria may affect the Sp and Se of the assay. An estimated median Se of 87.6% (73–100%) and Sp of 96.6% (85–99.6%) were reported for the Bovigam TB kit based on 15 field studies conducted over a 15-year period (7). However, the median Sp value (96.6%) published by de la Rua-Domenech and colleagues (7) differs from the Sp values (6.9–74%) observed in further studies (21–23). These discrepancies may be the result of different testing conditions, laboratory procedures, and evaluation criteria and, most of all, may depend on the TB prevalence and the presence of nontuberculous mycobacteria (NTM), leading to cross-reactivity in the tested populations (24). Moreover, the IFN-γ production of specific breeds such as French bullfight cattle has been shown to be significantly lower than classical diary animals (4, 24).

Recently, a new IFN-γ assay has become commercially available (ID Screen Bovine Tuberculosis IFN-γ, IDvet, Grabels, France), and it has already been extensively used in different countries including Switzerland. However, independent evaluations on the test accuracy under field conditions are either not publicly available or scarce, showing low Se (36.7%) when applying the cutoff recommended by the manufacturer or slightly better values (49.0–56.0%) using more stringent cutoff thresholds (25).

In their scientific opinion, the expert panel convened on the use of the IFN-γ test for the diagnosis of bTB highlighted the necessity to harmonize the assay protocol (20). In this regard, various critical points need to be evaluated, such as the time between blood collection and stimulation, antigens used and their concentrations, interpretation criteria including cutoff values, and finally, the inclusion of stimulation control and EIA control. Nevertheless, specific epidemiological conditions, such as exposure to environmental mycobacteria in certain geographical areas, possibly negatively influence the test accuracy (26–28).

Besides the members of the MTBC, over 190 species of NTM have been described (www.bacterio.net/mycobacterium.html). Several NTMs are commonly encountered in the environment and have been isolated from a variety of sources, such as water, feed, soil, dust, aerosol, protozoa, and animals, including cattle (29, 30). Of these, more than 60 species are known to be opportunistic pathogenic to humans and other mammals, and human infections with these emerging pathogens are now more common than tuberculosis in industrialized countries (31–33).

To avoid cross-reactive immune responses in cattle exposed to NTM, PPDA is injected in the SICCT or included in first-generation IFN-γ assays. However, in geographical areas where the dominant NTM shares epitopes with MTBC members, more specific diagnostic markers have been identified (34–36) and implemented in second-generation IFN-γ assays and subsequent versions (37, 38). Among these, antigen cocktails containing the 6-kDa early secretory antigenic target- and 10-kDa culture filtrate protein-derived peptides have gained great importance for their presumptive MTBC specificity (39). Despite earlier evidence to the contrary, orthologs of 6-kDa early secretory antigenic target and 10-kDa culture filtrate protein have now been shown to be present in frequently isolated NTM, such *Mycobacterium smegmatis*, *Mycobacterium kansasii*, *Mycobacterium persicum*, *Mycobacterium marinum*, *Mycobacterium szulgai*, *Mycobacterium gastri*, and *Mycobacterium flavescens* (34, 40–43). The specificity of the available commercial IFN-γ assays is therefore questionable in geographical areas where cattle may be exposed to NTM, influencing the test accuracy. An increased number of false-positive (FP) tested animals can result in reduced stakeholders' acceptance of control measurements, undermining the credibility of the involved authorities.

This study aimed to describe, based on the epidemiological situation (bTB-free status) in Switzerland, the difference of applying a cutoff point of 0.05 compared with 0.1 and considering the ethical implications, i.e., if a more stringent cutoff is ethically acceptable for bTB surveillance and import/export of livestock. Additionally, the effect of time between blood

collection and stimulation, culture results, and OD values were evaluated.

MATERIALS AND METHODS

Selection Criteria and Collection of Blood Samples

From a total of 118 randomly selected healthy cows older than 6 months originating from 101 different premises and 14 Swiss Cantons, two blood samples were collected *antemortem*. No more than two cows originating from the same premise were included in the study. Three different breeds covered ∼90% of the animals, with Holstein/Red Holstein ($n = 36$) being the most represented group, followed by Swiss Fleckvieh/Simmental ($n = 35$) and Swiss Brown ($n = 32$). The remaining animals were Montbéliard ($n = 8$) Normande ($n = 2$), one Charolais, one Limousin, and three mixed breeds. Of these, 90% were regularly moved to pastures in mountain regions during the summer months. Before sampling, animals were stabled in the proximity of the abattoir during the morning of the day before being killed, and heparinized blood was collected by trained personnel from the caudal vein ≥3 h after delivering. Each sample was immediately transported unchilled to the laboratory.

Culture and Identification of Mycobacteria

To confirm the bTB-free status of the tested 118 animals and to detect potential cross-reactions with NTM species, a pool of pulmonary lymph nodes (left bronchial and caudal mediastinal) and a pool of intestinal tissues (ileal mucosa and jejunal/cecal lymph nodes) from each cattle were collected immediately after killing. The pulmonary lymph nodes were cultured at 37°C for 8 weeks as described elsewhere (30). The pool of intestinal tissues was cultured at 37°C for 16 weeks on Herrold's Egg Yolk Agar with mycobactin J and ANV (BD, Basel, Switzerland), on BBL Stonebrink agar slants (BD) and on liquid MGIT supplemented with PANTA (BD) and mycobactin J (IDvet) as culture media.

All tubes showing growth of presumptive mycobacterial colonies were investigated for acid-fast bacilli after Ziehl–Neelsen staining. The colonies were identified using matrix-assisted laser desorption/ionization-time of flight mass spectrometry, and presumptive positive *Mycobacterium avium* subsp. *paratuberculosis* (MAH) colonies were confirmed by the ID Gene Paratuberculosis Duplex PCR (IDvet). For three isolates, sequencing of two housekeeping genes (*hsp65* and 16S rRNA) was performed (30). DNA sequencing was performed at Microsynth (Balgach, Switzerland). The resulting sequences were assembled using CLC Genomics Workbench 7.5.1 (Qiagen), and BLAST similarity searching for multiple sequence alignment was performed (https://blast.ncbi.nlm.nih.gov/Blast.cgi).

Interferon-γ Assays

The commercial IFN-γ kits Bovigam TB (Thermo Fisher Scientific), Bovigam 2G (Thermo Fisher Scientific), and ID Screen Bovine Tuberculosis IFN-γ (ID Screen) were tested for each blood sample according to the manufacturers' instructions. The blood samples were divided into four aliquots and incubated with PPDB, PPDA, both in addition to pokeweed mitogen

(PWM) (Prionics, Lelystad, The Netherlands for Thermo Fisher Scientific; CZ Veterinaria, Porriño, Spain for IDvet) and phosphate-buffered saline (NIL) as positive and negative stimulation controls, respectively. Two different stimulations times for each blood sample were performed, and these occurred within 6 and 22–24 h after collection, respectively. Released IFN-γ was measured using the enzyme-linked immunosorbent assay kit provided by the respective manufacturer.

Interpretation of the three kits was performed using the following criteria, with the mentioned ODs representing mean values:

- Criterion 1: positive test outcome = $OD_{PPDB} - OD_{NIL} \geq 0.05$ and $OD_{PPDB} - OD_{PPDA} \geq 0.05$
- Criterion 2: positive test outcome = $OD_{PPDB} - OD_{NIL} \geq 0.1$ and $OD_{PPDB} - OD_{PPDA} \geq 0.1$

The results of the ID Screen kit were additionally evaluated using the S/P ratio, as recommended by the manufacturer.

- Positive test outcome:
$$\frac{S}{P} = \left(\frac{OD_{PPDB} - OD_{PPDA}}{OD_{ELISA\ positive\ control} - OD_{ELISA\ negative\ control}} \right) * 100 \geq 35\%.$$

To assess the viability of T cells, stimulation with PWM was included for each test, and OD values of samples that not fulfilled the following criteria were interpreted as invalid. For the ID Screen kit, the following interpretation was adopted: $\frac{OD_{PWM}}{OD_{ELISA\ positive\ control} - OD_{ELISA\ negative\ control}} \geq 0.5$, whereas for both Bovigam variants, mean values of $OD_{PWM} - OD_{NIL}$ were supposed to be ≥ 0.5.

Moreover, animals responding to unspecific stimulation where excluded if their mean OD_{NIL} was ≥ 0.3.

Statistical Methods

With the aim to assess if the proportion of FP test results (i) differed between the three IFN-γ assays, (ii) was affected by the time elapsed between sampling and stimulation (6 and 22–24 h), (iii) and accounting for two different cutoffs (0.05 and 0.1), a model was fit with generalized estimating equations with the function geeglm from the package geepack in R (44). To account for potential within-animal clustering, an exchangeable correlation was chosen in the marginal model. Adjustment for multiple comparisons between the three IFN-γ assays was performed with Tukey's approach from the multcomp package (45). The resulting effect sizes are presented in the form of odds ratios (ORs) with their corresponding 95% confidence intervals (CIs) and p-values, adjusted for multiple comparisons.

Based on culture outcome, three different groups were defined as follows: MAP ($n = 6$), MAH ($n = 14$), and culture-negative animals ($n = 94$). Responses to PPDA (OD_{PPDA}) of the three groups were investigated for the different kits and stimulation within 6 h using a linear mixed-effects model with animals as a random effect (nlme-package) (46). The differences of the mean ODs PPDA-NIL of the three groups were compared for each kit. In addition, the effect of time between blood collection and stimulation (6 and 22–24 h) on the mean OD_{PWM} values was assessed for the three kits using the same model as for PPDA. Fisher's exact test using GraphPad Prism 9.1.0 (GraphPad

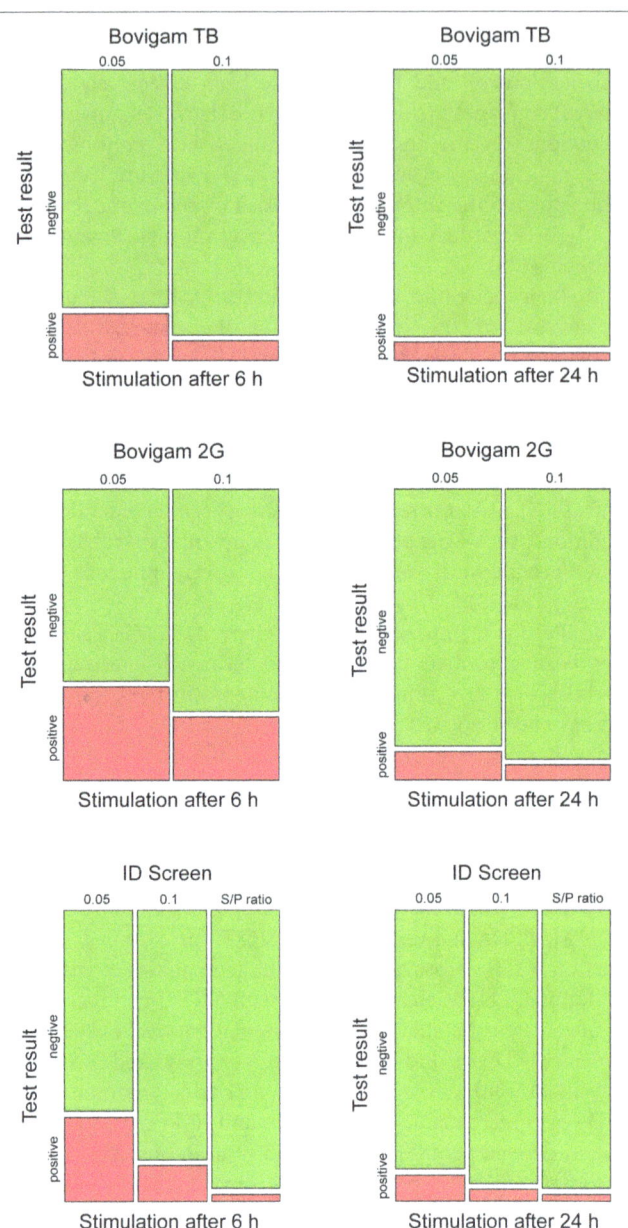

FIGURE 1 | Mosaic plots for the test outcomes using three different kits (Bovigam TB, Bovigam 2G, ID Screen), stimulation times (6 and 24 h), and cutoffs (0.05, 0.1, S/P ratio). Results are displayed in green and red for negative and positive responses, respectively.

Software) was performed to evaluate a possible association between positive test outcome and animal breed for the three major breed groups after 6 h stimulation.

RESULTS

Culture and Identification of Mycobacteria

All the tissue samples were negative for MTBC, whereas NTM was found in 17 of the 118 cultured pulmonary lymph node pools with MAH as the predominant species ($n = 14$). In the remaining three pools, *M. persicum*, *Mycobacterium lentiflavum*, and a member of the *Mycobacterium chimaera/intracellulare* group were isolated. In six of the 118 intestine tissue pools, MAP was cultured, and one animal was positive for *Mycobacterium engbaekii*.

Interferon-γ Assays

The test outcomes for each kit, stimulation time, and cutoffs are resumed in **Figure 1**. The animal positive for *M. persicum* showed a clear positive result with all three kits, stimulation times, and cutoffs. Cattle tested positive for MAP were negative with all kits and test conditions except for two FP results with the lower cutoff of 0.05 (all three kits). The majority of the MAH-positive animals showed negative results with the IFN-γ assay; only two animals were positive using the stricter cutoff of 0.05 (Bovigam 2G and ID Screen), whereas one animal was also positive using the cutoff of 0.1 and the Bovigam 2G kit.

Taken the culture as a gold standard and assuming the likelihood of an MTBC infection in Swiss cattle as very unlikely, every positive test result was assumed to be an FP result. The false-positive rate (FPR) for the three kits, stimulation times, and cutoff were evaluated. The ID Screen kit with the S/P ratio evaluation showed the best performance with an FPR of 2.5% (95% CI 0.8–7.2), independently from the stimulation times. The other two kits showed high amounts of FP results, especially when applying the more stringent cutoff (criterion 1) and the stimulation time of 6 h after blood collection, e.g., FPR 32.7% (95% CI 24.2–41.3) for the Bovigam 2G (**Table 1**).

Comparison of Kits, Cutoffs, and Stimulation Time

The applied statistical models enabled a comparison of the three kits, taking into account the two different cutoffs and stimulation times. Based on the results of the generalized equation estimates, significant differences regarding the proportion of FP between the two Bovigam tests and between Bovigam 2G and ID Screen were found. Samples analyzed with Bovigam 2G were 2.5 (95% CI 1.6–3.9) times more likely to yield an FP test result than samples analyzed with Bovigam TB. Similarly, the OR for testing samples FP with ID Screen compared with Bovigam TB was 1.9 (95% CI 1.21–2.9). The OR for testing with ID Screen compared with Bovigam 2G was 0.75 (95% CI 0.5–1.1). When using a cutoff of 0.05 instead of 0.1, the OR for an FP test result was 2.2 (95% 1.6–3.1). For samples with a stimulation time of 6 h compared with 22–24 h, the OR of testing FP was 3.9 (95% CI 2.7–5.6).

Culture Outcome and OD$_{PPDA}$ Values

The OD values in response to PPDA of the MAP-($n = 6$) and MAH-($n = 14$) infected animals were compared with the corresponding values of the culture-negative animals. No significant variation could be observed between the three groups ($p = 0.166$). Because the number of animals with MAP is low, this result should be considered with caution due to power.

Stimulation Time and OD$_{PWM}$ Values

Delay in blood stimulation (22–24 h) caused a significant reduction of the mean OD$_{PWM}$ obtained. This phenomenon was particularly evident for the ID Screen kit (overall mean OD$_{PWM6h}$ 2.94 and OD$_{PWM22-24h}$ 2.36). The smallest effect of time stimulation was observed for the Bovigam TB kit (overall mean OD$_{PWM6h}$ 1.40 and OD$_{PWM22-24h}$ 1.29); this kit had the lowest mean OD values and also the most invalid results ($n = 10$; 8.5%) compared with the other two kits (**Table 1**). The Bovigam 2G kit had two invalid results because of low mean OD$_{PWM22-24h}$ values (overall mean OD$_{PWM6h}$ 2.58 and OD$_{PWM22-24h}$ 2.17), by contrast, five invalid result for this kit were observed due to high mean OD$_{NIL6h/22-24h}$ values (≥ 0.3). Using the described interpretation criteria, the ID Screen kit showed one invalid result due to a high mean OD$_{NIL6h}$ value (≥ 0.3) in one animal.

Association Between Positive Test Outcome and Animal Breed Groups

Three major animal breed groups were investigated, with Holstein/Red Holstein ($n = 36$) being the most represented group, followed by Swiss Fleckvieh/Simmental ($n = 35$) and Swiss Brown ($n = 32$). As shown in **Figure 2**, by using a 0.1 cutoff and the Bovigam 2G kit, animals classified as Swiss Brown were more likely to test positive compared with Swiss Fleckvieh/Simmental (37.50 and 14.29%, respectively, $P < 0.05$). This difference was even more evident by applying the more stringent 0.05 cutoff, with 43.75 and 17.14% positive Swiss Brown and Swiss Fleckvieh/Simmental, respectively ($P < 0.05$). The opposite effect was observed by using the ID Screen kit (0.1 cutoff), with 25.71% of the Swiss Fleckvieh/Simmental animals resulting positive compared with 3.13% of the Swiss Brown. This phenomenon was exacerbated by applying the more stringent 0.05 cutoff, with 45.71 and 6.25% positive Swiss Fleckvieh/Simmental and Swiss Brown, respectively ($P < 0.001$). No statistically significant difference was observed between the test outcome and the three breed groups for the Bovigam TB kit.

DISCUSSION

According to the Swiss technical instruction for bTB, the IFN-γ assay is applied in specific epidemiologically relevant situations where the intradermal tuberculin skin test leads to inconclusive results. Cattle are the major livestock species in Switzerland, with roughly 1.5 million animals (Federal Statistical Office, census 2019). Approximately two-thirds of the Swiss cattle industry is dedicated to dairy production, and the average lifespan of a dairy cow in Switzerland is 6.2 years, giving birth on average 3.7 calves in a lifetime (47).

The agents causing bTB have been isolated from numerous different domestic and wild animal species, with the latter possibly covering long distances and spreading the disease (48, 49). This results in continuous interspecies transmissions from wild animals to livestock and *vice versa*, hindering national and international eradication programs (16, 50–52). Badger (*Meles meles*), free-ranging red deer (*Cervus elaphus*), and wild boar (*Sus scrofa*) are the most relevant known wild animals acting as a reservoir of bTB in Europe.

Accuracy of the IFN-γ assay for diagnosis of bTB varies considerably according to the literature and depends on the

TABLE 1 | Specificity of the three commercial kits assessed with two different times after stimulation and OD cutoffs. Specificity (95% CI), time after stimulation shown in hours after blood collection, and OD cutoffs including criterion 1 (0.05), criterion 2 (0.1), and S/P ratio for the ID Screen kit were evaluated.

Kit	Stimulation time	Criterion 1	Criterion 2	S/P ratio
Bovigam TB	6 h	83.33 (75.20–89.66) [4][†]	92.98 (86.64–96.92) [4]	/
	22–24 h	93.52 (87.10–97.35) [10]	97.22 (92.10–99.42) [10]	/
Bovigam 2G	6 h	67.26 (57.79–75.79) [5]	77.88 (69.10–85.14) [5]	/
	22–24 h	90.09 (82.96–94.95) [7]	94.59 (88.61–97.99) [7]	/
ID screen	6 h	70.34 (61.23–78.39) [1]	87.29 (79.90–92.71) [1]	97.46 (92.75–99.47) [1]
	22–24 h	90.68 (83.93–95.25) [0]	95.76 (90.39–98.61) [0]	97.46 (92.75–99.47) [0]

[†]Number of invalid tests results excluded from the analysis according to the interpretation criteria described in the Materials and Methods section are displayed in square brackets.

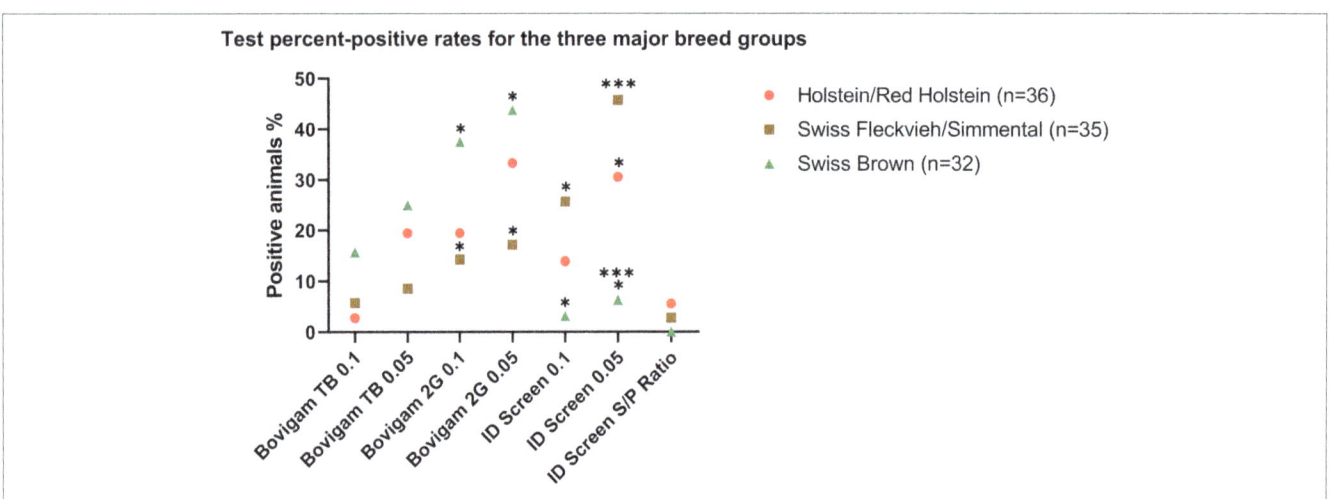

FIGURE 2 | Test percent-positive rates for the three major breed groups. Data are shown as a positive percentage of each breed group for the tested kits at 6 h stimulation. Fisher's exact test was used to evaluate the different groups. *$P < 0.05$; ***$P < 0.001$.

epidemiological settings of the tested population, the laboratory procedure, and the evaluation criteria adopted. The use of more stringent cutoff thresholds can increase the Se of the assay but may negatively influence the Sp. To date, different evaluation criteria, including thresholds, are currently used by European Member States (20). In our hands, statistically significant differences were observed for the different kits concerning the test outcome (Bovigam TB vs. Bovigam 2G and ID Screen vs. Bovigam TB), whereas the mean OD values in response to PPDA of the three culture groups (MAP, MAH, and culture-negative animals) showed no statistically significant differences.

Delay in the stimulation of the blood samples >6–8 h has been described to negatively affect IFN-γ assay performance, significantly decreasing ODs of tuberculin skin-test reactor and non-reactor animals (9, 53). The mentioned delay was deliberately included in the project to simulate a sample delivery overnight in comparison with immediate blood stimulation. Statistically significant reduction of the OD values obtained from samples PWM-stimulated within 6 h and after 22–24 h was observed for all three kits tested in the present study. This is in line with previous observations in cattle and goats (53, 54) and could negatively affect the Se of the assay due to the reduction of viable T cells in the sample.

As previously shown for M. kansasii (55), exposure to M. persicum may lead to FP results, independently from the assay used, whereas, based on the present findings, MAH and MAP seem to play a minor role in the cross-reaction. Hence, contrary to our expectations, no significant effect on the PPDA median OD values was observed between the three groups (MAP, MAH, and culture-negative) analyzed. This may be due to previous contacts of the negative culture group with mycobacteria sharing common antigens with those included in the PPDA cocktail. Among these, MAH, a ubiquitous environmental saprophyte frequently isolated from water, soil, and various animal species, including cattle, is to be mentioned and possibly plays a crucial role (30, 56).

Similar to M. kansasii, M. persicum shows marked homologies in surface protein expression, e.g., CFP-10 and ESAT-6, to MTBC members (42). Based on these findings, the inclusion of more specific antigens as proposed by second-generation assays may not overcome cross-reactivity issues due to NTM.

Alarming high amounts of FP results were observed using the two Bovigam assays, especially when applying the more stringent cutoff (criterion 1) and the stimulation time of 6 h after collection. For instance, using the Bovigam 2G kit, an FPR of 32.7% (95% CI 24.2–41.3) was determined, meaning that one-third of the tested animals are supposed to be classified as positive, although MTBC was not cultured in the tested population.

According to the manufacturer's recommendations, 8.5% ($n = 10$) and 5.9% ($n = 7$) of the cattle showed an invalid result when blood samples were stimulated 22–24 h after collection and tested with the Bovigam TB and the Bovigam 2G, respectively. For the ID Screen kit, one invalid result was observed. Under realistic conditions, an invalid result would require an additional farm visit for blood sample collection, resulting in increased time and cost efforts. Previous reports showed that the collection of blood samples before stunning or even at the commencement of exsanguination is a reliable method for accessing bTB infection using the IFN-γ assay (57). A negative effect on the IFN production due to holding and handling procedures in the present study, however, cannot be excluded (24). Thus, the number of invalid results should be interpreted with caution.

Genetic influence of the breed and the outcome of the SICCT test have been reported (58). A similar impact on the Bovigam TB test result, however, has only been demonstrated in particular cases (4). Although the present findings need further confirmation with larger animal numbers, specific breeds might show an increased risk to result in FP in the Bovigam 2G and the ID Screen assays, whereas, in accordance with previous observations (59), this was not seen for the Bovigam TB kit.

Epidemiological aspects, such as farming conditions, have been shown to play a pivotal role in the *antemortem* bTB diagnostic (4, 24). Swiss cattle spend the summer months grazing on Alpine and pre-Alpine pastures, possibly resulting in prolonged close contact with environmental NTM. Considering the particular epidemiological context of the present study, similar low individual Sp values of the IFN-γ assay were observed in neighboring countries such as France and Germany (22, 23). This suggests that the observed local cross-reactivity of NTM and possibly the negative effect on the assay due to specific breeds may not be restricted to Switzerland.

In conclusion, the general application of the IFN-γ assay and, in particular, the use of more stringent interpretation criteria should be carefully evaluated. Under specific settings such as testing animals originating from herds with bTB-positive cases or import from endemic areas, the assay ensures the detection of additional infected animals and, in some cases, permits their earlier recognition compared with the tuberculin test (12). In the authors' opinion, despite the unsatisfactory Sp observed in the present study, interpretation criteria should be adapted depending on the epidemiological context. For bTB-epidemiologically linked herds, Se should be prioritized over Sp, applying the more stringent cutoff. Conversely, for surveillance purposes within a cattle population with low bTB prevalence, however, Sp should be prioritized using a more suitable cutoff or an alternative test. Within the context of a notifiable and zoonotic disease such as bTB, however, culling of infected animals to stop the spread of the causative pathogen and to reduce animal suffering is considered necessary for disease control. Preemptive culling and culling due to compromised welfare due to transport restrictions raised ethical concerns. These concerns are resumed in the EU directive 2003/85/EC: "One of the Community's tasks in the veterinary field is to improve the state of health of livestock,

thereby increasing the profitability of livestock farming and facilitating trade in animals and animal products. At the same time the Community is also a Community of values, and its policies to combat animal diseases must not be based purely on commercial interests but must also take genuine account of ethical principles" (46). Still, it is not clear what according to the EU legislation is meant by "taking ethical principles into genuine account." One possible approach to gain clarity is to consider three standard ethical principles, which are respect for well-being, autonomy, and fairness or justice (47). Thus, the ethical question here is to assess if applying a more stringent cutoff for IFN-γ tests negatively affects the well-being, autonomy, and fairness of cows, farmers, and other potential stakeholders. Although the arbitrary value of the culled animals is currently reimbursed by the Swiss Government, the individual value of single animals for their farmers is often higher and results from decades of meticulous genetic selection. Briefly sketched, when applying a more stringent cutoff threshold, the well-being of the cows and the farmers will be affected because—based on the present OR of 2.2 (95% CI 1.6–3.1)—the odds or chance of an FP test result is two times more likely when reducing the cutoff from 0.1 to 0.05. A harmonized or generally prescribed cutoff of 0.05—irrespective of the local epidemiological situation, which is determined by the local prevalence of bovine TB, the occurrence of other cross-reacting NTM, and the tested cattle breed—might affect the principle of autonomy, presumably mostly relevant for the local veterinary authorities. As cows living in geographical areas with a higher occurrence of certain NTM species, they might be more likely to obtain an FP test result, which would affect the principle of fairness and justice. Briefly summarized, following the principles approach, the general application of a stringent cutoff of 0.05 compared with 0.1 is ethically questionable. Still, based on the results of our study, with a cutoff of 0.1 and the stimulation time of 6 h, the point estimates of the specificities of ID Screen and Bovigam 2G are below 90%. For the purpose of illustration, in an epidemiological setting with a true TB prevalence of 10%, assumed test sensitivity and specificity of 95 and 90%, the probability that a cow with a positive test result is truly infected is 51%. If the true prevalence is 5%, this probability is reduced to 33.3%.

Modifying the cutoff with the aim to increase the specificity is also not a feasible solution, as this would potentially lead to a decrease in sensitivity. A potential TB outbreak might be detected later, affecting subsequently more cows, causing more welfare losses in both cows and farmers. The application of a more stringent cutoff during the clarification of an outbreak may result in a significantly high number of animals with negative *postmortem* tests, such as RT-PCR or culture, greatly diminishing the reliability of positive IFN-γ results and consequently the long-term compliance of farmers. Based on our results regarding the proportion of FP and the presence of NTM potentially causing FP test results, we suggest evaluating the IFN-γ assay in light of the local epidemiological situation (20). Thus, a better understanding of the local epidemiological situation, including the identification of breeds that are more likely to react FP with specific test assay, is crucial. Monitoring programs such as LyMON provide essential data on the possible reoccurrence of bTB, and the present findings highlight an alarmingly high number of FP reactors. Moreover, transparency of data generated from surveillance studies is essential for the establishment of an international standard based on OD-values.

Within the context of One Health, the well-being, autonomy, and fairness of the involved parties such as dairy farmers, consumers, and cows should be considered. Among others, single aspects including food safety, animal welfare, and the intrinsic value of animals are some of the interests to be evaluated before more stringent diagnostic tests are officially approved.

CONCLUSION

The application of a more stringent threshold leads to a questionable high number of FP results. Depending on the epidemiological context, including cross-reactive NTM in specific geographic areas, expected bTB prevalence, consequences of a positive test, the tested cattle breed, and the assay threshold should be carefully selected. If necessary, the inclusion of more specific antigens is to be considered.

ETHICS STATEMENT

All animals included in this study were sampled in accordance with the Swiss Act SR 455. The animal testing was approved by the Animal Welfare Committee of the Canton of Zurich.

AUTHOR CONTRIBUTIONS

GG, SS, and RS designed and coordinated the study. PL, MM, GG, and UF performed the experiments. SH and GG conceived and carried out the statistical analyses. GG, SS, and SH drafted the manuscript. All authors read and approved the final manuscript.

ACKNOWLEDGMENTS

The authors would like to thank Marianne Schneeberger, Ella Hübschke, and Fenja Rademacher for their support. We thank Thermo fisher Scientific for kindly providing the kits (Bovigam TB and Bovigam 2G) free of charge.

REFERENCES

1. More S, Botner A, Butterworth A, Calistri P, Depner K, Edwards S, et al. Assessment of listing and categorisation of animal diseases within the framework of the animal health law (Regulation (EU) No2016/429): bovine tuberculosis. *EFSA J.* (2017) 15. doi: 10.2903/j.efsa.2017.4959

2. World Organisation for Animal Health. *Bovine Tuberculosis.* (2020). Available online at: https://www.oie.int/en/disease/bovine-tuberculosis/ (accessed April 27, 2021).

3. Buddle BM, Mackintosh CG. Improving the diagnosis of bovine tuberculosis in farmed deer. *Vet Rec.* (2017) 180:66–7. doi: 10.1136/vr.j270

4. Keck N, Boschiroli ML, Smyej F, Vogler V, Moyen JL, Desvaux S. Successful application of the gamma-interferon assay in a bovine tuberculosis eradication program: the French bullfighting herd experience. *Front Vet Sci.* (2018) 5:27. doi: 10.3389/fvets.2018.00027

5. Kelley HV, Waibel SM, Sidiki S, Tomatis-Souverbielle C, Scordo JM, Hunt WG, et al. Accuracy of two point-of-care tests for rapid diagnosis of bovine tuberculosis at animal level using non-invasive specimens. *Sci Rep.* (2020) 10:5441. doi: 10.1038/s41598-020-62314-2

6. World Organisation for Animal Health. *Manual of Diagnostic Tests and Vaccines for Terrestrial Animals.* (2019). Available online at: https://www. oie.int/en/what-we-do/standards/codes-and-manuals/terrestrial-manual-online-access/ (accessed April 27, 2021).

7. de la Rua-Domenech R, Goodchild AT, Vordermeier HM, Hewinson RG, Christiansen KH, Clifton-Hadley RS. Ante mortem diagnosis of tuberculosis in cattle: a review of the tuberculin tests, gamma-interferon assay and other ancillary diagnostic techniques. *Res Vet Sci.* (2006) 81:190–210. doi: 10.1016/j.rvsc.2005.11.005

8. Faye S, Moyen JL, Gares H, Benet JJ, Garin-Bastuji B, Boschiroli ML. Determination of decisional cut-off values for the optimal diagnosis of bovine tuberculosis with a modified IFN gamma assay (Bovigam) in a low prevalence area in France. *Vet Microbiol.* (2011) 151:60–7. doi: 10.1016/j.vetmic.2011.02.026

9. Rothel JS, Jones SL, Corner LA, Cox JC, Wood PR. A sandwich enzyme-immunoassay for bovine interferon-gamma and its use for the detection of tuberculosis in cattle. *Aust Vet J.* (1990) 67:134–7. doi: 10.1111/j.1751-0813.1990.tb07730.x

10. Wood PR, Jones SL. BOVIGAM (TM): an *in vitro* cellular diagnostic test for bovine tuberculosis. *Tuberculosis.* (2001) 81:147–55. doi: 10.1054/tube.2000.0272

11. Buddle BM, Delisle GW, Pfeffer A, Aldwell FE. Immunological responses and protection against *Mycobacterium bovis* in calves vaccinated with a low-dose of BCG. *Vaccine.* (1995) 13:1123–30. doi: 10.1016/0264-410X(94)00055-R

12. Gormley E, Doyle MB, Fitzsimons T, McGill K, Collins JD. Diagnosis of *Mycobacterium bovis* infection in cattle by use of the gamma-interferon (Bovigam) assay. *Vet Microbiol.* (2006) 112:171–9. doi: 10.1016/j.vetmic.2005.11.029

13. Lilenbaum W, Schettini JC, Souza GN, Ribeiro ER, Moreira EC, Fonseca LS. Comparison between a gamma-IFN assay and intradermal tuberculin test for the diagnosis of bovine tuberculosis in field trials in Brazil. *J Vet Med B Infect Dis Vet Public Health.* (1999) 46:353–8. doi: 10.1111/j.1439-0450.1999.tb01240.x

14. World Organisation for Animal Health. *OIE Procedure for Registration of Diagnostic Kits.* (2015). Available online at: https://www.oie.int/fileadmin/ Home/eng/Our_scientific_expertise/docs/pdf/OIE_Register_Bovigam_Abstract_v1_05.2015.pdf (accessed April 27, 2021).

15. Ghielmetti G, Scherrer S, Friedel U, Frei D, Suter D, Perler L, et al. Epidemiological tracing of bovine tuberculosis in Switzerland, multilocus variable number of tandem repeat analysis of *Mycobacterium bovis* and *Mycobacterium caprae*. *PLoS ONE.* (2017) 12:e0172474. doi: 10.1371/journal.pone.0172474

16. Fink M, Schleicher C, Gonano M, Prodinger WM, Pacciarini M, Glawischnig W, et al. Red deer as maintenance host for bovine tuberculosis, Alpine region. *Emerg Infect Dis.* (2015) 21:464–7. doi: 10.3201/eid2103.141119

17. Schoepf K, Prodinger WM, Glawischnig W, Hofer E, Revilla-Fernandez S, Hofrichter J, et al. A two-years' survey on the prevalence of tuberculosis caused by *Mycobacterium caprae* in red deer (*Cervus elaphus*) in the Tyrol, Austria. *ISRN Vet Sci.* (2012) 2012:245138. doi: 10.5402/2012/245138

18. FSVO FFSaVO. *LyMON – Lymphknoten-Monitoring bei Rindern am Schlachthof.* (2020). Available online at: https://www.blv.admin.ch/blv/de/ home/tiere/tiergesundheit/frueherkennung/lymon.html (accessed April 27, 2021).

19. FSVO FFSaVO. *Gesundheitsmonitoring Wild.* (2020). Available online at: https://www.blv.admin.ch/blv/de/home/tiere/tiergesundheit/ frueherkennung/gm-wild.html (accessed April 27, 2021).

20. EFSA Panel on Animal Health and Welfare (AHAW). Scientific opinion on the use of a gamma interferon test for the diagnosis of bovine tuberculosis. *EFSA J.* (2012) 10. doi: 10.2903/j.efsa.2012.2975

21. Buddle BM, McCarthy AR, Ryan TJ, Pollock JM, Vordermeier HM, Hewinson RG, et al. Use of mycobacterial peptides and recombinant proteins for the diagnosis of bovine tuberculosis in skin test-positive cattle. *Vet Rec.* (2003) 153:615–20. doi: 10.1136/vr.153.20.615

22. Praud A, Boschiroli ML, Meyer L, Garin-Bastuji B, Dufour B. Assessment of the sensitivity of the gamma-interferon test and the single intradermal comparative cervical test for the diagnosis of bovine tuberculosis under field conditions. *Epidemiol Infect.* (2015) 143:157–66. doi: 10.1017/S0950268814000338

23. Pucken VB, Knubben-Schweizer G, Dopfer D, Groll A, Hafner-Marx A, Hormansdorfer S, et al. Evaluating diagnostic tests for bovine tuberculosis in the southern part of Germany: a latent class analysis. *PLoS ONE.* (2017) 12:e0179847. doi: 10.1371/journal.pone.0179847

24. Schiller I, Waters WR, Vordermeier HM, Nonnecke B, Welsh M, Keck N, et al. Optimization of a whole-blood gamma interferon assay for detection of *Mycobacterium bovis*-infected cattle. *Clin Vaccine Immunol.* (2009) 16:1196–202. doi: 10.1128/CVI.00150-09

25. de la Cruz ML, Branscum AJ, Nacar J, Pages E, Pozo P, Perez A, et al. Evaluation of the performance of the IDvet IFN-Gamma test for diagnosis of bovine tuberculosis in Spain. *Front Vet Sci.* (2018) 5:229. doi: 10.3389/fvets.2018.00229

26. Hermansen TS, Thomsen VO, Lillebaek T, Ravn P. Non-tuberculous mycobacteria and the performance of interferon gamma release assays in Denmark. *PLoS ONE.* (2014) 9:e93986. doi: 10.1371/journal.pone.0093986

27. Jenkins AO, Gormley E, Gcebe N, Fosgate GT, Conan A, Aagaard C, et al. Cross reactive immune responses in cattle arising from exposure to *Mycobacterium bovis* and non-tuberculous mycobacteria. *Prev Vet Med.* (2018) 152:16–22. doi: 10.1016/j.prevetmed.2018.02.003

28. Michel AL. *Mycobacterium fortuitum* infection interference with *Mycobacterium bovis* diagnostics: natural infection cases and a pilot experimental infection. *J Vet Diagn Invest.* (2008) 20:501–3. doi: 10.1177/104063870802000415

29. Falkinham JO, 3rd. Environmental sources of nontuberculous mycobacteria. *Clin Chest Med.* (2015). 36:35–41. doi: 10.1016/j.ccm.2014.10.003

30. Ghielmetti G, Friedel U, Scherrer S, Sarno E, Landolt P, Dietz O, et al. Non-tuberculous mycobacteria isolated from lymph nodes and faecal samples of healthy slaughtered cattle and the abattoir environment. *Transbound Emerg Dis.* (2018) 65:711–8. doi: 10.1111/tbed.12793

31. Biet F, Boschiroli ML. Non-tuberculous mycobacterial infections of veterinary relevance. *Res Vet Sci.* (2014) 97:S69–77. doi: 10.1016/j.rvsc.2014.08.007

32. Griffith DE, Aksamit T, Brown-Elliott BA, Catanzaro A, Daley C, Gordin F, et al. An official ATS/IDSA statement: diagnosis, treatment, and prevention of nontuberculous mycobacterial diseases. *Am J Respir Crit Care Med.* (2007) 175:367–416. doi: 10.1164/rccm.200604-571ST

33. Tortoli E. Microbiological features and clinical relevance of new species of the genus *Mycobacterium. Clin Microbiol Rev.* (2014) 27:727–52. doi: 10.1128/CMR.00035-14

34. Arend SM, de Haas P, Leyten E, Rosenkrands I, Rigouts L, Andersen P, et al. ESAT-6 and CFP-10 in clinical versus environmental isolates of *Mycobacterium kansasii. J Infect Dis.* (2005) 191:1301–10. doi: 10.1086/428950

35. Lein AD, von Reyn CF, Ravn P, Horsburgh CR, Alexander LN, Andersen P. Cellular immune responses to ESAT-6 discriminate between patients with pulmonary disease due to *Mycobacterium avium* complex and those with pulmonary disease due to *Mycobacterium tuberculosis. Clin Diagn Lab Immunol.* (1999) 6:606–9. doi: 10.1128/CDLI.6.4.606-609.1999

36. Schiller I, Waters RW, Vordermeier HM, Jemmi T, Welsh M, Keck N, et al. Bovine tuberculosis in Europe from the perspective of an officially tuberculosis free country: trade, surveillance and diagnostics. *Vet Microbiol.* (2011) 151:153–9. doi: 10.1016/j.vetmic.2011.02.039

37. Aagaard C, Govaerts M, Meikle V, Vallecillo AJ, Gutierrez-Pabello JA, Suarez-Guemes F, et al. Optimizing antigen Cocktails for detection of *Mycobacterium bovis* in herds with different prevalences of bovine tuberculosis: ESAT6-CFP10 mixture shows optimal sensitivity and specificity. *J Clin Microbiol.* (2006) 44:4326–35. doi: 10.1128/JCM.01184-06

38. Hoffmann H, Avsar K, Gores R, Mavi SC, Hofmann-Thiel S. Equal sensitivity of the new generation QuantiFERON-TB Gold plus in direct comparison with the previous test version QuantiFERON-TB Gold IT. *Clin Microbiol Infect.* (2016) 22:701–3. doi: 10.1016/j.cmi.2016.05.006

39. Millington KA, Fortune SM, Low J, Garces A, Hingley-Wilson SM, Wickremasinghe M, et al. Rv3615c is a highly immunodominant RD1 (Region of Difference 1)-dependent secreted antigen specific for *Mycobacterium tuberculosis* infection. *Proc Natl Acad Sci U S A.* (2011) 108:5730–5. doi: 10.1073/pnas.1015153108

40. Colangeli R, Spencer JS, Bifani P, Williams A, Lyashchenko K, Keen MA, et al. MTSA-10, the product of the Rv3874 gene of *Mycobacterium tuberculosis*, elicits tuberculosis-specific, delayed-type hypersensitivity in guinea pigs. *Infect Immun.* (2000) 68:990–3. doi: 10.1128/IAI.68.2.990-993.2000

41. Harboe M, Oettinger T, Wiker HG, Rosenkrands I, Andersen P. Evidence for occurrence of the ESAT-6 protein in *Mycobacterium tuberculosis* and virulent *Mycobacterium bovis* and for its absence in *Mycobacterium bovis* BCG. *Infect Immun.* (1996) 64:16–22. doi: 10.1128/IAI.64.1.16-22.1996

42. Scherrer S, Landolt P, Friedel U, Stephan R. Distribution and expression of *esat-6* and *cfp-10* in non-tuberculous mycobacteria isolated from lymph nodes of slaughtered cattle in Switzerland. *J Vet Diagn Invest.* (2019) 31:217–21. doi: 10.1177/1040638718824074

43. van Ingen J, de Zwaan R, Dekhuijzen R, Boeree M, van Soolingen D. Region of difference 1 in nontuberculous *Mycobacterium* species adds a phylogenetic and taxonomical character. *J Bacteriol.* (2009) 191:5865–7. doi: 10.1128/JB.00683-09

44. Halekoh U, Hojsgaard S, Yan J. The R package geepack for generalized estimating equations. *J Stat Softw.* (2006) 15:1–11. doi: 10.18637/jss.v015.i02

45. Hothorn T, Bretz F, Westfall P. Simultaneous inference in general parametric models. *Biom J.* (2008) 50:346–63. doi: 10.1002/bimj.2008 10425

46. Pinheiro J, Bates D, DebRoy S, Sarkar D, R Core Team (2020). Available online at: https://CRAN.R-project.org/package=nlme (accessed April 27, 2021).

47. Scharrer S, Presi P, Hattendorf J, Chitnis N, Reist M, Zinsstag J. Demographic model of the Swiss cattle population for the years 2009-2011 stratified by gender, age and production type. *PLoS ONE.* (2014) 9:e109329. doi: 10.1371/journal.pone.0109329

48. Gortazar C, Torres MJ, Vicente J, Acevedo P, Reglero M, de la Fuente J, et al. Bovine tuberculosis in donana biosphere reserve: the role of wild ungulates as disease reservoirs in the last Iberian lynx strongholds. *PLoS ONE.* (2008) 3:e2776. doi: 10.1371/journal.pone.0002776

49. Rodwell TC, Whyte IJ, Boyce WM. Evaluation of population effects of bovine tuberculosis in free-ranging African buffalo (*Syncerus caffer*). *J Mammal.* (2001) 82:231–8. doi: 10.1644/1545-1542(2001)082<0231:EOPEOB>2.0.CO;2

50. Atkins PJ, Robinson PA. Bovine tuberculosis and badgers in Britain: relevance of the past. *Epidemiol Infect.* (2013) 141:1437–44. doi: 10.1017/S095026881200297X

51. Garcia-Jimenez WL, Cortes M, Benitez-Medina JM, Hurtado I, Martinez R, Garcia-Sanchez A, et al. Spoligotype diversity and 5-year trends of bovine tuberculosis in extremadura, southern Spain. *Trop Anim Health Prod.* (2016) 48:1533–40. doi: 10.1007/s11250-016-1124-4

52. Nigsch A, Glawischnig W, Bago Z, Greber N. *Mycobacterium caprae* infection of red deer in Western Austria-optimized use of pathology data to infer infection dynamics. *Front Vet Sci.* (2019) 5:350. doi: 10.3389/fvets.2018.00350

53. Gormley E, Doyle MB, McGill K, Costello E, Good M, Collins JD. The effect of the tuberculin test and the consequences of a delay in blood culture on the sensitivity of a gamma-interferon assay for the detection of *Mycobacterium bovis* infection in cattle. *Vet Immunol Immunopathol.* (2004) 102:413–20. doi: 10.1016/j.vetimm.2004.08.002

54. Bezos J, Alvarez J, Juan L, Romero B, Rodriguez S, Castellanos E, et al. Factors influencing the performance of an interferon-gamma assay for the diagnosis of tuberculosis in goats. *Vet J.* (2011) 190:131–5. doi: 10.1016/j.tvjl.2010.09.026

55. Waters WR, Palmer MV, Thacker TC, Payeur JB, Harris NB, Minion FC, et al. Immune responses to defined antigens of *Mycobacterium bovis* in cattle experimentally infected with *Mycobacterium kansasii. Clin Vaccine Immunol.* (2006) 13:611–9. doi: 10.1128/CVI.00054-06

56. Lahiri A, Kneisel J, Kloster I, Kamal E, Lewin A. Abundance of *Mycobacterium avium* ssp. hominissuis in soil and dust in Germany - implications for the infection route. *Lett Appl Microbiol.* (2014) 59:65–70. doi: 10.1111/lam.12243

57. Okafor CC, Grooms DL, Bolin SR, Averill JJ, Kaneene JB. Evaluation of the interferon-gamma assay on blood collected at exsanguination of cattle under field conditions for surveillance of bovine tuberculosis. *Transbound Emerg Dis.* (2014) 61:E68–75. doi: 10.1111/tbed.12080

58. Amos W, Brooks-Pollock E, Blackwell R, Driscoll E, Nelson-Flower M, Conlan AJ. Genetic predisposition to pass the standard SICCT test for bovine tuberculosis in British cattle. *PLoS ONE.* (2013) 8:e58245. doi: 10.1371/journal.pone.0058245

59. Gormley E, Doyle M, Duignan A, Good M, More SJ, Clegg TA. Identification of risk factors associated with disclosure of false positive bovine tuberculosis reactors using the gamma-interferon (IFN gamma) assay. *Vet Res.* (2013) 44:117. doi: 10.1186/1297-9716-44-117

Mycobacterial Infection of Precision-Cut Lung Slices Reveals Type 1 Interferon Pathway is Locally Induced by *Mycobacterium bovis* but not *M. tuberculosis* in a Cattle Breed

Aude Remot[1]*, Florence Carreras[1], Anthony Coupé[1], Émilie Doz-Deblauwe[1], Maria L. Boschiroli[2], John A. Browne[3], Quentin Marquant[4], Delphyne Descamps[4], Fabienne Archer[5], Abraham Aseffa[6], Pierre Germon[1], Stephen V. Gordon[7] and Nathalie Winter[1]

[1] INRAE, Université de Tours, Nouzilly, France, [2] Paris-Est University, National Reference Laboratory for Tuberculosis, Animal Health Laboratory, Anses, Maisons-Alfort, France, [3] UCD School of Agriculture and Food Science, University College Dublin, Dublin, Ireland, [4] INRAE, Université Paris-Saclay, UVSQ, Jouy-en-Josas, France, [5] INRAE, UMR754, Viral Infections and Comparative Pathology, IVPC, Univ Lyon, Université Claude Bernard Lyon 1, EPHE, Lyon, France, [6] Armauer Hansen Research Institute, Addis Ababa, Ethiopia, [7] UCD School of Veterinary Medicine and UCD Conway Institute, University College Dublin, Dublin, Ireland

*Correspondence:
Aude Remot
aude.remot@inrae.fr

Tuberculosis exacts a terrible toll on human and animal health. While *Mycobacterium tuberculosis* (Mtb) is restricted to humans, *Mycobacterium bovis* (Mb) is present in a large range of mammalian hosts. In cattle, bovine TB (bTB) is a noticeable disease responsible for important economic losses in developed countries and underestimated zoonosis in the developing world. Early interactions that take place between mycobacteria and the lung tissue early after aerosol infection govern the outcome of the disease. In cattle, these early steps remain poorly characterized. The precision-cut lung slice (PCLS) model preserves the structure and cell diversity of the lung. We developed this model in cattle in order to study the early lung response to mycobacterial infection. *In situ* imaging of PCLS infected with fluorescent Mb revealed bacilli in the alveolar compartment, in adjacent or inside alveolar macrophages, and in close contact with pneumocytes. We analyzed the global transcriptional lung inflammation signature following infection of PCLS with Mb and Mtb in two French beef breeds: Blonde d'Aquitaine and Charolaise. Whereas, lungs from the Blonde d'Aquitaine produced high levels of mediators of neutrophil and monocyte recruitment in response to infection, such signatures were not observed in the Charolaise in our study. In the Blonde d'Aquitaine lung, whereas the inflammatory response was highly induced by two Mb strains, AF2122 isolated from cattle in the UK and Mb3601 circulating in France, the response against two Mtb strains, H37Rv, the reference laboratory strain, and BTB1558, isolated from zebu in Ethiopia, was very low. Strikingly, the type I interferon pathway was only induced by Mb but not Mtb strains, indicating that this pathway may be involved in mycobacterial virulence and host tropism. Hence, the PCLS model in cattle is a valuable tool to deepen our understanding of early interactions between lung host cells and mycobacteria. It revealed striking differences between cattle breeds and mycobacterial strains. This model could help in deciphering biomarkers of resistance vs. susceptibility to bTB in cattle as such information is still critically needed for bovine genetic selection programs and would greatly help the global effort to eradicate bTB.

Keywords: cattle, *Mycobacterium bovis*, *ex vivo*, precision cut lung slices, alveolar macrophages, type I interferon

INTRODUCTION

Bovine tuberculosis (bTB) caused by *Mycobacterium bovis* (Mb) remains one of the most challenging infections to control in cattle. Because of its zoonotic nature, this pathogen and its associated noticeable disease in cattle are under strict surveillance and regulation in the European Union. When bTB cases are detected through surveillance, culling of these reactor cattle is mandatory. In spite of intensive eradication campaigns, bTB is still prevalent in European cattle (1, 2) and has significant economic, social, and environmental implications. Since 2001, France is an officially bTB-free country, a status that was achieved through costly surveillance programs. However, each year, around 100 Mb foci of infection are identified (3), with certain geographical areas showing a constant rise in disease prevalence since 2004.

bTB eradication is an unmet priority that faces two major difficulties: the persistence of undetected infected animals in herds because of the lack of diagnostic sensitivity and the risk of transmission from infected sources (4). Moreover, the poor understanding of bTB pathophysiology in cattle and the lack of correlates of protection are substantial knowledge gaps that must be resolved so as to better tackle the disease (DISCONTOOLS, https://www.discontools.eu/).

Both Mb and *Mycobacterium tuberculosis* (Mtb) belong to the same genetic complex. Mtb is responsible for tuberculosis (TB) in humans, which displays similar features with bTB. It is estimated that one-third of the global human population are latently infected with Mtb, which kills 1.4 million people each year (5). Despite the high degree of identity that Mtb and Mb share both at the genetic level as well as during the infection process, the two pathogens display distinct tropism and virulence depending on the host. While Mb is highly virulent and pathogenic for cattle and a range of other mammals, Mtb is restricted to sustain in humans. An experimental infection of cattle with the widely used Mtb laboratory strain H37Rv, which was genome-sequenced in 1998 (6), shows a strong attenuation compared to Mb (7, 8). However, the natural infection of cattle with Mtb has been reported, and the strain Mtb BTB1558 was once such a case, isolated from a zebu bull in Ethiopia (9, 10). In comparison to the original UK Mb strain AF2122/97, the first genome-sequenced Mb isolate (11, 12), the Mtb strain BTB1558 displayed a much lower virulence in European cattle (13).

The Mb strains that circulate in France today are phylogenetically distant from the UK Mb reference strain. While AF2122 belongs to the European 1 clonal complex (14), the European 3 clonal complex is widespread in France, (15). The Eu3 genetic cluster is composed of field strains that

share the SB0120 spoligotype with the attenuated Bacillus-Calmette-Guerin (BCG) vaccine strain (16, 17). In our study, we used Mb3601 as the representative strain of this widespread French cluster. Originally, Mb3601 was isolated from the tracheobronchial lymph node of an infected bovine in a bTB highly enzootic area in France (16). However, despite the widespread circulation in its original area, nothing is known today of the pathophysiology of Mb3601 infection.

Indeed greater knowledge is available on Mtb infection process and disease development both in humans and mouse models compared to Mb infection in cattle. With both mycobacteria, the alveolar macrophage (AMP) is the frontline cell that first presents the first niche for mycobacteria entering the lung, and the role of the AMP in early-stage infection is well established (8). Both Mtb and Mb have established their lifestyle in AMPs: they can escape its bactericidal mechanisms and multiply within this niche. During the infection process, bacilli disseminate to different anatomical sites and establish new infection foci both in the lungs and secondary lymphoid organs (18, 19). During Mtb infection, lung epithelial cells also play key roles in host defense [reviewed in (20–22)]. Type II pneumocytes are infected by Mtb (23) and produce pro-inflammatory cytokines which augment the AMP innate resistance mechanisms (24). The role of type II pneumocytes during Mb infection in cattle is not well known. Most of the available knowledge on the role of bovine macrophages (MPs) during Mb infection also comes from studies conducted with monocytes sampled from blood and derived as MPs during *in vitro* culture (25, 26).

In our study, we wanted to investigate the bovine innate response following Mb or Mtb infection in a preserved lung environment to allow the resident lung cells to interact with bacilli and crosstalk. Precision cut lung slices (PCLS) are an experimental model in which resident lung cell types are preserved and remain alive for at least 1 week (27). The tissue architecture and the interactions between the different cells are maintained. PCLS have already been validated for the study of various respiratory pathogens (27–29). In chicken PCLS, mononuclear cells are highly motile and actively phagocytic (30). This model is well designed to study complex interactions taking place early after the host–pathogen encounter. During Mb infection in cattle, important differences in the production of key proinflammatory cytokines such as IFNγ or TNFα by peripheral blood mononuclear cells are observed, depending on the clinical status of the animal. Interestingly, such differences are observed at early time points (31), indicating that the innate phase of the host response is key to the establishment of the pathological outcome of the infection.

Therefore, the PCLS model is ideally suited to investigate early host–pathogen interactions in the bovine lung during Mb infection and may help to find clues to the impact of the innate response on the outcome of infection. This model, which fully mimics the early environment of the bacillus entering the lung (compared to monocyte-derived MPs), may also aid in understanding the molecular basis of mycobacterial host preference (32). To this end, we decided to compare four mycobacterial strains: two Mtb species—namely, the Mtb H37Rv reference strain for human TB and the cattle derived Mtb BTB1558—and two Mb species—namely, Mb AF2122 as representative of the EU1 clonal complex and Mb3601 as the hallmark EU3 strain. Since the host genetic background also has a profound impact on the outcome of bTB disease (33), we decided to compare PCLS from two prevalent beef breeds in France—Charolaise and Blonde d'Aquitaine—and conducted a thorough characterization of the lung responses to Mb and Mtb during ex vivo infection. The PCLS allowed us to decipher important differences in the transcriptomic and cytokine profile during the innate response to infection, depending both on the breed, i.e., between Blonde d'Aquitaine and Charolaise cows, and on the mycobacterial species, i.e., between Mtb and Mb.

MATERIALS AND METHODS

Animal Tissue Sampling
Lungs from 15 Blonde d'Aquitaine and nine Charolaise cows were collected post-mortem at a commercial abattoir. The animals were between 3 and 11 years old and originated from eight different French departments where no recent bTB outbreak had been noticed (**Supplementary Figure 1**). No ethical committee approval was necessary as no animal underwent any experimental procedure. After slaughter by professionals following the regulatory guidelines from the abattoir, the lungs from each cow were systematically inspected by veterinary services at the abattoir. The origin of each animal was controlled, and its sanitary status was recorded on its individual passport: the animals were certified to be free of bTB, leucosis, brucellosis, and infectious bovine rhinotracheitis.

Bacterial Strains and Growth Conditions
Strains Mb AF2122/97 and Mb MB3601 had previously been isolated from infected cows in Great Britain and France, respectively (12, 15). The Mb3601-EGFP fluorescent strain was derived by electroporation with an integrative plasmid expressing EGFP and selected with Hygromycin B (50 μg/ml) (Sigma, USA) as described previously (34). Mtb BTB1558 had been previously isolated from a zebu bull in Ethiopia (13). Bacteria were grown in Middlebrook 7H9 broth (Difco, UK) supplemented with 10% BBLTM Middlebrook albumin–dextrose–catalase (BD, USA) and 0.05% Tween 80 (Sigma-Aldrich, St Louis, USA). At mid-log phase, the bacteria were harvested, aliquoted, and stored at −80°C. Batch titers were determined by plating serial dilutions on Middlebrook 7H11 agar supplemented with 10% oleic acid–albumin–dextrose–catalase (BD, USA), with 0.5% glycerol or 4.16 g/L sodium pyruvate (Sigma, USA) added for Mtb or Mb strains, respectively. The plates were incubated at 37°C for 3–4 weeks

(H37Rv, BTB558, and AF2122) and up to 6 weeks for Mb3601 before colony-forming unit (CFU) numeration. The inocula were prepared from one frozen aliquot (titer determined by CFU numeration) that was thawed in 7H9 medium without glycerol and incubated overnight at 37°C. After centrifugation for 10 min at $3,000 \times g$, the concentration was adjusted to 10^6 CFU/ml in RPMI medium.

Obtention and Infection of Precision-Cut Lung Slices
PCLS were obtained from fresh lungs using a tissue slicer, MD 6000 (Alabama Research and Development). For each animal, the right accessory lobe was filled via the bronchus with RPMI containing 1.5% low-melting-point (LMP) agarose (Invitrogen) warmed at 39°C. After 20 min at 4°C, the solidified lung tissue was cut in 1.5-cm slices with a scalpel. A 0.8-mm diameter-punch was used to obtain biopsies that were placed in the microtome device of the Krumdieck apparatus, filled with cold phosphate-buffered saline (PBS), and 100-μm-thick PCLS were cut. One PCLS was introduced in each well of a 24-well plate (Nunc); 1 ml of RPMI 1640 (Gibco) supplemented with 10% heat-inactivated fetal calf serum (FCS, Gibco), 2 mM L-glutamine (Gibco), and PANTA™ antibiotic mixture (polymyxin B, amphotericin B, nalidixic acid, trimethoprim, and azlocillin; Becton Dickinson) was added to the well, and the plate was incubated at 37°C with 5% CO_2. The medium was changed every 30 min during the first 2 h to remove all traces of LMP agarose. At 24 h later, after the last medium change, ciliary activity was observed under a microscope to ensure tissue viability.

The PCLS were infected for 2 days with 10^5 CFU of Mb or Mtb strains. As indicated, the PCLS were either fixed in formalin for imaging or lysed with a Precellys in lysing matrix D tubes in 800 μl Tri-reagent for RNA extraction. The bacillary load of each strain present in the PCLS was compared after the transfer of the PCLS to a new plate at 1 day after infection (dpi), two washes in 1 ml of PBS, and homogenization in 1 ml of PBS in lysing matrix D tubes (MP Biomedicals) with a Precellys (Ozyme). To determine CFUs, serial dilutions were plated as described above.

Alveolar Macrophages
To harvest alveolar macrophages (AMPs) from Blonde d'Aquitaine cows, broncho-alveolar lavages (BAL) were performed on the left basilar lobe of the lung at a local abattoir after culling the animal. The lobe was filled with 2×500 ml of cold PBS containing 2 mM EDTA (Sigma-Aldrich). After the massage, the BAL was collected and transported at 4°C to the laboratory. BAL was filtered with a 100-μm cell strainer (Falcon) and centrifuged for 10 min at $300 \times g$. The cells were washed in RPMI medium supplemented with 10% heat-inactivated fetal calf serum (Gibco), 2 mM L-glutamine (Gibco), and PANTA™ Antibiotic Mixture. Then, 10^7 BAL cells per milliliter were suspended in 90% FCS and 10% dimethyl sulfoxide (Sigma-Aldrich) and cryopreserved in liquid nitrogen. At 1 day before infection, the BAL cells were thawed at 37°C, washed in complete RPMI medium, and transferred to a 75-cm² culture flask with a ventilated cap. After 2 h at 37°C and 5% CO_2, non-adherent cells were removed, and adherent AMPs were incubated 2×10 min

at 4°C with 10 ml of cold PBS to detach and enumerate them in a Malassez chamber. Then, 5×10^5 AMPs/well were distributed in a 24-well plate and incubated overnight at 37°C and 5% CO_2. The medium was changed once, and AMPs were infected with Mb3601 or Mtb H37Rv at a multiplicity of infection (MOI) of 1. At 6 and 24 h post-infection, the supernatants were filtered through a 0.2-μm filter, and the cells were lysed in 800 μl of Tri-reagent for RNA extraction. The MOI was checked by CFU determination at 24 h after infection.

Cell Supernatant Collection and Lactate Dehydrogenase Assay

In order to evaluate cytotoxicity, supernatants from infected PCLS or AMPs were passed through a 0.2-μm filter at indicated time points, and cells were lysed in 1 ml of lysis buffer (5 mM EDTA, 150 mM NaCl, 50 mM Tris-HCl, Triton 1%, pH 7.4), containing anti-proteases (Roche), in a lysing matrix D tube, with a Precellys apparatus. The homogenates were clarified by centrifugation for 10 min at $10,000 \times g$, filtered through 0.2 μm, and collected on microplates. The cytotoxicity of infection in PCLS was assessed using the Non-radioactive Cytotoxicity Assay kit (Promega) according to the manufacturer's instructions. The cytotoxicity was calculated as cytotoxicity (%) = [OD_{490} of lactate dehydrogenase (LDH) in the supernatant]/(OD_{490} of LDH in the supernatant + OD_{490} of LDH in the PCLS homogenates) × 100.

Immunohistochemistry on PCLS

The infected PCLS were fixed 24 h at 4°C with 4% formalin and then transferred to a 48-well culture plate in PBS. All steps that will be described below were done under gentle agitation at room temperature (RT). The PCLS were incubated for 2 h with 100 μl of PBS, 0.25% Triton X-100, and 10% horse serum for permeabilization and saturation (saturation buffer). They were incubated overnight at 4°C with primary Ab (anti-bovine MHCII clone MCA5655 from BioRad and anti-bovine pancytokeratine clone BM4068 from Acris) diluted in saturation buffer. The PCLS were washed four times with 300 μl of PBS (two times for 5 min and then two times for 10 min) and then incubated for 3 h with fluorescent-conjugated secondary antibodies diluted in saturation buffer (goat anti-mouse IgG1-APC and goat anti-mouse IgG2a A555 from Invitrogen). The PCLS were washed four times with 300 μl of PBS (two times for 5 min and then two times for 10 min), transferred on cover slides which were mounted with Fluoromount-G™ mounting medium containing DAPI (Invitrogen), and sealed with a transparent nail polish. Z-stack imaging was performed at ×63 enlargement with a confocal microscope (LEICA) and analyzed with LAS software. The presence/absence of Mb and number of macrophages per alveoli were numerated by eye at the confocal microscope, with one person counting and the other confirming and reporting the data.

Quantification of Cytokines and Chemokines Released by PCLS and AMPs

The cytokine and chemokine levels produced by PCLS after 2 dpi were assessed in a Multiplex assay in supernatants (dilution 1:2) with MILLIPLEX® Bovine cytokine/chemokine panel 1 (BCYT1-33K-PX15, Merck) according to the manufacturer's

instructions. IFNγ, IL-1α, IL-1β, IL-4, IL-6, IL-8 (CXCL8), IL-10, IL-17A, IL-36RA (IL-1F5), IP-10 (CXCL10), MCP-1 (CCL2), MIP-1α (CCL3), MIP-1β (CCL4), TNFα, and VEGF-A were measured. Data were acquired using a MagPix instrument (Luminex) and analyzed with Bio-Plex Manager software (Bio-Rad). IL-8 was out of range in the Multiplex, so we performed a sandwich ELISA with the following references: goat anti-bovine interleukin-8 Ab AHP2817, recombinant bovine interleukin-8 PBP039, and goat anti-bovine interleukin-8 Ab conjugated to biotin AHP2817B (all from Bio-Rad), following the protocol according to the manufacturer's instructions.

RNA Extraction and Gene Expression Analysis

The total RNA from two pooled PCLS was extracted using a MagMAX™-96 Total RNA isolation kit (ThermoFisher). For AMPs, we used the Nucleospin RNA isolation kit (Macherey Nagel). After DNase treatment (ThermoFisher or Macherey Nagel), the mRNAs were reverse-transcribed with iScript™ Reverse Transcriptase mix (Biorad) according to the manufacturer's instructions. The primers (Eurogenetec; **Supplementary Table 1**) were validated, using a serially diluted pool of cDNA mix obtained from bovine lung, lymph nodes, blood, and bone marrow, with a LightCycler® 480 Real-Time PCR System (Roche). Gene expression was then assessed with the BioMark HD (Fluidigm) in 96 × 96-well integrated fluidic circuit plate according to the manufacturer's instructions. The annealing temperature was 60°C. The data were analyzed with Fluidigm RealTime PCR software to determine the cycle threshold (Ct) values. The messenger RNA (mRNA) expression was normalized to the mean expression of three housekeeping genes (*PPIA*, *GAPDH*, and *ACTB*) to obtain the ΔCt value. For each animal, values from infected PCLS were normalized to the uninfected PCLS gene expression (ΔΔCt value and relative quantity = $2^{-\Delta\Delta Ct}$). Principal component analysis (PCA) was performed using ΔΔCt values in R studio (version 1.1.456, ©2009–2018 RStudio, PBC) using the FactoMineR packages (version R 3.5.3).

Statistical Analysis

The individual data and the median and interquartile range are presented in the figures, except for **Figure 2** where the mean and standard error of the mean (SEM) are presented. Statistical analyses were performed with Prism 6.0 software (GraphPad). Analyses were performed on data from two to six independent experiments, with two-way ANOVA or Wilcoxon non-parametric tests for paired samples used. The represented p-values were $*p < 0.05$, $**p < 0.01$, and $***p < 0.001$.

RESULTS

Ex vivo Infection With Mycobacteria of Live Bovine Lung Tissue in PCLS Allows Bacilli Uptake by AMPs and Their Recruitment to the Alveoli

The early events of bTB pathophysiology in the bovine lung remain poorly defined due to the complexity of biocontained experimental infection in large animals. Since PCLS have been

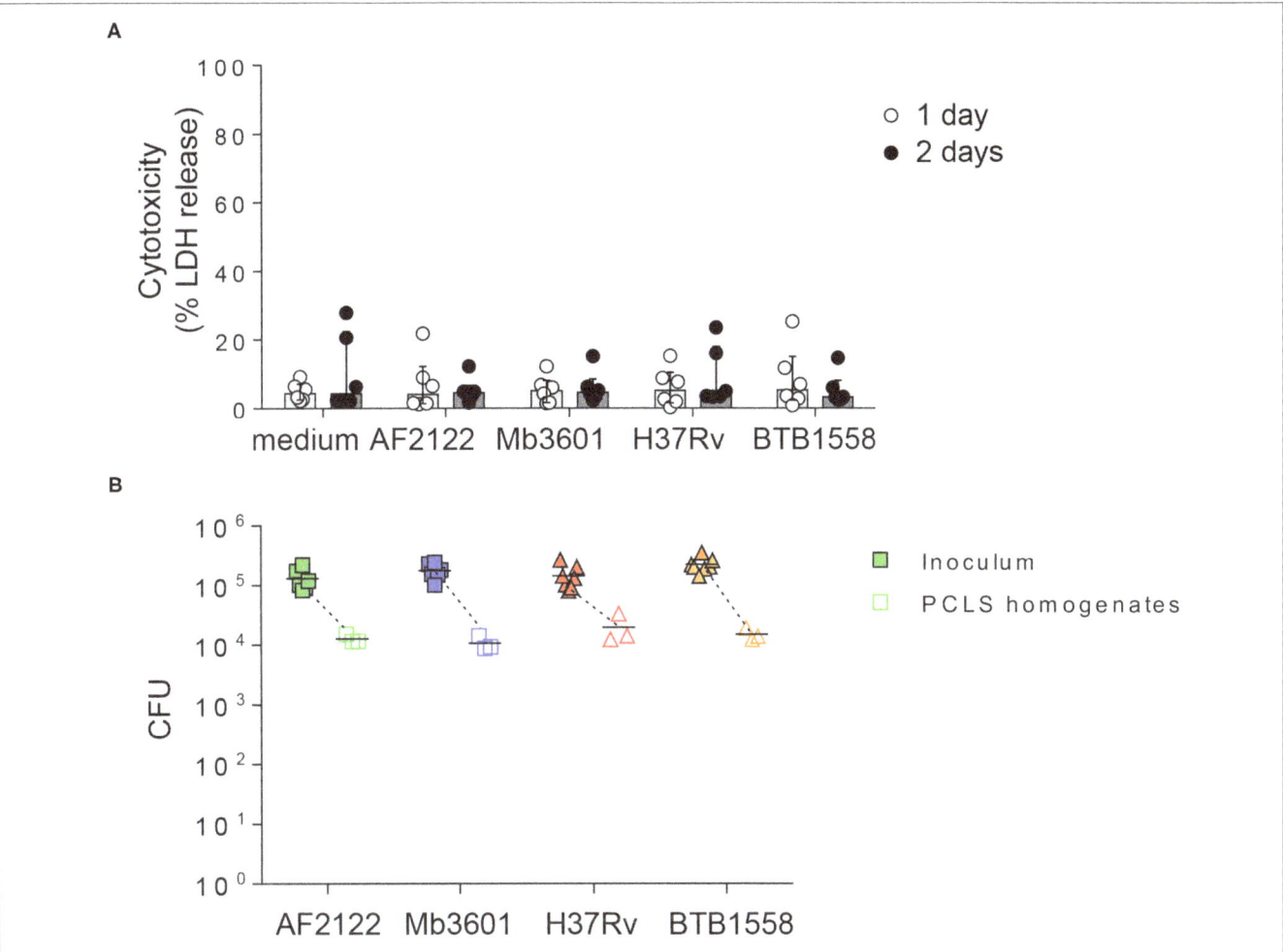

FIGURE 1 | Precision-cut lung slice (PCLS) infection with four different Mb or Mtb strains does not induce lung tissue cytotoxicity, and equivalent numbers of bacilli are recovered 24 h post-infection. **(A)** PCLS prepared from Blonde d'Aquitaine lungs post-mortem were infected with 10^5 CFU of two Mb strains (AF2122 or Mb3601) or two Mtb strains (H37Rv or BTB1558). After 1 and 2 days post-infection, the PCLS supernatants were harvested, and tissue was homogenized. Lactate dehydrogenase (LDH) was measured in both compartments using the "non-radioactive cytotoxicity assay" kit. Cytotoxicity was determined as (%) = (O.D. 490 nm LDH in supernatant)/(O.D. 490 nm LDH in supernatant + O.D. 490 nm LDH in PCLS homogenates) × 100. Individual data and the median and interquartile range in each group are presented ($n = 6$ animals from six independent experiments). **(B)** At 24 h post-infection, the PCLS were washed and homogenized to recover bacilli. The inoculum and PCLS homogenates were serially diluted and plated with colony-forming units numerated after 3–6 weeks of incubation. Individual data and the mean in each group are presented ($n = 6$ independent inocula prepared; PCLS homogenates data represent the mean of technical duplicates from $n = 3$ animals from three independent experiments).

used to study viral respiratory infections in the bovine (27), we decided to use this model to assess early events taking place following entry of Mb into the lung. We infected bovine PCLS obtained *ex vivo* with the four mycobacterial strains: Mb AF2122, Mb3601, Mtb H37Rv, or BTB1558.

We first monitored tissue cytotoxicity at 1 and 2 dpi using a LDH release assay. The mean percentage of cytotoxicity remained below 10%, and no difference was observed between infected and non-infected PCLS (**Figure 1A**). The ciliary activity from the PCLS bronchial cells monitored every day under a light microscope remained vigorous and stable after infection (data not shown). We calibrated our model and inocula to use 10^5 CFUs for each of the four different strains. We analyzed CFUs still present in PCLS at 24 h later and observed an equivalent

1 log decrease for all strains (**Figure 1B**). This indicated an equivalent infection by all strains, allowing them to be directly compared. Therefore, with a similar bacterial load and excellent tissue viability in all experimental conditions, we validated PCLS as a model to study the early events taking place in the bovine lung after infection with mycobacteria.

In order to visualize the interactions taking place between bacilli and lung cells, we infected the PCLS with a fluorescent version of the Mb3601 strain, and at 1 and 2 dpi, we analyzed the cells by *in situ* immunohistochemistry. The lung structure was visualized by DAPI and pancytokeratine staining, and we used confocal microscopy to image 10–15-μm sections and localize Mb3601-EGFP (**Figure 2A**). We observed Mb in 27 ± 3% of PCLS alveoli (**Figures 2A,B**) and almost always in

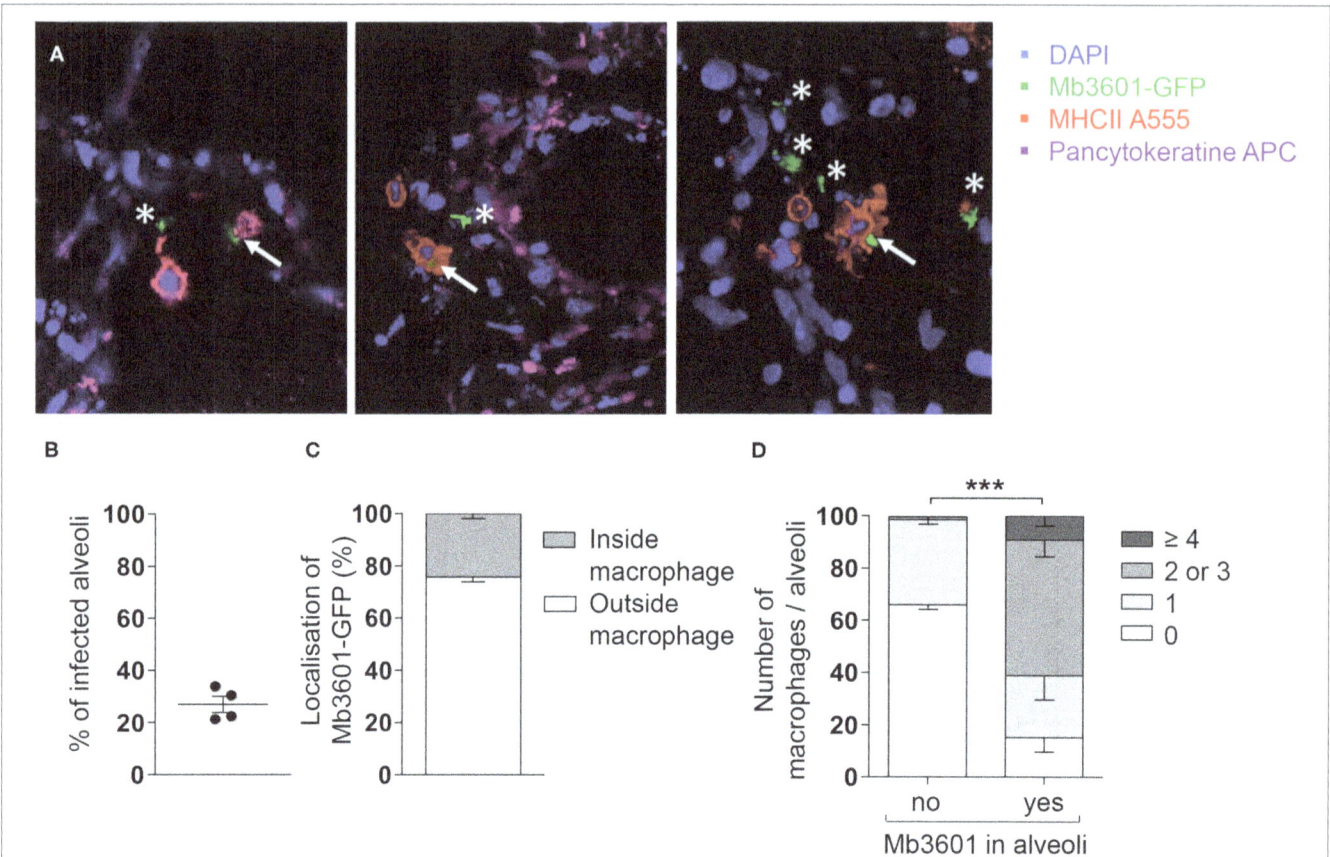

FIGURE 2 | Mb3601 is internalized by alveolar macrophages (AMPs) in the preserved lung structure from precision-cut lung slice (PCLS), and the infected alveoli contain higher numbers of AMPs compared to non-infected alveoli. The PCLS were infected with 10^5 colony-forming units of the green fluorescent protein Mb3601-GFP recombinant strain and fixed 2 days later. After labeling with anti-pancytokeratine (magenta) and anti-MHCII antibodies (Alexa 555, red), the PCLS were mounted with Fluoromount-G^{TM} mounting medium containing DAPI (blue) and analyzed under a Leica confocal microscope **(A)**; 3D images were analyzed with Leica LAS software. Z-stack imaging was performed at ×63 enlargement (10–15 μm in thickness, step size of 0.5–1 μm). The white asterisks indicate extracellular bacilli, and the white arrows indicate bacilli inside MHC-II^{pos} AMPs. **(B)** The graph represents the percentage of infected alveoli per PCLS among the 55–80 alveoli that were observed under the microscope (*n* = 4 PCLS from two different Blonde d'Aquitaine cattle). **(C)** Stack histogram of the mean percentage ± SEM of intra- or extracellular bacilli among a minimum of 15 infected alveoli that were observed (*N* = 4 PCLS). **(D)** The number of MHC-II^{pos} AMPs per alveoli was counted in infected or non-infected alveoli. The data presented as percent are the mean ± SEM of *n* = 4 PCLS from two different Blonde d'Aquitaine cattle. Between 55 and 80 alveoli were observed to obtain these data (two-way ANOVA, ***p < 0.001).

close contact with large MHC-II-positive AMPs. The bacilli were localized outside AMPs in 76 ± 2% observations and resided intracellularly in AMPs in 24 ± 2% (**Figures 2A,C** and **Supplementary Video 1**). Interestingly, the number of AMPs per alveoli differed upon bacilli presence or absence (**Figure 2D**). In uninfected PCLS, lung alveoli generally contained one AMP (data not shown). However, in Mb-infected PCLS, we either observed no AMPs in 66 ± 2% of alveoli or one AMP in 33 ± 2% of alveoli in the absence of any Mb. On the contrary, the number of AMPs significantly increased in alveoli where at least one Mb was observed (**Figure 2D**, p < 0.001). The number of AMPs varied among infected alveoli, with 24 ± 9% containing one AMP, 52 ± 6% containing two or three AMPs, and 9 ± 4% containing more than four AMPs. Such observations indicated that, during the 2 days of infection, AMPs were recruited from one alveolus to another in response to signals linked to Mb infection. In conclusion, even though Mb infection

was performed *ex vivo*, bacilli were observed in the alveoli, close or inside their target host cell, i.e., the AMP. Moreover, the PCLS model was physiological enough to allow AMPs to crawl in response to signals linked to bacilli entry.

The Lung Response to Mycobacterial Infection Vastly Differs Between Blonde d'Aquitaine and Charolaise Cows

Two bovine beef breeds are widely used in France: Blonde d'Aquitaine and Charolaise. We decided to compare how these two breeds respond to mycobacterial infection, using our PCLS system. We measured 15 cytokines and chemokines secreted by the lung tissue at 2 dpi with the four mycobacterial strains and performed a PCA. As depicted in **Figure 3A**, the PCA revealed important differences in the immune response of the lung tissue between the two breeds. The group samples clearly

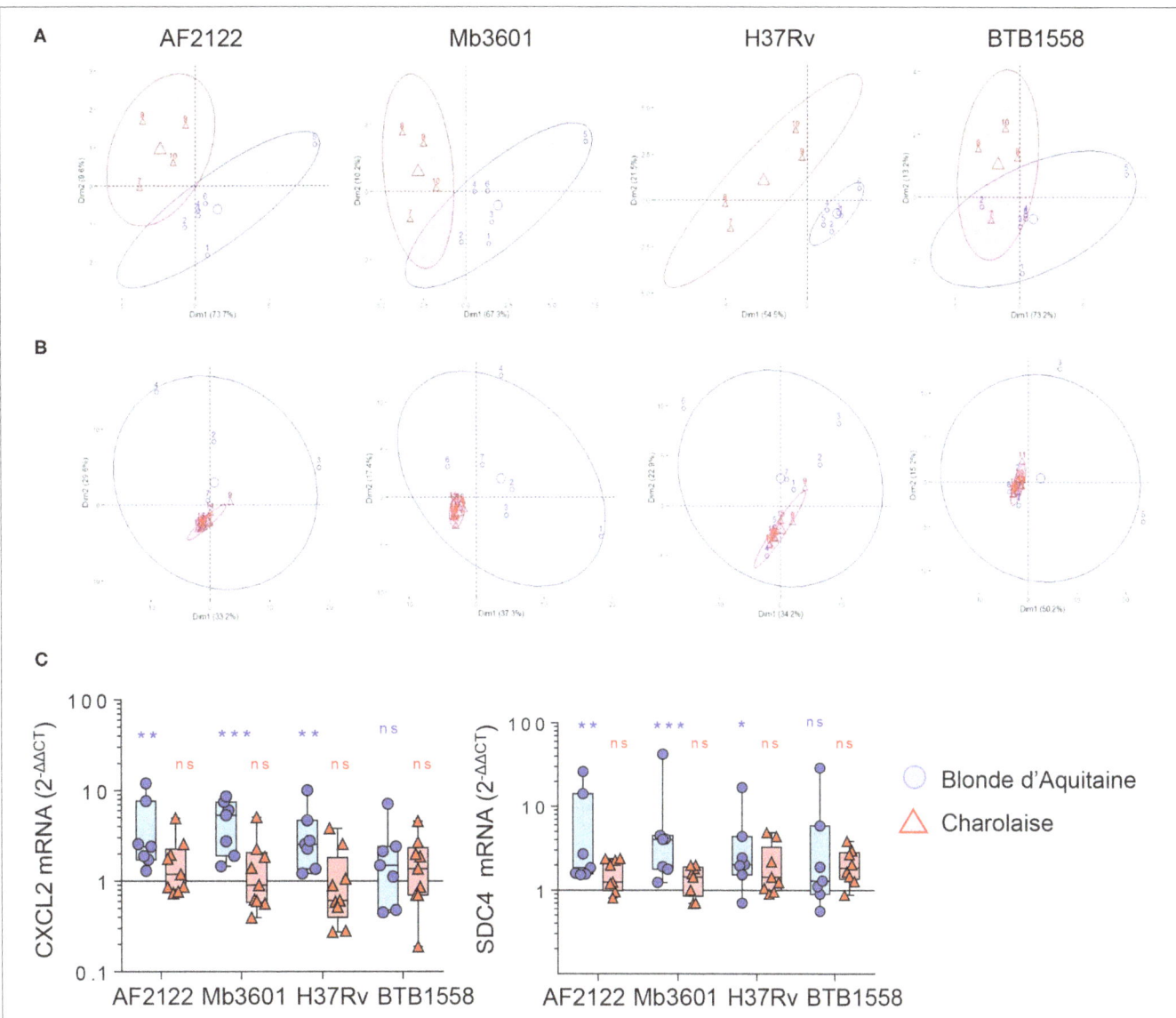

FIGURE 3 | Principal component analysis (PCA) of inflammatory lung tissue signature reveals differences between two beef cattle breeds after 2 days of infection by Mb or Mtb. **(A)** Fifteen cytokines and chemokines were measured in PCLS supernatants from Blonde d'Aquitaine or Charolaise cows 2 days after infection with four different mycobacterial strains. Raw data were used to run PCA in R studio. Individual data are shown ($n = 4$ for Charolaise, red; $n = 6$ for Blonde d'Aquitaine, blue). The ellipses represent a confidence range of 90%. **(B)** PCA were built from the expression data of 96 genes ($2^{-\Delta\Delta Ct}$) obtained from precision-cut lung slice total RNA extracted 2 days after infection. Individual data are shown ($n = 9$ for Charolaise, red; $n = 7$ for Blonde d'Aquitaine, blue). The ellipses represent a confidence range of 90%. **(C)** Two examples of differentially expressed genes. Individual data and the median and interquartile range in each group are presented ($n = 7$ Blonde d'Aquitaine and $n = 9$ Charolaise) $*p < 0.05$; $**p < 0.01$; $***p < 0.001$. Two-way ANOVA test.

plotted apart, and their ellipses showed either a small overlay (AF2122 and Mb360A) or no overlay at all (H37Rv). The results for the BTB1558 group showed less clustering of samples due to higher individual variations. We then extracted total RNA from PCLS after 1 or 2 dpi and analyzed the expression of 96 genes related to innate immunity and inflammation (see the full list in **Supplementary Table 1**). The RT-qPCR data were normalized and expressed as fold change compared to uninfected PCLS control for each cow. Gene expression was higher at 2 days after infection compared to that at 1 dpi (data not shown). We

therefore decided to focus our analysis on this 2-dpi time point. Remarkably, the transcriptomic signature induced by infection was very low for the Charolaise breed, whichever mycobacterial strain was used, which explains the clustering of Charolaise samples (**Figure 3B**). Increasing the inoculum in the Charolaise PCLS up to 5×10^6 CFU did not induce gene expression (**Supplementary Figure 2**). The response of the lung tissue to mycobacterial infection in Blonde d'Aquitaine was very different compared to that in Charolaise as revealed by a PCA (**Figure 3B**). Whereas, in PCLS from Charolaise the gene expression from

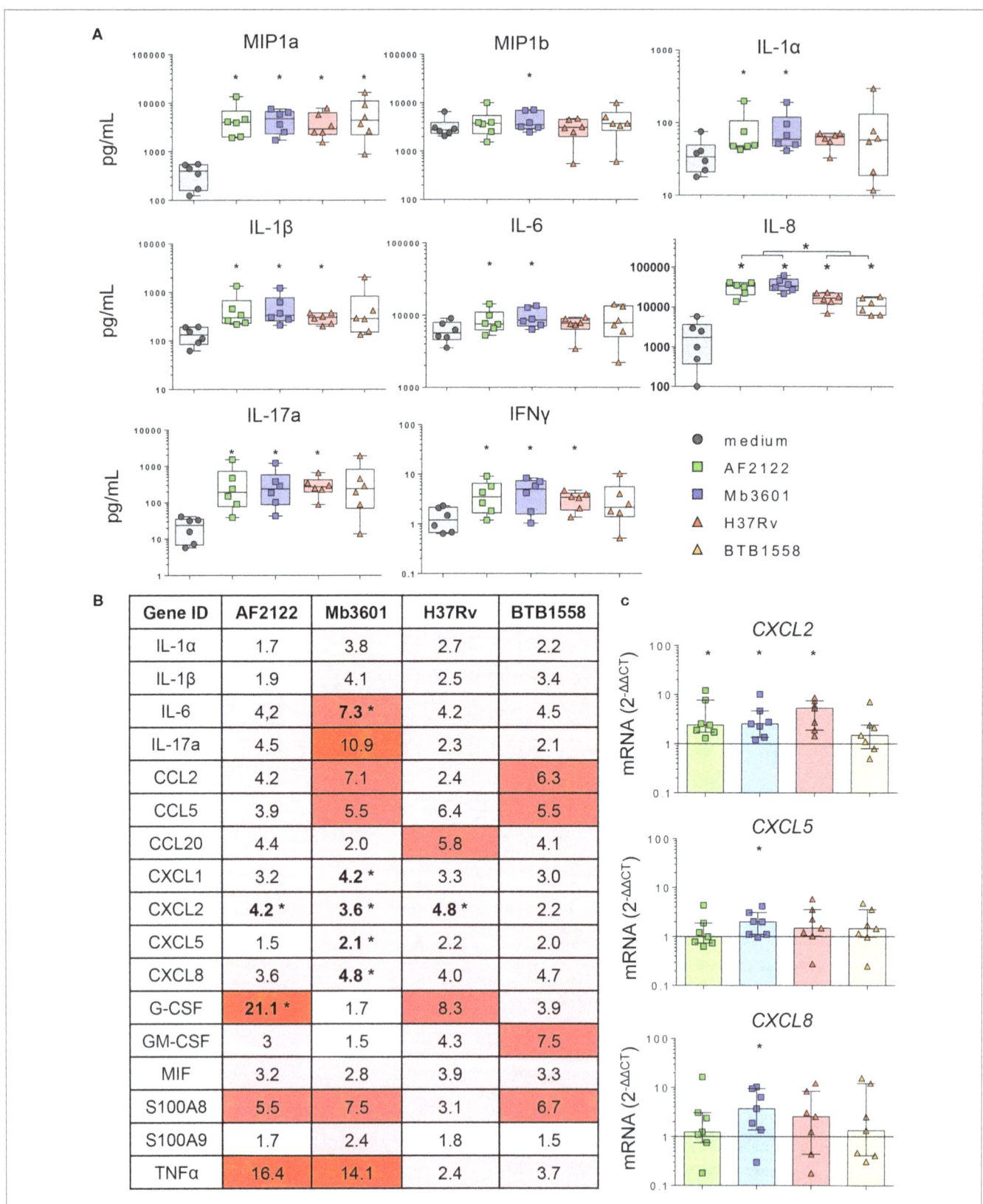

FIGURE 4 | The lung inflammatory neutrophil and monocyte recruitment signature induced by infection in precision-cut lung slice (PCLS) from Blonde d'Aquitaine cows is more efficiently triggered by *Mycobacterium bovis* than *Mycobacterium tuberculosis*. **(A)** The cytokine and chemokine levels were measured in PCLS

(Continued)

FIGURE 4 | supernatant by Multiplex ELISA 2 days after infection with two Mb or two Mtb strains. Individual data and the median and interquartile range in each group are presented ($n = 6$ cows). **(B)** Table of the mean of fold change ($2^{-\Delta\Delta CT}$) for each group ($n = 7$ cows) of 17 major genes involved in neutrophil and monocyte recruitment and inflammation. The graduated red box coloring represents levels of gene expression, and the asterisks mark significant differences compared to non-infected controls. **(C)** CXCL2, CXCL5, and CXCL8 gene expression at 2 days post-infection. Individual data and the median and interquartile range in each group are presented ($n = 7$ cows). **(B,C)** *$p < 0.05$ (Wilcoxon nonparametric test).

infected and non-infected controls clustered, in PCLS from Blonde d'Aquitaine, the gene expression levels were significantly more dispersed after infection compared to those of controls (**Figure 3B**). We compared the individual gene expression between the two breeds for a number of genes. For instance, both the CXCL2 chemokine and the mycobacteria receptor syndecan 4 SDC4 were significantly upregulated after PCLS infection with AF2122, Mb3601, or H37Rv in Blonde d'Aquitaine, but not in Charolaise (**Figure 3C**). Our data altogether revealed important differences in the early lung response to mycobacterial infection, depending on the breed of the animals, that could be measured both at the gene expression and protein production level in the PCLS system.

The Overall Inflammation Signature in the Lung Tissue Is Triggered More Efficiently by *M. bovis* Than *M. tuberculosis*

We then focused our analysis on Blonde d'Aquitaine to determine how the lung tissue responded to different mycobacterial strains. We analyzed 15 cytokines and chemokines produced in the PCLS supernatants 2 days following an infection. No IL-4 was detected, and the production of TNFα, IL-36RA, IL-10, VEGFA or MCP-1 was not different between infected PCLS and controls (**Supplementary Figure 3A**). We observed that *ex vivo* infection of PCLS with mycobacteria triggered an inflammatory response that contrasted between the strains (**Figure 4A**). At the protein level, the Mtb strain BTB1558 induced the most heterogenous response, and due to high individual variation, differences in chemokine/cytokine production between infected PCLS and controls only reached a statistical significance for MIP-1a (CCL3) and IL-8 (**Figure 4A**). These two inflammatory mediators were also strongly induced by all strains. IL-17A, IL-1β, and IFNγ were efficiently induced by mycobacterial infection, and no significant difference was observed between Mtb and Mb. By contrast, IL-6 and IL-1α were significantly induced after Mb, but not Mtb, infection, and IL-8 production was also significantly higher after Mb than Mtb infection (**Figure 4A**). The only strain able to induce a significant production of MIP-1b was Mb3601. We then analyzed the inflammatory transcriptomic signature using a panel of 17 genes involved in monocyte/macrophage and neutrophil recruitment (**Figure 4B**). A number of these genes was significantly upregulated upon PCLS infection even though significant differences were not always reached due to inter-individual variation. Remarkably, Mb3601 induced the strongest inflammatory response, with five out of 17 genes significantly upregulated compared to non-infected controls. Focusing on chemokines involved in neutrophil recruitment, we observed that CXCL2 expression was induced by all strains—except

BTB1558—whereas CXCL1, CXCL5, and CXCL8 were only upregulated by Mb3601 (**Figures 4B,C**). IL-6 expression was also high after Mb3601 infection. Therefore, the *ex vivo* infection of PCLS efficiently triggered signals involved in monocyte and neutrophil recruitment. Infection by Mb strains, more specifically the Mb3601 strain circulating in France, triggered inflammation in the bovine lung more efficiently than Mtb.

The Type I Interferon Pathway Is Induced in the Bovine Lung by Infection With *M. bovis*, but Not *M. tuberculosis*

Because in humans and mouse models susceptibility to mycobacterial infection and disease progression is driven by type I IFN (35–37), we decided to compare the induction of this pathway by Mtb and Mb strains in bovine lung tissue. We measured the expression of different genes involved in the type I IFN pathway in Blonde d'Aquitaine PCLS infected by the four mycobacterial strains (**Figure 5**). The gene expression of both IFNβ and the IFNAR1 receptor was significantly increased after Mb but not Mtb infection (**Figures 5A,C**). Similarly, the major IFN-stimulated genes (ISG) MX1, OAS1, ISG15, and CXCL10 were induced only after Mb infection (**Figures 5A,C**), and this difference was also detected at the protein level for CXCL10 (**Figures 5A,B**). Therefore, we observed the induction of a number of genes of the type I IFN pathway, recapitulated in **Figure 5D**, after infection with Mb, but not Mtb, strains. Strikingly, strain Mb3601 was the highest inducer of this pathway in the lung from Blonde d'Aquitaine cows.

Because AMPs are the most prominent host cells interacting with Mb (8), which we also observed in PCLS (**Figure 2**), we next decided to decipher if AMPs contributed to the induction of the type I IFN pathway after Mb3601 or H37Rv infection. At 1 day after the infection of AMPs with these two strains, similar bacterial levels were recovered (data not shown). At 6 h post-infection, no cell cytotoxicity was observed, and we analyzed the expression of genes from the type 1 IFN pathway at this early time point. While we did not observe differences in IFNAR1, IRF3, STAT1, nor ISG15 expression induced by the two strains (**Figure 6A**), IFNβ, LPG2, RIG1, and OAS1 were significantly induced after infection with Mb3601, but not H37Rv (**Figure 6B**). Regarding MX1, the same trend was observed, although statistical significance was not reached (**Figure 6B**, $p = 0.07$).

Interestingly, while CXCL10 was detected both at the mRNA and protein levels in PCLS infected with Mb (**Figure 5**), we did not detect the expression of this gene by AMPs in our analysis. These results altogether demonstrate that AMPs globally contribute to the type I IFN pathway in the lung after Mb infection, although other cells present in PCLS may also

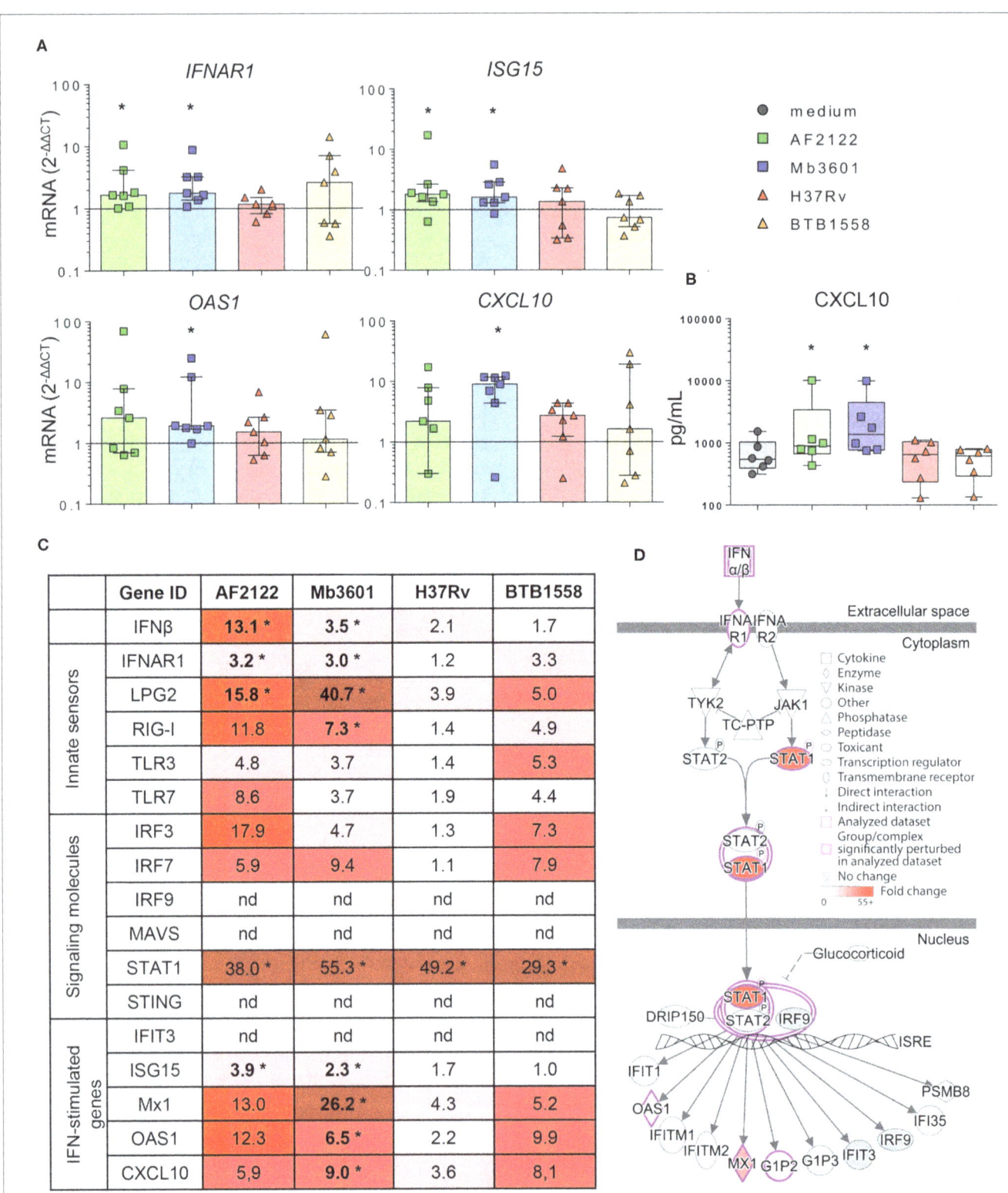

FIGURE 5 | Mb but not Mtb infection in the lung tissue from Blonde d'Aquitaine cows induces the type I interferon pathway. The precision-cut lung slice (PCLS) was infected as described in **Figure 1**. **(A)** *IFNAR*, ISG15, *CXCL10*, and *OAS1* gene expression at 2 dpi. Individual data and the median and interquartile range in each group are presented (*n* = 7). **(B)** CXCL10 protein level was measured in PCLS supernatant at 2 dpi. Individual data and the median and interquartile range in each group are presented (*n* = 6). **(C)** The table represents the mean of fold change (2^{-dCT}) for each group (*n* = 7) of major genes involved in type I interferon pathway. The graduated red box coloring is for higher gene expression, and the asterisks mark significant differences compared to uninfected PCLS. nd, not detected. **(D)** Ingenuity pathway analysis drawing of the type I interferon pathway under IFNAR in the Mb3601 group. The graduated red box coloring is for higher gene expression. **(A–C)** *p* < 0.05 (Wilcoxon nonparametric test).

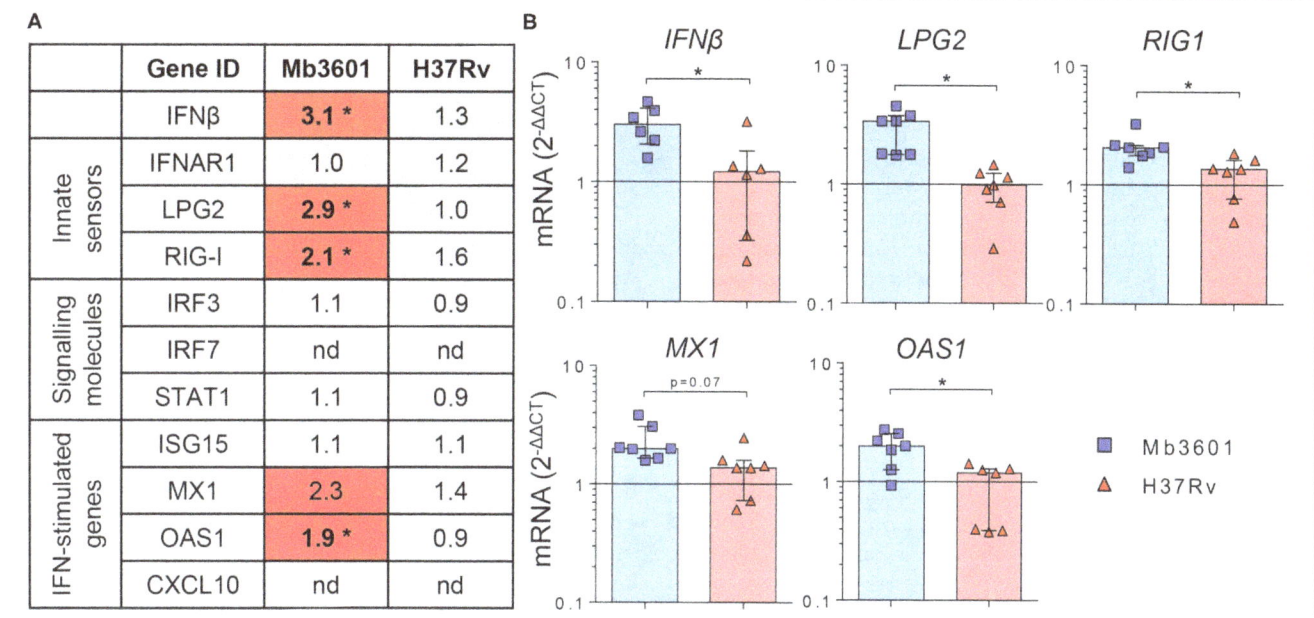

FIGURE 6 | Alveolar macrophages (AMP) from Blonde d'Aquitaine contribute to the type I IFN signature in the lung induced by Mb infection. AMPs from Blonde d'Aquitaine lungs were infected with 10^5 CFU of Mb3601 or Mtb H37Rv. At 6 h later, mRNA was extracted, and the expression of major genes from the type 1 IFN pathway was analyzed. **(A)** Mean fold change ($2^{-\Delta\Delta CT}$) of gene expression normalized to three housekeeping genes was calculated in each group ($n = 7$). The graduated red box coloring represents gene expression, and the asterisks mark significant differences compared to non-infected controls (nd, not detected). **(B)** *IFNβ*, *LPG2*, *RIG1*, *MX1*, and *OAS1* gene expression in AMPs was analyzed by RT-qPCR at 6 h post-infection. Individual data and the median and interquartile range in each group are presented ($n = 7$). **(A,B)** *$p < 0.05$ (Wilcoxon nonparametric test).

specifically induce some genes, such as *CXCL10* or *IRF7*, for example (**Figures 5C, 6A**).

DISCUSSION

The lung is the main organ targeted by Mb infection in cattle (38), and early interactions between the different lung cell types and the bacillus that govern the pathophysiology of the disease need to be better understood. In this study, we used PCLS for the first time to monitor the early bovine lung response to Mb infection and validated this model as a means to measure the local innate response at the protein and mRNA level. A main advantage of PCLS is conservation of the complex lung tissue both in structure and diversity of cell types. After infection with mycobacteria, the ciliary activity of bronchial cells was maintained. The AMP main function is to patrol the lung, crawling in and between alveoli; they sensed, chemotaxed, and phagocytosed debris or inhaled bacteria (39). We observed increased numbers of AMPs in alveoli where Mb was present, indicating AMP mobility inside the tissue. In chicken, PCLS allowed the observation of the movement of macrophages and phagocytosis (30). The AMP is well established as the main host cell for Mtb infection in humans (40) and Mb infection in cattle (41). Accordingly, in PCLS, we observed Mb inside AMPs in 20% of infected alveoli. We sometimes observed several bacilli inside one AMP. Although Mb is able to replicate inside this hostile cell, it is difficult to know if this observation was due to bacillary multiplication or the phagocytosis of several

bacilli. This issue would need live imaging of PCLS to follow the fate of fluorescent Mb, an approach which remains challenging under BSL3 conditions.

In uninfected PCLS, we observed generally one AMP for two to three alveoli [**Supplementary Figure 4**; in good correlation with the observations of Neupane et al. (39)]. After Mb infection, we observed several AMPs inside the same alveolus in 50% of cases. Moreover, when the alveoli contained more than four AMPs, they were in close contact. Multinucleated giant cells are formed by the fusion of several MPs and are a hallmark of TB pathophysiology. It has recently been demonstrated that, after infection of human or bovine blood-derived MPs by Mb or Mtb, only Mb was able to induce the formation of multinucleated cells (26). Although at 2 dpi we did not observe the formation of such cells in PCLS, it would be interesting to analyze if such events could be detected after longer infection periods. Goris et al. have maintained bovine PCLS during 1 week to study viral infections (27).

One other advantage of our model is the preserved diversity of lung cell composition. PCLS contain type I and II pneumocytes, endothelial cells, and bronchial cells (**Supplementary Figure 4**) and also produce key molecules like surfactant, which has an established role in Mtb uptake (42). Mtb is also capable of invading type II alveolar epithelial cells (23) that play important roles in host defense (20–22). In our study, we did not observe intraepithelial Mb, but specific labeling of bovine epithelial cells would be required to investigate interactions between bovine lung pneumocytes and Mb in more detail. However, as we have observed that infected AMPs were in close contact with epithelial cells in PCLS, this model will allow a more refined analysis of the crosstalk between AMPs and pneumocytes during Mb infection (24).

One limitation of the PCLS model is the lack of recruitment of immune cells from circulating blood. During mycobacterial infection, in response to local signals, a variety of immune cells are recruited to the infection site to form the mature granuloma that constrains bacillary multiplication. How this response is orchestrated at the level of the lung tissue in cattle remains poorly established. Neutrophils, together with other innate cells, such as macrophages, γδ-T lymphocytes, and natural killer cells, were recently identified as key immune cells in the early containment of infection (43) and development of early lesions (44). Moreover, humans regularly exposed to Mtb or cattle exposed to Mb do not always develop signs of infection, i.e., remain negative in IFNg-release assay or skin testing. In humans, such resistance to infection through the successful elimination of bacilli could be mediated by neutrophils (45). Similarly, in cattle experimentally infected with Mb, some contact animals resist infection, while others develop lesions due to productive infection (46). It is possible that neutrophils could also play an important role in the early elimination of Mb in cattle (43). Immune signals involved in the early recruitment of neutrophils to the lung after the entry of Mb need to be better understood in cattle. It is known that epithelial cells secrete, among other cytokines and chemokines, MIP1 and CXCL8 that attract MPs and neutrophils to the site of infection. Interestingly, we measured important differences in the production of such mediators by PCLS in response to different strains of mycobacteria that could be linked to variable virulence. Although one cattle type II pneumocyte cell line has been described (47), such transformed cells are less physiologically relevant than primary cells. Recently, immortalized type II cells were co-cultured with endothelial cells as a model of the bovine alveolus to study mycobacterial interactions with BCG. In this study, the authors detected the production of IL-8, TNFα, IL-22, and IL-17a. One limitation of this model was epithelial cell death, which occurred shortly after infection (48). As a physiological model, PCLS could help in understanding the early orchestration of the local inflammatory response in the lung in response to mycobacterial infection.

Resistance to bTB is linked to the host genetics. Zebu breeds (*Bos indicus*) are more resistant to bTB disease than *Bos taurus*-derived breeds (49). Our results with PCLS, as a physiological model of the early lung response to infection, demonstrated striking differences between Blonde d'Aquitaine and Charolaise, emphasizing the importance of host genetics in response to Mb. It is not known whether the stronger inflammatory response of the Blonde d'Aquitaine tissue is associated with a greater sensitivity or resistance to Mb infection. While robust immunological responses are associated with an increased pathology at the level of the animal (31), at the cellular level, blood-derived MPs from animals with greater resistance to bTB (and that kill BCG more efficiently than cells from susceptible animals) produce higher levels of the pro-inflammatory mediators iNOS, IL-1β, TNFα, MIP1, and MIP3 (25). Although genetic selection of cattle would greatly complement bTB management and

surveillance programs to control and ultimately eradicate the disease, especially in countries with the highest burden (50, 51), biomarkers to evaluate the resistance or susceptibility of cattle to Mb infection are critically missing. Some genomic regions and candidate genes have been identified in Holstein-Friesian cows, the most common dairy breed (52), and not surprisingly, these candidates are often involved in inflammation. A genomic region on chromosome 23, containing genes involved in the TNFα/NFκ-B signaling pathway, was strongly associated with host susceptibility to bTB infection (53). However, large within-breed analyses of Charolaise, Limousine, and Holstein-Friesian cattle identified 38 SNPs and 64 QTL regions associated with bTB susceptibility to infection (54). The genotyping of 1966 Holstein-Friesian dairy cows that were positive by skin test and either did or did not harbor visible bTB lesions, together with their skin test negative matched controls, led to the conclusion that these variable phenotypes following Mb exposure were governed by distinct and overlapping genetic variants (55). Thus, variation in the pathology of Mb seems to be controlled by a large number of loci and a combination of small effects. Similar conclusions were drawn from the genetic studies of human tuberculosis (56). In areas where Mb is highly prevalent, recurrent exposure to Mb may also imprint the bovine genome, and epigenetics could also contribute to the immune response in certain breeds. In France, the Nouvelle Aquitaine region accounted for 80% of Mb outbreaks last year. Interestingly, Blonde d'Aquitaine breed is very abundant in this area (**Figure 7**). Together with Limousine, another very abundant beef breed in this region, they contribute to most bTB outbreaks in Nouvelle Aquitaire (bovine tuberculosis national reference laboratory communication). In the future, comparisons between Blonde d'Aquitaine and Limousine would be interesting. In our study, Blonde d'Aquitaine or Charolaise cows were sampled from eight different French departments, none with recurrent Mb outbreaks, rendering previous exposure to Mb unlikely. Moreover, the breeding management was similar for the two breeds, as far as we could ascertain, suggesting that exposure to environment and possible wildlife sources would be comparable. We nevertheless observed striking differences in the early lung response to Mb infection between these two breeds, pointing to the possible control of Mb infection at the genetic or epigenetic level. Whether some cattle breeds are more susceptible to bTB than others remains an open question that deserves future studies with more consequent animal sampling. We furthermore believe that the PCLS model could greatly contribute to unraveling the role of tissue-level protective responses that would, in turn, reveal important biomarkers.

In addition to the cattle breed, our study pointed toward differences in the host response to distinct mycobacterial strains. The Mb strains were better inducers of a lung immune response than Mtb in cattle, which is in agreement with a previous work showing that Mtb H37Rv was attenuated *in vivo* in cattle compared to Mb AF2122 (13). *In vitro* studies with bovine AMPs infected with AF2122 or H37Rv revealed differences in the innate cytokine profiles: the CCL4, IL-1β, IL-6, and TNFα levels were more elevated in response to AF2122 than H37Rv (8), which is in agreement with our data. Interestingly, Mb3601,

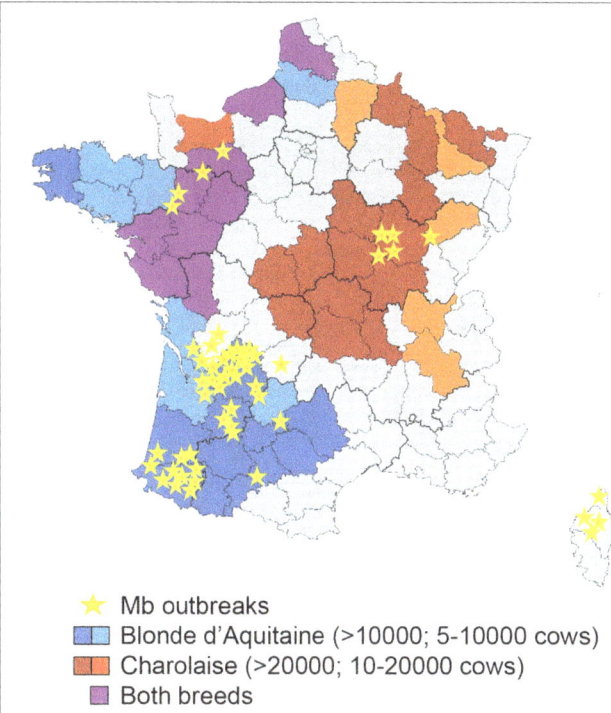

FIGURE 7 | Superposition of Blonde d'Aquitaine and Charolaise beef breeds in French counties where Mb outbreaks were declared between December 2019 and 2020. This map of France shows the counties where Mb outbreaks were declared between December 2019 and December 2020 (yellow stars) and was obtained with data extracted from https://www.plateforme-esa.fr/. Herd densities of Blonde d'Aquitaine (blue), Charolaise (red), or both breeds (violet) were extracted from data obtained from https://www.racesdefrance.fr/ (cows above 3 years old have been considered).

a representative strain of a highly successful genetic cluster that circulates both in cattle and wildlife in France (16), induced an inflammatory signature in the lung more efficiently than Mb AF2122. Whether this correlates with differences in Mb virulence in cattle or other mammals remains to be investigated; but, if this were the case, the PCLS model would be a practical tool to study and compare the virulence of Mb field strains compared to the *in vivo* experimental infection of cattle. Contrary to Mtb which is mostly restricted to humans, Mb is adapted to sustain across a large host range through repeated cycles of infection and transmission (57, 58). This remarkable trait is due to pathogen molecular genetic changes (59) that allow adapted bacilli to manipulate the host immune response to establish infection and disease and ultimately transmit infection to new, susceptible hosts (60, 61). We observed a weaker inflammation in the bovine lung after infection with Mtb compared to Mb, and it will be interesting to compare the ability of Mtb and Mb to induce inflammation in human PCLS obtained post-surgery. This latter comparative analysis could give clues on the links between lung innate inflammatory responses and host adaptation during TB.

Our most striking observation was the Mb-restricted induction of the type I IFN pathway in the bovine lung. This is in agreement with previous studies in bovine AMPs where cytosolic

DNA-sensing pathways, in particular, RIG-I, were activated after 48 h of infection by Mb AF2122, but not Mtb H37Rv (32). In agreement with our data, these authors also demonstrated an induction of the RIG-I signaling pathway by Mb in AMPs (62). Therefore, AMPs contribute to type I IFN signaling in the lung. However, we also noticed differences between PCLS and AMPs in the induction of the IFN signature by Mb: for example, CXCL10 was detected in PCLS, but not in AMPs, in our study, which may be due to the time point used (63). However, it is also possible that other cells involved in crosstalk with AMPs contributed to CXCL10 production in response to Mb infection. Since CXCL10 has been proposed as a diagnostic biomarker of Mb infection in cattle (64), it will be interesting to better understand how this key mediator is regulated. Type I interferon favors Mb survival, and its induction may be a good manipulation strategy for the maintenance of infection. This manipulation mechanism, deciphered *in vitro* in murine bone marrow monocyte-derived MPs, involves the triggering of autophagy by cytosolic Mb DNA, in turn inducing IFNβ production. Autophagy antagonizes inflammasome activation to the benefit of Mb survival (65, 66). In C57BL/6 mice treated with IFNAR1 blocking Ab and infected with Mb, the recruitment of neutrophils was reduced, but the pro-inflammatory profile of MPs was increased, leading to a reduced bacillary burden (67). No impact on T-cells was observed in this *in vivo* model, revealing a role of type I IFN signaling during the innate phase of the host response to infection. Therefore, Mb exploits type I IFN signaling in many ways, and this pathway seems an important avenue to better understand Mb virulence. The PCLS model will greatly help to better dissect out this pathway in the lung during bTB. This could lead to new biomarkers to help genomic selection programs for cattle that are more resistant to bTB as well as new immunostimulation strategies counteracting the type I IFN pathway. This new knowledge will ultimately improve bTB control, a goal which is so greatly needed at the global level (68).

ETHICS STATEMENT

Ethical review and approval was not required for the animal study because We only used post-mortem sampling at commercial abattoir.

AUTHOR CONTRIBUTIONS

AR designed and did most of the experiments, obtained funding, analyzed the data, prepared all the figures, and wrote the manuscript. FC performed experiments and prepared the inocula for experimental infections under BSL3 conditions. AC cultured AMPs and performed ELISA and q-RT-PCR. ED-D helped in PCLS experiments and revised the figures. MB provided the

Mb3601 strain and revised the manuscript. AA provided the strain Mtb BTB1558. JB improved the RNA extraction protocol. DD and QM performed multiple experiments, and revised the manuscript. FA provided Ab and critically reviewed the imaging data. PG helped with transcriptomic analysis and revised the manuscript. SG obtained funding, designed the experiments, and revised the manuscript. NW obtained funding, supervised all aspects of the work, critically analyzed the data, and wrote the manuscript. All the authors read and approved the manuscript before publication.

FUNDING

This work was supported by the Veterinary Biocontained research facility Network (VETBIONET), the ANR EpiLungCell (grant ANR-17-CE20-0018), and FEDER/Region Centre Val de Loire ANIMALT grant (FEDER convention number EX007516, Region Centre convention number 2019-00134936, research program number AE-2019-1850). Mobilities between France and Ireland were supported by the ONE-TB project (PHC Ulysses, funded by Campus France and the Irish Research Council) and the Fédération de Recherche en Infectiologie du Centre Val de Loire (FéRI).

ACKNOWLEDGMENTS

We thank the staff from the Abattoir du Perche Vendômois for valuable access to and assistance for bovine post-mortem sampling. We thank Dr. Bojan Stokjovic for his assistance for some PCLS experiment. We are very grateful to Gillian P. McHugo for the drawing of the type I interferon pathway with Ingenuity Pathway analysis.

SUPPLEMENTARY MATERIAL

Supplementary Table 1 | Sequences of primers used in this study. The primers were designed, using Geneious software, in intron-spanning regions when possible. The annealing temperature was set at 60°C. Housekeeping genes used as the reference to calculate ΔCT are indicated in the gray boxes.

Supplementary Figure 1 | Age and geographical origin of the cows used in the study. The Charolaise and Blonde d'Aquitaine cows used were between 3 and 11 years old and came from eight different French departments. Two Blonde d'Aquitaine cows came from the same farm in Indre et Loire, and three Charolaise cows came from the same farm in Sarthe. All the other animals are from distinct farms. The data represent the age of individual animals and the median and interquartile range.

Supplementary Figure 2 | Transcriptomic signature after infection with different doses of mycobacteria. Bovine precision-cut lung slices were obtained as described in **Figure 1** and infected with 10^5, 5×10^5, 10^6, or 5×10^6 colony-forming units. The RNA was extracted 2 days post-infection, and *SDC4*, *CXCL1*, *HIF1*, and *OAS1* gene expressions were assessed with the Fluidigm Biomark. Individual data and the mean and standard deviation in each group are presented ($n = 3$ Charolaise). The dotted line represents the level of expression in the uninfected group.

Supplementary Figure 3 | Cytokines/chemokines in precision-cut lung slice (PCLS) supernatants. The protein levels were measured in PCLS supernatant at 2 days post-infection with Multiplex. Individual data and the median and interquartile range in each group are presented ($n = 6$). *$p < 0.05$ (Wilcoxon nonparametric test).

Supplementary Figure 4 | Structure of the bovine precision-cut lung slices (PCLS) under a light microscope. The PCLS were observed under a light microscope (enlargement ×40 to ×200). The PCLS contain numerous alveoli and between one to three bronchioles, with thick and wavy epithelium that can be easily recognized (black asterisk, two views from the same area under two enlargements). Thin blood vessels (red dotted lines) were localized next to the bronchioles and diffused between the alveoli. No blood cells remained inside the endothelium (the cows were bled out at the abattoir). Alveolar macrophages can be seen inside the alveoli (black arrows).

Supplementary Figure 5 | Localization of Mb3601-GFP in bovine precision-cut lung slices (PCLS). The PCLS were fixed at 2 days post-infection with 10^5 colony-forming units of Mb3601-GFP recombinant strain and labeled with anti-pancytokeratine and anti-MHCII antibodies, which, respectively, revealed anti-pancytokeratine and Alexa 555 conjugated secondary Ab. The PCLS were transferred on cover slides and mounted with Fluoromount-G™ mounting medium containing DAPI. **(A)** The 3D images were analyzed with Leica LAS software. Z-stack imaging was performed at ×63 enlargement with a confocal microscope (10–15 μm in thickness, step size of 0.5–1 μm). Dotted white lines are drawn on the alveoli structure. **(B,C)** Crosshead sections illustrating Mb3601 inside **(B)** or near **(C)** an alveolar macrophage. X and Y projections are seen on the bottom and to the right of the picture; the intracellular localization of Mb3601-GFP is indicated by color merging (green + red = yellow). The results from one representative animal are shown (a total of $n = 4$ animals were analyzed).

Supplementary Video 1 | Internalization of Mb3601 in alveolar macrophages after precision-cut lung slice (PCLS) *ex vivo* infection. The PCLS was fixed at 2 dpi with 10^5 colony-forming units of Mb3601-GFP recombinant strain and labeled with anti-pancytokeratine and anti-MHCII antibodies, which, respectively, revealed anti-pancytokeratine and Alexa 555 conjugated secondary Ab. The PCLS was transferred on cover slides and mounted with Fluoromount-G™ mounting medium containing DAPI. Z-stack imaging was performed at ×63 enlargement with a confocal microscope. The 3D images were analyzed with Leica LAS software.

REFERENCES

1. Downs SH, Prosser A, Ashton A, Ashfield S, Brunton LA, Brouwer A, et al. Assessing effects from four years of industry-led badger culling in England on the incidence of bovine tuberculosis in cattle, 2013-2017. *Sci Rep.* (2019) 9:14666. doi: 10.1038/s41598-019-49957-6

2. Pereira A, Reis A, Ramos B, Cunha M. Animal tuberculosis:Impact of disease heterogeneity in transmission, diagnosis and control. *Transbound Emerg Dis.* (2020) 67:1828–46 doi: 10.1111/tbed.13539

3. Hauer A, De Cruz K, Cochard T, Godreuil S, Karoui C, Henault S, et al. Genetic evolution of *Mycobacterium bovis* causing tuberculosis in livestock and wildlife in France since 1978. *PLoS ONE.* (2015) 10:e0117103. doi: 10.1371/journal.pone.0117103

4. Reveillaud E, Desvaux S, Boschiroli ML, Hars J, Faure E, Fediaevsky A, et al. Infection of wildlife by *Mycobacterium bovis* in france assessment through a national surveillance system, sylvatub. *Front Vet Sci.* (2018) 5:262. doi: 10.3389/fvets.2018.00262

5. Harding E. WHO global progress report on tuberculosis elimination. *Lancet Respir Med.* (2020) 8:19. doi: 10.1016/S2213-2600(19)30418-7

6. Cole S, Brosch R, Parkhill J, Garnier T, Churcher C, Harris D, et al. Deciphering the biology of *Mycobacterium tuberculosis* from the complete genome sequence. *Nature.* (1998) 393:537–44. doi: 10.1038/31159

7. Whelan AO, Coad M, Cockle PJ, Hewinson G, Vordermeier M, Gordon SV. Revisiting host preference in the *Mycobacterium tuberculosis* complex:experimental infection shows *M. tuberculosis* H37Rv to be avirulent in cattle. *PLoS One.* (2010) 5:e8527. doi: 10.1371/journal.pone.0008527

8. Magee DA, Conlon K, Nalpas NC, Browne JA, Pirson C, Healy C, et al. Innate cytokine profiling of bovine alveolar macrophages reveals commonalities and divergence in the response to *Mycobacterium bovis* and *Mycobacterium tuberculosis* infection. *Tuberculosis (Edinb).* (2014) 94:441–50. doi: 10.1016/j.tube.2014.04.004

9. Ameni G, Vordermeier M, Firdessa R, Aseffa A, Hewinson G, Gordon SV, et al. *Mycobacterium tuberculosis* infection in grazing cattle in central Ethiopia. *Vet J.* (2011) 188:359–61. doi: 10.1016/j.tvjl.2010.05.005

10. J.M. van den Berg, van Koppen E, Ahlin A, Belohradsky BH, Bernatowska E, Corbeel L, et al. Chronic granulomatous disease:the European experience. *PLoS ONE.* (2009) 4:e5234. doi: 10.1371/journal.pone.0005234

11. Garnier T, Eiglmeier K, Camus JC, Medina N, Mansoor H, Pryor M, et al. The complete genome sequence of *Mycobacterium bovis. Proc Natl Acad Sci USA.* (2003) 100:7877–82. doi: 10.1073/pnas.1130426100

12. Malone KM, Farrell D, Stuber TP, Schubert OT, Aebersold R, Robbe-Austerman S, et al. Updated Reference Genome Sequence and Annotation of *Mycobacterium bovis* AF2122/97. *Genome Announc.* (2017) 5:e00157-17. doi: 10.1128/genomeA.00157-17

13. Villarreal-Ramos B, Berg S, Whelan A, Holbert S, Carreras F, Salguero FJ, et al. Experimental infection of cattle with *Mycobacterium tuberculosis* isolates shows the attenuation of the human tubercle bacillus for cattle. *Sci Rep.* (2018) 8:894. doi: 10.1038/s41598-017-18575-5

14. Smith N, Berg S, Dale J, Allen A, Rodriguez S, Romero B, et al. European 1:a globally important clonal complex of *Mycobacterium bovis. Infect Genet Evol.* (2011) 11:1340–51. doi: 10.1016/j.meegid.2011.04.027

15. Branger M, Loux V, Cochard T, Boschiroli M, Biet F, Michelet L. The complete genome sequence of *Mycobacterium bovis* Mb3601, a SB0120 spoligotype strain representative of a new clonal group. *Infect Genet Evol.* (2020) 82:104309. doi: 10.1016/j.meegid.2020.104309

16. Hauer A, Michelet L, Cochard T, Branger M, Nunez J, Boschiroli ML, et al. Accurate phylogenetic relationships among *Mycobacterium bovis* strains circulating in france based on whole genome sequencing and single nucleotide polymorphism analysis. *Front Microbiol.* (2019) 10:955. doi: 10.3389/fmicb.2019.00955

17. Brosch R, Gordon SV, Garnier T, Eiglmeier K, Frigui W, Valenti P, et al. Genome plasticity of BCG and impact on vaccine efficacy. *Proc Natl Acad Sci USA.* (2007) 104:5596–601. doi: 10.1073/pnas.0700869104

18. Cosma C, Humbert O, Ramakrishnan L. Superinfecting mycobacteria home to established tuberculous granulomas. *Nat Immunol.* (2004) 5:828–35. doi: 10.1038/ni1091

19. Cassidy J, The pathogenesis and pathology of bovine tuberculosis with insights from studies of tuberculosis in humans and laboratory animal models. *Vet Microbiol.* (2006) 112:151–61. doi: 10.1016/j.vetmic.2005.11.031

20. Scordo JM, Knoell DL, Torrelles JB. Alveolar epithelial cells in *Mycobacterium tuberculosis* infection:active players or innocent bystanders? *J Innate Immun.* (2016) 8:3–14. doi: 10.1159/000439275

21. Li Y, Wang Y, Liu X. The role of airway epithelial cells in response to mycobacteria infection. *Clin Dev Immunol.* (2012) 2012:791392. doi: 10.1155/2012/791392

22. Ryndak MB, Laal S. *Mycobacterium tuberculosis* primary infection and dissemination:a critical role for alveolar epithelial cells. *Front Cell Infect Microbiol.* (2019) 9:299. doi: 10.3389/fcimb.2019.00299

23. Thacker VV, Dhar N, Sharma K, Barrile R, Karalis K, McKinney JD. A lung-on-chip model of early *Mycobacterium tuberculosis* infection reveals an essential role for alveolar epithelial cells in controlling bacterial growth. *Elife.* (2020) 9:e59961. doi: 10.7554/eLife.59961

24. Sato K, Tomioka H, Shimizu T, Gonda T, Ota F, Sano C. Type II alveolar cells play roles in macrophage-mediated host innate resistance to pulmonary mycobacterial infections by producing proinflammatory cytokines. *Journal of Infectious Disease.* (2002) 185:1139–47. doi: 10.1086/340040

25. Castillo-Velázquez U, Gomez-Flores R, Tamez-Guerra R, Tamez-Guerra P, Rodríguez-Padilla C. Differential responses of macrophages from bovines naturally resistant or susceptible to *Mycobacterium bovis* after classical and alternative activation. *Vet Immunol Immunopathol.* (2013) 154:8–16. doi: 10.1016/j.vetimm.2013.04.010

26. Queval CJ, Fearns A, Botella L, Smyth A, Schnettger L, Mitermite M, et al. Macrophage-specific responses to human- and animal-adapted tubercle bacilli reveal pathogen and host factors driving multinucleated cell formation. *PLoS Pathog.* (2021) 17:e1009410. doi: 10.1371/journal.ppat.1009410

27. Goris K, Uhlenbruck S, Schwegmann-Wessels C, Kohl W, Niedorf F, Stern M, et al. Differential sensitivity of differentiated epithelial cells to respiratory viruses reveals different viral strategies of host infection. *J Virol.* (2009) 83:1962–8. doi: 10.1128/JVI.01271-08

28. Marquant Q, Laubreton D, Drajac C, Mathieu E, Bouguyon E, Noordine ML, et al. The microbiota plays a critical role in the reactivity of lung immune components to innate ligands. *FASEB J.* (2021) 35:e21348. doi: 10.1096/fj.202002338R

29. Carranza-Rosales P, Carranza-Torres IE, Guzman-Delgado NE, Lozano-Garza G, Villarreal-Trevino L, Molina-Torres C, et al. Modeling tuberculosis pathogenesis through ex vivo lung tissue infection. *Tuberculosis (Edinb).* (2017) 107:126–132. doi: 10.1016/j.tube.2017.09.002

30. Bryson KJ, Garrido D, Esposito M, McLachlan G, Digard P, Schouler C, et al. Precision cut lung slices:a novel versatile tool to examine host-pathogen interaction in the chicken lung. *Vet Res.* (2020) 51:2. doi: 10.1186/s13567-019-0733-0

31. Thacker T, Palmer M, Waters W. Associations between cytokine gene expression and pathology in *Mycobacterium bovis* infected cattle. *Vet Immunol Immunopathol.* (2007) 119:204–13. doi: 10.1016/j.vetimm.2007.05.009

32. Malone KM, Rue-Albrecht K, Magee DA, Conlon K, Schubert OT, Nalpas NC, et al. Comparative 'omics analyses differentiate *Mycobacterium tuberculosis* and *Mycobacterium bovis* and reveal distinct macrophage responses to infection with the human and bovine tubercle bacilli. *Microb Genom.* (2018) 4:. doi: 10.1099/mgen.0.000163

33. Allen AR, Minozzi G, Glass EJ, Skuce RA, McDowell SW, Woolliams JA, et al. Bovine tuberculosis:the genetic basis of host susceptibility. *Proc Biol Sci.* (2010) 277:2737–45. doi: 10.1098/rspb.2010.0830

34. Abadie V, Badell E, Douillard P, Ensergueix D, Leenen PJ, Tanguy M, et al. Neutrophils rapidly migrate via lymphatics after *Mycobacterium bovis* BCG intradermal vaccination and shuttle live bacilli to the draining lymph nodes. *Blood.* (2005) 106:1843–50. doi: 10.1182/blood-2005-03-1281

35. Berry MPR, Graham CM, McNab FW, Xu Z, Bloch SAA, Oni T, et al. An interferon-inducible neutrophil-driven blood transcriptional signature in human tuberculosis. *Nature.* (2010) 466:973–977. doi: 10.1038/nature09247

36. Moreira-Teixeira L, Mayer-Barber K, Sher A, O'Garra A. Type I interferons in tuberculosis: foe and occasionally friend. *J Exp Med.* (2018) 215:1273–1285. doi: 10.1084/jem.20180325

37. Ji DX, Yamashiro LH, Chen KJ, Mukaida N, Kramnik I, Darwin KH, et al. Type I interferon-driven susceptibility to *Mycobacterium tuberculosis* is mediated by IL-1Ra. *Nat Microbiol.* (2019) 4:2128–35. doi: 10.1038/s41564-019-0578-3

38. Menzies F, Neill S. Cattle-to-cattle transmission of bovine tuberculosis. *Vet J.* (2000) 160:92–106. doi: 10.1016/S1090-0233(00)90482-9

39. Neupane A, Willson M, Krzysztof Chojnacki A, F. Patrolling alveolar macrophages conceal bacteria from the immune system to maintain homeostasis. *Cell.* (2020) 183:110–25. doi: 10.1016/j.cell.2020.08.020

40. Queval CJ, Brosch R, Simeone R. The macrophage: a disputed fortress in the battle against *Mycobacterium tuberculosis. Front Microbiol.* (2017) 8:2284. doi: 10.3389/fmicb.2017.02284

41. Wedlock D, Kawakami R, Koach J, Buddle B, Collins D. Differences of gene expression in bovine alveolar macrophages infected with virulent and attenuated isogenic strains of *Mycobacterium bovis. Int Immunopharmacol.* (2006) 6:957–61. doi: 10.1016/j.intimp.2006.01.003

42. Ferguson J, Schlesinger L. Pulmonary surfactant in innate immunity and the pathogenesis of tuberculosis. *Tuber Lung Dis.* (2000) 80:173–84. doi: 10.1054/tuld.2000.0242

43. Cassidy J, Martineau A. Innate resistance to tuberculosis in man, cattle and laboratory animal models:nipping disease in the bud? *Comp Pathol.* (2014) 151:291–308. doi: 10.1016/j.jcpa.2014.08.001

44. Palmer MV, Wiarda J, Kanipe C, Thacker TC. Early pulmonary lesions in cattle infected via aerosolized *Mycobacterium bovis. Vet Pathol.* (2019) 56:544–554. doi: 10.1177/0300985819833454

45. Martineau AR, Newton SM, Wilkinson KA, Kampmann B, Hall BM, Nawroly N, et al. Neutrophil-mediated innate immune resistance to mycobacteria. *J Clin Invest.* (2007) 117:1988–94. doi: 10.1172/JCI31097

46. McCorry T, Whelan A, Welsh M, McNair J, Walton E, Bryson D, et al. Shedding of *Mycobacterium bovis* in the nasal mucus of cattle infected experimentally with tuberculosis by the intranasal and intratracheal routes. *Vet Record.* (2005) 157:613–8. doi: 10.1136/vr.157.20.613

47. Su F, Liu X, Liu G, Yu Y, Wang Y, Jin Y, et al. Establishment and evaluation of a stable cattle type II alveolar epithelial cell line. *PLoS ONE.* (2013) 8:e76036. doi: 10.1371/journal.pone.0076036

48. Lee DF, Stewart GR, Chambers MA. Modelling early events in *Mycobacterium bovis* infection using a co-culture model of the bovine alveolus. *Sci Rep.* (2020) 10:18495. doi: 10.1038/s41598-020-75113-6

49. Ameni G, Aseffa A, Engers H, Young D, Gordon S, Hewinson G, et al. High prevalence and increased severity of pathology of bovine tuberculosis in Holsteins compared to zebu breeds under field cattle husbandry in central Ethiopia. *Clin Vaccine Immunol.* (2007) 14:1356–61. doi: 10.1128/CVI.00205-07

50. Raphaka K, Sanchez-Molano E, Tsairidou S, Anacleto O, Glass EJ, Woolliams JA, et al. Impact of genetic selection for increased cattle resistance to bovine tuberculosis on disease transmission dynamics. *Front Vet Sci.* (2018) 5:237. doi: 10.3389/fvets.2018.00237

51. Banos G, Winters M, Mrode R, Mitchell AP, Bishop SC, Woolliams JA, et al. Genetic evaluation for bovine tuberculosis resistance in dairy cattle. *J Dairy Sci.* (2017) 100:1272–1281. doi: 10.3168/jds.2016-11897

52. Raphaka K, Matika O, Sanchez-Molano E, Mrode R, Coffey MP, Riggio V, et al. Genomic regions underlying susceptibility to bovine tuberculosis in Holstein-Friesian cattle. *BMC Genet.* (2017) 18:27. doi: 10.1186/s12863-017-0493-7

53. Richardson IW, Berry DP, Wiencko HL, Higgins IM, More SJ, McClure J, et al. A genome-wide association study for genetic susceptibility to *Mycobacterium bovis* infection in dairy cattle identifies a susceptibility QTL on chromosome 23. *Genet Sel Evol.* (2016) 48:19. doi: 10.1186/s12711-016-0197-x

54. Ring SC, Purfield DC, Good M, Breslin P, Ryan E, Blom A, et al. Variance components for bovine tuberculosis infection and multi-breed genome-wide association analysis using imputed whole genome sequence data. *PLoS ONE.* (2019) 14:e0212067. doi: 10.1371/journal.pone.0212067

55. Wilkinson S, Bishop SC, Allen AR, McBride SH, Skuce RA, Bermingham M, et al. Fine-mapping host genetic variation underlying outcomes to *Mycobacterium bovis* infection in dairy cows. *BMC Genomics.* (2017) 18:477. doi: 10.1186/s12864-017-3836-x

56. Abel L, Fellay J, Haas DW, Schurr E, Srikrishna G, Urbanowski M, et al. Genetics of human susceptibility to active and latent tuberculosis:present knowledge and future perspectives. *Lancet Infect Dis.* (2018) 18:e64–e75. doi: 10.1016/S1473-3099(17)30623-0

57. Allen A. One bacillus to rule them all?-Investigating broad range host adaptation in *Mycobacterium bovis*. *Infect Genet Evol.* (2017) 53:68–76. doi: 10.1016/j.meegid.2017.04.018

58. J. Sabio Y García, Bigi MM, Klepp LI, García EA, Blanco FF, Bigi F. Does *Mycobacterium bovis* persist in cattle in a non-replicative latent state as *Mycobacterium tuberculosis* in human beings? *Vet Microbiol.* (2020) 247:108758. doi: 10.1016/j.vetmic.2020.108758

59. Gonzalo-Asensio J, Malaga W, Pawlik A, Astarie-Dequeker C, Passemar C, Moreau F, et al. Evolutionary history of tuberculosis shaped by conserved mutations in the PhoPR virulence regulator. *Proc Natl Acad Sci USA.* (2014) 111:11491–6. doi: 10.1073/pnas.1406693111

60. Huynh K, Joshi S, Brown E. A delicate dance:host response to mycobacteria. *Curr Opin Immunol.* (2011) 23:464–72. doi: 10.1016/j.coi.2011.06.002

61. Russell DG. *Mycobacterium tuberculosis* and the intimate discourse of a chronic infection. *Immunol Rev.* (2011) 240:252–68. doi: 10.1111/j.1600-065X.2010.00984.x

62. Nalpas NC, Magee DA, Conlon KM, Browne JA, Healy C, McLoughlin KE, et al. RNA sequencing provides exquisite insight into the manipulation of the alveolar macrophage by tubercle bacilli. *Sci Rep.* (2015) 5:13629. doi: 10.1038/srep13629

63. Jensen K, Gallagher IJ, Johnston N, Welsh M, Skuce R, Williams JL, et al. Variation in the early host-pathogen interaction of bovine macrophages with divergent *Mycobacterium bovis* Strains in the United Kingdom. *Infect Immun.* (2018) 86:e00385-17. doi: 10.1128/IAI.00385-17

64. Palmer M, Thacker T, Rabideau M, Jones G, Kanipe C, Vordermeier H, et al. Biomarkers of cell-mediated immunity to bovine tuberculosis. *Vet Immunol Immunopathol.* (2020) 220:109988. doi: 10.1016/j.vetimm.2019.109988

65. Chunfa L, Xin S, Qiang L, Sreevatsan S, Yang L, Zhao D, et al. The Central Role of IFI204 in IFN-beta Release and Autophagy Activation during *Mycobacterium bovis* Infection. *Front Cell Infect Microbiol.* (2017) 7:169. doi: 10.3389/fcimb.2017.00169

66. Liu C, Yue E, Yang Y, Cui Y, Yang L, Zhao D, et al. AIM2 inhibits autophagy and IFN-β production during *M. bovis* infection. *Oncotarget.* (2016) 7:46972–87. doi: 10.18632/oncotarget.10503

67. Wang J, Hussain T, Zhang K, Liao Y, Yao J, Song Y, et al. Inhibition of type I interferon signaling abrogates early *Mycobacterium bovis* infection. *BMC Infect Dis.* (2019) 19:1031. doi: 10.1186/s12879-019-4654-3

68. Olea-Popelka F, Muwonge A, Perera A, Dean A, Mumford E, Erlacher-Vindel E, et al. Zoonotic tuberculosis in human beings caused by *Mycobacterium bovis*-a call for action. *Lancet Infect Dis.* (2017) 17:e21–e25. doi: 10.1016/S1473-3099(16)30139-6

Human-to-Cattle *Mycobacterium tuberculosis* Complex Transmission in the United States

Jason E. Lombard [1]*, Elisabeth A. Patton [2], Suzanne N. Gibbons-Burgener [3], Rachel F. Klos [3], Julie L. Tans-Kersten [3], Beth W. Carlson [4], Susan J. Keller [4], Delora J. Pritschet [5], Susan Rollo [6], Tracey V. Dutcher [1], Cris A. Young [1], William C. Hench [7], Tyler C. Thacker [8], Claudia Perea [8], Aaron D. Lehmkuhl [8] and Suelee Robbe-Austerman [8]

[1] United States Department of Agriculture: Animal and Plant Health Inspection Service, Veterinary Services, Field Epidemiologic Investigation Services, Fort Collins, CO, United States, [2] Wisconsin Department of Agriculture, Trade and Consumer Protection, Madison, WI, United States, [3] Wisconsin Department of Health Services, Division of Public Health, Madison, WI, United States, [4] North Dakota Department of Agriculture, State Board of Animal Health, Bismarck, ND, United States, [5] North Dakota Department of Health, Bismarck, ND, United States, [6] Texas Animal Health Commission, Austin, TX, United States, [7] United States Department of Agriculture: Animal and Plant Health Inspection Service, Veterinary Services, Ruminant Health Center, Fort Collins, CO, United States, [8] United States Department of Agriculture: Animal and Plant Health Inspection Service, Veterinary Services, National Veterinary Services Laboratories, Ames, IA, United States

*Correspondence:
Jason E. Lombard
jason.e.lombard@usda.gov

The *Mycobacterium tuberculosis* complex (MTBC) species includes both *M. tuberculosis*, the primary cause of human tuberculosis (TB), and *M. bovis*, the primary cause of bovine tuberculosis (bTB), as well as other closely related *Mycobacterium* species. Zoonotic transmission of *M. bovis* from cattle to humans was recognized more than a century ago, but transmission of MTBC species from humans to cattle is less often recognized. Within the last decade, multiple published reports from around the world describe human-to-cattle transmission of MTBC. Three probable cases of human-to-cattle MTBC transmission have occurred in the United States since 2013. In the first case, detection of active TB disease (*M. bovis*) in a dairy employee in North Dakota prompted testing and ultimate detection of bTB infection in the dairy herd. Whole genome sequencing (WGS) demonstrated a match between the bTB strain in the employee and an infected cow. North Dakota animal and public health officials concluded that the employee's infection was the most likely source of disease introduction in the dairy. The second case involved a Wisconsin dairy herd with an employee diagnosed with TB disease in 2015. Subsequently, the herd was tested twice with no disease detected. Three years later, a cow originating from this herd was detected with bTB at slaughter. The strain in the slaughter case matched that of the past employee based on WGS. The third case was a 4-month-old heifer calf born in New Mexico and transported to Texas. The calf was TB tested per Texas entry requirements and found to have *M. tuberculosis*. Humans are the suspected source of *M. tuberculosis* in cattle; however, public health authorities were not able to identify an infected human associated with the cattle operation. These three cases provide strong evidence of human-to-cattle transmission of MTBC organisms and highlight human infection as a potential source of introduction of MTBC into dairy herds in the United States. To better understand and address the issue, a multisectoral One Health approach is needed, where industry, public health, and animal health work together to better understand the epidemiology and identify preventive measures to protect human and animal health.

Keywords: *Bovine tuberculosis*, zoonotic disease, human-to-cattle transmission, public health, dairy employees

INTRODUCTION

The primary causative agents of human and bovine tuberculosis (bTB) in North America, *Mycobacterium tuberculosis* and *Mycobacterium bovis*, respectively, are included in the *Mycobacterium tuberculosis* complex (MTBC). Other members of the MTBC include *Mycobacterium orygis, Mycobacterium caprae, Mycobacterium microti, Mycobacterium pinnipedii, Mycobacterium mungi,* and *Mycobacterium suricattae* (1). The MTBC species are so closely related that they are now considered a single species, *M. tuberculosis*, with variants (1, 2).

Worldwide, tuberculosis is the leading cause of human deaths by any single infectious agent and responsible for approximately 1.2 M deaths in HIV-negative people in 2019 (3). Tuberculosis was a leading cause of human morbidity and mortality in the United States at the beginning of the twentieth century. A study conducted in 1912 reported that 66% of New York children diagnosed with tuberculosis (TB) in 1910 were infected with *M. bovis* (4). Based on the transmission of *M. bovis* to children through milk, multiple jurisdictions enacted laws requiring pasteurization. Cincinnati was the first city to establish pasteurization requirements in 1897; New York City followed in 1898 (5). Michigan became the first state to require pasteurization of milk in 1948 and all states have since followed suit. In addition to milk, meat from *M. bovis*-affected cattle is also a potential risk for human infection. Accordingly, the Federal Meat Inspection Act of 1906 (6, 7) gave the U.S. Department of Agriculture (USDA) the authority to inspect cattle before, during, and after slaughter as another tool for preventing zoonotic transmission of *M. bovis*. Lesions detected during this inspection, or entire carcasses if necessary, could be removed from the food chain. Not only did this reduce the risk of human infection, but also cattle with bTB could be identified and trace-back investigations to the herd of origin allowed for identification of bTB-infected herds. Slaughter inspection is the primary means of bTB surveillance in the United States today.

In addition to implementing these two mitigation strategies to reduce human exposure to *M. bovis*, state and federal authorities designed and implemented the U.S. Cooperative State-Federal Bovine TB Eradication Program to reduce the prevalence in cattle populations. The program officially began in 1917; at that time, approximately 1 in 20 cattle were infected with *M. bovis* (8). Reviews of the program and its progress have been published (9–12). Current estimates of animal- and herd-level prevalence of *M. bovis* in the United States are <0.002 and <0.006%, respectively (12). The partnership between State and Federal Animal Health Officials to conduct testing, share data, and conduct disease investigations has been critical to these advancements. In other parts of the world, including parts of Mexico and Central and South America, *M. bovis* infection rates in cattle and other hoof stock are much higher and serve as an important source for human disease (13). Additionally, consumption of unpasteurized dairy products remains a primary cause of human infections with *M. bovis* in North America (14–16).

Despite the early success of the program in the United States, the number of newly identified bTB-affected herds each year has remained relatively steady for the past 30 years (17). The advent of whole genome sequencing (WGS) has markedly advanced our ability to link sources of infection based on genetic similarities. For example, in Michigan WGS routinely supports wildlife as a source of infection. However, for cases outside of Michigan, even after extensive epidemiological investigations, including WGS and trace-back of purchased cattle, the source of disease and method of introduction into a herd is determined only about 40% of the time (17). Without a source of infection, risk mitigation, and disease eradication remain elusive.

Humans are considered the primary host for *M. tuberculosis* and animals are considered accidental hosts (18, 19). Human-to-animal transmission of MTBC organisms, primarily *M. tuberculosis*, is well-documented in many countries around the world. Many of these reports confirm finding *M. tuberculosis* in tissues and fluids from cattle (20–32) and also other animals, including dogs (33), non-human primates (34), elephants (35, 36), and parrots (37, 38). Most reports of cattle with *M. tuberculosis* are from countries where human *M. tuberculosis* prevalence is very high and likely to have been the source of introduction into the cattle populations.

With the technology now available to obtain DNA sequences of *M. bovis* isolates found in U.S. cattle, it is easier to discern the origin of certain *M. bovis* strains. This information may provide possible modes of transmission based on the most common ancestor in the genomic database and similarity of DNA sequences over time. Sharing isolate DNA sequence data between animal and public health will further our understanding of the complex transmission of MTBC organisms between humans and animals.

The objectives of this paper are to present the identified cases of human-to-cattle MTBC transmission in the United States and to highlight the importance of a multisectoral One Health approach in detecting and addressing human-to-cattle transmission of these important human and animal pathogens.

MATERIALS AND METHODS

Case Selection

Records from the 174 bTB affected livestock herds identified in the USA between 1998 and 2020 were reviewed. As part of the State Federal Cooperative Bovine Tuberculosis program, each herd had been extensively investigated under that cooperative umbrella and if possible, the likely source of the infection was identified and investigated. Also included in this review were 422 records for tuberculous confirmed animals between 2001 and 2020 not associated with a herd, such as feedlot and dairy heifer development facilities.

Inclusion criteria were as follows: All *Mycobacterium tuberculosis* cases detected in livestock; and zoonotic tuberculosis (all were *M. bovis*) cases where humans associated with livestock were identified with active tuberculosis prior to the detection within the herd.

Public Health Investigations

Public health authorities in the U.S. investigate all reported cases of TB disease in humans to ensure patients quarantine until non-infectious and receive and complete appropriate antimicrobial treatment. Contact investigations are routinely performed when patients have pulmonary TB and are considered infectious. Close contacts are screened for exposure risk and tested to determine their TB infection and disease status. The public health investigation may identify animals (especially livestock and captive wildlife) with an epidemiological link to the infectious patient. In North Dakota and Wisconsin, the public health agency alerts their animal health partners and a One Health investigation may be deemed necessary. All information on the human cases contained in this paper was collected during the normal process that occurs in these states when humans with TB are detected.

Phylogenetic Analysis

Whole genome sequences were obtained from both animal health and public health investigations. NVSL's in-house vSNP pipeline was used for the analysis (see https://github.com/USDA-VS/vSNP). vSNP is a reference based, two-step pipeline. Briefly in step one, sequences were aligned to a reference; those identified as *M. bovis* were aligned to the reference genome AF2122/97 (GenBank accession NC_002945.4), and those identified as *M. tuberculosis* were aligned to the reference genome H37Rv (GenBank accession NC_000962.3). The alignment was performed using Burrows-Wheeler Aligner (BWA) (39) and SNPs were called using Freebayes (40). The variant call format (vcf) files created in step one were then added to a database of vcf files and step two was initiated which filters or flags unreliable and low quality variant calls, as well as groups sequences into user defined clades according to relatedness by identifying common SNPs. For each user defined group, step two outputs SNP tables in Excel, an aligned FASTA file and phylogenetic trees constructed with RAxML (41) using the aligned whole-genome SNP sequences under a GTR-CAT model of substitution and a maximum-likelihood algorithm. The annotated and position referenced SNP tables allow for quick error identification and correction. The trees were then manually compared to the SNP table to ensure accuracy of the model.

Tree visualization, annotation, and editing was performed with FigTree (http://tree.bio.ed.ac.uk/software/figtree/) and iTOL (42). **Supplementary File 1** lists the accession numbers for the publicly available sequences from previous studies (17, 43, 44).

RESULTS

Three cases met the criteria for inclusion, two *M. bovis* affected dairy herds, and one *M. tuberculosis* infected 4-month-old calf at a dairy heifer development facility. Those cases are described in detail below.

Case 1: North Dakota Dairy Herd

In October 2013, the North Dakota Department of Agriculture (NDDA), State Board of Animal Health was notified by the North Dakota Department of Health (NDDOH) that an employee at a North Dakota dairy was diagnosed with pulmonary TB with cavitary lung lesions. The case-patient, a man born in Mexico, had been recently diagnosed with another medical condition that likely suppressed his immune system resulting in active TB disease. The case-patient worked for the dairy for at least 3 years prior to his diagnosis. During this time, he worked for 9 consecutive months then returned to Mexico for the remaining 3 months each year. During his employment, the case-patient worked with all ages of dairy cattle. NDDOH tested three household contacts to the case-patient. All were latently infected with TB (LTBI) and were treated prophylactically with a 4-month course of antibiotics per CDC guidelines to prevent future disease.

The North Dakota operation housed 400 dairy cattle and 160 beef cattle. Beef and dairy heifers were often commingled for a few months each year. While the operation had no record of TB skin testing in the dairy or beef herds in the recent past, cull dairy and beef cattle from this operation were slaughtered at abattoirs with high granuloma submission rates for TB surveillance.

After meeting with the NDDOH's TB controller and state animal health officials, the herd owner agreed to herd testing in November 2013. North Dakota Department of Agriculture veterinarians conducted whole-herd testing in consultation with the USDA. All cows and heifers 6 months of age and older were tested using standard protocol of the caudal fold tuberculin (CFT) test in series with the comparative cervical tuberculin (CCT) test.

A 19-month-old pregnant heifer (ND1) was declared a reactor based on CCT testing. Upon necropsy, multiple micro abscesses were identified in a normal appearing mediastinal lymph node that was culture-positive for *M. bovis* at USDA's National Veterinary Services Laboratories (NVSL). Ten additional cows were CCT-negative and sent to slaughter in WI. Samples were collected from all 10 cows and although no gross lesions were identified, samples were submitted for culture at NVSL. Two of the 10 cows (ND2 and ND3) were determined to be infected with *M. bovis*. Microscopic granulomas in a lymph node that contained acid-fast bacteria from ND2 were PCR positive for MTBC but no *mycobacteria* were identified on culture. Representative, normal appearing lymph nodes from the head and thorax were submitted from ND3; these tissues were histologically negative for evidence of mycobacterial infection, but *M. bovis* was isolated from culture. Tissue from the post-mortem exam and the ear tags were DNA tested to confirm they were from the same animal and no errors were made during sampling, labeling, or processing. Over the course of testing, approximately 40 cattle were removed from the herd and no additional infected cattle identified.

Whole genome sequencing was conducted and the infected pregnant heifer (ND1) had the identical strain to the dairy employee with active TB disease (**Figure 1**; see **Supplementary File 1** for SNP table). The isolate from ND3 had seven single nucleotide polymorphisms (SNPs) compared with the isolates from ND1 and the case-patient. *Mycobacterium bovis* was not detected in the beef cattle. The infected dairy cattle were born and raised on the dairy operation. Two herds with fence line contact were tested and no infected animals were detected. Additionally, surveillance was conducted on barn cats, wild rodents, and hunter harvested deer with no disease detected. North Dakota Game and Fish Department conducted surveillance in the fall of 2014 on hunter-harvested deer and no lesions were identified. After a thorough investigation, no other possible sources of *M. bovis* were found.

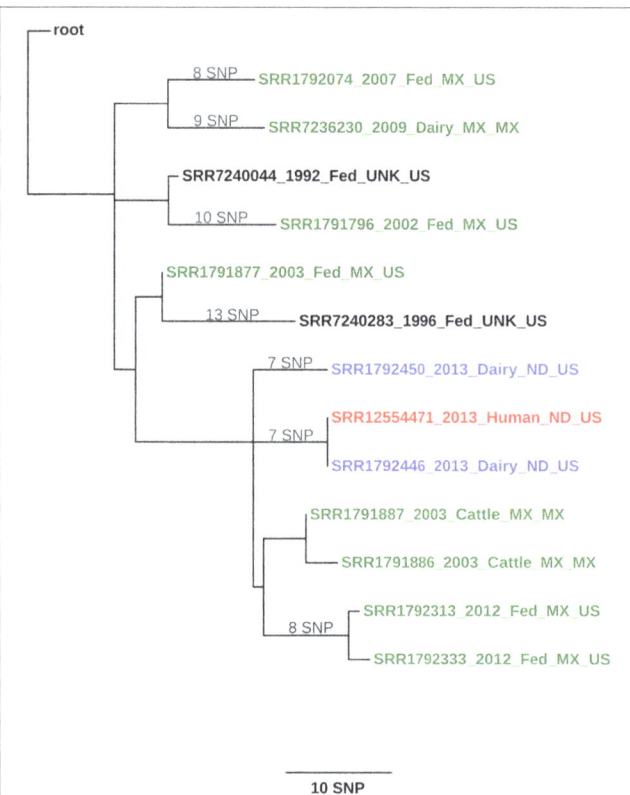

FIGURE 1 | Maximum likelihood phylogenetic tree illustrating the genetic relationship between *M. bovis* isolates from a cattle herd in North Dakota (United States) and a human. The color key indicates the origin of the cattle from which *M. bovis* was isolated: green, Mexico; blue, United States; and black, cattle whose origin could not be traced (unknown). The human isolate is shown in red. Sequences are identified using the following syntax: NCBI SRA accession number_year of isolation_ production type (dairy, fed, cattle [unknown])_geographical origin of the animal (state, country or unknown)_country of detection. The scale bar represents a branch length of 10 SNPs. The tree is rooted to the reference genome *M. bovis* AF2122/97.

Case 2: Wisconsin Dairy Herd

Similar to the identification of the North Dakota herd, the Wisconsin Department of Agriculture, Trade and Consumer Protection (DATCP) was contacted in late April 2015 by the Wisconsin Department of Health Services (WIDHS) about a case-patient with TB disease that worked on a dairy from January to March 2015. The case-patient reportedly became ill in March 2015 before seeking medical care in early April. The case-patient presented in the emergency room with night sweats, cough, and fever. Sputum smears were positive for acid fast bacteria and nucleic acid amplification test (NAAT) was positive for MTBC. Culture revealed the case-patient was infected with *M. bovis*. The case-patient was placed in respiratory isolation and started on a standard four-drug regimen (45). After drug susceptibility testing was complete and pyrazinamide (PZA) resistance detected, PZA was discontinued. Due to severe cavitary disease, the case-patient was treated with TB medications for a full year, with directly observed therapy for the entire course. The case-patient was released from isolation in July 2015 when determined to no longer be contagious. The individual is believed to have become infected while previously living in a Latin-American country where *M. bovis* infections of humans and cattle are prevalent. Public health conducted a routine contact investigation that included TB risk assessment and testing of close contacts to the patient. No additional cases of infectious TB were identified in household or farm employee contacts.

In May 2015, DATCP conducted herd testing, in accordance with USDA guidance, of the 1,500-head herd. Like the ND herd, all cows and heifers 6 months of age and older were testing using the CFT test and CCT-test in series, with no infected animals detected. A single CCT-suspect cow from this first test was euthanized and necropsied with no lesions identified. In September 2015, the herd was tested a second time and was again test negative for bTB with no CCT-positive animals detected. In September 2018, slaughter plant surveillance detected tuberculosis in a carcass from a cow that traced back to this herd, and *M. bovis* was isolated. DATCP conducted another round of whole-herd testing using the CFT and CCT tests in series beginning in October 2018. Seven infected cows were identified during this initial test based on culture of *M. bovis*. Two additional infected cattle were detected during herd testing in March 2019, one infected cow was identified at slaughter in April 2020, and one cow was detected following herd testing in June 2020. Since the detection of the herd as infected, more than 1,500 cows have been examined for bTB by either necropsy or slaughter surveillance. One of the infected cows was test-negative and detected at slaughter. Additionally, surveillance was conducted on wildlife surrounding the premises and included white tailed deer ($n = 232$), raccoons ($n = 10$), and opossums ($n = 6$). One dairy that had heifers housed on the same premises as heifers from the affected dairy including fence line contact will be tested a total of three annual tests (2/3 have been completed and were negative).

At the time of this writing, the herd has had a total of 12 cows, including the slaughter case, detected as infected with *M. bovis*; and the isolates were within a 1–4 SNP difference from the human isolate (**Figure 2**; see **Supplementary File 1** for

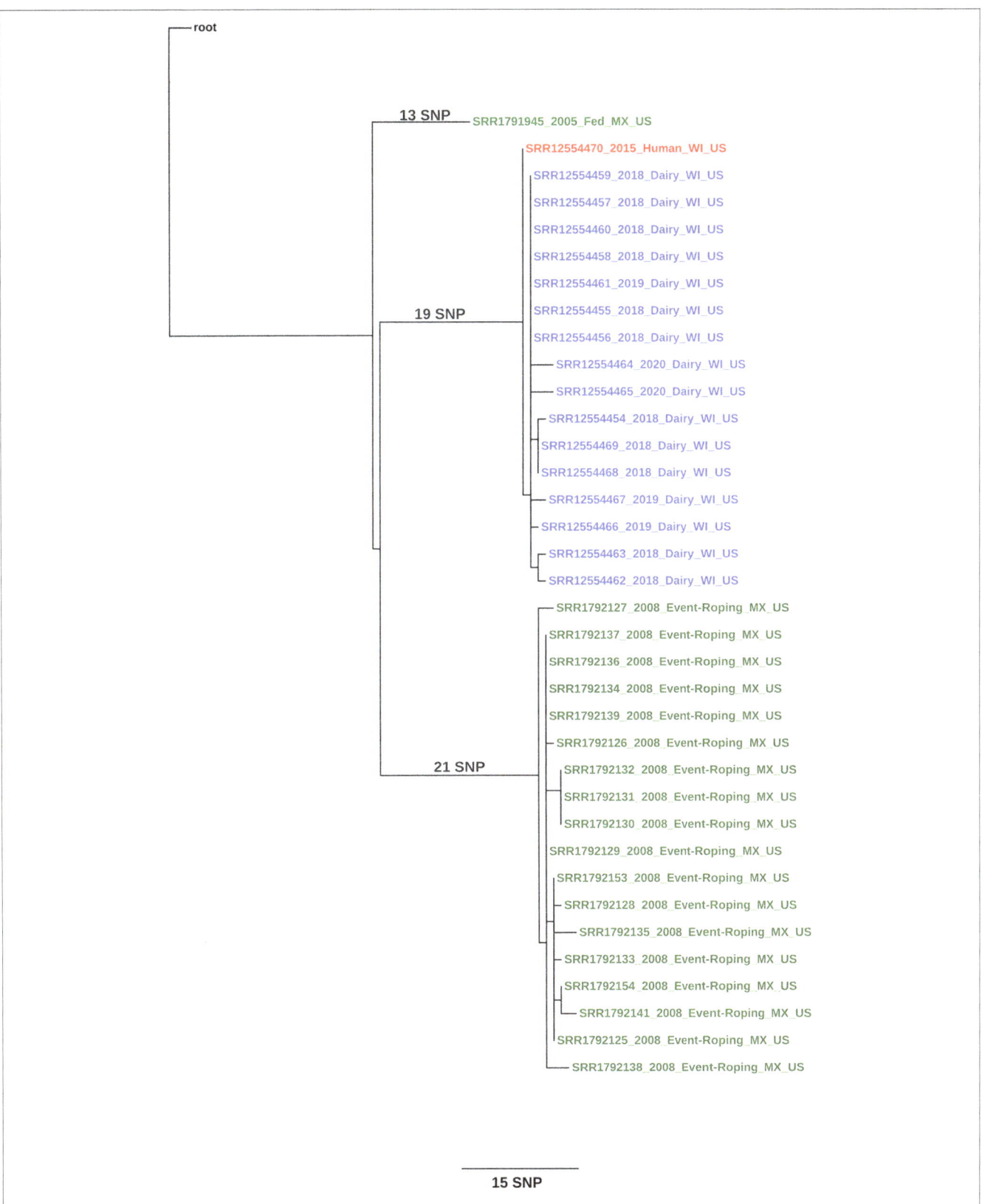

FIGURE 2 | Maximum likelihood phylogenetic tree illustrating the genetic relationship between *M. bovis* isolates a herd in Wisconsin (United States) and a human. The color key indicates the origin of the cattle from which *M. bovis* was isolated: green, Mexico and blue, United States. The human isolate is shown in red. Sequences are identified using the following syntax: NCBI SRA accession number_year of isolation_ production type (dairy, fed, event-roping)_geographical origin of the animal (state, country)_country of detection. The scale bar represents a branch length of 15 SNPs. The tree is rooted to the reference genome *M. bovis* AF2122/97.

SNP table). The public health follow-up with farm employees continues until the farm is released from quarantine. Testing of source herds for purchased cattle added to the Wisconsin herd were not conducted since the epidemiologic investigation and WGS supported the human case-patient as the source of introduction into the herd.

Case 3: Texas Dairy Heifer

In early 2018, a 1-day-old heifer calf from a dairy in New Mexico was transported to Texas where import regulations require post-import TB testing of cattle younger than 2 months of age that move into the state. The heifer was raised at a facility in Texas and was TB test positive in April 2018 at approximately 4 months of age. The heifer was euthanized and necropsied in late April 2018, and tissue samples were sent to NVSL for additional TB testing. There were no gross or microscopic lesions suggestive of MTBC infection. *Mycobacterium tuberculosis* was cultured from the retropharyngeal lymph node collected at necropsy and results were reported in June 2018. The heifer calf isolate grouped with sublineage 4.2.2 (43) and is in NCBI as accession SRR12481506.

The Texas Department of State Health Services (DSHS) conducted a source case investigation to determine if an infectious TB suspect had been identified by public health; however, a source case was not identified. Personnel from DSHS discussed the situation with dairy management, and a dairy employee was identified who exhibited signs and symptoms of TB but was no longer employed at the dairy. Whole genome sequencing of human cases was just being implemented by the Centers of Disease Control and Prevention, and consequently, the previous human cases in this area had not been sequenced. However, both the calf and three adults in the region that were diagnosed in 2017 and 2018 (46) had a matching, rather rare spoligotype for Texas, with an octal code 007000024000000. No employees were tested, but DSHS conducted symptom screening and provided education for the current employees. We were unable to retrospectively obtain WGS from any of the Texas human cases to include in this report.

DISCUSSION

The three cases presented here are the first formal reports of MTBC transmission from humans to cattle in the United States since 1968 (47). In both the North Dakota and Wisconsin cases, the human TB case-patients were exposed to cattle on the operation prior to or at the time bTB was discovered in the cattle. In the North Dakota case, bTB was detected in three dairy cattle within 2 months after the human was diagnosed; in the Wisconsin herd, it was 3 years between the human TB detection and the herd detection.

When bTB-affected herds in the United States are identified, state, and federal animal health agencies conduct epidemiologic investigations to determine the probable source of disease and trace any animals that left the herd to control disease spread. Historically, in the United States the most common sources for bTB infection in cattle have been other infected cattle. The exception to this is in several counties in Michigan where bTB is endemic in the wild white-tailed deer population. Investigations

in Michigan have identified deer as the most common source of infection in cattle (48). Animal health authorities conduct interviews with herd owners to determine all potential routes of exposure, including sources of all purchased cattle over a multiyear period and any contact with cattle from other operations, including fence-line contact. These exposures are investigated, and all cattle contacts are tested to determine their bTB status per Bovine tuberculosis eradication uniform methods and rules (49). Additionally, most adult cattle that leave dairies undergo inspection at slaughter for bTB, which is the method by which most infected herds are identified.

Inspection of carcasses at slaughter, or slaughter surveillance has been an effective method of detecting bTB in cattle in the United States. This is highlighted by the WI herd being detected by slaughter surveillance and subsequently, having a test-negative, infected cow that was detected at slaughter. Both the ND and WI herds sent animals to slaughter prior to bTB detection and they continue to do so on a routine basis, providing additional surveillance for bTB. Although infected animals can be missed with slaughter surveillance, 47% of bTB affected herds are detected through slaughter surveillance, excluding herds in the endemic are of Michigan and a localized outbreak in Minnesota (17, 50).

The results of the North Dakota investigation suggest it is highly unlikely that cattle in the herd could have transmitted *M. bovis* to the human. The progression of disease in ND1 appeared to be relatively recent given the finding of *M. bovis* in a single mediastinal lymph node. In the Wisconsin case, the case-patient was diagnosed with TB within 2–3 months of employment. Although *M. bovis* infections in humans have been reported to progress from infection to clinical disease within a few months, more often this progression in humans takes much longer (51, 52). Most of the knowledge of TB in humans is based on infection with *M. tuberculosis* but it might not be the same for *M. bovis* infections.

Additionally, the ND patient's housemates were all tested and considered as LTBI, while the farm family were all negative for bTB. If the cattle were the source of the human infection, one would expect the farm family members to be exposed and potentially infected. The housemates of the patient were exposed to the patient and so it was expected that some or all of them would be infected. None of the patient's housemates were actively shedding *M. bovis* and considered as LTBI.

The North Dakota dairy herd has been tested 9 times since 2013, with only the three infected cows detected at the first herd test, despite this additional testing. Only one of those three infected cows (ND1) had a small gross lesion associated with bTB infection. The WGS of the *M. bovis* strain from the North Dakota case-patient and ND1 were an exact match. Significant epidemiological evidence supports the transmission of *M. bovis* from the employee to the heifer. Evidence includes the degree of illness in the employee with active TB disease (e.g., lung cavitation); the very small lesion in the infected heifer, possibly indicating recent infection; the lack of movement of animals on or off the farm; and the fact that the employee was born in Mexico, a TB-endemic country, and returned annually. Based on the epidemiological and laboratory evidence, the human was considered the most likely source of disease in the cattle by both animal and public health officials investigating the case.

One of the three bTB-infected cattle, ND2 was PCR positive but culture negative, and no isolate was available for WGS. The last cow, ND3, had normal appearing lymph nodes that were histologically negative but culture positive. The WGS revealed 7 SNP changes from the case-patient and ND1 strain. It is difficult to explain this finding based on the current data but we believe the human patient was likely infected with this strain variation. Humans and cattle have been found to be infected with multiple strains of MTBC, so it is possible the human was infected with more than 1 strain but only 1 was isolated. Unless a more closely related strain is identified in the future, the source of infection for ND3 will remain unknown. Based on the small size of the lesions, however, it is unlikely that ND3 was shedding *M. bovis*. An evaluation of the phylogenetic tree (and **Supplementary File 1**, SNP Table) shows that both ND1 and ND3 share a common ancestor with other Mexican cattle in the region that the dairy worker was known to previously reside and visit on an annual basis. This provides further support that the initial exposure of the case-patient was likely in their home country.

The Wisconsin case report provides the strongest epidemiologic evidence for human-to-cattle transmission, as the case-patient was diagnosed 3 years before the herd was detected. The individual was a very recent addition to the dairy's workforce and was diagnosed with TB disease within 3 months of beginning employment. Collectively, this provides strong evidence that the case-patient's exposure to *M. bovis* occurred prior to employment on the dairy. All cattle having potential contact with the case-patient were tested 2 and 6 months after the employee was no longer working on the dairy, and bTB was not detected. It is highly unlikely that infection was present and circulating in the herd and transmitted from cattle to the case-patient. Further, the WGS from the infected cows had at least 1 SNP change difference from the human and most recent common ancestor, or root sequence, suggesting the cattle isolates were closely related, direct descendants of the human isolate.

Results of testing of other dairy employees and family members continue to be negative since the initial tests in 2015. If the dairy cattle were the source of infection, we would have expected other employees or family members to be infected. The public health investigators were adamant that the employee with TB disease was very sick at the time of diagnosis and could not have progressed to this stage of disease in two months. They were confident the employee was infected prior to entering the dairy's workforce.

Investigators also found no evidence suggesting latent infection in the Wisconsin cattle. Three of the 12 infected cows were purchased additions (WI2, WI3, WI4), while the remaining cows were born and raised on the operation. One of the purchased cows (WI2) was brought on the operation in January 2015, roughly the same time the case-patient began employment. This cow was test negative in May and September 2015 suggesting she was not infected at the time of introduction into the herd. In October 2018, WI2 was found to be infected. The other two purchased cows were brought into the herd in 2016 after the case-patient was no longer present. Their infections are consistent with cattle-to-cattle transmission within the herd. Other than these two cows, the remaining 10 infected cows were all test negative at least once during the 2015 testing.

For both the North Dakota and Wisconsin cases, WGS supports that the TB case-patients were infected in their home country, possibly through contact with infected cattle or consumption of raw dairy products, and subsequently infected cattle on these farms after their disease became active. Others have reported similar scenarios where *M. bovis* infection makes the complete cycle from cow to human and back to cow (20).

While the Texas *M. tuberculosis* case lacks a confirmed case of human TB directly linking a human to the calf, the epidemiologic investigation and evidence of the matching spoligotype circulating in the local community strongly supports human to cattle transmission. Furthermore, a review of the literature found that, with one reported exception, humans are the direct source of *M. tuberculosis* infection for cattle. There is one report of a calf from an experimentally infected cow that was infected via colostrum or milk (53). To our knowledge, that has not been replicated in a naturally infected dairy. This is the first modern reported case *M. tuberculosis* infection in a U.S. bovine.

In addition to the three cases presented here, there have been at least 10 other U.S. bovine cases (i.e., affected herds) since 2009 that investigators were very suspicious of human-to-cattle *M. bovis* transmission as the source of introduction into these herds. These suspicions were based on both epidemiologic data collected, and WGS conducted by animal health officials, but all lacked the active, prospective identification of human cases.

Often, lesions are not present in young cattle diagnosed with *M. tuberculosis* (54–56). Although cattle without gross lesions are not considered a risk for transmission of disease to cattle or humans, *M. tuberculosis* has been found in cows' milk (57–59) and in granulomatous lesions from infected cattle, suggesting infected cattle may be a risk to other cattle and humans (23). Published reports suggest that humans are the primary source of *M. tuberculosis* infections in cattle with transmission occurring via the respiratory route (60). Although evidence for direct human-to-cattle transmission is not always present, *M. tuberculosis* has been found in cattle in multiple countries. Worldwide, human-to-cattle transmission of *M. tuberculosis* has been documented more frequently than *M. bovis,* likely due to the increased prevalence of *M. tuberculosis* in humans. More evaluations are needed to determine the importance of livestock in the transmission of *M. tuberculosis* between cattle and humans. The U.S has been characterizing MTBC isolates in livestock for over 40 years, and the last documented case of *M. tuberculosis* that occurred in U.S. livestock was a llama in 1991, associated with exotic animal trade (unpublished data).

Human-to-cattle transmission of *M. bovis* has infrequently been reported (20, 28, 47, 61–63) and there is only a single report of human-to-cattle *M. orygis* transmission (64). The finding of human-to-cattle transmission of *M. bovis* in the United States may be related to the increased risk of *M. bovis* infection among non-U.S.-born livestock workers compared to U.S.-born workers.

The prevalence of *M. bovis* in humans in the United States has declined from at least 10% of MTBC cases in 1900 to <2% of all

MTBC cases in 2005 (65). Another publication demonstrated that human cases of *M. bovis* in the United States were more likely to be of Hispanic/Latino origin and born outside the United States (66). More recently, Scott et al. (67) reported human *M. bovis* prevalence in the United States with a similar prevalence of 1.3–1.6% of all MTBC cases, and a higher prevalence in children, Hispanics/Latinos, and females.

Although the number of human cases of MTBC infection in the United States has decreased about 90% since 1953 (68), some areas of the United States have reported an increase, especially along the southern U.S. border. A review of pediatric tuberculosis cases in San Diego, CA, from 1980 to 1997 revealed *M. bovis* was responsible for 10.8% of all TB cases and 33.9% of culture-positive cases (14). Hispanics represented 78.9% of the cases. More than half the *M. bovis* culture-positive case-patients (55.2%) had only extra-pulmonary bTB. This study highlights the concern of foodborne exposure via unpasteurized dairy products. Since dairy products appear to be the main source of human *M. bovis* infection in Mexico (17), efforts to eradicate bTB from the Mexican dairy industry must be strengthened to improve human and animal health in both the United States and Mexico.

Although the North Dakota and Wisconsin herds were most likely infected via the respiratory route, given active pulmonary disease in the workers, other publications suggest that extrapulmonary infections are more common with *M. bovis* infection. The authors concluded that the prevalence of extra-pulmonary disease in young, U.S.- or Mexican-born Hispanic/Latino populations suggested recent infection due to foodborne exposure (66). Extra-pulmonary disease was nine times more frequent among those with *M. bovis* than those with *M. tuberculosis*. Since transmission via urine has been reported in the literature in *M. bovis* cases (55), this possible extrapulmonary route of disease spread should be investigated when testing high-risk groups.

The median herd size of U.S. dairies has increased from 80 cows in 1987 to 1,300 cows in 2017 (69). The increase in the average size of dairy operations over the past few decades, in terms of the number of cows per herd, has resulted in dramatic needs for on-farm labor. Non-U.S.-born employees make up a significant portion of the workforce on U.S. dairy farms (70). A 2015 National Milk Producers Federation survey of 1,000 dairies (>50 cows) across the United States reported that 93% of operations hired outside labor and over 51% of employees were immigrants (71). A 2007 Wisconsin survey of dairy farms revealed that 40% of hired labor were immigrants; of these, 88.5% were from Mexico and most of the remainder of employees were from Central and South America (72). Based on the higher risk of MTBC infection in many non-U.S.-born employees compared with U.S. born workers, the Centers for Disease Control and Prevention recommends TB screening testing the high-risk groups (45).

Access to medical care can be challenging for non-U.S.-born employees. Often English language skills are limited, and employees may not have the documentation necessary to reside legally in the United States (71). A pilot project developed at the University of Wisconsin-Eau Claire School of Nursing was developed to immerse nursing students into Hispanic and rural culture. The focus of the program is to provide preventive healthcare and routine health screenings to a population that might not otherwise have access. Tuberculosis screening is included as one of the health screenings offered (73). Although this is a pilot project, it serves as a model that could be used in developing health-care programs that improve dairy employee health and safety.

The case reports presented here provide additional epidemiological support for human-to-cattle MTBC transmission and were largely the result of strong working relationships between animal health and public health in both North Dakota and Wisconsin. The communication and collaboration between animal health and public health officials to investigate cases of zoonotic diseases are crucial for gathering the information necessary to evaluate risk and identify effective preventive measures. While the actions of these two states can serve as a model, there are collaborative opportunities to establish additional best practices for issues important to both animal and human health.

Currently, the U.S. Cooperative State-Federal Bovine TB Eradication Program does not include mitigation strategies to address the risk of human introduction of MTBC into U.S. cattle herds, and these findings could change the paradigm of the program. A collaborative One Health approach is needed to address the health of the dairy workers and the animals. The U.S. government has defined One Health as "a collaborative, multisectoral, and transdisciplinary approach—working at the local, regional, national, and global levels—with the goal of achieving optimal health outcomes recognizing the interconnection between people, animals, plants, and their shared environment." (74). In response, the U.S. dairy industry convened a multisectoral working group of state and federal animal and public health officials to address this challenge.

CONCLUSION

This is this first published report using epidemiological and genotype evidence to establish human-to-cattle *M. bovis* transmission in the United States. This is also the first report of *M. tuberculosis* infection of cattle in the United States. In order to advance eradication of bTB in the U.S. cattle herd, the program must incorporate and address humans as another potential source of *M. bovis* or other MTBC species for cattle. This effort can only be achieved with a collaborative One Health approach that includes federal and state animal, public health, and wildlife agencies, livestock industries, producers, and healthcare workers and is focused on safeguarding both human and animal health.

ETHICS STATEMENT

Ethical review and approval was not required for the study on human participants in accordance with the local legislation and institutional requirements. Written informed consent for participation was not required for this study in accordance with the national legislation and the institutional requirements. Ethical review and approval was not required for the animal study because this is a case series involving client owned cattle and is not a research project. Written informed consent for participation was not obtained from the owners because Regulatory procedures were performed that didn't necessarily require written consent. Written consent was obtained for animals removed based on results of regulatory testing.

AUTHOR CONTRIBUTIONS

JL, TD, CY, and SR-A contributed to the conception of the paper. EP, SG-B, RK, JT-K, BC, SK, DP, SR, WH, TT, and SR-A performed the investigations. JL, EP, TD, and SR-A wrote the first draft. CP constructed the phylogenetic trees. All authors contributed to manuscript revisions, read, and approved the submitted version.

ACKNOWLEDGMENTS

The authors thank the dairy producers for their cooperation in these investigations and federal, state, and local animal and public health officials for conducting the investigations and herd testing. We also thank Dr. Brian McCluskey, Anne Berry, and Mary Foley for technical assistance, and Dr. Kathy Orloski for manuscript review.

REFERENCES

1. Garcia-Betancur JC, Menendez MC, Del Portillo P, Garcia MJ. Alignment of multiple complete genomes suggests that gene rearrangements may contribute towards the speciation of Mycobacteria. *Infect Genet Evol.* (2012) 12:819–26. doi: 10.1016/j.meegid.2011.09.024

2. Riojas MA, Mcgough KJ, Rider-Riojas CJ, Rastogi N, Hazbon MH. Phylogenomic analysis of the species of the *Mycobacterium tuberculosis* complex demonstrates that *Mycobacterium africanum, Mycobacterium bovis, Mycobacterium caprae, Mycobacterium microti* and *Mycobacterium pinnipedii* are later heterotypic synonyms of *Mycobacterium tuberculosis. Int J Syst Evol Microbiol.* (2018) 68:324–32. doi: 10.1099/ijsem.0.002507

3. WHO. *Global Tuberculosis Report 2020.* Geneva: World Health Organization (2020). Available online at: https://apps.who.int/iris/bitstream/handle/10665/336069/9789240013131-eng.pdf (accessed May 23, 2021).

4. Park WH, Krumwiede C. The relative importance of the bovine and human types of tubercle bacilli in the different forms of tuberculosis: (Final summary of cases investigated.). *J Med Res.* (1912) 27:109–14.

5. Steele JH. History, trends, and extent of pasteurization. *J Am Vet Med Assoc.* (2000) 217:175–8. doi: 10.2460/javma.2000.217.175

6. USDA. *Federal Meat Inspection Act. USDA Food Safety Inspection Service* (updated January 21, 2016; cited 2021) (2021). Available online at: https://www.fsis.usda.gov/policy/food-safety-acts/federal-meat-inspection-act (accessed March 31, 2021).

7. USDA. *Our History. USDA Food Safety Inspection Service* (updated February 21, 2018; cited 2022) (2021). Available online at: https://www.fsis.usda.gov/about-fsis/history (accessed March 31, 2021).

8. United States Department of Agriculture. (1956). *The Yearbook of Agriculture 1956: Animal Diseases.* Washington, DC: Gov't Print. Ofc.

9. Essey MA, Koller MA. Status of bovine tuberculosis in North America. *Vet Microbiol.* (1994) 40:15–22. doi: 10.1016/0378-1135(94)90043-4

10. Olmstead AL, Rhode PW. An impossible undertaking: the eradication of bovine tuberculosis in the United States. *J Econ Hist.* (2004) 64:734–72. doi: 10.1017/S0022050704002955

11. Palmer MV, Waters WR. Bovine tuberculosis and the establishment of an eradication program in the United States: role of veterinarians. *Vet Med Int.* (2011) 2011:816345. doi: 10.4061/2011/816345

12. Naugle AL, Schoenbaum M, Hench CW, Henderson OL, Shere J. Bovine tuberculosis eradication in the United States. In: Thoen CO, Steele JH, Kaneene JB, editors. *Zoonotic Tuberculosis.* Chichester: Wiley; Blackwell (2014). p. 235–51. doi: 10.1002/9781118474310.ch21

13. Thoen CO, Steele JH, Kaneene JB. *Zoonotic Tuberculosis: Mycobacterium bovis and Other Pathogenic Mycobacteria.* Chichester: John Wiley and Sons (2014). doi: 10.1002/9781118474310

14. Dankner WM, Davis CE. *Mycobacterium bovis* as a significant cause of tuberculosis in children residing along the United States-Mexico border in the Baja California region. *Pediatrics.* (2000) 105:E79. doi: 10.1542/peds.105.6.e79

15. Anonymous. Human tuberculosis caused by *Mycobacterium bovis*–New York City, 2001-2004. *Morbid Mortal Week Rep.* (2005). 52:605–8.

16. Rodwell TC, Kapasi AJ, Moore M, Milian-Suazo F, Harris B, Guerrero LP, et al. Tracing the origins of *Mycobacterium bovis* tuberculosis in humans in the USA to cattle in Mexico using spoligotyping. *Int J Infect Dis.* (2010) 14:e129–35. doi: 10.1016/j.ijid.2009.11.037

17. Orloski K, Robbe-Austerman S, Stuber T, Hench B, Schoenbaum M. Whole genome sequencing of *Mycobacterium bovis* isolated from livestock in the United States, 1989-2018. *Front Vet Sci.* (2018) 5:253. doi: 10.3389/fvets.2018.00253

18. Steele JH. Human tuberculosis in animals. In: Steele JH, Stoenner H, Kaplan W, Torten M, editors. *CRC Handbook Series in Zoonoses. Section A: Bacterial, Rickettsial, and Mycotic Diseases. Vol. II.* Boca Raton, FL: CRC Press, Inc. (1980). p. 141–59.

19. Thoen C, Steele JH. *Mycobacterium bovis Infections in Animals and Humans.* Ames, IA: Iowa State University Press (1995).

20. Fritsche A, Engel R, Buhl D, Zellweger JP. *Mycobacterium bovis* tuberculosis: from animal to man and back. *Int J Tuberc Lung Dis.* (2004) 8:903–4.

21. Ocepek M, Pate M, Zolnir-Dovc M, Poljak M. Transmission of *Mycobacterium tuberculosis* from human to cattle. *J Clin Microbiol.* (2005) 43:3555–7. doi: 10.1128/JCM.43.7.3555-3557.2005

22. Prasad HK, Singhal A, Mishra A, Shah NP, Katoch VM, Thakral SS, et al. Bovine tuberculosis in India: potential basis for zoonosis. *Tuberculosis (Edinb).* (2005) 85:421–8. doi: 10.1016/j.tube.2005.08.005

23. Chen Y, Chao Y, Deng Q, Liu T, Xiang J, Chen J, et al. Potential challenges to the stop TB plan for humans in China; cattle maintain *M. bovis* and *M tuberculosis. Tuberculosis (Edinb).* (2009) 89:95–100. doi: 10.1016/j.tube.2008.07.003

24. Romero B, Rodríguez S, Bezos J, Díaz R, Copano MF, Merediz I, et al. Humans as source of *Mycobacterium tuberculosis* infection in cattle, Spain. *Emerg Infect Dis.* (2011) 17:2393–5. doi: 10.3201/eid1712.101476

25. Gumi B, Schelling E, Berg S, Firdessa R, Erenso G, Mekonnen W, et al. Zoonotic transmission of tuberculosis between pastoralists and their livestock in South-East Ethiopia. *Ecohealth.* (2012) 9:139–49. doi: 10.1007/s10393-012-0754-x

26. Krajewska M, Kozińska M, Zwolska Z, Lipiec M, Augustynowicz-Kopeć E, Szulowski, K. Human as a source of tuberculosis for cattle. first evidence of transmission in Poland. *Vet Microbiol.* (2012). 159:269–71. doi: 10.1016/j.vetmic.2012.04.001

27. Špičić S, Duvnjak S, Deždek D, Kompes G, Habrun B, Cvetnić Z, et al. Molecular epidemiology of *Mycobacterium tuberculosis* transmission between cattle and man - a case report. *Vet Arhiv.* (2012) 82:303–10.

28. Ameni G, Tadesse K, Hailu E, Deresse Y, Medhin G, Aseffa A, et al. Transmission of *Mycobacterium tuberculosis* between farmers and cattle in central Ethiopia. *PLoS ONE*. (2013) 8:e76891. doi: 10.1371/journal.pone.0076891

29. Malama S, Munyeme M, Mwanza S, Muma JB. Isolation and characterization of non tuberculous mycobacteria from humans and animals in Namwala District of Zambia. *BMC Res Notes*. (2014) 7:622. doi: 10.1186/1756-0500-7-622

30. Mittal M, Chakravarti S, Sharma V, Sanjeeth BS, Churamani CP, Kanwar NS. Evidence of presence of *Mycobacterium tuberculosis* in bovine tissue samples by multiplex PCR: possible relevance to reverse zoonosis. *Transbound Emerg Dis*. (2014) 61:97–104. doi: 10.1111/tbed.12203

31. Hlokwe TM, Said H, Gcebe N. *Mycobacterium tuberculosis* infection in cattle from the Eastern Cape Province of South Africa. *BMC Vet Res*. (2017) 13:299. doi: 10.1186/s12917-017-1220-3

32. Adesokan HK, Akinseye VO, Streicher EM, Van Helden P, Warren RM, Cadmus SI. Reverse zoonotic tuberculosis transmission from an emerging Uganda I strain between pastoralists and cattle in South-Eastern Nigeria. *BMC Vet Res*. (2019) 15:437. doi: 10.1186/s12917-019-2185-1

33. Parsons SD, Warren RM, Ottenhoff TH, Gey Van Pittius NC, Van Helden PD. Detection of *Mycobacterium tuberculosis* infection in dogs in a high-risk setting. *Res Vet Sci*. (2012) 92:414–9. doi: 10.1016/j.rvsc.2011.03.026

34. Shipley ST, Coksaygan T, Johnson DK, Mcleod CG Jr, Detolla LJ. Diagnosis and prevention of dissemination of tuberculosis in a recently imported rhesus macaque (*Macaca mulatta*). *J Med Primatol*. (2008) 37(Suppl 1):20–4. doi: 10.1111/j.1600-0684.2007.00266.x

35. Mikota SK, Peddie L, Peddie J, Isaza R, Dunker F, West G, et al. Epidemiology and diagnosis of *Mycobacterium tuberculosis* in captive Asian elephants (*Elephas maximus*). *J Zoo Wildl Med*. (2001) 32:1–16. doi: 10.1638/1042-7260(2001)032[0001:EADOMT]2.0.CO;2

36. Payeur JB, Jarnagin JL, Marquardt JG, Whipple DL. Mycobacterial isolations in captive elephants in the United States. *Ann N Y Acad Sci*. (2002) 969:256–8. doi: 10.1111/j.1749-6632.2002.tb04388.x

37. Hoop, R. K. (2002). *Mycobacterium tuberculosis* infection in a canary (*Serinus canana* L.) and a blue-fronted Amazon parrot (*Amazona amazona* aestiva). *Avian Dis*. 46:502–4. doi: 10.1637/0005-2086(2002)046[0502:MTIIAC]2.0.CO;2

38. Schmidt V, Schneider S, Schlomer J, Krautwald-Junghanns ME, Richter E. Transmission of tuberculosis between men and pet birds: a case report. *Avian Pathol*. (2008) 37:589–92. doi: 10.1080/03079450802428901

39. Li H, Durbin R. Fast and accurate short read alignment with Burrows-Wheeler transform. *Bioinformatics*. (2009) 25:1754–60. doi: 10.1093/bioinformatics/btp324

40. Garrison E, Marth G. Haplotype-based variant detection from short-read sequencing. *arXiv:1207.3907* (2012).

41. Stamatakis A. RAxML version 8: a tool for phylogenetic analysis and post-analysis of large phylogenies. *Bioinformatics*. (2014) 30:1312–3. doi: 10.1093/bioinformatics/btu033

42. Letunic I, Bork P. Interactive Tree Of Life (iTOL) v4: recent updates and new developments. *Nucleic Acids Res*. (2019) 47:W256–9. doi: 10.1093/nar/gkz239

43. Coll F, Mcnerney R, Guerra-Assuncao JA, Glynn JR, Perdigao J, Viveiros M, et al. A robust SNP barcode for typing *Mycobacterium tuberculosis* complex strains. *Nat Commun*. (2014) 5:4812. doi: 10.1038/ncomms5812

44. Broeckl S, Krebs S, Varadharajan A, Straubinger RK, Blum H, Buettner M. Investigation of intra-herd spread of *Mycobacterium caprae* in cattle by generation and use of a whole-genome sequence. *Vet Res Commun*. (2017) 41:113–28. doi: 10.1007/s11259-017-9679-8

45. CDC. Recommendations for prevention and control of tuberculosis among foreign-born persons. Report of the Working Group on Tuberculosis among Foreign-Born Persons. Centers for Disease Control and Prevention. *MMWR Recomm Rep*. (1998) 47:1–29.

46. Edriss H, Lee M, Nugent K. *Mycobacterium tuberculosis* in a calf in West Texas: a rare pathology. *Southwest Respir Crit Care Chron*. (2020) 8:63–7. doi: 10.12746/swrccc.v8i33.643

47. Baldwin JH. Pulmonary bovine tuberculosis in an owner and in his dairy herd. *Cornell Vet*. (1968) 58:81–7.

48. Salvador LCM, O'brien DJ, Cosgrove MK, Stuber TP, Schooley AM, Crispell J, et al. Disease management at the wildlife-livestock interface: using whole-genome sequencing to study the role of elk in *Mycobacterium bovis* transmission in Michigan, USA. *Mol Ecol*. (2019) 28:2192–205. doi: 10.1111/mec.15061

49. USDA. *Bovine Tuberculosis Eradication Uniform Methods and Rules, APHIS 91-4, 91-45-011*. (2005). Available online at: https://www.aphis.usda.gov/animal_health/animal_diseases/tuberculosis/downloads/tb-umr.pdf (accessed May 21, 2021).

50. Ahola, S. 2019 National bovine tuberculosis eradication program update. In: *United States Animal Health Association Annual Meeting*. Washington, DC (2019).

51. Sjögren I, Hillerdal O. Bovine tuberculosis in man—reinfection or endogenous exacerbation. *Scand J Respir Dis*. (1978) 59:167–70.

52. Davidson JA, Loutet MG, O'connor, C, Kearns C, Smith RMM, Lalor MK, et al. Epidemiology of *Mycobacterium bovis* disease in humans in England, Wales, and Northern Ireland, 2002–2014. *Emerg Infect Dis*. (2017) 23:377–86. doi: 10.3201/eid2303.161408

53. Griffith AS. Human tubercle bacilli in the milk of a vaccinated cow. *J Pathol Bacteriol*. (1912) 17:323–8. doi: 10.1002/path.1700170304

54. Lesslie IW. Tuberculosis in attested herds caused by the human type tubercle bacillus. *Vet Rec*. (1960) 72:218–24.

55. Huitema H. The eradication of bovine tuberculosis in cattle in the Netherlands and the significance of man as a source of infection for cattle. *Select Pap R Netherl Tubercul Assoc*. (1969) 12:62–7.

56. Ibrahim S, Abubakar UB, Danbirni S, Usman A, Ballah FM, Kudi AC, et al. Molecular identification of *Mycobacterium tuberculosis* transmission between cattle and man: a case report. *J Microbiol Exp*. (2016) 3:00091. doi: 10.15406/jmen.2016.03.00091

57. Srivastava K, Chauhan DS, Gupta P, Singh HB, Sharma VD, Yadav VS, et al. Isolation of *Mycobacterium bovis* and *M. tuberculosis* from cattle of some farms in north India–possible relevance in human health. *Indian J Med Res*. (2008) 128:26–31.

58. Bezerra AV, Dos Reis EM, Rodrigues RO, Cenci A, Cerva C, Mayer FQ. Detection of *Mycobacterium tuberculosis* and *Mycobacterium avium* complexes by real-time PCR in bovine milk from Brazilian dairy farms. *J Food Prot*. (2015) 78:1037–42. doi: 10.4315/0362-028X.JFP-14-365

59. Bhanurekha V, Gunaseelan L, Pawar G, Nassiri R, Bharathy S. Molecular detection of *Mycobacterium tuberculosis* from bovine milk samples. *J Adv Vet Anim Res*. (2015) 2:80–3. doi: 10.5455/javar.2015.b44

60. Lepper AWD, Corner LA. Naturally occuring mycobacterioses of animals. In: Ratledge C, Stanford J, editors. *The Biology of Mycobacteria, Vol. 2, Immunological and Environmental Aspects*. London: Academic Press (1983). p. 417–521.

61. Tice FJ. Man, a source of bovine TB in cattle. *Cornell Vet*. (1944) 34:363–5.

62. Black H. The association of tuberculosis in man with a recurrent infection in a dairy herd. *N Z Vet J*. (1972) 20:14–5. doi: 10.1080/00480169.1972.33991

63. Alemayehu R, Girmay M, Gobena A. Bovine tuberculosis is more prevalent in cattle owned by farmers with active tuberculosis in central Ethiopia. *Vet J*. (2008) 178:119–25. doi: 10.1016/j.tvjl.2007.06.019

64. Dawson KL, Bell A, Kawakami RP, Coley K, Yates G, Collins DM. Transmission of *Mycobacterium orygis* (*M. tuberculosis* complex species) from a tuberculosis patient to a dairy cow in New Zealand. *J Clin Microbiol*. (2012) 50:3136–8. doi: 10.1128/JCM.01652-12

65. Hlavsa MC, Moonan PK, Cowan LS, Navin TR, Kammerer JS, Morlock GP, et al. Human tuberculosis due to *Mycobacterium bovis* in the United States, 1995-2005. *Clin Infect Dis*. (2008) 47:168–75. doi: 10.1086/589240

66. Lobue PA, Betacourt W, Peter C, Mosert KS. Epidemiology of *Mycobacterium bovis* disease in San Diego County, 1994-2000. *Int J Tuberc Lung Dis*. (2003) 7:180–5.

67. Scott C, Cavanaugh JS, Pratt R, Silk BJ, Lobue P, Moonan PK. Human tuberculosis caused by *Mycobacterium bovis* in the United States, 2006-2013. *Clin Infect Dis*. (2016) 63:594–601. doi: 10.1093/cid/ciw371

68. CDC. *TB Incidence in the United States, 1953-2019*. (2020). Available online at: https://www.cdc.gov/tb/statistics/tbcases.htm (accessed March 31, 2021).

69. Macdonald JM, Law J, Mosheim R. *Consolidation in U.S. Dairy Farming*. USDA (2020).

70. Harrison J, McReynolds J, O'kane T, Valentine B. "Hired labor on Wisconsin dairy farms: trends and implications. In: Jesse E, editor. *Status of Wisconsin Agriculture, 2008*. Madison, WI: University of Wisconsin (2008). p. 58–68.

71. Adcock F, Anderson D, Rosson P. The economic impacts of immigrant labor on U.S. dairy farms. In: *Center for North American Studies Report*. Center for North American Studies (2015).

72. Harrison J, Lloyd S, O'kane T, Turnquist A. Immigrant labor holds 40 percent market share. In: *Hoard's Dairyman*. (2009). p. 749–50.

73. Schiller L. *Nurses Reaching into the Rural Community - What's Happening at UWEC?* Univeristy of Wisconsin-Eau Claire (2015). Available online at: http://umash.umn.edu/wp-content/uploads/2015/09/nursing-schiller.pdf (accessed March 31, 2021).

74. USDA. (2020). *One Health 2020. USDA One Health*. (updated November 18, 2020; cited 2020). Available online at: https://www.aphis.usda.gov/aphis/ourfocus/animalhealth/sa_one_health (accessed March 31, 2021).

17

Enhanced Detection of *Mycobacterium bovis*-Specific T Cells in Experimentally-Infected Cattle

Paola M. Boggiatto [1]*, Carly R. Kanipe [1,2,3] and Mitchell V. Palmer [1]

[1] Infectious Bacterial Diseases Research Unit, National Animal Disease Center, Agricultural Research Service, United States Department of Agriculture, Ames, IA, United States, [2] Immunobiology Program, Iowa State University, Ames, IA, United States, [3] Oak Ridge Institute for Science and Education (ORISE), Oak Ridge, TN, United States

*Correspondence:
Paola M. Boggiatto
paola.boggiatto@usda.gov

Bovine tuberculosis (bTB), caused by infection with *Mycobacterium bovis*, continues to be a major economic burden associated with production losses and a public health concern due to its zoonotic nature. As with other intracellular pathogens, cell-mediated immunity plays an important role in the control of infection. Characterization of such responses is important for understanding the immune status of the host, and to identify mechanisms of protective immunity or immunopathology. This type of information can be important in the development of vaccination strategies, diagnostic assays, and in predicting protection or disease progression. However, the frequency of circulating *M. bovis*-specific T cells are often low, making the analysis of such responses difficult. As previously demonstrated in a different cattle infection model, antigenic expansion allows us to increase the frequency of antigen-specific T cells. Moreover, the concurrent assessment of cytokine production and proliferation provides a deeper understanding of the functional nature of these cells. The work presented here, analyzes the T cell response following experimental *M. bovis* infection in cattle via *in vitro* antigenic expansion and re-stimulation to characterize antigen-specific CD4, CD8, and γδ T cells and their functional phenotype, shedding light on the variable functional ability of these cells. Data gathered from these studies can help us better understand the cellular response to *M. bovis* infection and develop improved vaccines and diagnostic tools.

Keywords: Bovine tuberculosis, *Mycobacterium bovis*, T cell responses, proliferation, IFN-g, functional potential

INTRODUCTION

Bovine tuberculosis (bTB), is a chronic bacterial infection caused primarily by *Mycobacterium bovis*, a member of the *Mycobacterium tuberculosis* complex (1). This group of genetically-related mycobacteria also includes *M. tuberculosis*, *M. cannetii*, *M. africanum*, *M. pinnipeii*, *M. microti*, *M. caprae*, and *M. mungi*, which are known to infect and result in similar disease pathology in multiple hosts (2). Worldwide, bTB is a major cause of economic hardship. In 1995, it was estimated that bTB causes >50 million cattle infections resulting in $3 billion of losses annually (3, 4). The number of infected cattle and associated economic loss are likely higher today and its zoonotic nature poses a legitimate public health risk.

As with other intracellular pathogens, protective immune responses against tuberculosis (TB)

are associated with interferon gamma (IFN-γ) production derived from T helper 1 (T$_H$1) CD4 T cells (5–9). Delayed-type hypersensitivity reactions and IFN-γ release assays (IGRA) are commonly used to assess Mycobacterial reactivity or infection in various species [reviewed in Schiller et al. (10), Walzl et al. (11)]. However, these responses may not necessarily correlate with protection. In cattle, vaccination against bTB results in the induction of IFN-γ responses that can be measured *ex vivo* following overnight antigen stimulation, yet neither the presence nor the levels of IFN-γ induced translate into levels of protection afforded by vaccination (4, 11, 12).

Immune protection from future infections is mediated by the induction and maintenance of memory responses. Memory T cells are a heterogenous population of cells including T effector memory (T$_{EM}$), T central memory (T$_{CM}$), and T resident memory (T$_{RM}$) cells, which display distinct functional, effector, and migratory phenotypes (13). T$_{EM}$ tend to have a fast response to antigen, retain their effector function (i.e., cytokine production), and are relatively short-lived. In contrast, T$_{CM}$ respond slower to antigen, show increased proliferative capabilities, can generate T effector and T$_{EM}$ cells, and are long-lived. Previously, our laboratory demonstrated that following *M. bovis* infection in cattle, both T$_{EM}$ and T$_{CM}$ CD4 T cells are generated (14). In addition, we demonstrated that following *M. bovis* infection, bovine T$_{CM}$ are highly proliferative to antigen stimulation, and that T$_{CM}$ cells can revert in phenotype to generate T$_{EM}$ and T effector phenotypes (14).

While IFN-γ may not serve as a correlate of protection, it nevertheless plays a central role in the response to TB. Long-term culture systems, that measure IFN-γ from T$_{CM}$ cells, appear to be better predictors of vaccine efficacy as compared to *ex vivo* IFN-γ production (15–17). These data would suggest that perhaps the T cell source of IFN-γ is a better predictor of protection rather than the overall levels of IFN-γ. Since proliferation is another characteristic feature of memory responses, typically associated with T$_{CM}$, we wondered if the concurrent assessment of proliferation and IFN-γ production would allow us to better understand the source of IFN-γ and the overall functional phenotype of memory responses following *M. bovis* infection.

In the work presented here, we utilize an *in vitro* recall response assay, whereby antigen-specific cells are expanded, and proliferation and IFN-γ production are assessed concurrently. Additionally, we assess the potential of these antigen-specific cells to produce IFN-γ via restimulation, thereby enhancing their detection.

MATERIALS AND METHODS

Animals and *Mycobacterium bovis* Aerosol Challenge

Holstein steers ($\sim$6 months of age) were obtained from a tuberculosis-free source and housed at the National Animal Disease Center, agricultural biosafety level 3 (AgBSL3) animal facility. Animals were allowed to acclimate for 2 weeks prior to challenge. All animal studies were conducted with approval from

the Institutional Animal Care and Use Committee (AICUC) at the National Animal Disease Center in Ames, Iowa.

Mycobacterium bovis strain 10-7428, a field strain of low passage (<3), which has been shown to be virulent in a calf aerosol model (18). The inoculum was prepared using standard techniques (19) in Middlebrook's 7H9 liquid media (Becton Dickinson, Franklin Lakes, NJ) supplemented with 10% oleic acid-albumin-dextrose complex (OADC) (Difco, Detroit, MI) plus 0.05% Tween 80 (Sigma Chemical Co., St. Louis, MO). Mid log-phase growth bacilli were pelleted by centrifugation at 750x g, washed twice with phosphate buffered saline (PBS) (0.01 M, pH 7.2) and stored at -80° C until used. Frozen stock was warmed to room temperature and diluted to the appropriate cell density in 2 ml of PBS. Bacilli were enumerated by serial dilution plate counting on Middlebrook's 7H11 selective media (Becton Dickinson). A single dose was determined to be 1.12×10^4 CFU per steer.

M. bovis aerosol infection in cattle has been previously described (18, 20, 21). Briefly, eight (8) steers were infected with a single dose of virulent *M. bovis* strain 10-7428 by nebulization of inoculum into a mask (Equine AeroMask®, Trudell Medical International, London, ON, Canada) covering the nostrils and mouth. Six (6) age-matched steers were used as non-infected controls. All experimental animal procedures were conducted in accordance with recommendations in the Care and Use of Laboratory Animals of the National Institutes of Health and the Guide for the Care and Use of Agricultural Animals in Research and Teaching (22, 23). All animal-related procedures were also approved by the USDA-National Animal Disease Center Animal Care and Use Committee.

Isolation of Peripheral Blood Mononuclear Cells

Whole blood was collected via venipuncture of the jugular vein into EDTA tubes. Blood was processed for isolation of PBMC as described earlier (24), with some modifications. Briefly, 10 ml of blood were diluted 1:2 in sterile, culture grade, Dubelcco's phosphate-buffered saline (DPBS) (Gibco, Thermo Fisher, Waltham, MA) and centrifuged at 1,200 $\times$ g for 30 min at room temperature (RT). The buffy coats were harvested and overlayed onto 5 ml of 1.077 Ficoll (Sigma-Aldrich, St. Louis, MO), and centrifuged again at 1,200 $\times$ g for 30 min at RT. PBMC were then harvested and washed once in sterile PBS at 300 $\times$ g for 10 min. Cells were then counted on a hemocytometer using trypan blue staining to determine number and viability. Cells were then resuspended to the desired concentration using complete RPMI 1640 (Gibco Life Tech, Thermo Fisher) media, as described previously (24).

PBMC Labeling, *in vitro* Antigen Stimulation, and Restimulation

In order to assess antigen-specific responses, PBMC were first labeled using the CellTrace® violet proliferation kit (Invitrogen, Thermo Fisher), according to manufacturer's recommendations. Following labeling, 1×10^6 cells were plated onto 96-well, flat bottom plates and left unstimulated, or stimulated with

PPDb (5 μg/well), or Concanavalin A (ConA, 0.5μg/well, Sigma-Aldrich), in a total volume of 200 μl. Cells were then incubated at 37°C with 5% CO_2 for 7 days. In order to assess intracellular cytokine production, cultured PBMC were treated with either a 1× solution of eBioscience™ Protein transport inhibitor (500× Brefeldin A, Thermo Fisher) or with a 1× solution of eBioscience™ Cell Stimulation cocktail plus Protein transport inhibitor [500× phorbol 12-myristate 13-acetate (PMA), ionomycin, Brefeldin A] (Thermo Fisher) and incubated overnight for ~16 h prior to harvest on day 7 (24).

Surface and Intracellular Staining

For surface and intracellular cytokine staining, PBMC were harvested on day 7 of culture and washed with DPBS via centrifugation at 300 × g for 5 min at RT. Staining was performed as described previously (24). Briefly, cells were incubated with a fixable viability dye (eBioscience™, Thermo Fisher) and then stained for surface markers using FITC-labeled anti-bovine CD4 (CC8, Bio-Rad, Hercules, CA), APC-labeled anti-bovine CD8 (CC63, Bio-Rad), and anti-bovine γδ (IgG2b, TCR1-N24, Washington State University, Pullman, WA; BUV-labeled anti-IgG2b, BD Bioscience, San Jose, CA) antibodies. Cells were then fixed and permeabilized using BD Cytofix/Cytoperm™ kit (BD Bioscience) according to manufacturer's recommendation and stained with an anti-bovine, PE-labeled IFN-γ antibody (CC302, Bio-Rad). Cells were resuspended in FACS buffer and then analyzed using a BD FACSymphony™ A5 flow cytometer (BD Bioscience). Data was analyzed using FlowJo® software (Tree Star, Inc., San Diego, CA).

Statistical Analysis

Statistical analyses were performed using GraphPad Prism 8 (GraphPad software, San Diego, CA). Pair-wise comparisons of means were performed using t-tests, and multiple comparisons mixed-effects analysis were performed using Sidak's multiple comparisons test. $P \leq 0.05$ were considered statistically-significant.

RESULTS

T Cell Population Subsets

Analysis of T cell population subsets from cultured PMBC from control and M. bovis-infected animals at various time points post-challenge was performed; gating scheme for the analysis is shown in **Supplementary Figure 1**. Frequencies of CD4, CD8, and γδ T cells did not differ significantly between control and infected animals at all time points analyzed (**Figures 1A–C**). Overall, frequencies of all three subsets were relatively stable through the course of infection, with γδ T cells comprising the majority of the circulating pool of T cells (**Figure 1C**).

T Cell Proliferative Responses Following M. bovis Infection

In order to assess antigen-specific responses, PBMC from control and M. bovis-infected animals were stimulated in vitro with PPDb and the frequency of proliferating CD4, CD8, and γδ T cells were determined. Representative histograms for assessment of

proliferation can be seen in **Supplementary Figure 2**. Following antigen stimulation, we observed a significant increase in the frequency of proliferating CD4 T cells from M. bovis-infected animals as compared to controls at 4, 8-, and 48-weeks post-infection (**Figure 2A**). CD8 T cells from infected animals at 4- and 8-weeks post-infection showed an increase in the frequency of proliferating cells, as compared to control animals, however, this change was not statistically significant (**Figure 2B**). Similarly, proliferation was observed in γδ T cells from M. bovis-infected animals, however, the frequency of proliferating cells was only statistically different from control animals at 4 weeks post-infection (**Figure 2C**). Altogether, these data indicate that the majority of the proliferative response to PPDb antigens occurred within the CD4 T cell compartment of PBMCs from M. bovis-infected animals.

T Cell IFN-γ Responses Following *M. bovis* Infection

The frequency of IFN-γ-producing cells following in vitro stimulation of PBMC from control and infected animals was also assessed. Similar to the proliferation data, IFN-γ production was predominantly observed within the CD4 T cell compartment of infected animals, at all time points analyzed (**Figure 3**). However, despite observing an increased frequency of IFN-γ-producing CD4 T cells from M. bovis-infected animals as compared to controls, these differences were not statistically significant ($p = 0.09$, 0.08, and 0.30, respectively, for each time point) (**Figure 3A**). At 4- and 8-weeks post-infection, we observed an increase in the frequency of IFN-γ-producing CD8 T cells as compared to controls, however, this increase was not statistically significant (**Figure 3B**). The IFN-γ contribution from γδ T cells was relatively minimal, and no differences were seen between infected and control animals (**Figure 3C**). Congruent with the proliferation findings from above, the majority of IFN-γ produced in response to PPDb antigens is derived from CD4 T cells following M. bovis infection.

Concurrent Assessment of Proliferation and IFN-γ Responses to Mycobacterial Antigens

Assessing proliferation and cytokine production concurrently, allows for further characterization of the functional potential of antigen-specific cells. By analyzing cells in this fashion, four distinct functional subsets were identified: cells that proliferate and produce IFN-γ (double function), cells that only produce IFN-γ, cells that only proliferate, and cells that neither proliferate nor produce IFN-γ (double negative) in response to antigen (**Supplementary Figure 3**). These functional subsets were identifiable for CD4 (**Figure 4**), CD8 (**Supplementary Figure 4**), and γδ (**Supplementary Figure 5**) T cells. However, not unexpectedly, these subsets were more discernable within the CD4 T cell compartment, as this is the T cell population with the greatest frequency of cells responding to antigen stimulation. Functionally, antigen-specific CD4 T cells are primarily capable of either proliferating or both proliferating and producing IFN-γ. At 4, 8-, and 48-weeks post-infection, CD4 T cells that

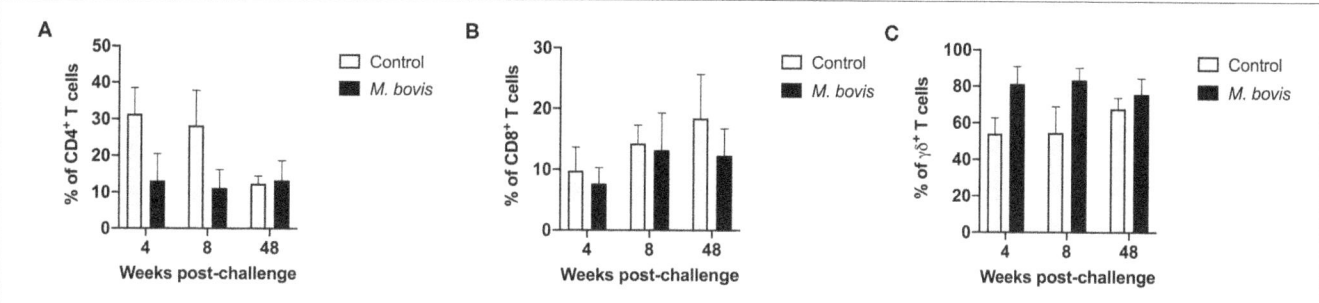

FIGURE 1 | Frequency of T cell subsets in control and *M. bovis* infected animals following challenge and *in vitro* antigen stimulation. PBMC from control (gray bars) and *M. bovis*-infected (black bars) animals were isolated at different time points after infection and stimulated *in vitro* with PPDb. Shown are the frequency of CD4 **(A)**, CD8 **(B)**, and γδ **(C)** T cells following *in vitro* stimulation. Presented are mean frequency values ± S.D.

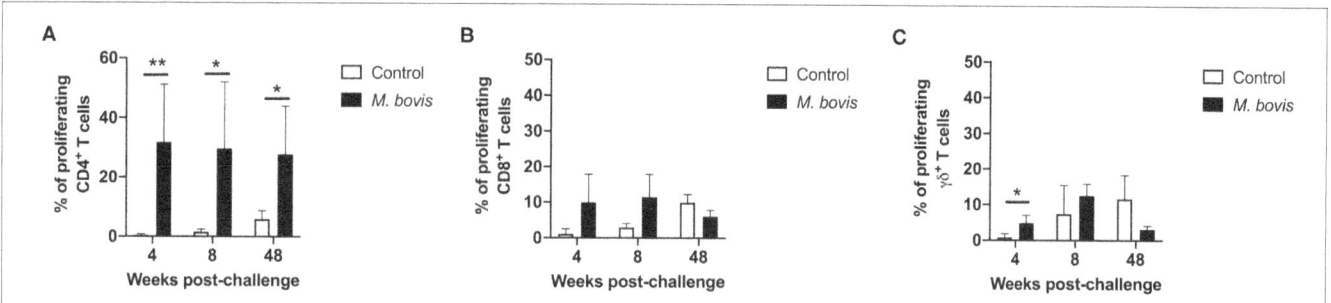

FIGURE 2 | Proliferation responses of T cell subsets from control and *M. bovis*-infected animals, following challenge and *in vitro* antigen stimulation. Shown are the frequencies of proliferating CD4 **(A)**, CD8 **(B)**, and γδ **(C)** T cells for control (gray bars) and *M. bovis* infected (black bars) animals at 4, 8, and 48 weeks post-infection in response to PPDb *in vitro* stimulation. Presented are mean frequency values ± S.D. Statistically significant differences are indicated; $^*p \leq 0.05$ and $^{**}p \leq 0.01$.

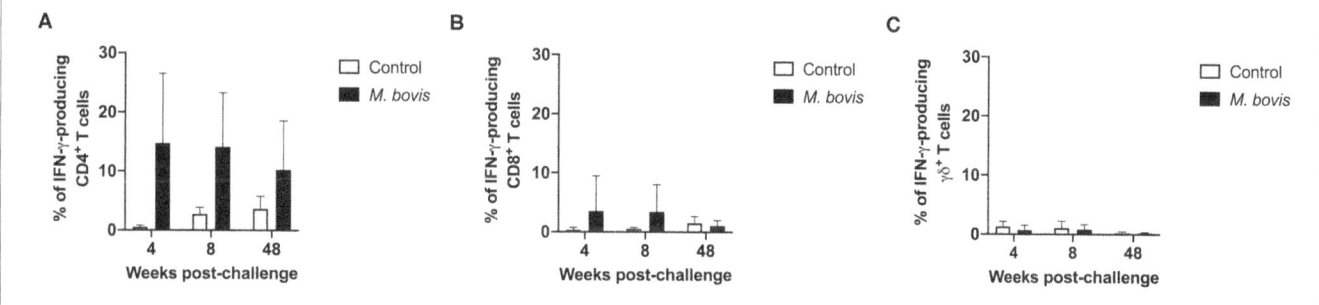

FIGURE 3 | Frequency of IFN-γ responses of T cell subsets from control and *M. bovis*-infected animals following *in vitro* antigen stimulation. Shown are the frequencies of IFN-γ-producing CD4 **(A)**, CD8 **(B)**, and γδ **(C)** T cells from control (gray bars) and *M. bovis*-infected (black bars) animals at 4-, 8-, and 48-weeks post-infection, following *in vitro* PPDb stimulation. Presented are mean frequency values ± S.D.

proliferate and produce IFN-γ to antigen stimulation comprise approximately 8.19, 11.91, and 9.74% of the total CD4 response, respectively (**Figure 4**, pie charts, green color). In comparison, cells that only proliferate in response to antigen stimulation make up 21.65, 17.78, and 18.03% at 4, 8-, and 48-weeks post-infection, respectively (**Figure 4**, pie charts, purple color). These data indicate that a smaller frequency of CD4 T cells display dual function at all times points analyzed. In fact, further analysis of the CD4 antigen-specific response, which excludes the double negative population (i.e., cells not responding to antigen stimulation), revealed that the proliferation-only population

comprised over 50% of the response at all time points analyzed (**Supplementary Figure 6**, top panel). CD4 T cells that showed dual function (i.e., proliferation and IFN-γ) comprised 25–37% of the antigen specific cells (**Supplementary Figure 6**, top panel, green), while single IFN-γ producers only made up a very small percentage of the population (1–6%) (**Supplementary Figure 6**, top panel, blue).

Despite the reduced frequency of responding CD8 T cells, a similar pattern of functional phenotype was observed for this subset (**Supplementary Figure 4**). Proliferative responses made up the majority of the functional potential of CD8 T

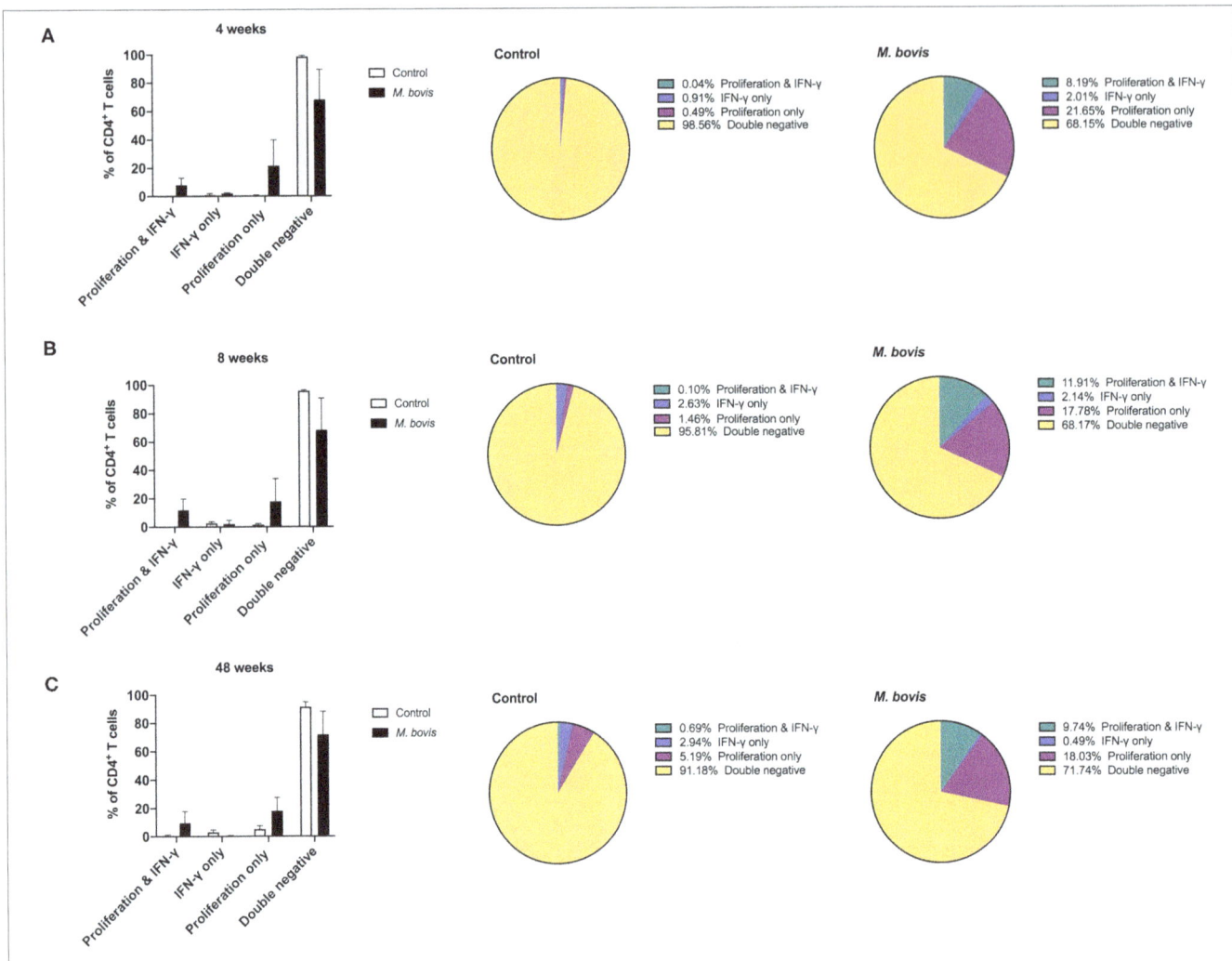

FIGURE 4 | Distinct functional subsets of *M. bovis*-specific CD4 T cells following concurrent assessment of proliferation and IFN-γ production. Bar graphs (left) and pie charts (right) showing the frequency of CD4 T cells with distinct functional phenotypes from control (gray bars) and *M. bovis*-infected animals (black bars) at 4-**(A)**, 8-**(B)**, and 48-**(C)** weeks post-infection. Functional phenotypes are denoted as CD4 T cells that in response to *in vitro* PPDb stimulation show proliferation and IFN-γ production (green), IFN-γ production only (blue), proliferation only (purple), or do not respond [double negative (gold)]. Shown are mean frequencies ± S.D.

cells, followed by double producers, and a smaller percentage of IFN-γ-only producing cells (**Supplementary Figures 4, 6**, middle panel). Interestingly, γδ T cells showed primarily a proliferative response (**Supplementary Figure 5**), making up over 90% of the antigen-specific response at all time points analyzed (**Supplementary Figure 6**, bottom panel). Altogether, these data showed that when functional phenotypes are assessed concurrently, proliferation appears to predominate for CD4, CD8, and γδ T cells. Additionally, CD4-, CD8-, and γδ-derived IFN-γ arises from cells that have also proliferated in response to antigen, with a much smaller contribution arising from non-proliferating cells.

Enhancing Cytokine Production Following Mycobacterial Antigen Stimulation

Above findings indicated that proliferation comprises the majority of the antigen-specific response, and that only a subset

of proliferating cells produced IFN-γ in response to PPDb stimulation. We wondered if the remainder of proliferating cells had the potential to make cytokines, when re-stimulation was provided *in vitro*. In order to determine if these cells had the potential to produce IFN-γ, 16 h prior to harvest on day 7, cells were re-stimulated with PMA/Ionomycin, a pan-T cell stimulator, in the presence of brefeldin A, as described previously (24). Indeed, following restimulation with PMA/Ionomycin, we observed a lower percentage of cells that only proliferated (**Supplementary Figure 3**, last column). This is particularly clear for CD4 T cells from *M. bovis*-infected animals, where cells displaying dual function (proliferation and IFN-γ) now constitute ∼44, 40, and 22% of the response at 4-, 8-, and 48-weeks post-infection, respectively (**Figure 5**). The frequency of proliferating-only CD4 T cells constitutes a mere 5, 0.15, and 2.13% of responding cells (**Figure 5**).

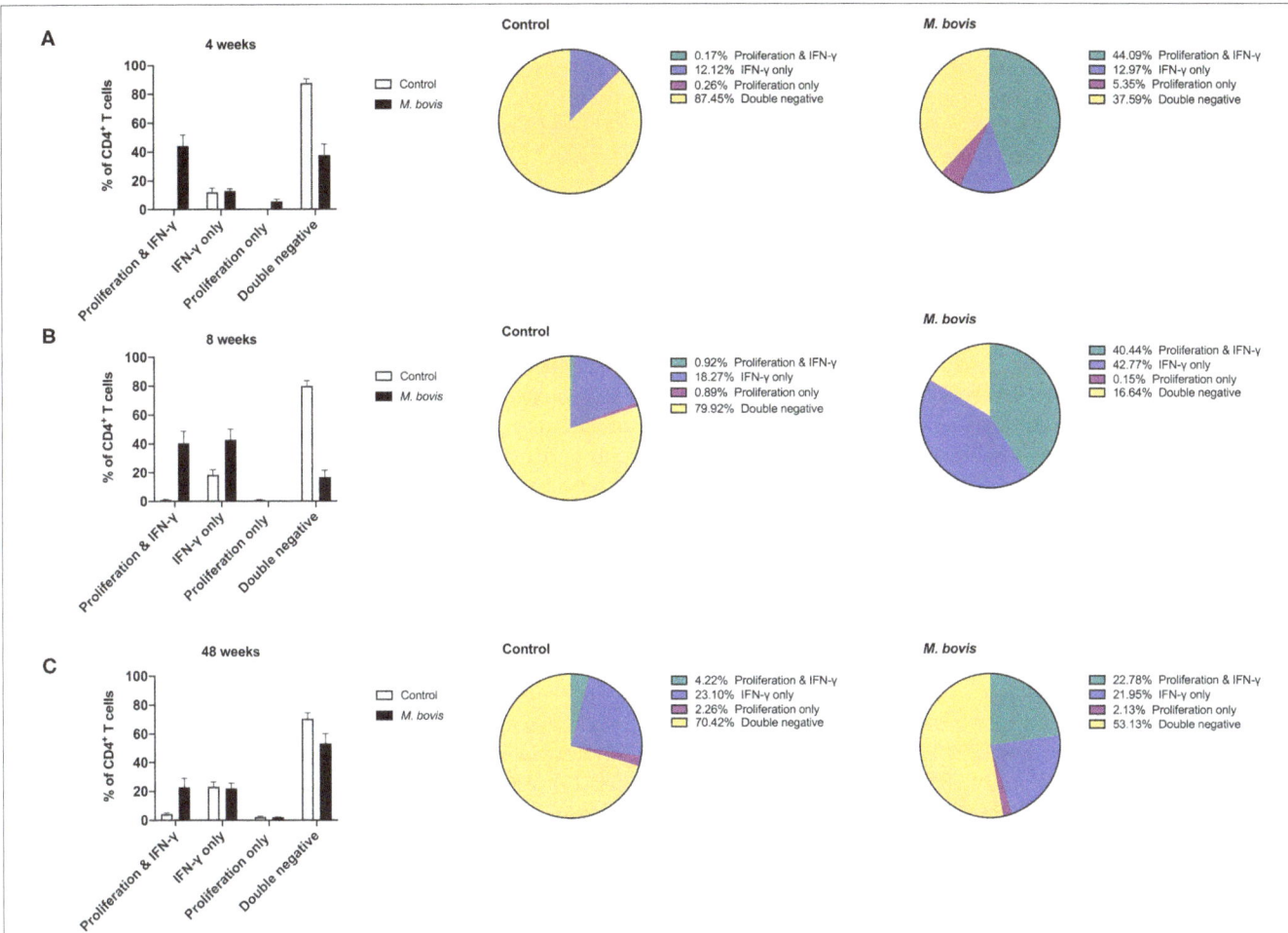

FIGURE 5 | Distinct functional subsets of *M. bovis*-specific CD4 T cells following concurrent assessment of proliferation and IFN-γ production following antigen stimulation and restimulation *in vitro*. Bar graphs (left) and pie charts (right) showing the frequency of CD4 T cells with distinct functional phenotypes from control (gray bars) and *M. bovis*-infected animals (black bars) at 4-**(A)**, 8-**(B)**, and 48-**(C)** weeks post-infection. PBMC were stimulated with PPDb for 7 days and restimulated with PMA/ionomycin overnight for the last 16 h of culture. Proliferation and IFN-γ production were then assessed concurrently via flow cytometry. Functional phenotypes are denoted as CD4 T cells that show proliferation and IFN-γ production (green), IFN-γ production only (blue), proliferation only (purple), or do not respond [double negative (gold)]. Shown are mean frequencies ± S.D.

This switch in the functional profile of antigen-specific T cells following restimulation is also observed in antigen-specific CD8 (**Supplementary Figure 7**) and γδ (**Supplementary Figure 8**) T cells, albeit not to the extent that was observed for CD4 T cells. When analyzing this response solely within the subset of cells responding to antigen, CD4 T cells that proliferate and produce IFN-γ constitute 70% of the response at 4 weeks post-infection and 48% at 8- and 48-weeks post infection (**Supplementary Figure 9**, top row). In comparison, antigen-responsive cells CD8 T cells that proliferate and produce IFN-γ consistently constitute ∼30% of the response at 4-, 8-, and 48-weeks post infection (**Supplementary Figure 9**, middle row, green). At 4- and 48-weeks post-infection, there remains a substantial population of CD8 T cells (33 and 23%, respectively), that only demonstrate proliferative potential despite the addition of restimulation (**Supplementary Figure 9**, middle row, purple). A similar pattern of response is observed for γδ T cells

responding to antigen stimulation; there is an increase in the frequency of proliferating and IFN-γ-producing cells at week 8 post-infection, yet at 4- and 48 weeks post infection proliferation predominates as the antigen-specific response (**Supplementary Figure 9**, bottom row, green and purple). Altogether, these data demonstrate that *M. bovis*-specific T cells that proliferate to antigen stimulation are all capable of producing IFN-γ, and that this response can be enhanced by providing restimulation.

CONCLUSIONS

Understanding the functional role of T cells following *M. bovis* infection in cattle will provide insights for the development of vaccine and diagnostic interventions. Proliferation and cytokine production are two major functional characteristics of activated, antigen-specific T cells. Production of IFN-γ from T cells is intimately tied with T_H1 responses, which are necessary for the clearance of intracellular pathogens, including mycobacteria. However, IFN-γ levels do not always correlate with protection (4, 11). In the work presented here, we sought to further dissect the functional potential of *M. bovis*-specific T cells by concurrently assessing two commonly-measured functional phenotypes: proliferation and IFN-γ production. In doing so, we were able to characterize three distinct functional subsets for all three T cell populations: cells with the potential to proliferate and produce IFN-γ (dual function), cells that only produce IFN-γ, and cells that only proliferate in response to antigen stimulation. Furthermore, we demonstrate that T cells with dual function and cells that proliferate-only make up the majority of the *M. bovis*-specific T cell response. We also demonstrate that when restimulated, antigen-specific cells that proliferate-only, are capable of producing IFN-γ.

The frequency of CD4, CD8, and γδ T cells remains relatively stable throughout the course of infection, or at least through the time points analyzed in this study (4, 8, and 48 weeks post-infection). In addition, we found that *M. bovis*-specific proliferative responses can be seen in all three T cell populations, yet significant increases in the frequency of proliferating cells were only observed for CD4 T cells at all three time points. Similarly, IFN-γ responses were primarily seen within CD4 T cells, and to a lesser extent with CD8 T cells. Interestingly, despite this increase in the frequency of IFN-γ-producing CD4 T cells in *M. bovis*-infected animals, these changes were not statistically significant when compared to CD4 T cells from control animals. We attribute this to the variability in responses observed for IFN-γ in outbred populations, such as cattle. It should be noted that moderate variability was also observed for proliferative responses. Cattle represent an outbred population, and while experimental infections provide some level of control, variability in animal responses are expected. Overall, however, we show that proliferation and IFN-γ responses following *M. bovis* infection are primarily found within the CD4 T cell compartment, with CD8 and γδ T cells providing minor contribution to these responses, consistent with previous observations from our laboratory (14).

Concurrent measurement of proliferation and IFN-γ provides another level of insight into the functional potential of antigen-specific T cells. As a result, we were able to identify three distinct antigen-specific T cell populations with functional potential. We observed that following *M. bovis* challenge, there are two proliferating populations, one that produces IFN-γ and one that only proliferates. These two populations could represent distinct effector or memory subsets. We have previously demonstrated that following *M. bovis* infection, cattle do develop T central memory (T_{CM}) and T effector memory (T_{EM}) responses (14). Furthermore, we have demonstrated that antigen stimulation not only results in proliferation of T_{CM}, but also in a switch from T_{CM} to T_{EM}, which are capable of producing IFN-γ (14). By measuring the functional phenotypes concurrently, we are likely seeing those distinct subsets. The work presented here did not include surface markers to corroborate memory phenotypes and only characterized proliferation and IFN-γ production. Despite

this, it should be noted that by measuring proliferation and cytokine production concurrently, we were able to identify two functionally-distinct populations of cells responding to antigen stimulation. This approach may allow further characterization into other memory and/or effector subsets, which cannot be identified using surface markers as they have either not yet been identified or are not available for cattle.

Concomitant immunity, is a mechanism of immunity whereby a persistent, low-grade infection results in protection from subsequent re-infection with the same pathogen. This type of protection has been shown in other infectious models such as *Leishmania* (25). Unlike the classical idea of "T cell memory," concomitant immunity is primarily driven by a unique subset of CD4 effector cells that are derived from T_{CM} cells, are non-proliferative, are high IFN-γ producers, and are long-lived but only under conditions of persistent antigen availability [reviewed in Reyed and Rafati (26)]. In the mouse, this subset of T effector cells can be characterized by expression of the surface marker Ly6C (26), but this marker has not been characterized in other species. Therefore, tracking of this specific cell type becomes difficult in other species. This phenomenon, and its potential role in mediating protection in tuberculosis, have been recently described in a non-human primate model (27). Further support for concomitant immunity is found in human cohort studies as well as epidemiological data suggesting that prior infection with *M. tuberculosis* provides protection against subsequent infections (28, 29). The role of concomitant immunity has not yet been explored for bTB. While we may be unable to characterize Ly6C-expressing T effector memory subset based on surface expression markers, it may be possible to characterize these cells based on their non-proliferative and high-IFN-γ expression profile, which this assay would facilitate. Additional surface and intracellular markers could be added in order to expand the profiling of memory subsets using this assay. We propose that by refining the concurrent analysis of functional phenotypes, we may be able to explore some of these questions in cattle, thus providing further insights into the cellular immune response to *M. bovis* in its natural host.

The presence of antigen-specific cells that proliferate but do not produce IFN-γ in response to antigen stimulation led us to ask the question about the functional potential of these cells. To address this, we stimulated these cells with PMA/Ionomycin and measured cytokine production. Interestingly, as seen with T cells from cattle vaccinated against brucellosis (24), this subset of proliferating T cells is capable of producing IFN-γ. These data beg the question as to why the distinction in functional phenotype. As mentioned earlier this could be related to memory subtypes (T_{CM} vs. T_{EM}), or perhaps this distinction is related to the nature of antigen stimulation. We assume that these antigen-specific T cells constitute a heterogenous populations of cells with a wide T cell repertoire and antigenic specificity. One hypothesis would be that the quantity and quality of the antigen may be responsible for driving function. Indeed, it has been previously shown that thresholds of T cell receptor signaling and duration of signaling determine T cell fate including functions such as cytokine production and proliferation [reviewed in Zikherman and Au-Yeung (30)]. We cannot discard the possibility that the antigen in this assay reaches varying degrees of stimulation for different T cell receptors. Further analysis utilizing defined antigens (i.e., single peptides or peptide cocktails) for stimulation using this assay, would allow us to determine if antigen-specificity and/or availability drives the functional distinction observed here.

Restimulation with PMA/ionomycin also allowed for the enhanced detection of antigen-specific, IFN-γ-producing CD4 cells (i.e., cells proliferating and producing IFN-γ). The restimulation step demonstrated that these proliferating cells are capable of producing IFN-γ when added stimulation is provided. However, we did not assess whether these cells could produce any other cytokines. Polyfunctional T cells (i.e., cells with the ability to produce multiple cytokines) have been shown to correlate with protection in various infectious models (31–33). However, the role of polyfunctional T cells in TB remains poorly understood, with conflicting data for their role in protection vs. active disease (34, 35). Work from our laboratory has shown that in cattle polyfunctional (IFN-γ/TNF-α/IL-2) CD4 T_{CM} cells are associated with protective responses following BCG vaccination, while IFN-γ/TNF-α T_{CM} cells are associated with higher bacterial burdens (36). The data presented here suggests that a large proportion of M. bovis-specific CD4 T cells only proliferate upon antigen stimulation, but are capable of producing cytokines in response to restimulation. It may be possible that a significant portion of antigen-specific cells are missed when cytokine analysis is performed in isolation. Assessment of cytokine polyfunctionality using restimulation, as described here, may provide a way to enhance our ability to detect these T cell subsets with polyfunctional phenotypes.

Altogether, the work presented here utilized an *in vitro* assay relying on enrichment of M. bovis-specific T cells via antigen stimulation to characterize functional phenotypes of proliferation and/or IFN-γ-production. The data demonstrate that the majority of antigen-responsive CD4 T cells proliferate in response to antigen, followed by cells capable of proliferating and producing cytokine. This type of approach, concurrent assessment of two major functions of activated T cells, along with further phenotypic analysis, are likely to increase our fundamental understanding of T cell responses involved in bTB.

ETHICS STATEMENT

The animal study was reviewed and approved by National Animal Disease Center Institutional Animal Care and Use Committee (NADC IACUC).

AUTHOR CONTRIBUTIONS

PB, CK, and MP: experiment design, sample collection, experiments, and manuscript editing. PB: data analysis and manuscript preparation. All authors contributed to the article and approved the submitted version.

FUNDING

Financial support for these studies were provided by the United States Department of Agriculture, Agricultural Research Service (ARS) and Animal and Plant Health Inspection Service (APHIS).

ACKNOWLEDGMENTS

We would like to thank the National Animal Disease Center's Animal Research Unit (NADC-ARU) clinical veterinarian Dr. Rebecca Cox and the High Containment Team animal care staff Jacob Fritz, Hannah Schroeder, Kolby Stallman, Derek Vermeer, Tiffany Williams, and Robin Zeisneiss for excellent animal care. We thank Hahley Wiltse and Shelly Zimmerman for excellent technical assistance. We would also like to thank Dr. Lauren Crawford and Lilia Walther for reading and editing the manuscript.

SUPPLEMENTARY MATERIAL

Supplementary Figure 1 | Flow cytometry gating scheme for T cell subsets. Shown are representative dot plots demonstrating gating strategies for lymphocytes and singlet discrimination based on FSC and SSC. Also shown are live/dead discrimination based on uptake of a fixable viability dye, and CD4, CD8, and γδ gating based on SSC and fluorescent signal.

Supplementary Figure 2 | Flow cytometry analysis of proliferating cells based on CellTrace™ violet dilution. Shown are representative histograms for determination of the frequency of proliferating CD4, CD8, and γδ T cells without stimulation (first column), PPD-B antigen stimulation (middle column), and ConA stimulation (last column).

Supplementary Figure 3 | Flow cytometry gating for the concurrent assessment of proliferation and IFN-γ responses for T cell subsets. Shown are representative dot plots for cells gated on CD4 (top row), CD8 (middle row), and γδ (bottom row) following *in vitro* culture without stimulation (first column), with PPDb stimulation (middle column) and PPDb + PMA/Ionomycin (last column), for the assessment of proliferation (CellTrace dilution, y-axis), and IFN-γ production (x-axis).

Supplementary Figure 4 | Distinct functional subsets of M. bovis-specific CD8 T cells following concurrent assessment of proliferation and IFN-γ production. Bar graphs (left) and pie charts (right) showing the frequency of CD4 T cells with distinct functional phenotypes from control (gray bars) and M. bovis-infected animals (black bars) at 4-**(A)**, 8-**(B)**, and 48-**(C)** weeks post-infection. Functional phenotypes are denoted as CD8 T cells that in response to *in vitro* PPDb stimulation show proliferation and IFN-γ production (green), IFN-γ production only (blue), proliferation only (purple), or do not respond [double negative (gold)]. Shown are mean frequencies ± S.D.

Supplementary Figure 5 | Distinct functional subsets of M. bovis-specific γδ T cells following concurrent assessment of proliferation and IFN-γ production. Bar graphs (left) and pie charts (right) showing the frequency of CD8 T cells with distinct functional phenotypes from control (gray bars) and M. bovis-infected animals (black bars) at 4-**(A)**, 8-**(B)**, and 48-**(C)** weeks post-infection. Functional phenotypes are denoted as γδ T cells that in response to *in vitro* PPDb stimulation show proliferation and IFN-γ production (green), IFN-γ production only (blue), proliferation only (purple), or do not respond [double negative (gold)]. Shown are mean frequencies ± S.D.

Supplementary Figure 6 | Breakdown of M. bovis-specific T cell subsets by functional phenotype. Shown are pie charts showing the distribution of CD4 (top row), CD8 (middle row), and γδ (bottom row) T cells responding to antigen stimulation from M. bovis-infected animals via proliferation and IFN-γ production (green), IFN-γ production only (blue), and proliferation only (purple).

Supplementary Figure 7 | Distinct functional subsets of *M. bovis*-specific CD8 T cells following concurrent assessment of proliferation and IFN-γ production following antigen stimulation and restimulation *in vitro*. Bar graphs (left) and pie charts (right) showing the frequency of CD4 T cells with distinct functional phenotypes from control (gray bars) and *M. bovis*-infected animals (black bars) at 4-**(A)**, 8-**(B)**, and 48-**(C)** weeks post-infection. PBMC were stimulated *in vitro* with PPDb for 7 days and restimulated with PMA/ionomycin overnight for the last 16 h of culture. Proliferation and IFN-γ production were then assessed concurrently via flow cytometry. Functional phenotypes are denoted as CD8 T cells that show proliferation and IFN-γ production (green), IFN-γ production only (blue), proliferation only (purple), or do not respond [double negative (gold)]. Shown are mean frequencies ± S.D.

Supplementary Figure 8 | Distinct functional subsets of *M. bovis*-specific γδ T cells following concurrent assessment of proliferation and IFN-γ production following antigen stimulation and restimulation *in vitro*. Bar graphs (left) and pie

charts (right) showing the frequency of CD4 T cells with distinct functional phenotypes from control (gray bars) and *M. bovis*-infected animals (black bars) at 4-**(A)**, 8-**(B)**, and 48-**(C)** weeks post-infection. PBMC were stimulated *in vitro* with PPDb for 7 days and restimulated with PMA/ionomycin overnight for the last 16 h of culture. Proliferation and IFN-γ production were then assessed concurrently via flow cytometry. Functional phenotypes are denoted as γδ T cells that show proliferation and IFN-γ production (green), IFN-γ production only (blue), proliferation only (purple), or do not respond [double negative (gold)]. Shown are mean frequencies ± S.D.

Supplementary Figure 9 | Breakdown of *M. bovis*-specific T cell subsets by functional phenotype following restimulation. Shown are pie charts showing the distribution of CD4 (top row), CD8 (middle row), and γδ (bottom row) T cells responding to *in vitro* PPDb stimulation from *M. bovis*-infected animals via proliferation and IFN-γ production (green), IFN-γ production only (blue), and proliferation only (purple).

REFERENCES

1. Langer A, LoBue PA. Public health significance of zoonotic tuberculosis in animals and humans. In: Thoen CO, Steele JH, and Kaneene JB, editors. *Zoonotic Tuberculosis: Mycobacterium bovis and Other Pathogenic Mycobacteria*. Ames, IA: Wiley Blackwell (2014). p. 21–34. doi: 10.1002/9781118474310.ch3
2. Rodriguez-Campos S, Smith NH, Boniotti MB, Aranaz A. Overview and phylogeny of *Mycobacterium tuberculosis* complex organisms: implications for diagnostics and legislation of bovine tuberculosis. *Res Vet Sci*. (2014) 97 (Suppl):S5–19. doi: 10.1016/j.rvsc.2014.02.009
3. Steele J. Introduction (part 2 regional and country status reports). In: Steele COTJH, editor. *Mycobacterium bovis Infection in Animals and Humans*. Steele. IA: University Press (1995).
4. Waters WR, Palmer MV, Buddle BM, Vordermeier HM. Bovine tuberculosis vaccine research: historical perspectives and recent advances. *Vaccine*. (2012) 30:2611–22. doi: 10.1016/j.vaccine.2012.02.018
5. Flynn JL, Chan J, Triebold KJ, Dalton DK, Stewart TA, Bloom BR. An essential role for interferon gamma in resistance to *Mycobacterium tuberculosis* infection. *J Exp Med*. (1993) 178:2249–54. doi: 10.1084/jem.178.6.2249
6. Vordermeier HM, Chambers MA, Cockle PJ, Whelan AO, Simmons J, Hewinson RG. Correlation of ESAT-6-specific gamma interferon production with pathology in cattle following *Mycobacterium bovis* BCG vaccination against experimental bovine tuberculosis. *Infect Immun*. (2002) 70:3026–32. doi: 10.1128/IAI.70.6.3026-3032.2002
7. Bold TD, Banaei N, Wolf AJ, Ernst JD. Suboptimal activation of antigen-specific CD4+ effector cells enables persistence of *M. tuberculosis in vivo*. *PLoS Pathog*. (2011) 7:e1002063. doi: 10.1371/journal.ppat.1002063
8. Pollock KM, Whitworth HS, Montamat-Sicotte DJ, Grass L, Cooke GS, Kapembwa MS, et al. T-cell immunophenotyping distinguishes active from latent tuberculosis. *J Infect Dis*. (2013) 208:952–68. doi: 10.1093/infdis/jit265
9. Waters WR, Maggioli MF, McGill JL, Lyashchenko KP, Palmer MV. Relevance of bovine tuberculosis research to the understanding of human disease: historical perspectives, approaches, immunologic mechanisms. *Vet Immunol Immunopathol*. (2014) 159:113–32. doi: 10.1016/j.vetimm.2014.02.009
10. Schiller I, Oesch B, Vordermeier HM, Palmer MV, Harris BN, Orloski KA, et al. Bovine tuberculosis: a review of current and emerging diagnostic techniques in view of their relevance for disease control and eradication. *Transbound Emerg Dis*. (2010) 57:205–20. doi: 10.1111/j.1865-1682.2010.01148.x
11. Walzl G, Ronacher K, Hanekom W, Scriba TJ, Zumla A. Immunological biomarkers of tuberculosis. *Nat Rev Immunol*. (2011) 11:343–54. doi: 10.1038/nri2960
12. Wedlock DN, Denis M, Vordermeier HM, Hewinson RG, Buddle BM. Vaccination of cattle with Danish and Pasteur strains of *Mycobacterium bovis* BCG induce different levels of IFNgamma post-vaccination, but induce similar levels of protection against bovine tuberculosis. *Vet Immunol Immunopathol*. (2007) 118:50–8. doi: 10.1016/j.vetimm.2007.04.005

13. Jameson SC, Masopust D. Understanding subset diversity in T cell memory. *Immunity*. (2018) 48:214–26. doi: 10.1016/j.immuni.2018.02.010
14. Maggioli MF, Palmer MV, Thacker TC, Vordermeier HM, Waters WR. Characterization of effector and memory T cell subsets in the immune response to bovine tuberculosis in cattle. *PLoS ONE*. (2015) 10:e0122571. doi: 10.1371/journal.pone.0122571
15. Whelan AO, Wright DC, Chambers MA, Singh M, Hewinson RG, Vordermeier HM. Evidence for enhanced central memory priming by live *Mycobacterium bovis* BCG vaccine in comparison with killed BCG formulations. *Vaccine*. (2008) 26:166–73. doi: 10.1016/j.vaccine.2007.11.005
16. Vordermeier HM, Villarreal-Ramos B, Cockle PJ, McAulay M, Rhodes SG, Thacker T, et al. Viral booster vaccines improve *Mycobacterium bovis* BCG-induced protection against bovine tuberculosis. *Infect Immun*. (2009) 77:3364–73. doi: 10.1128/IAI.00287-09
17. Waters WR, Palmer MV, Nonnecke BJ, Thacker TC, Scherer CF, Estes DM, et al. Efficacy and immunogenicity of *Mycobacterium bovis* DeltaRD1 against aerosol *M. bovis* infection in neonatal calves. *Vaccine*. (2009) 27:1201–9. doi: 10.1016/j.vaccine.2008.12.018
18. Waters WR, Thacker TC, Nelson JT, DiCarlo DM, Maggioli MF, Greenwald R, et al. Virulence of two strains of *Mycobacterium bovis* in cattle following aerosol infection. *J Comp Pathol*. (2014) 151:410–9. doi: 10.1016/j.jcpa.2014.08.007
19. Larsen MH, Biermann K, Jacobs WR. Laboratory maintenace of *Mycobacterium tuberculosis*. *Curr Protoc Microbiol*. (2007) Chapter 10:Unit 10A.1. doi: 10.1002/9780471729259.mc10a01s6
20. Palmer MV, Waters WR, Whipple DL. Aerosol delivery of virulent *Mycobacterium bovis* to cattle. *Tuberculosis*. (2002) 82:275–82. doi: 10.1054/tube.2002.0341
21. Palmer MV, Thacker TC, Waters WR. Analysis of cytokine gene expression using a novel chromogenic in-situ hybridization method in pulmonary granulomas of cattle infected experimentally by aerosolized *Mycobacterium bovis*. *J Comp Pathol*. (2015) 153:150–9. doi: 10.1016/j.jcpa.2015.06.004
22. FASS. Guide for the care and use of agricultural animals in research and teaching. Champaign, IL: Federation of Animal Science Societies (2010).
23. Garber JC. *Guide for the Care and Use of Laboratory Animals*. Washington, D.C: The National Academies Press (2011).
24. Boggiatto PM, Schaut RG, Olsen SC. Enhancing the detection of brucella-specific CD4(+) T cell responses in cattle via *in vitro* antigenic expansion and restimulation. *Front Immunol*. (2020) 11:1944. doi: 10.3389/fimmu.2020.01944
25. Sacks DL. Vaccines against tropical parasitic diseases: a persisting answer to a persisting problem. *Nat Immunol*. (2014) 15:403–5. doi: 10.1038/ni.2853
26. Seyed N, Rafati S. Th1 concomitant immune response mediated by IFN-gamma protects against sand fly delivered leishmania infection: implications for vaccine design. *Cytokine*. (2020) 155247. doi: 10.1016/j.cyto.2020.155247
27. Cadena AM, Hopkins FF, Maiello P, Carey AF, Wong EA, Martin CJ, et al. Concurrent infection with *Mycobacterium tuberculosis*. confers robust protection against secondary infection in macaques. *PLoS Pathog*. (2018) 14:e1007305. doi: 10.1371/journal.ppat.1007305

28. Andrews JR, Noubary F, Walensky RP, Cerda R, Losina E, Horsburgh CR. Risk of progression to active tuberculosis following reinfection with *Mycobacterium tuberculosis*. *Clin Infect Dis.* (2012) 54:784–91. doi: 10.1093/cid/cir951

29. Blaser N, Zahnd C, Hermans S, Salazar-Vizcaya L, Estill J, Morrow C, et al. Tuberculosis in cape town: an age-structured transmission model. *Epidemics.* (2016) 14:54–61. doi: 10.1016/j.epidem.2015.10.001

30. Zikherman J, Au-Yeung B. The role of T cell receptor signaling thresholds in guiding T cell fate decisions. *Curr Opin Immunol.* (2015) 33:43–8. doi: 10.1016/j.coi.2015.01.012

31. Darrah PA, Patel DT, De Luca PM, Lindsay RW, Davey DF, Flynn BJ, et al. Multifunctional TH1 cells define a correlate of vaccine-mediated protection against leishmania major. *Nat Med.* (2007) 13:843–50. doi: 10.1038/nm1592

32. Kannanganat S, Ibegbu C, Chennareddi L, Robinson HL, Amara RR. Multiple-cytokine-producing antiviral CD4 T cells are functionally superior to single-cytokine-producing cells. *J Virol.* (2007) 81:8468–76. doi: 10.1128/JVI.00228-07

33. Ciuffreda D, Comte D, Cavassini M, Giostra E, Buhler L, Perruchoud M, et al. Polyfunctional HCV-specific T-cell responses are associated with effective control of HCV replication. *Eur J Immunol.* (2008) 38:2665–77. doi: 10.1002/eji.200838336

34. Kalsdorf B, Scriba TJ, Wood K, Day CL, Dheda K, Dawson R, et al. HIV-1 infection impairs the bronchoalveolar T-cell response to mycobacteria. *Am J Respir Crit Care Med.* (2009) 180:1262–70. doi: 10.1164/rccm.200907-1011OC

35. Day CL, Abrahams DA, Lerumo L, Janse van Rensburg E, Stone L, O'Rie T, et al. Functional capacity of *Mycobacterium tuberculosis*-specific T cell responses in humans is associated with mycobacterial load. *J Immunol.* (2011) 187:2222–32. doi: 10.4049/jimmunol.1101122

36. Maggioli MF, Palmer MV, Thacker TC, Vordermeier HM, McGill JL, Whelan AO, et al. Increased TNF-α/IFN-γ/IL-2 and decreased TNF-α/IFN-γ production by central memory T cells are associated with protective responses against bovine tuberculosis following BCG vaccination. *Front Immunol.* (2016) 7:421. doi: 10.3389/fimmu.2016.00421

18

Whole Genome Sequencing Links *Mycobacterium bovis* from Cattle, Cheese and Humans in Baja California, Mexico

Alejandro Perera Ortiz [1,2], Claudia Perea [3], Enrique Davalos [4], Estela Flores Velázquez [5], Karen Salazar González [5], Erika Rosas Camacho [5], Ethel Awilda García Latorre [2], Citlaltepetl Salinas Lara [6], Raquel Muñiz Salazar [7], Doris M. Bravo [3], Tod P. Stuber [3], Tyler C. Thacker [3] and Suelee Robbe-Austerman [3]*

[1] United States Embassy, U.S. Department of Agriculture, Animal and Plant Health Inspection Service, Mexico City, Mexico, [2] Programa de Doctorado en Ciencias Quimicobiológicas, Departamento de Inmunología, Escuela Nacional de Ciencias Biológicas, Instituto Politécnico Nacional, Ciudad de México, Mexico, [3] National Veterinary Services Laboratories, U.S. Department of Agriculture, Animal and Plant Health Inspection Service, Veterinary Services, Ames, IA, United States, [4] United States Embassy, U.S. Department of Agriculture, Animal and Plant Health Inspection Service, Mexicali, Mexico, [5] Dirección de Campañas Zoosanitarias de la Dirección General de Salud Animal Servicio Nacional de Sanidad, Inocuidad y Calidad Agroalimentaria, Ciudad de México, Mexico, [6] Unidad de Investigación, Facultad de Estudios Superiores de Iztacala, Universidad Autónoma Nacional de México, Ciudad de México, Mexico, [7] Laboratorio de Epidemiología y Ecología Molecular, Escuela Ciencias de la Salud, Universidad Autónoma de Baja California, Ensenada, Baja California, Mexico

*Correspondence:
Suelee Robbe-Austerman
suelee.robbe-austerman@usda.gov

Mycobacterium bovis causes tuberculosis (TB) in cattle, which in turn can transmit the pathogen to humans. Tuberculosis in dairy cattle is of particular concern where the consumption of raw milk and dairy products is customary. Baja California (BCA), Mexico, presents high prevalence of TB in both cattle and humans, making it important to investigate the molecular epidemiology of the disease in the region. A long-term study was undertaken to fully characterize the diversity of *M. bovis* genotypes circulating in dairy cattle, cheese and humans in BCA by whole-genome sequencing (WGS). During a 2-year period, 412 granulomatous tissue samples were collected from local abattoirs and 314 cheese samples were purchased from local stores and vendors in BCA and sent to the laboratory for mycobacterial culture, histology, direct PCR and WGS. For tissue samples *M. bovis* was recovered from 86.8%, direct PCR detected 90% and histology confirmed 85.9% as mycobacteriosis-compatible. For cheese, *M. bovis* was recovered from 2.5% and direct PCR detected 6% of the samples. There was good agreement between diagnostic tests. Subsequently, a total of 345 whole-genome SNP sequences were obtained. Phylogenetic analysis grouped these isolates into 10 major clades. SNP analysis revealed putative transmission clusters where the pairwise SNP distance between isolates from different dairies was ≤3 SNP. Also, human and/or cheese isolates were within 8.45 (range 0–17) and 5.8 SNP (range 0–15), respectively, from cattle isolates. Finally, a comparison between the genotypes obtained in this study and those reported previously suggests that the genetic diversity of *M. bovis* in BCA is well-characterized, and can be used to determine if BCA is the likely source of *M. bovis* in humans and cattle in routine epidemiologic investigations and future studies. In conclusion, WGS provided evidence of ongoing local transmission of *M. bovis* among the dairies in this high-TB burden region of BCA, as well as show close relationships between isolates recovered from humans, cheese, and cattle. This confirms the need for a coordinated One Health approach in addressing the elimination of TB in animals and humans. Overall, the study contributes to the knowledge of the molecular epidemiology of *M. bovis* in BCA, providing insight into the pathogen's dynamics in a high prevalence setting.

Keywords: whole genome sequencing, Baja California, bovine tuberculosis, single nucleotide polymorphism, *M. bovis*, cheese

INTRODUCTION

Bovine tuberculosis (bTB), most commonly caused by *Mycobacterium bovis*, is characterized by the formation of granulomas in the lymph nodes and lungs of infected individuals, though other organs may also be affected (1, 2). It is an OIE (World Organization for Animal Health) reportable disease that infects a broad variety of mammals including humans. Infection in cattle can occur through direct contact by the inhalation of infected aerosols from sick animals and through oral ingestion of contaminated milk, fodder and pastures (3). Humans can acquire the infection also by direct contact with infected animals and through the consumption of contaminated unpasteurized milk and dairy products (4). Due to the significant impact this disease can have on public health and international trade of cattle and their byproducts, programs for the control and eradication of bTB have been implemented in many countries. In developed countries, significant success has been achieved, but wildlife reservoirs have challenged total eradication (5, 6); in least-developed or developing countries, however, the lack of economic compensation for culled animals due to test and slaughter strategies, or the absence of such strategies, complicates control (7, 8).

In Mexico, the bTB National Program classifies geographic territories into two zones (eradication or control) based on the regional bTB herd prevalence over a 12-month period. The program's strategies are to reduce or eliminate the prevalence of the disease in "eradication" zones, which have a bTB prevalence of <0.5%, as well as to prevent reinfection by applying mitigation measures in the movement of cattle from control zones to eradication zones. Eradication zones are primarily populated by beef cattle and currently 86.02% of the country is recognized as being an eradication zone. The bTB prevalence in the remaining control zones (13.98%) is >0.5% (range of 0.1–14.2%) or is unknown and contain primarily dairy cattle (9). The state of Baja California (BCA) is divided into two zones: an eradication zone with <0.5% of bTB herd prevalence and a control zone to the north, which borders California in the US, that is mainly populated by dairy cattle and has reported prevalence rates as high as 40% (10). As previously reported in the literature (11), there is very high prevalence of tuberculosis in cattle and humans in BCA and although *M. tuberculosis* is the main causative agent of TB in humans, *M. bovis* may play an important role in areas where bTB is endemic and even more so where bTB prevalence rates in cattle are high (12). In Mexico there is limited information available with respect to human TB caused by *M.*

bovis and some studies have reported a median percentage of 7.6% (range 0–31.6%) (13, 14). However, due to a lack of species identification in the diagnosis, cases of bTB in humans are likely underestimated (15). Additionally, in the US, 90% of human bTB cases are usually traced to people of Hispanic communities, most of which have origins in Mexico (16). Interestingly, San Diego County in California is the only county in the US which borders a control zone and reports the highest levels of *M. bovis* infection in people (17, 18). Consequently, this high TB burden dairy region of BCA may be contributing to that high level of *M. bovis* detection. Furthermore, isolation of *M. bovis* from cheese has been reported (19) and the association of human bTB cases in Hispanic people from Mexico has been attributed to the consumption of contaminated cheese produced with unpasteurized milk (20). The production of artisanal cheese is customary in Mexico and is often carried out by traditional "cheese-makers" in the rural areas of the country, to be later sold at the open markets and small stores (21). Comparably, cases of human bTB in the US have also been associated to fresh cheese brought into the US from Mexico (22).

Recovery of *M. bovis* from raw milk and cheese is challenging and relies on decontamination methods that can maintain the delicate balance between inactivation of undesirable microorganisms and the viability of mycobacteria, thus appropriate processing procedures such as homogenization, decontamination, concentration and culture media, must be selected to facilitate optimum recovery of mycobacteria (23). Previous studies at the National Veterinary Services Laboratories (NVSL) have evaluated the isolation of *M. bovis* and *M. avium* subsp. *paratuberculosis* from milk and cheese using various combinations of decontamination processes and have eventually settled on a chemical combination of N-acetyl-l-cysteine–sodium hydroxide (NALC-NaOH) for decontamination (19, 24, 25). Furthermore, comparisons of different types of media for the optimal recovery of *M. bovis* have yielded the best results for 7H11P (Middlebrook 7H11 agar supplemented with sodium pyruvate, calf serum, lysed sheep blood and malachite green) and BACTEC MGIT 960 (Becton Dickinson Diagnostic Systems, Sparks, MD) supplemented with an antibiotic mixture (BBL MGIT PANTA, Becton Dickinson) (26–28).

In contrast to the bTB prevalence in BCA dairy cattle, the US cattle herd has a very low prevalence of bTB (<0.001%) and several studies have suggested most new cattle herd detections are the result of new introductions and not continued spread within local cattle (29, 30). While many sources of bTB introduction remain unknown, some of the genotypes have closely matched isolates recovered from previous studies in BCA (11). Since dairy cattle movements are strictly controlled in Mexico, humans and fomites may be a likely source as this region serves as a major port of transit for people and goods, including fresh cheese. To address this issue, a binational collaboration was initiated with three overall objectives: (1) fully characterize the diversity of *M. bovis* genotypes circulating in BCA by whole-genome sequencing, (2) to determine the role of fresh cheese from the region as a potential source of infection to humans and (3) compare the genotypes identified in BCA to those previously reported for the region, the rest of Mexico and the US.

MATERIALS AND METHODS

Study Area

The study was performed in the control zone of Baja California, Mexico, which is the dairy region located in the far northwest of the state (**Figure 1**). The location of the dairy herds from which the sampled cattle originated was mapped and clusters were formed based on a maximum distance (radius) of 5 km between the dairies. Thirteen clusters were assigned as follows: Ensenada 1 (ENS-1), Ensenada 2 (ENS-2), Ensenada 3 (ENS-3), Ensenada 4 (ENS-4), Mexicali 1 (MEX-1), Rosarito 1 (ROS-1), Rosarito 2 (ROS-2), Tecate 1 (TEC-1), Tecate 2 (TEC-2), Tijuana 1 (TIJ-1), Tijuana 2 (TIJ-2), Tijuana 3 (TIJ-3) and Tijuana 4 (TIJ-4). A full list of the dairies that corresponded to each cluster is in **Supplementary File 1**.

Tissue Samples

From October 2016 to November 2018, tissue samples with bTB-suspicious lesions (granulomas) were collected by an accredited veterinarian during post-mortem inspection of dairy cull cattle, under the supervision of the abattoir's official veterinarian. Three abattoirs, each in the municipalities of Ensenada, Tecate and Tijuana, were targeted. Based on estimations by the Mexican Secretariat of Agriculture and Rural Development (Secretaría de Agricultura y Desarrollo Rural, SADER), these three abattoirs receive over 90% of the cull dairy cows in the region. The abattoirs were visited 2–3 times per week on days in which the volume of animals was highest. Each sample was divided in two: one half was stored in formalin for histopathological analysis and the second half was frozen for bacteriological analysis. Epidemiological data associated to each animal's official identification tag (SINIIGA) was collected, such as owner, farm of origin (location, production unit), dealer, transit document number (movement authorization), etc. (https://www.siniiga.org.mx/identifica.html). Finally, samples were submitted to the USDA's National Veterinary Services Laboratories (NVSL) in Ames, Iowa for analysis.

Cheese Samples

Fresh cheese samples were collected throughout the region of Ensenada, Rosarito, Tecate and Tijuana in BCA from October 2016 to December 2019. Approximately 250 g pieces were purchased from informal sellers, small stores and markets, 2–4 times per week. Samples were stored in sterile, airtight containers and shipped in styrofoam coolers with icepacks to NVSL for analysis.

Mycobacterial Isolation and Identification
Tissues

Prior to culture, a pea-sized sample was obtained for direct PCR. Then, granuloma samples were trimmed of excess fat and connective tissue and soaked for 20–30 min in a 1:100 solution of bleach and R/O water, then tissues were homogenized. Seven mL of macerated tissue were placed in 5 mL of 1 N NaOH and decontaminated for 7–10 min and neutralized to effect with the MycoDDR Neutralization Buffer B (Immuno-Mycologics, Inc., US) to a final volume of 35 ± 5 mL. Specimens were centrifuged at 4,700xg for 25 ± 2 min at 10°C and the supernatant decanted off. Pellet was resuspended in 2–3 mL of PBS and was inoculated into BACTEC MGIT 960 (Becton Dickinson, Sparks, Md.) for up to 42 days and two tubes of Middlebrook 7H11 media with sodium pyruvate and incubated at 37°C for up to 8 weeks.

Cheese

Mycobacterial isolation from cheese samples was performed following a previously described methodology (19). Briefly, 5 g portions of cheese were weighed and aseptically transferred into a blender jar containing 45 mL of 2% sodium citrate. The cheese was homogenized and the jars were placed in a 37°C water bath for 1 h to help liquefy the specimen. The cheese suspension was decontaminated using the N-acetyl-L-cysteine (NALC)-NaOH method (31). 10 mL of the liquefied and homogenized sample was mixed with 10 mL of digestant containing NaOH-Sodium citrate and NALC. The mixture was allowed to stand at room temperature for 15–20 min. 30 mL of phosphate buffer was then added. The mixture was then centrifuged at 4,700xg for 25 min at 10°C and the supernatant decanted off. Pellet was resuspended in 2–3 mL of PBS and was inoculated into BACTEC MGIT 960 (Becton Dickinson, Sparks, Md.) and incubated for up to 42 days and two tubes of Middlebrook 7H11 media with sodium pyruvate (7H11P) and incubated at 37°C for up to 8 weeks.

Isolate Identification by PCR and Sanger Sequencing

Real-time PCR against *IS*1081was performed on DNA extracted from acid fast colonies either from solid media or MGIT media. If the Ct value was below 14, the DNA was sent for whole genome sequencing. If the PCR was above 14, the isolate was subcultured on to fresh 7H11P solid media and allowed to grow. If the PCR was negative, the DNA was sent for Sanger sequencing using both universal primers against 16S rDNA and mycobacterial specific primers for rpoB and the sequences were blasted against GenBank.

Direct PCR

Direct real-time PCR was performed directly from tissue as previously described (32), with modifications. Direct PCR was performed on a pea-sized sample obtained from the tissue used for culture. Briefly, tissues were examined for granulomatous lesions and dissected to obtain a pea-sized subsample. Subsamples were transferred into 2 mL screw-cap microcentrifuge tubes with a glass bead mixture of approximately

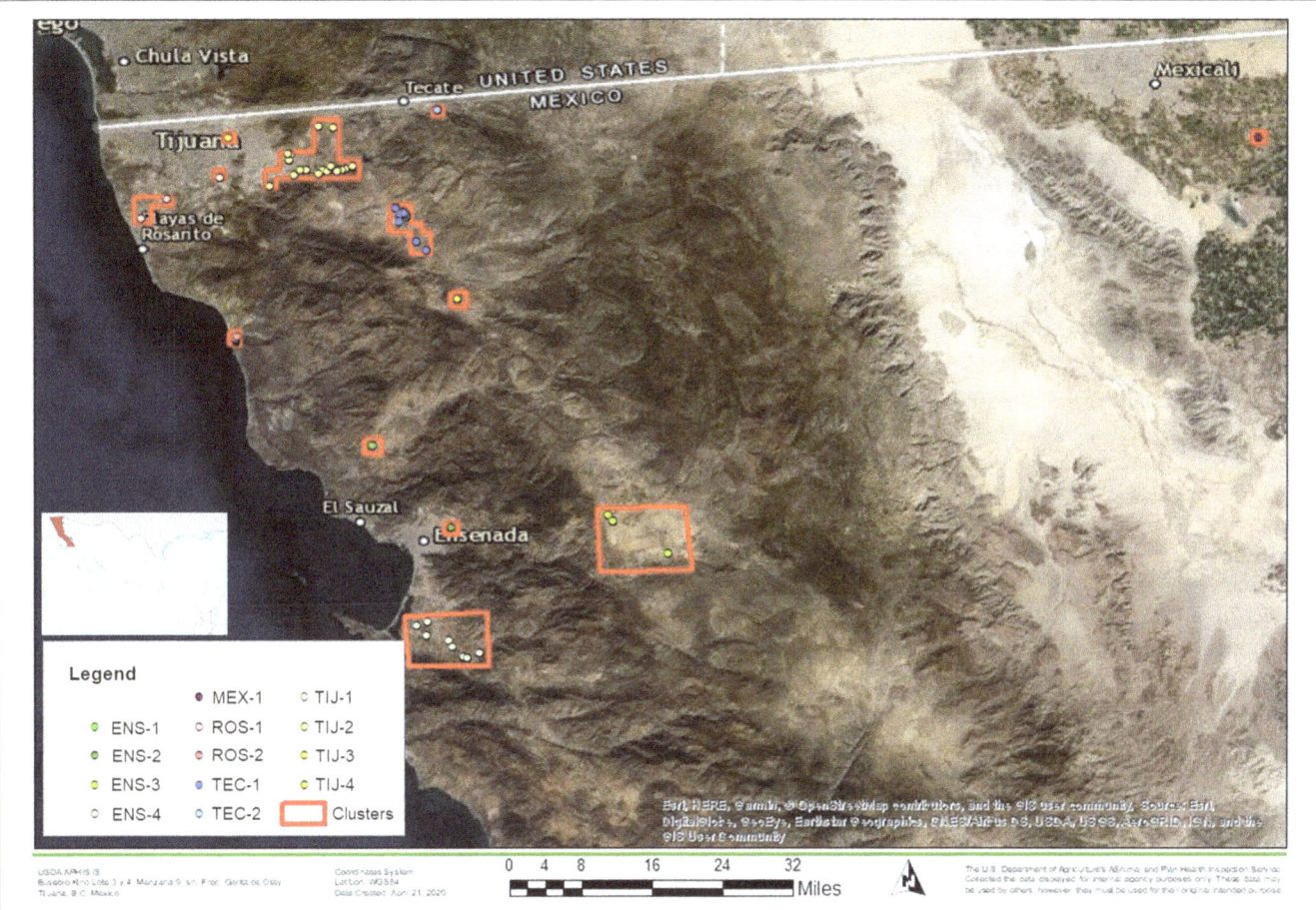

FIGURE 1 | Map of the northern region of Baja California. The location of BCA with respect to Mexico is shown on the left. Red squares represent dairy clusters (n = 13) formed based on a maximum distance of 5 km (radius) between dairies. Clusters' names are indicated in the legend. The map was built using ArcGIS software (basemap WGS1984).

125 μL of 1.0 mm and 125 μL of 0.1 mm beads. 400 μL of a buffer solution containing approximately 400 μL 1X TE buffer and 2.5 μL of DNA Extraction Control 670 were added per sample. Samples were heat-inactivated in a heat-block at 100°C for 30 min and posteriorly bead-disrupted at full speed for 2 min using a mini-bead beater. Samples were then centrifuged at 16,000xg for 5 min. The top aqueous layer was used to extract mycobacterial DNA using the MagMax CORE nucleic acid purification kit (Applied Biosystems, ThermoFisher Scientific, US) and a KingFisher Flex System (Thermo Fisher Scientific, Waltham, MA, USA). Real time PCR was performed on the QuantStudio or Viia7 instruments (Applied Biosystems, California, USA).

For cheese, 400 μL of the homogenate were transferred into 2 mL screw-cap microcentrifuge tubes with a glass bead mixture of approximately 125 μL of 1.0 mm and 125 μL of 0.1 mm beads. PCR tubes contained a total volume of 500 μL: 98.5 μL of 1X TE buffer, 2.5 μL of DNA Extraction Control 670 and 400 μL of phenol/chloroform. After inactivation with the phenol/chloroform, samples were bead-disrupted and processed the same as for tissue as mentioned above.

Whole Genome Sequencing and Data Analysis

DNA from colonies was extracted using the MagMax CORE nucleic acid purification kit (Applied Biosystems, ThermoFisher Scientific, US) and a KingFisher Flex System (Thermo Fisher Scientific, Waltham, MA. USA). Real time PCR was performed on the QuantStudio or Viia7 instruments (Applied Biosystems, California, USA). A minimum of 20 μL of DNA sample with a minimum concentration of 5 ng/μL was required for sequencing. Sequencing was performed in an Illumina MiSeq device (Illumina, San Diego, CA, USA), according to manufacturer's instructions, using 250 bp paired-end read chemistry and libraries were prepared using the Nextera XT Library Preparation Kit (Illumina, San Diego, CA, USA) also according to manufacturer's instructions. Raw FASTQ files were analyzed with the vSNP pipeline (https://github.com/USDA-VS/vSNP). Quality check is done as part of the vSNP package (see **Supplementary File 5** for sequencing metrics). Briefly, FASTQ files were used to align reads against the reference genome *M. bovis* AF2122/97 (NCBI RefSeq Accession NC_002945.4) using BWA-mem (33). 80X depth of coverage was targeted. SNPs were called using FreeBayes (34) and visually validated with IGV (35). Phylogenetic trees were constructed based on whole genome concatenated SNP sequences using RAxML (36) under a GTR-CAT model of substitution. Tree visualization, annotation and editing was performed with FigTree (37). As output from the vSNP pipeline, SNP tables for each major clade were generated; these are formatted Excel tables that group and sort isolates and SNP according to relatedness and reflect exactly what is shown by the phylogenetic tree, which provides transparency of the results. In the SNP tables the columns identify the genome location of the SNP calls and the isolates are listed in the rows. The reference (*M. bovis* AF2122/97, NC_002945.4) is listed across the top and is identified as the "reference call." All SNP are highlighted. Map-quality for each SNP is indicated and is an average of the map quality scores of each isolate at that position. A score of 60 is the highest possible. Finally, the annotation of the position is listed at the bottom of the SNP table.

The complete analysis involved the sequences generated in this study and sequences from the NVSL database generated by previous studies (11, 30, 38), which are publicly available in the NCBI Sequence Read Archive under Bioprojects PRJNA384996, PRJNA251692 and PRJNA449507, respectively (**Supplementary File 4**).

Cluster Analysis
A cut-off value for pairwise SNP distances between isolates of 12 SNP has been widely used for *M. tuberculosis* transmission studies (39–41). Here, a cut-off value of 10 SNP was used based on patterns observed in the data by the careful visual inspection of the SNP matrices (Excel tables) obtained from the vSNP pipeline. Each cluster was identified and labeled based on the defining SNP for that cluster according to its genome position with respect to the reference genome (*M. bovis* AF2122/97, RefSeq accession number NC002945.4). Additionally, a cut-off value of 3 SNP was also used for identifying putative transmission between the dairies.

Statistical Analysis
To evaluate concordance between laboratory tests for the diagnosis of *M. bovis* (culture, histology and PCR), Cohen's kappa coefficient was determined for histology and culture and for PCR and culture, as culture remains the gold standard for *M. bovis* confirmatory diagnosis. The following formula was applied:

$$K = (Po - Pe)/(1 - Pe) \quad (1)$$

where Po refers to the observed agreement between tests and Pe refers to the expected agreement. For this, Pe was determined with the following formula:

$$Pe = [(n1/n) * (m1/n)] + [(n0/n) * (m0/n)] \quad (2)$$

where the values n1, n, m1, n0 and m0 are based on the following:

Histology/PCR	Culture Positive	Negative	Total
Positive	a	b	m_1
Negative	C	d	m_0
Total	n_1	n_0	n

Cohen suggested the Kappa result be interpreted as follows: values ≤ 0 as indicating no agreement and 0.01–0.20 as none to slight, 0.21–0.40 as fair, 0.41–0.60 as moderate, 0.61–0.80 as substantial and 0.81–1.00 as almost perfect agreement (42).

RESULTS
Source Herd Information
Based on cattle census data by Mexico (43), over 95% of the dairies that were larger than 100 head were sampled during the study. Animals were housed in open-air dry-lot dairies where modern management practices are in place, similar to what can be seen in developed countries such as the US. The main breeds in these dairies were Holstein and Swedish Red, with an average milk production of 25 liters per day. This region of the country is an ideal environment for dairy production and upon observation, the animals appear healthy and with adequate body condition and clinical tuberculosis is not typically recognized.

Tissue Samples
A total of 445 tissue samples with TB-suspicious lesions were obtained from dairy cattle, which represented a total of 90 dairies. Unfortunately, 33 samples failed to make it to the laboratory in acceptable condition for testing due to shipping logistics. Consequently, 412 samples were included in the analysis, representing a final total of 61 dairies. Ten samples could not be traced back to a dairy, so they were labeled as "Unknown." Of the total, 363 (88.1%) samples corresponded to lymph nodes (superficial cervical, mandibular, parotid, retropharyngeal, tracheobronchial, mediastinal and hepatic), 10 were from lung (2.4%) and 39 from liver (9.5%). The number of granulomas collected per dairy varied widely between 0 and 35. The overall detection rate for *M. bovis* from tissue samples was 86.9%, with lymph nodes achieving the highest rate at 91.7% (**Table 1**).

Cheese Samples
A total of 314 cheese samples were included in the analysis (**Supplementary File 6**). Overall, 22 (7%) were reported out as contaminated (overgrowth of non-acid fast bacteria); 262 (83.4%) were reported as no isolation made, and 30 (9.6%) contained acid fast bacteria, of which 8 (2.5%) were *M. bovis*. Other acid fast bacteria recovered from the cheese included 17 *M. porcinum* isolates, and one each of *M. bolletii*, *M. fortuitum* and *M. neoaurum*; and two atypical, likely unnamed mycobacteria with sequences that did not match close enough for species determination.

A total of 85 stores were visited throughout the four municipalities. *M. bovis* was cultured from all four municipalities, one store in Tecate, two different stores in Rosarito, one store

TABLE 1 | Total tissue samples obtained from dairy cattle in Baja California, Mexico for the detection of *M. bovis*.

Type of tissue	Total number of samples	Samples detected with *M. bovis*	Proportion detected (%)
Lymph nodes	363	333	91.7
Superficial cervical	1	1	100.0
Hepatic	12	12	100.0
Mandibular	8	6	75.0
Mediastinal	24	21	87.5
Parotid	12	12	100.0
Retropharyngeal	217	196	90.3
Tracheobronchial	89	85	95.5
Lung	10	6	60.0
Liver	39	19	48.7
Total	412	358	86.9

TABLE 2 | Distribution of culture, histology and direct PCR results for the detection of *M. bovis* from tissue from dairy cattle from Baja California, Mexico.

	Culture		
Direct PCR	Positive	Negative	Total
Detected	351	20	371
Not Detected	6	34	40
Inconclusive	1	0	1
Total	358	54	412
Histology			
Mycobacteriosis compatible	345	9	354
Other diagnosis	13	45	58
Total	358	54	412

TABLE 3 | Comparison between histology and culture results for the detection of *M. bovis* from granulomas obtained from dairy cattle in Baja California, Mexico.

	Culture results		
	M. bovis isolated	No isolation	Total
Histology diagnosis			
Mycobacteriosis-compatible	345	9	354
Abscess	0	4	4
Actinobacillosis or mycosis	0	9	9
Chronic pneumonia	0	2	2
Coccidioidomycosis	0	2	2
Eosinophilic granuloma	1	0	1
Granuloma, unknown etiology	2	1	3
Hepatitis	0	1	1
Lymphoid hyperplasia	1	1	2
Lymphoplasmitic hepatitis	1	0	1
Lymphosarcoma	0	2	2
Microgranuloma	0	1	1
Mycotic granuloma	0	1	1
No significant findings	2	5	7
Pyogranuloma	6	16	22
Total	358	54	412

in Tijuana (two samples collected at different times), and one store in Ensenada (three samples collected at different times). Even though the number of samples for "fresh" cheese (188) was greater than "panela" cheese (126), the isolation rate of *M. bovis* by culture was the same for both (2.7 and 2.4%, respectively). Similarly, the detection rate of *M. bovis* from fresh and panela cheese by direct PCR was not significantly different between the two types, having obtained detection rates of 5.8% (11/188) and 6.3% (8/126), respectively. Overall, the detection rate was higher for direct PCR (5.7%) compared to culture (2.5%). All the *M. bovis* isolates recovered from these cheese samples had different WGS sequences, suggesting different cow sources despite several obtained from the same store.

Culture, Histology, and Direct PCR

For *M. bovis* detection, cattle tissues were processed by direct PCR, culture and histology. A comparison of culture, histology and direct PCR results is shown in **Table 2**. Of the 412 tissue samples, 358 were positive for culture, 354 were positive for histology (mycobacteriosis-compatible) and 345 were detected by both. Direct PCR alone detected 371 samples and 351 were detected by both PCR and culture. Six culture-positive samples were not detected by direct PCR and 20 culture-negative were detected by direct PCR. For culture and PCR, the kappa obtained was 0.6774 (CI 95% 0.6398–0.7149), indicating substantial agreement between these tests. For histology and culture, 345 samples were detected by both tests, nine were "mycobacteriosis compatible" but culture-negative and 13 identified as "other diagnosis" by histology were positive for culture. Thereby, a kappa statistic of 0.7727 (CI 95% 0.7449–0.8004) was obtained for culture and histology, also indicating a substantial level of concordance between the two tests (**Table 2**).

Additionally, **Table 3** details the various diagnosis classified as "other diagnosis," representing the samples identified as negative by histology. Thirteen samples fell under this classification and included eosinophilic granuloma ($n = 1$), granuloma of unknown etiology ($n = 2$), lymphoid hyperplasia ($n = 1$), lymphoplasmitic hepatitis ($n = 1$), pyogranuloma ($n = 6$) and no significant findings ($n = 2$).

WGS and SNP Clusters

Of the 61 final total dairies, 58 (93.5%) were confirmed to contain animals infected with *M. bovis*, having obtained at least one isolate from an animal in the dairy (**Figure 2**). The highest number of isolates obtained from a single dairy was 31 (Dairy001) and a single isolate was recovered for 17 dairies. Also, at least one and up to 12 SNP clusters were identified for a single dairy (Dairy039), only Dairy053 and Dairy059 were not associated to a SNP cluster. Additionally, 20 isolates that corresponded to 13 dairies were indicative of mixed infection due to their

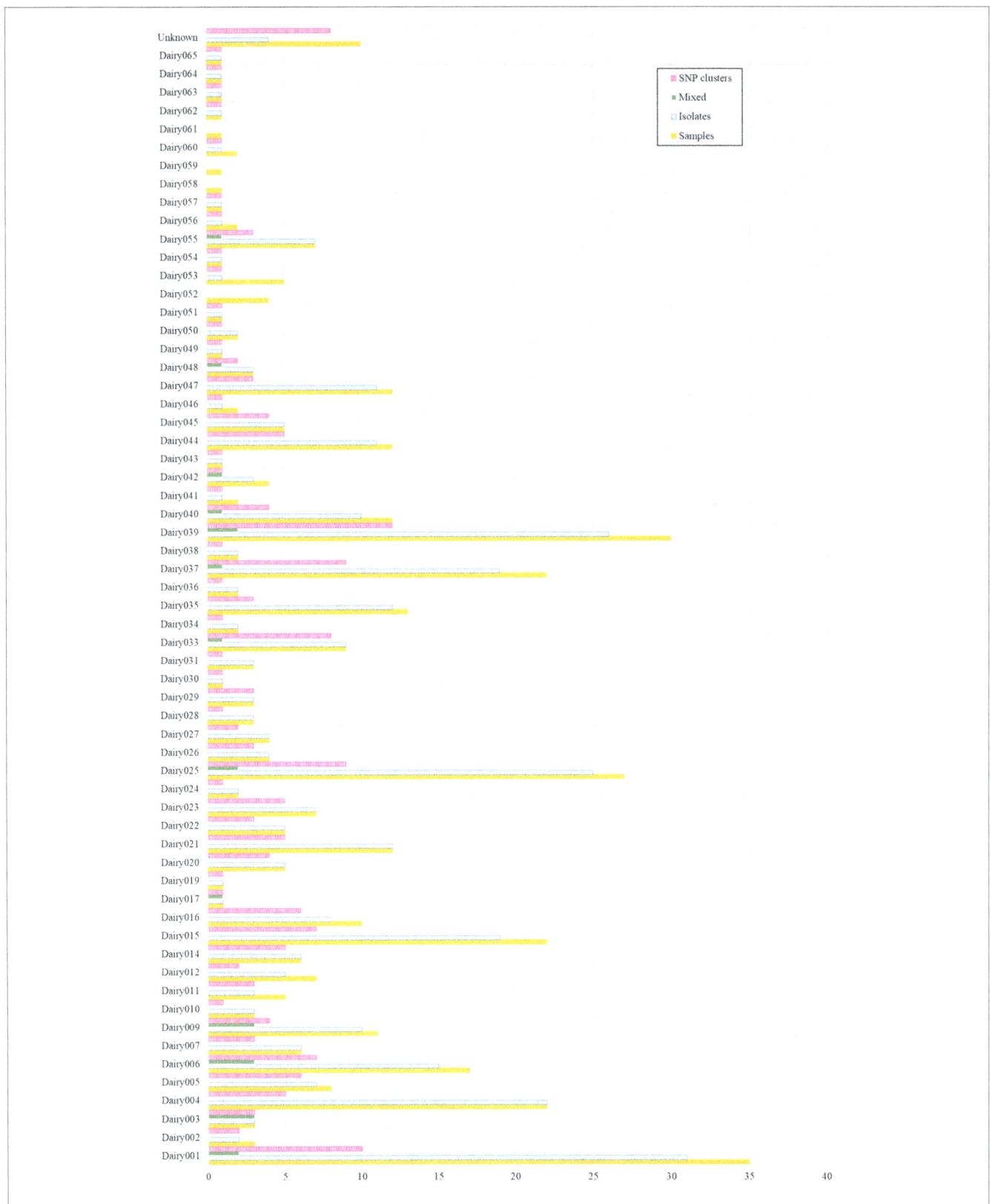

FIGURE 2 | Baja California dairies with positive detection of *M. bovis*. For each dairy, the figure indicates the total number of samples, isolates and SNP clusters. "Mixed" refers to isolates that had a high proportion (≥50%) of ambiguous SNP calls, indicating the presence of more than one genotype. "Unknown" refers to dairies that were not possible to trace back.

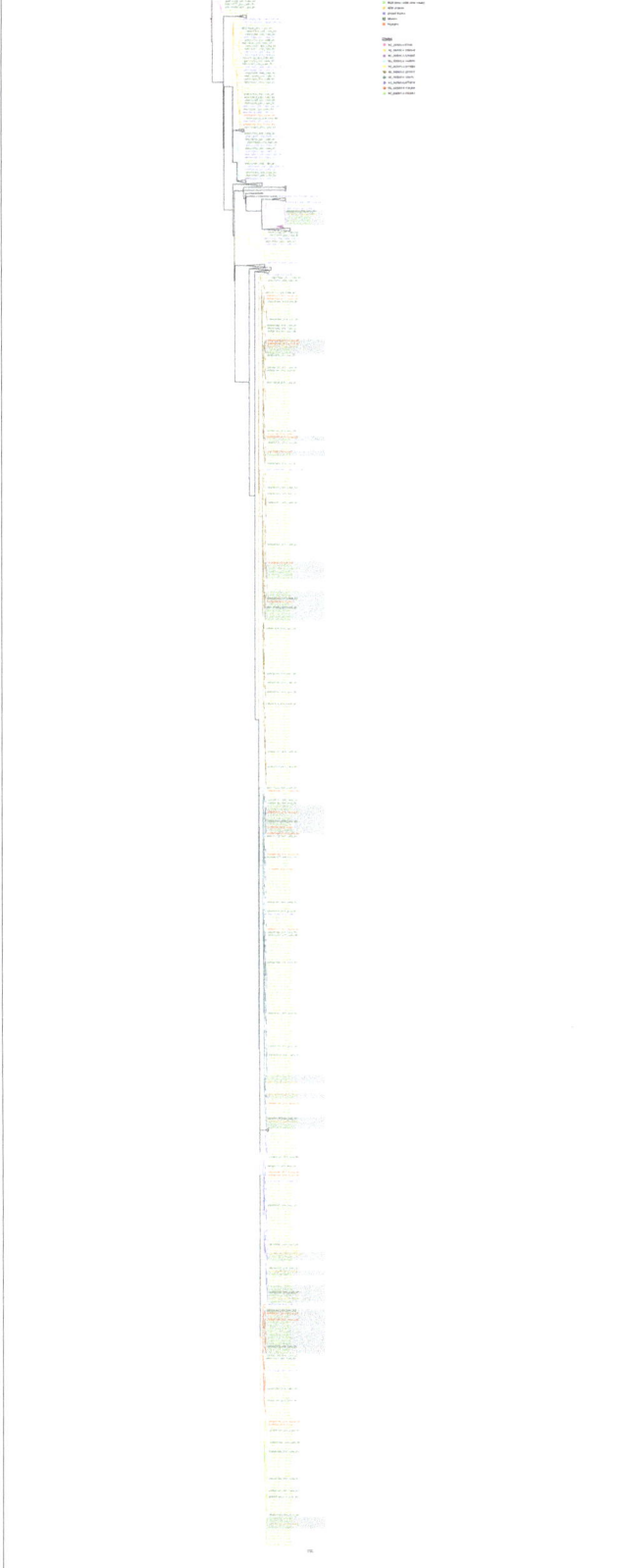

FIGURE 3 | and the US. The BCA isolates from dairy cattle and cheese obtained from this study correspond to 10 main clades, as indicated in the legend. Each clade is labeled according to the genome position of the defining SNP for that clade, with respect to the reference genome *M. bovis* AF2122/97 (NC002945.4). Gray-shaded areas indicate clusters of human and/or cheese isolates that are within 10 SNPs of a recent common shared ancestor. Some clades (of unrelated isolates to BCA) were collapsed for to improve visibility. The scale bar represents a distance of 40 SNPs (branch length).

FIGURE 3 | Whole-genome SNP-based phylogeny of 642 *M. bovis* isolates obtained from cattle, cheese and humans from Baja California, Mexico (BCA)
(Continued)

high proportion of ambiguous calls ($\geq 50\%$), which suggests the presence of more than one genotype.

A total of 642 whole genome SNP sequences were included for analysis: 346 from this study (eight from cheese and 338 from dairy cattle) and 297 obtained from GenBank from previous studies (26 human—Mexico, four cheese—Mexico and 267 cattle—from USA and Mexico) (11, 30, 44). Overall, 26 main groups/clades were identified, of which 10 corresponded to the isolates from this study and were labeled according to the defining SNP for each clade (with respect to its genome position in the reference) (**Figure 3**).

Final alignments (SNP matrices) for each clade are shown in **Supplementary File 2**. Most of the isolates from this study fell in clades NC_002945.4:4219410 (38%, 132/345) and NC_002945.4:389472 (26%, 90/345). Clades NC_002945.4:57046 and NC_002945.4:1945505 included the least number isolates with 2 and 1, respectively. All the clades included cattle isolates, five clades included cheese isolates (NC_002945.4:389472 = 3; NC_002945.4:2778919 = 5; NC_002945.4:4219410 = 1; NC_002945.4:1254487 = 1; and NC_002945.4:1622803 = 1) and seven clades included human isolates (NC_002945.4:389472 = 8; NC_002945.4:2778919 = 2; NC_002945.4:4219410 = 9; NC_002945.4:1295549 = 2; NC_002945.4:1790349 = 2; NC_002945.4:2232592; and NC_002945.4:1622803 = 2), one of which does not include any isolates from this study.

In general, all the cheese and human isolates had genotypes that were also found in cattle. On average, human and/or cheese isolates were within 8.45 (range 0–17) and 5.8 SNPs (range 0–15), respectively, from cattle isolates (**Figure 3**, gray shaded clusters). Consequently, nine out of 11 of the cheese isolates were ≤ 10 SNPs from a cattle isolate from a BCA dairy and this was also true for 11 out of 26 of the human isolates. Within the global context of the *M. bovis* phylogeny, most of the isolates belonged to the European 1 Clonal Complex (Eu1) and only isolates from clade NC_002945.4:1254487 belonged to the European 2 Clonal Complex (Eu2).

To determine how much of the diversity of *M. bovis* in BCA has been captured, the genotypes identified in this study were compared to those from previous reports (**Figure 4A**). From a total of 97 SNP clusters, only two were exclusive to this study (BCA-P), while none were exclusive to what was previously reported in other studies (BCA-O). In total, 19 SNP clusters were identified as specific to the BCA region, while 29 were common to other regions in Mexico (MEX). A total of 49 SNP clusters were found for other regions of Mexico only and not in BCA. Additionally, a comparison between the genotypes isolated from

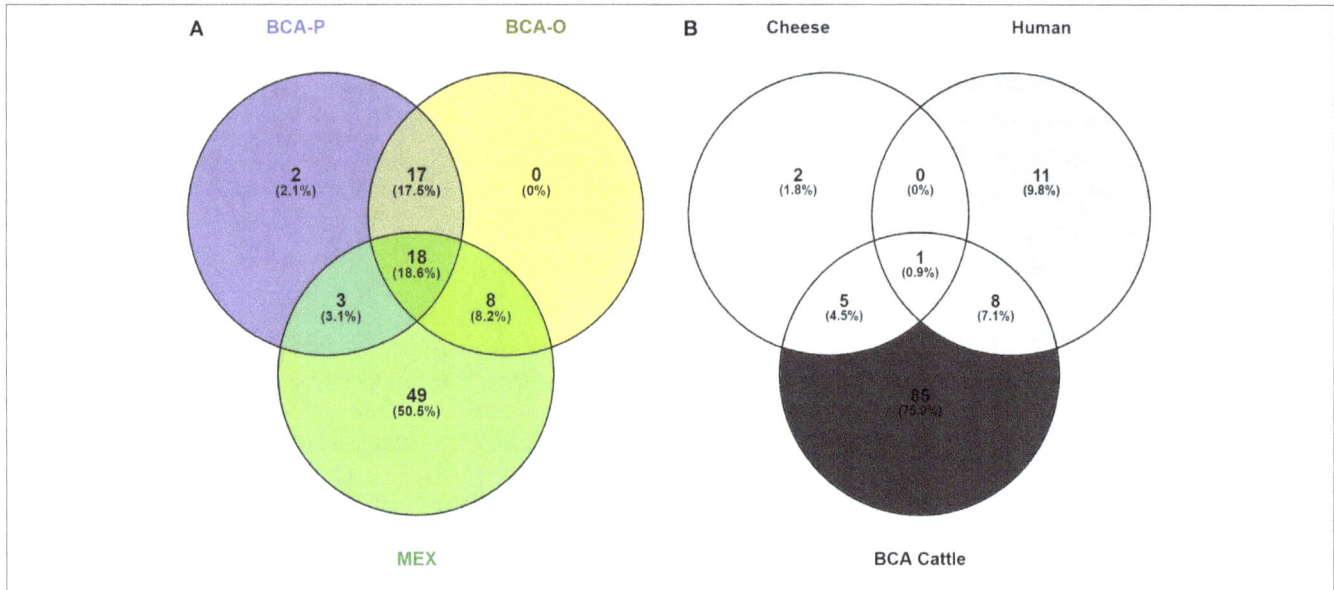

FIGURE 4 | Venn diagrams representing comparisons of *M. bovis* genotypes **(A)** identified in Baja California in this study (BCA-P) and previously (BCA-O, MEX) **(B)** from cattle, humans and cheese.

cheese, humans and cattle revealed that one was common to all three sources, five were common to both cattle and cheese and eight were common to cattle and humans (**Figure 4B**). The larger proportion of SNP clusters (75.9%) belonged only to cattle. A list of the SNP clusters identified in this study can be consulted in **Supplementary File 3**.

Putative Transmission Among Dairies

A total of 64 isolates were found that had a pairwise SNP distance of ≤3 SNP to at least one other isolate and the dairies of origin were identified (**Table 4**). Thirty-three out of the total 61 dairies, which represents 54% of the dairies included in this study, were found to have very closely related isolates, thereby suggesting epidemiological associations between dairies. Most of these associations involved only two dairies and in two instances there were three dairies involved. Moreover, nine pairs of these closely related isolates had identical SNP profiles. Dairy001 was found to have the most associations ($n = 8$), four of which involved isolates with identical SNP profiles (**Supplementary File 2**). Dairy039 followed closely with a total of six associations, while Dairies 004, 025 and 037 had four each. The rest had only one or two associations.

These dairies belonged to nine of the 13 previously defined dairy clusters: ROS-1, ROS-2, TIJ-2, TIJ-4, TEC-1, TEC-2, ENS-2, ENS-3 and ENS-4. The frequency at which genotypes were common to two or more dairy clusters is represented in **Figure 5**. At least one genotype was common to all clusters and each cluster had at least one genotype in common with another cluster. Cluster TIJ-2 had SNP clusters in common with at least six other clusters; of these, ROS-2 had the most shared SNP clusters. Cluster TEC-1 had genotypes in common with at least four other clusters (TIJ-2, TIJ-4, TEC-2 and ROS-2). The rest of the clusters shared genotypes with at least two others and three clusters

(ENS-2, ENS-3 and ROS-1) only shared genotype(s) with one other cluster.

DISCUSSION

The state of Baja California borders the United States, more specifically the state of California, and contains San Ysidro, the busiest border port in the world. Consequently, a high level of cooperation between the governments of Mexico and the US in both human and animal disease surveillance is necessary to address the transmission of the disease between animals, dairy products or people. Tuberculosis is particularly problematic as BCA is one of the states with the highest incidence of TB in cattle and humans in Mexico (10, 45). This study was carried out as a binational effort between the US and Mexico to use WGS to characterize the bTB genotypes circulating in BCA, determine the role of fresh cheese from the region as a potential source of infection to humans and compare the genotypes identified here to those previously reported in the region, Mexico and the US.

Overall, the detection of *M. bovis* from granulomatous tissue at abattoirs in BCA was high, with 84% from histology/culture and 85% from direct PCR/culture. In contrast, the bordering Mexican State of Sonora, which has strict controls to prevent cattle movement from BCA, has an *M. bovis* detection rate of ~1.5% from granulomatous lesions sampled in abattoirs (46). In this study, histology and direct PCR performed nearly the same as culture, which is regarded as the gold standard. Only six and 13 culture positive samples were negative by direct PCR and histology, respectively. Several factors can affect the sensitivity of histopathologic diagnosis, including the multifocal distribution of small granulomas, which may prevent histopathologic identification. On the other hand, 20 and nine samples were negative to culture, but detected by the direct

TABLE 4 | Possible epidemiological associations between BCA dairies based on isolates with a difference of ≤3 SNP.

Dairies with closely related isolates (≤3 SNP)		Total matches within 3 SNPs	Total genomes per dairy
Dairy001*	Dairy003*, Dairy004, Dairy005*, Dairy007*, Dairy011, Dairy047, Dairy050*, Dairy057	8	29
Dairy002	Dairy062	1	2
Dairy003	Dairy001, Dairy004, Dairy025	3	3
Dairy004	Dairy001, Dairy003, Dairy015, Dairy037	4	22
Dairy005*	Dairy001*, Dairy014*	2	7
Diary006*	Dairy064*	1	12
Dairy007*	Dairy001*	1	6
Dairy009	Dairy039, Dairy053	2	7
Dairy010	Dairy037	1	3
Dairy011	Dairy001, Dairy039	2	3
Dairy012	Dairy028, Dairy044	2	5
Dairy014	Dairy005	1	6
Dairy015	Dairy004, Dairy026	2	19
Dairy016	Dairy039	1	8
Dairy023	Dairy025	1	7
Dairy025*	Dairy003, Dairy023, Dairy039*, Dairy040	4	23
Dairy026	Dairy015, Dairy037	2	4
Dairy028*	Dairy012*	I	3
Dairy029*	Dairy037*	1	3
Dairy033	Dairy041	1	8
Dairy037*	Dairy004, Dairy010, Dairy026, Dairy029*	4	18
Dairy039	Diary006, Dairy009, Dairy011, Dairy016, Dairy025, Dairy053	6	24
Dairy040	Dairy025	1	9
Dairy041	Dairy033	1	1
Dairy044	Dairy012	1	11
Dairy047	Dairy001	1	11
Dairy050	Dairy001	1	2
Dairy053	Dairy009, Dairy039	2	1
Dairy055	Unknown	1	6
Dairy057	Dairy001	1	1
Dairy062	Dairy002	1	1
Dairy064*	Diary006*	1	4
Unknown	Dairy055	1	4

Total associations found for each dairy and total number of high-quality genomes for the specific dairy are indicated. An asterisk indicates associations based on a 0 SNP difference (identical SNP profiles).

PCR and histology. For PCR, this could reflect amplification of mycobacterial DNA from non-viable organisms; and the absence of acid-fast bacteria upon histological examination may be because of degradation of bacteria or scarcity of bacteria in lesions. Nonetheless, correlation between diagnostic tests (culture vs. PCR and culture vs. histology) was substantial based on kappa coefficients of 0.6774 and 0.7727, respectively.

Genotype characterization of pathogens is essential for disease surveillance, epidemiology and the development of proper control strategies. Previous studies on the diversity of *M. bovis* in cattle in BCA used spoligotyping and VNTR (47, 48) and one study also used WGS (11) to characterize the strains in the region. In comparison to (11), which evaluated 155 *M. bovis* WGS from BCA cattle, our study, which contained 338 WGS, only identified two additional groups, for a total of 10 main *M. bovis* genetic groups circulating in the region (**Figure 4A**). Overall, 726 WGS sequences, including cattle and cheese have been collected from this region, and based on the significant overlap, we suggest that the genetic diversity of *M. bovis* in BCA is now well-represented. In comparison to other Mexican states, about 30% of the genotypes were common to both BCA and the rest of the country, 20% were exclusive to BCA and 50% were exclusive to the rest of Mexico (**Figure 4A**). Due to its proximity to the US, it is possible that heifers that were historically imported into BCA may have introduced the disease, as the genotypes found here coincided with those once dominant in the US cattle population (29). Current normativity in Mexico restricts the movement of animals from high-prevalence to low-to-zero prevalence regions, which may explain why the genotypes exclusive to BCA have not been spread. In this regard, the state of Sonora, which separates BCA from the rest of Mexico, is classified as "Advanced Modified Accredited" due to the extremely low prevalence, which may act as a deterrent (or geographical barrier) against the movement of dairy cattle to-and-from BCA and the rest of Mexico through this region (49).

The recovery of *M. bovis* from 2.5% of cheese samples collected from local markets is startling and has far reaching consequences. This suggests that routine consumption of fresh cheese by the local population on both sides of the boarder will likely result in the exposure of infectious tuberculous bacteria by most regular consumers of this product over time. Such a claim does require a high level of evidence and merits further discussion. **Supplementary File 6** contains in-depth details of collection date, type of cheese, municipality and store code. While some stores had multiple culture positive samples, all isolates recovered had different WGS profiles, and were collected at different times. Also of note, the isolates recovered from cheese samples most closely matched the diaries located within the same municipality.

Isolation of *M. bovis* from raw milk and cheese is known to present complications due to their complex matrix (high protein and lipid components), as well-susceptibility to contamination by background microflora (50). NVSL has extensive experience developing methods to improve the rate of recovery from these difficult sample types. A contamination rate between 5 and 10%, and a 9.6% recovery rate of acid-fast bacteria suggests decontamination was optimal. Despite this, it is likely that recovery of *M. bovis* does not fully capture the overall prevalence of cheese containing infectious *M. bovis*. This is indicated by the total PCR positivity rate of 6% (19/314). However, because PCR only detects the presence of DNA, the conservative approach is to focus on the samples proven to have live bacteria.

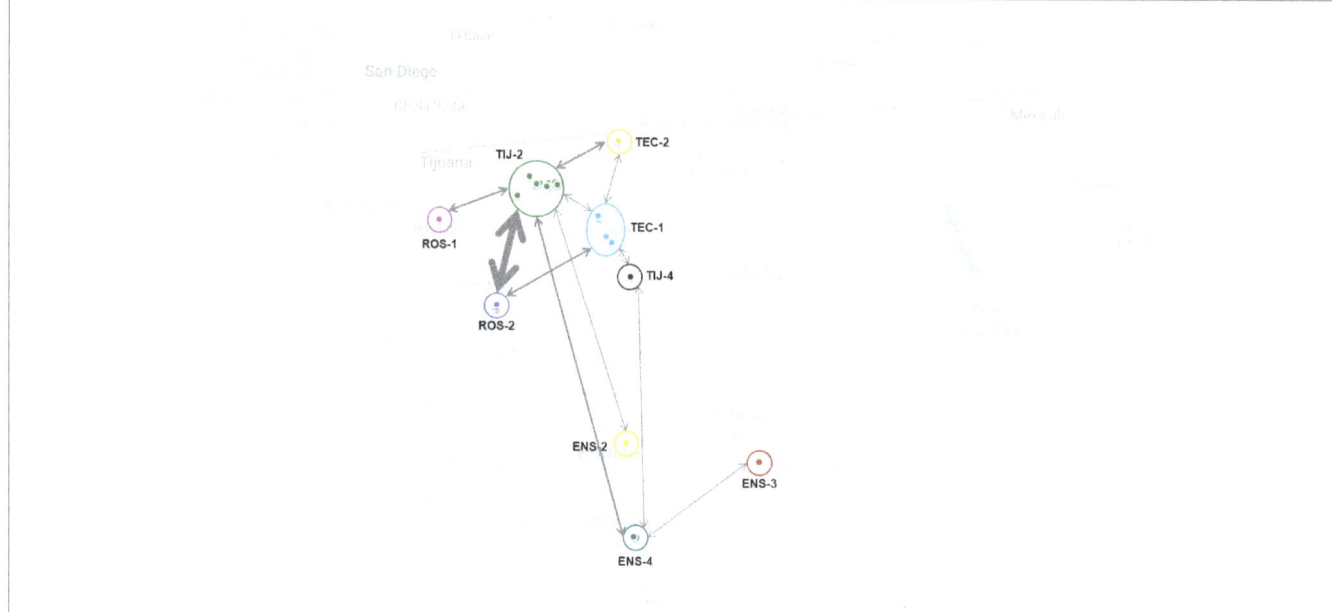

FIGURE 5 | Putative interaction among dairies based on the identification of one or more shared genotypes. Dairies' clusters are indicated and labeled accordingly (ROS-1, ROS-2, TIJ-2, TIJ-4, TEC-1, TEC-2, ENS-2, ENS-3 and ENS-4). Bidirectional arrows are indicative of shared genotypes between dairy clusters and thickness is directly related to the number of shared genotypes (the thicker the arrow, the more shared genotypes). Map was built using GoogleMaps.

Previous studies have established a relationship between *M. bovis* genotypes found in cattle and humans (51) and positive correlations between the consumption of Mexican fresh cheese and cases of zoonotic tuberculosis (20, 52, 53). Through WGS, this study was able to find a direct relationship (transmission clusters) between *M. bovis* infected dairy cattle in BCA, fresh cheese that originated from the same region, *M. bovis* isolates from humans also from BCA and sporadic dairy cattle in California (**Figure 3**). Only one previous study, also performed in BCA, used WGS to determine relationships between cases of zoonotic tuberculosis and cattle from the region, also finding positive results (11). The fact that the cheese contains *M. bovis* from the local dairy cattle suggests it is in fact being made with unpasteurized milk from these infected herds. The official norm NOM-243-SSA1-2010 states that milk destined for human consumption is required to undergo "a thermal treatment of a determined time and temperature that guarantees its innocuity," such as boiling, pasteurization, ultra-pasteurization, sterilization or dehydration, but it exempts the milk that is used for making cheese "whose typical characteristics may not allow it to be made from milk that has undergone thermal treatment" (54). Additionally, NOM-031-ZOO-1995, which is the official norm for the control of bTB in Mexico, states that only 50% of the total national milk production is pasteurized and the rest is consumed [as raw milk] or transformed into dairy products. Consequently, the threat of raw [unpasteurized] milk and its derivatives, possibly from bTB infected cattle, is apparent. Fresh cheeses are a staple food in Mexican households, making them an important source of infection to humans. If pasteurization is not a viable option due to the intrinsic organoleptic characteristics of these types of cheese, cheese-makers must make sure that the

raw milk they use comes from healthy animals as to guarantee the innocuity of the product, as stipulated in the official norm for the sanitary requirements of milk and its derivatives (54). In addition to this, education to the public regarding the risks of consuming unpasteurized dairy products could have an impact on their decision to continue to consume these products (55, 56).

For bTB control programs to be successful, strict quarantine measures and animal movement restrictions of infected animals are key. In this study, WGS of *M. bovis* isolates obtained from different dairies throughout the area of study revealed that at least 50% of these dairies were identified with the same SNP clusters or very closely related SNP clusters. This is indicative of herd-to-herd transmission either through the exchange of infected animals or by the acquisition of animals from a same infected source, among other possible causes (57–59). For this study, many dairy owners reported no testing was routinely performed (such as tuberculin skin test for bTB) when introducing new cattle into their herd. In Mexico, the bTB National Program implemented in 1995 has had great success in the beef cattle sector, with most of the focus being on cattle for export to the US. Unfortunately, due to the characteristics of the dairy production systems (longer life/production cycle, higher density of animals, cost of replacement animals, etc.) and relaxed herd management practices (such as lack of testing for newly introduced animals), as well as no compensation of culled animals for farmers, it has been more difficult to reduce the prevalence in dairy regions, where it has been reported at up to 16% (60). Based on experience of the authors, there is a strong and widespread misconception amongst dairy farmers regarding the risk of bTB to human health: because they believe that the milk will ultimately be pasteurized, they don't consider the status of bTB in their herd to be critical.

Another important aspect observed in this study regarding the burden of infection in these BCA dairies is the presence of mixed infections. A mixed infection refers to the simultaneous presence of multiple strains (i.e., genotypes, variants, etc.) of the same pathogen in an individual host. In this study, based on the identification of 20 isolates that presented a high proportion of ambiguous (heterozygous) SNP calls (>50%), nearly 6% of the infected animals had a mixed infection. The high number of heterogenous SNPs point to clearly distinct DNA fingerprints, which support co-infection with different genotypes acquired either at a single point in time or as separate events. This could be indicative of multiple introductions of bTB into the diaries and highlights the lack of control in the movement of animals in the region. Previous studies in *M. tuberculosis* have also found mixed infections in humans more frequently in high-TB burden regions (61). Though a well-studied occurrence in humans, information on identification of mixed *M. bovis* infections in cattle through WGS is scarce; thus, the results shown here may be useful for future comparisons.

A limitation of the study was that sampling only focused on granulomatous lesions observed at carcass inspection. This may have led to the exclusion of animals with an early stage of infection and thus an underestimation of further micro diversity within the herds. However, the large number of animals sampled and the long-term sampling period, as well as the comparison to previously published genomes, support the overall diversity of *M. bovis* seen in the region. Another limitation of the study was the lack of *M. bovis* isolates recovered from humans. In Mexico, mycobacterial culture is not commonly performed in humans, as diagnosis and treatments are initiated using acid fast staining of sputum and PCR. Typically, only cases refractory to treatment are cultured and further characterized. A better understanding of the TB strains infecting humans in the region is needed.

CONCLUSIONS

Despite the well-managed dairy production of this region, a high proportion (93.5%) of the dairies sampled was found infected with bovine tuberculosis. WGS provided evidence of ongoing local transmission of *M. bovis* among these dairies as several of them shared at least one genotype with at least one other dairy in the region. This study was successful at characterizing the diversity of *M. bovis* circulating in the region. This will allow future studies to evaluate the regional and global spread of these genotypes

in humans and animals, allowing for a coordinated One Health approach to be used in animal and human TB elimination programs.

ETHICS STATEMENT

Ethical review and approval was not required for the animal study because all samples were collected as part of authorized regulatory surveillance (NOM-031-ZOO-1995) on animals after harvesting. Written informed consent for participation was not obtained from the owners because all samples were collected as part of authorized regulatory surveillance.

AUTHOR CONTRIBUTIONS

SR-A, AP, RM, and EF conceived and designed the study. ED, ER, and KS collected the samples. All authors analyzed the data, wrote, and reviewed the manuscript.

ACKNOWLEDGMENTS

A special thanks to Dr. Giber Alain Sandoval Milán (State Committee for Livestock Promotion and Protection in Baja California) for the invaluable support, sample collection and expertise during the execution of this project. This project was supported in part by an appointment to the Science Education and Workforce Development Programs at Oak Ridge National Laboratory, administered by ORISE through the U.S. Department of Energy Oak Ridge Institute for Science and Education.

SUPPLEMENTARY MATERIAL

Supplementary File 1 | Total dairies and dairy-clusters included in this study.

Supplementary File 2 | SNP tables for the 10 clades associated to *M. bovis* isolates obtained from dairy cattle, humans and cheese in Baja California.

Supplementary File 3 | List of *M. bovis* SNP clusters (genotypes) identified in BCA dairies.

Supplementary File 4 | List of accessions retrieved from NCBI's Sequence Read Archive.

Supplementary File 5 | Sequencing metrics for the genomes obtained in this study.

Supplementary File 6 | Metadata and results associated to the cheese samples obtained from Baja California Mexico.

REFERENCES

1. Neill SD, Pollock JM, Bryson DB, Hanna J. Pathogenesis of *Mycobacterium bovis* infection in cattle. *Vet Microbiol.* (1994) 40:41–52. doi: 10.1016/0378-1135(94)90045-0

2. OIE. *Terrestrial Animal Health Code.* 23rd ed. Paris: World Organisation for Animal Health (2019).

3. Neill SD, Bryson DG, Pollock JM. Pathogenesis of tuberculosis in cattle. *Tuberculosis.* (2001) 81:79–86. doi: 10.1054/tube.2000.0279

4. Thoen CO, Kaplan B, Thoen TC, Gilsdorf MJ, Shere JA. Zoonotic tuberculosis. A comprehensive ONE HEALTH approach. *Medicina.* (2016) 76:159–65.

5. Allen AR, Skuce RA, Byrne AW. Bovine tuberculosis in Britain and Ireland – a perfect storm? The confluence of potential ecological and epidemiological impediments to controlling a chronic infectious disease. *Front Vet Sci.* (2018) 5:109. doi: 10.3389/fvets.2018.00109

6. Price-Carter M, Brauning R, de Lisle GW, Livingstone P, Neill M, Sinclair J, et al. Whole genome sequencing for determining the source of *Mycobacterium bovis* infections in livestock herds and wildlife in New Zealand. *Front Vet Sci.* (2018) 5:272. doi: 10.3389/fvets.2018.00272

7. de Kantor IN, Ritacco V. Bovine tuberculosis in Latin America and the Caribbean: current status, control and eradication programs. *Vet Microbiol.* (1994) 40:5–14. doi: 10.1016/0378-1135(94)90042-6

8. Areda DB, Muwonge A, Dibaba AB. Status of Bovine Tuberculosis in Ethiopia: challenges Opportunities for Future Control Prevention. In: Dibaba AB, Kriek NPJ, Thoen CO, editors. *Tuberculosis in Animals: An African Perspective.* Cham: Springer International Publishing (2019). p. 317–37. doi: 10.1007/978-3-030-18690-6_14

9. SENASICA. *Situacion Actual de la Tuberculosis Bovina en Mexico.* Mexico (2020). Available online at: https://www.gob.mx/senasica/documentos/situacion-actual-de-tuberculosis-bovina?state=published (accessed March 2, 2021).

10. Lopez-Valencia G, Renteria-Evangelista T, Williams JdJ, Licea-Navarro A, Mora-Valle ADl, Medina-Basulto G, et al. Field evaluation of the protective efficacy of *Mycobacterium bovis* BCG vaccine against bovine tuberculosis. *Res Vet Sci.* (2010) 88:44–9. doi: 10.1016/j.rvsc.2009.05.022

11. Sandoval-Azuara SE, Muñiz-Salazar R, Perea-Jacobo R, Robbe-Austerman S, Perera-Ortiz A, López-Valencia G, et al. Whole genome sequencing of *Mycobacterium bovis* to obtain molecular fingerprints in human and cattle isolates from Baja California, Mexico. *Int J Infect Dis.* (2017) 63:48–56. doi: 10.1016/j.ijid.2017.07.012

12. WHO F, OIE. *Roadmap for Zoonotic Tuberculosis.* Geneva, Switzerland: WHO Press (2017).

13. Zumárraga MJ, Arriaga C, Barandiaran S, Cobos-Marín L, de Waard J, Estrada-Garcia I, et al. Understanding the relationship between *Mycobacterium bovis* spoligotypes from cattle in Latin American Countries. *Res Vet Sci.* (2013) 94:9–21. doi: 10.1016/j.rvsc.2012.07.012

14. Torres-Gonzalez P, Cervera-Hernandez ME, Martinez-Gamboa A, Garcia-Garcia L, Cruz-Hervert LP, Bobadilla-del Valle M, et al. Human tuberculosis caused by *Mycobacterium bovis*: a retrospective comparison with *Mycobacterium tuberculosis* in a Mexican tertiary care centre, 2000–2015. *BMC Infect Dis.* (2016) 16:657. doi: 10.1186/s12879-016-2001-5

15. Olea-Popelka F, Muwonge A, Perera A, Dean AS, Mumford E, Erlacher-Vindel E, et al. Zoonotic tuberculosis in human beings caused by *Mycobacterium bovis*—a call for action. *Lancet Infect Dis.* (2017) 17:e21–5. doi: 10.1016/S1473-3099(16)30139-6

16. CDC. *Reported Tuberculosis in the United States.* Atlanta, GA: US Department of Health and Human Services (2018). Available online at: https://www.cdc.gov/tb/statistics/reports/2018/default.htm (accessed March 2, 2021).

17. LoBue PA, Betacourt W, Peter C, Moser KS. Epidemiology of *Mycobacterium bovis* disease in San Diego County, 1994–2000. *Int J Tuberc Lung Dis.* (2003) 7:180–5.

18. Rodwell TC, Moore M, Moser KS, Brodine SK, Strathdee SA. Tuberculosis from *Mycobacterium bovis* in binational communities, United States. *Emerg Infect Dis.* (2008) 14:909–16. doi: 10.3201/eid1406.071485

19. Harris NB, Payeur J, Bravo D, Osorio R, Stuber T, Farrell D, et al. Recovery of *Mycobacterium bovis* from soft fresh cheese originating in Mexico. *Appl Environ Microbiol.* (2007) 73:1025–8. doi: 10.1128/AEM.01956-06

20. Müller B, Dürr S, Alonso S, Hattendorf J, Laisse CJM, Parsons SDC, et al. Zoonotic *Mycobacterium bovis*–induced Tuberculosis in Humans. *Emerg Infect Dis J.* (2013) 19:899. doi: 10.3201/eid1906.120543

21. Díaz Galindo EP, Valladares Carranza B, Gutiérrez Castillo ADC, Arriaga Jordan CM, Quintero-Salazar B, Cervantes Acosta P, et al. Caracterización de queso fresco comercializado en mercados fijos y populares de Toluca, Estado de México. *Rev Mex Cienc Pecuarias.* (2017) 8:139–46. doi: 10.22319/rmcp.v8i2.4419

22. CDC. *Human Tuberculosis Caused by Mycobacterium bovis — New York City, 2001–2004.* Morbidity and Mortality Weekly Report 54. Centers for Disease Control and Prevention (2005). p. 3. doi: 10.1097/01.inf.0000180986.01284.df

23. Pfyffer GE, Palicova F. Mycobacterium: general characteristics, laboratory detection, and staining procedures. In: Versalovic J, Carroll K, Funke G, Jorgensen J, Landry M, Warnock D, editors. *Manual of Clinical Microbiology.* 10th ed. Washington, DC: ASM Press (2011). p. 472–502. doi: 10.1128/9781555816728.ch28

24. Kinde H, Mikolon A, Rodriguez-Lainz A, Adams C, Walker RL, Cernek-Hoskins S, et al. Recovery of *Salmonella, Listeria monocytogenes,* and *Mycobacterium bovis* from cheese entering the united states through a noncommercial land port of entry. *J Food Prot.* (2007) 70:47–52. doi: 10.4315/0362-028X-70.1.47

25. Bradner L, Robbe-Austerman S, Beitz DC, Stabel JR. Chemical decontamination with N-acetyl-L-cysteine-sodium hydroxide improves recovery of viable Mycobacterium avium subsp. paratuberculosis organisms from cultured milk. *J Clin Microbiol.* (2013) 51:2139. doi: 10.1128/JCM.00508-13

26. Hines N, Payeur JB, Hoffman LJ. Comparison of the recovery of *Mycobacterium bovis* isolates using the BACTEC MGIT 960 system, BACTEC 460 system, and Middlebrook 7H10 and 7H11 solid media. *J Vet Diagn Invest.* (2006) 18:243–50. doi: 10.1177/104063870601800302

27. Robbe-Austerman S, Bravo DM, Harris B. Comparison of the MGIT 960, BACTEC 460 TB and solid media for isolation of *Mycobacterium bovis* in United States veterinary specimens. *BMC Vet Res.* (2013) 9:74. doi: 10.1186/1746-6148-9-74

28. Forgrave R, Donaghy JA, Fisher A, Rowe MT. Optimization of modified Middlebrook 7H11 agar for isolation of *Mycobacterium bovis* from raw milk cheese. *Lett Appl Microbiol.* (2014) 59:384–90. doi: 10.1111/lam.12290

29. Tsao K, Robbe-Austerman S, Miller RS, Portacci K, Grear DA, Webb C. Sources of bovine tuberculosis in the United States. *Infect Genet Evol.* (2014) 28:137–43. doi: 10.1016/j.meegid.2014.09.025

30. Orloski K, Robbe-Austerman S, Stuber T, Hench B, Schoenbaum M. Whole genome sequencing of *Mycobacterium bovis* isolated from Livestock in the United States, 1989–2018. *Front Vet Sci.* (2018) 5:253. doi: 10.3389/fvets.2018.00253

31. Pfyffer GE, Brown-Elliot BA, Wallace J, Richard J. Mycobacterium: general characteristics, isolation, staining procedures. In: *Manual of Clinical Microbiology.* 8th ed. Washington, DC: A. Press (2003). p. 532–59.

32. Dykema P, Stokes K, Beckwith N, Mungin J, Xu L, Vickers D, et al. Development and validation of a direct real-time PCR assay for Mycobacterium bovis and implementation into the United States national surveillance program. *PeerJ PrePrints.* (2016) 4:e1703v1. doi: 10.7287/peerj.preprints.1703v1

33. Li H, Durbin R. Fast and accurate short read alignment with Burrows-Wheeler transform. *Bioinformatics (Oxford, England).* (2009) 25:1754–60. doi: 10.1093/bioinformatics/btp324

34. Garrison E, Marth G. Haplotype-based variant detection from short-read sequencing. *arXiv preprint* arXiv:1207.3907[q-bio.GN] (2012).

35. Robinson JT, Thorvaldsdóttir H, Winckler W, Guttman M, Lander ES, Getz G, et al. Integrative genomics viewer. *Nat Biotechnol.* (2011) 29:24–6. doi: 10.1038/nbt.1754

36. Stamatakis A. RAxML version 8: a tool for phylogenetic analysis and post-analysis of large phylogenies. *Bioinformatics (Oxford, England).* (2014) 30:1312–3. doi: 10.1093/bioinformatics/btu033

37. Rambaut A. FigTree, version 1.4.3. Computer program distributed by the author. Available online at: http://tree.bio.ed.ac.uk/software/figtree/

38. Perea Razo CA, Rodríguez Hernández E, Ponce SIR, Milián Suazo F, Robbe-Austerman S, Stuber T, et al. Molecular epidemiology of cattle tuberculosis in Mexico through whole-genome sequencing and spoligotyping. *PLoS ONE.* (2018) 13:e0201981. doi: 10.1371/journal.pone.0201981

39. Walker TM, Ip CLC, Harrell RH, Evans JT, Kapatai G, Dedicoat MJ, et al. Whole-genome sequencing to delineate *Mycobacterium tuberculosis* outbreaks: a retrospective observational study. *Lancet Infect Dis.* (2013) 13:137–46. doi,:10.1016/S.1473-3099(12)70277-3

40. Meehan CJ, Moris P, Kohl TA, Pečerska J, Akter S, Merker M, et al. The relationship between transmission time and clustering methods in *Mycobacterium tuberculosis* epidemiology. *EBioMedicine*. (2018) 37:410–6. doi: 10.1016/j.ebiom.2018.10.013

41. Lin D, Cui Z, Chongsuvivatwong V, Palittapongarnpim P, Chaiprasert A, Ruangchai W, et al. The geno-spatio analysis of *Mycobacterium tuberculosis* complex in hot and cold spots of Guangxi, China. *BMC Infect Dis*. (2020) 20:462. doi: 10.1186/s12879-020-05189-y

42. Cohen J. A coefficient of agreement for nominal scales. *Educ Psychol Meas*. (1960) 20:37–46. doi: 10.1177/001316446002000104

43. OEIDRUS. *Panorama General de la Produccion Lechera en Baja California*. G. Secretaria de Agricultura, Desarrollo Rural, Pesca y Alimentacion. Oficina Estatal de Informacion para el Desarrollo Rural Sustentable (2011). Available online at: https://www.nacionmulticultural.unam.mx/empresasindigenas/docs/1934.pdf (accessed February 20, 2021).

44. Perea Razo CA, Milian Suazo F, Barcenas Reyes I, Sosa Gallegos S, Rodriguez Hernandez E, Flores Villalva S, et al. Whole genome sequencing for detection of zoonotic tuberculosis in Queretaro, Mexico. *J Infect Dis Prevent Med*. (2017) 5:5. doi: 10.4172/2329-8731.1000158

45. Secretaria de Salud. *Mision de Evaluacion Externa del Programa de Control de Tuberculosis*. O.P.d.l. Salud. Organizacion Mundial de la Salud (2013). Available online at: http://www.cenaprece.salud.gob.mx/programas/interior/micobacteriosis/descargas/pdf/reporte_final_mexico.pdf (accessed February 22, 2021).

46. SENASICA. *Informe de Concordancia y Tiempo Promedio de Procesamiento de Muestras Granulomatosas*. D.G.d.S. Animal (2020). Available online at: https://www.gob.mx/cms/uploads/attachment/file/569824/9_TB_LAB_CONCORDANCIA_CIERRE_2019.pdf (accessed March 3, 2021).

47. Martínez-Vidal C, Hori-Oshima S, Mora-Valle ADl, Bermúdez-Hurtado RM, Rentería-Evangelista TB, López-Valencia G, et al. Genotipificación por VNTR de aislados de Mycobacterium bovis de ganado sacrificado en Baja California, México. *Rev Mexic Cienc Pecuarias*. (2011) 2:393–401. Available online at: http://www.scielo.org.mx/scielo.php?script=sci_arttext&pid=S2007-11242011000400004&lng=es&tlng=es (accessed January 19, 2021).

48. Bermúdez HR, Rentería ET, Medina BG, Hori-Oshima S, De la Mora Valle A, López VG. Evaluation of a lateral flow assay for the diagnosis of *Mycobacterium bovis* infection in dairy cattle. *J Immunoassay Immunochem*. (2012) 33:59–65. doi: 10.1080/15321819.2011.594473

49. NOM-031-ZOO-1995. Modificacion a la Norma Oficial Mexicana NOM-031-ZOO-1995, Campaña Nacional contra la Tuberculosis Bovina (Mycobacterium bovis). In: Gobernacion Sd, editor. *NOM-031-ZOO-1995*. Mexico: Diario Oficial de la Federacion (1998).

50. Rowe MT, Donaghy J. *Mycobacterium bovis*: the importance of milk and dairy products as a cause of human tuberculosis in the UK. A review of taxonomy and culture methods, with particular reference to artisanal cheeses. *Int J Dairy Technol*. (2008) 61:317–26. doi: 10.1111/j.1471-0307.2008.00433.x

51. Rodwell TC, Kapasi AJ, Moore M, Milian-Suazo F, Harris B, Guerrero LP, et al. Tracing the origins of *Mycobacterium bovis* tuberculosis in humans in the USA to cattle in Mexico using spoligotyping. *Int J Infect Dis IJID*. (2010) 3:e129–35. doi: 10.1016/j.ijid.2009.11.037

52. Besser RE, Pakiz B, Schulte JM, Alvarado S, Zell ER, Kenyon TA, et al. Risk Factors for positive mantoux tuberculin skin tests in children in San Diego, California: evidence for boosting and possible foodborne transmission. *Pediatrics*. (2001) 108:305. doi: 10.1542/peds.108.2.305

53. Silva MR, Rocha AdS, da Costa RR, de Alencar AP, de Oliveira VM, Fonseca Júnior AA, et al. Tuberculosis patients co-infected with *Mycobacterium bovis* and *Mycobacterium tuberculosis* in an urban area of Brazil. *Mem Inst Oswaldo Cruz*. (2013) 108:321–7. doi: 10.1590/S0074-02762013000300010

54. NOM-243-SSA1-2010. *Norma Oficial Mexicana NOM-243-SSA1-2010, Productos y Servicios. Leche, Fórmula Láctea, Producto Lácteo Combinado y Derivados Lácteos. Disposiciones y Especificaciones Sanitarias. Métodos de Prueba*. S.d. Salud. (2010). Available online at: http://dof.gob.mx/normasOficiales/4156/salud2a/salud2a.htm (accessed January 16, 2021).

55. Leal-Bohórquez AF, Castro-Osorio CM, Wintaco-Martínez LM, Villalobos R, Puerto-Castro GM. Tuberculosis por *Mycobacterium bovis* en trabajadores de fincas en saneamiento para tuberculosis bovina, de Antioquia, Boyacá y Cundinamarca. *Rev Salud Pública*. (2016) 18:727–37. doi: 10.15446/rsap.v18n5.51187

56. Silva MR, Rocha AdS, Araújo FR, Fonseca-Júnior AA, Alencar APd, Suffys PN, et al. Risk factors for human *Mycobacterium bovis* infections in an urban area of Brazil. *Mem Inst Oswaldo Cruz*. (2018) 113:e170445. doi: 10.1590/0074-02760170445

57. Broughan JA-O, Judge J, Ely E, Delahay RJ, Wilson G, Clifton-Hadley RS, et al. A review of risk factors for bovine tuberculosis infection in cattle in the UK and Ireland. *Epidemiol Infect*. (2016) 144:2899–2926. doi: 10.1017/S095026881600131X

58. Skuce RA, Allen AR, McDowell SWJ. Herd-level risk factors for bovine tuberculosis: a literature review. *Vet Med Int*. (2012) 2012:621210. doi: 10.1155/2012/621210

59. Pozo P, Romero B, Bezos J, Grau A, Nacar J, Saez JL, et al. Evaluation of risk factors associated with herds with an increased duration of bovine tuberculosis breakdowns in Castilla y Leon, Spain (2010-2017). *Front Vet Sci*. (2020) 7:545328. doi: 10.3389/fvets.2020.545328

60. Milian-Suazo F, Salman MD, Ramirez C, Payeur JB, Rhyan JC, Santillan M. Identification of tuberculosis in cattle slaughtered in Mexico. *Am J Vet Res*. (2000) 61:86–9. doi: 10.2460/ajvr.2000.61.86

61. Byrne AS, Goudreau A, Bissonnette N, Shamputa IC, Tahlan K. Methods for detecting mycobacterial mixed strain infections–a systematic review. *Front Genet*. (2020) 11:1590. doi: 10.3389/fgene.2020.600692

Evaluation of P22 ELISA for the Detection of *Mycobacterium bovis*-Specific Antibody in the Oral Fluid of Goats

Javier Ortega [1,2†], *José A. Infantes-Lorenzo* [3†], *Javier Bezos* [1,2*], *Álvaro Roy* [1],
Lucia de Juan [1,2], *Beatriz Romero* [1], *Inmaculada Moreno* [3], *Alberto Gómez-Buendía* [1],
Irene Agulló-Ros [4], *Lucas Domínguez* [1,2] *and Mercedes Domínguez* [3]

[1] VISAVET Health Surveillance Centre, Complutense University of Madrid, Madrid, Spain, [2] Departamento de Sanidad Animal, Facultad de Veterinaria, Universidad Complutense de Madrid, Madrid, Spain, [3] Unidad de Inmunología Microbiana, Centro Nacional de Microbiología, Instituto de Investigación Carlos III, Madrid, Spain, [4] Grupo de Investigación en Sanidad Animal y Zoonosis, Departamento de Anatomía y Anatomía Patológica Comparadas, Facultad de Veterinaria, Universidad de Córdoba, Córdoba, Spain

Correspondence:
Javier Bezos
jbezosga@visavet.ucm.es

[†] *These authors have contributed equally to this work*

The ante-mortem diagnosis of tuberculosis (TB) in ruminants is based mainly on the intradermal tuberculin test and the IFN-γ assay. Antibody (Ab)-based tests have emerged as potential tools for the detection of TB infected animals using serum, plasma, or even milk samples. Oral fluids have also been evaluated as alternative samples with which to detect specific Abs against *Mycobacterium bovis* in pigs or wild boars, but not in ruminants. The objective of this study was, therefore, to evaluate the performance of an in house-ELISA for TB diagnosis (P22 ELISA) in goats as an experimental model for the diagnosis of TB using oral fluid samples. Oral fluid samples from 64 goats from a TB-infected herd ($n = 197$) and all the animals from a TB-free herd ($n = 113$) were analyzed using the P22 ELISA. The estimated sensitivity (Se) and specificity (Sp) were 34.4% (95% CI: 22.4–45.6) and 100% (95% CI: 97.4–100), respectively. The optimal cut-off point was set at 100% according to the ROC analysis. Those animals with a higher level of Abs in their oral fluid attained a higher lesion score ($p = 0.018$). In fact, when taking into account only the setting of the animals with severe lesions ($n = 16$), the ELISA showed a Se of 75% (95% CI: 53.7–96.2). Results of the present study suggest that the P22 ELISA is highly specific but has a limited value detecting infected animals in oral fluid samples. Nevertheless, its performance is significantly higher in the presence of severe lesions.

Keywords: diagnosis, goat, tuberculosis, oral fluid, P22 ELISA

INTRODUCTION

Animal tuberculosis (TB) is a zoonotic infection that is caused mainly by *Mycobacterium bovis* and, more rarely, by other members of the *Mycobacterium tuberculosis* complex (MTBC) (1). The control programmes carried out for ruminants such as cattle and goats are based principally on a test and cull strategy using the single and comparative intradermal tuberculin (SIT and CIT) tests, both of which are based on cell-mediated immune response (2). The interferon-gamma release assay (IGRA), which is an official ancillary diagnostic test for bovine TB, is used to maximize the detection of infected animals and is also based on the cellular immune response (3).

Serological tests have, in recent years, emerged as a potential ancillary test for livestock, and may even be a first option for wildlife owing to their advantages when compared to cell-based tests (4, 5). Moreover, serological tests could be a valuable diagnostic tool in the form of screening tests with which to detect TB at the herd level and have been shown to maximize the detection of TB infected ruminants when they are used in combination with cellular-based tests (6–8). An ELISA based on the recently developed P22 protein complex (P22 ELISA) has shown high performance in terms of sensitivity (Se) and specificity (Sp) in ruminants (4, 6, 8, 9).

Non-invasive and easy-to-collect samples other than serum and plasma have also been evaluated for the detection of specific Abs against several diseases including TB, one of which is oral fluids (10–13). Previous studies have evaluated the performance of the ELISA by comparing milk samples with those of serum for TB diagnosis, and have obtained a similar Se and Sp (14, 15). The use of milk samples is, however, restricted to dairy animals. Oral fluid, which is a biological fluid, can, meanwhile, allow the routine monitoring of animals' health status owing to the minimally invasive and non-stressful method employed to collect it, which can be performed by personnel with minimal training. Moreover, unlike the case of milk samples, it is not necessary for the animal to be lactating and allows males and those animals that do not produce milk (kids, females not lactating or meat herds) to be sampled (11) Oral fluid samples have additionally been proposed as an alternative biological specimen by which to detect specific Abs against *M. bovis* in wild boar, attaining a Se and a Sp of 67.3 and 100%, respectively (13). In fact, oral fluid samples have been used in the fight against other swine diseases, such as classical swine fever, influenza, or porcine reproductive and respiratory syndrome (PRRS) (16–20), thus suggesting that oral fluids are valuable samples for the surveillance and control of TB and other diseases in suids through the use of Ab-based diagnostic platforms (21).

Despite their use in swine populations, few studies have evaluated serological tests by employing oral fluid samples in ruminants in order to detect antibodies against foot and mouth disease virus (FMDV) or Schmallenberg virus (SBV) in bovines (22, 23). With regard to TB, no studies using oral fluid samples for the antibody-based diagnosis of TB in domestic ruminants have, to the best of the authors' knowledge, been published previously.

Given the usefulness of oral fluid samples in other species, we have adapted a P22 ELISA in order to analyze oral fluid samples in goats. The main objective of the present study was to evaluate, for the first time, the usefulness of oral fluid samples as regards detecting specific antibodies against *M. bovis* in ruminants.

MATERIALS AND METHODS
Study Design and Herds of Study
The study was performed with two herds of Guadarrama-breed goats located in central Spain, one of which was *M. bovis*-infected (range: 1–7 year old animals) and one of which was TB-free

(range: 1–6 year old animals), which were used for Se and Sp estimations, respectively. The Se was evaluated in a herd ($n = 197$) in which *M. bovis* SB0121 was isolated. This herd was subjected to a SIT test, a CIT test and an IGRA, which showed an apparent prevalence of 87.5, 67.7, and 53.8%, respectively. Owing to the high proportion of reactors, all the animals were slaughtered and subjected to *post-mortem* analysis. The presence of TB-compatible lesions was evaluated during slaughtering, and tissue samples were collected for the bacteriological culture and isolation of bacteria in the laboratory. Culture positive (*M. bovis* SB0121 was isolated) animals and those with TB compatible lesions ($n = 64$) were included in the study in order to evaluate the Se of the P22 ELISA in oral fluid samples. The Sp was evaluated in a TB-free herd ($n = 113$), based on its history of TB-free status and the negative results obtained from the animals' SIT, CIT, and serological tests (P22 ELISA) in the last three testing events in the last 2 years. The Gudair vaccine (CZ Vaccines, Porriño, Spain) against *M. avium* subsp. *paratuberculosis* (MAP) had been administered to the animals in both herds at the age of 6 months as part of their vaccination programmes.

The animals included in the study were subjected to SIT and CIT tests and IGRA. Serum and oral fluid samples were collected before the intradermal test and analyzed using a P22 ELISA. The results obtained were compared with the *post-mortem* analysis.

The animals in the present study were not considered as experimental animals. All handling and sampling procedures were performed in compliance with Spanish legislation (Royal Decree 720.7/2011).

Serum and Oral Fluid Sample Collection
Blood samples were collected from the jugular vein by means of venipuncture, using plastic serum tubes (BD Vacutainer Becton, Dickinson and Company, Franklin Lakes, USA). The samples were stored at room temperature for 24 h and then centrifuged for 15 min at 650 g, after which sera were stored at $-20°C$ until assaying. Oral fluid samples were obtained from the same goats by dry swabbing the animals' mouths, which were cleaned beforehand. In the laboratory, the dry swabs were introduced into 2 ml tubes with a medium composed of 4 µl of azidiol (Panreac, Spain) and 1 ml of phosphate buffered saline (PBS). These dry swabs were conserved at 4°C for 8 h, after which the samples were centrifuged at 13,000 g for 5 min, and an aliquot of 500 µl of the supernatant was obtained and stored at $-20°C$ until the assay test.

P22 ELISA
Serum samples were analyzed by employing a P22 ELISA, as previously described by Infantes-Lorenzo et al. (4). The protocol was adapted to oral fluid samples as follows: the optimal dilution of oral fluid was determined by evaluating the reactivity of samples diluted from 1:2 to 1:128, and a dilution of 1:2 was eventually chosen. One hundred microliters of detection antibody at 1:2,000 were added, and the plates were incubated at room temperature for 30 min. As before, the secondary antibody [Rabbit anti sheep IgG(H/L)-HRP] (Southern Biotech, USA) was titrated from 1:500 to 1:8,000 in order to choose the optimal dilution.

The results were expressed as a P22 ELISA percentage (E%), which was calculated using the following formula:

$$E\% = [\text{mean sample OD}/(2 \times \text{mean of negative control OD})] \times 100$$

In the case of the serum samples, E% values of 100 or higher were considered positive, as described elsewhere (4), while in that of oral fluid samples, a cut-off was calculated using a receiver operating characteristic (ROC) analysis, and E% values of 100 or higher were considered positive.

Intradermal Tuberculin Tests

The SIT and CIT tests were carried out by means of the intradermal inoculation of 0.1 ml of bovine and avian PPDs (CZ Vaccines, Porriño, Spain) in the right and left site of the cervical region, respectively, using a Dermojet syringe (Akra Dermojet, Pau, France). All tests were performed according to Council Directive 64/432/EEC and Royal Decree RD2611/1996, and the reactions were interpreted as previously described (24).

Interferon-Gamma Release Assay

Blood samples were collected from the jugular vein using evacuated tubes (BD Vacutainer Becton, Dickinson and Company, Franklin Lakes, USA) with heparin in order to detect IFN-γ production. The blood samples were then processed as previously described (25). The blood was incubated at 37°C in a humidified atmosphere in the presence of antigens (PPD-B and PPD-A) for 18–20 h. The samples were then centrifuged at 2,500 rpm for 15 min, and the supernatant was collected. Interferon-gamma release was measured using a commercial IGRA designed for goats (Bovigam TB kit, Thermo Fisher Scientific, Waltham, USA), according to manufacturer's instructions, and the results were interpreted as described elsewhere (26).

Post-mortem Analysis

TB-compatible gross lesions (TBL) include nodular off-white lesions containing caseous material, which may be mineralized in the center and encapsulated by fibrous tissue (27, 28). The inspection and semi-quantitative scoring of the TBL present in the lung lobes and lymph nodes (LNs) of culled animals were carried out on the basis of a previous lesion valuation model proposed by Vordermeier et al. (29), with some modifications. This scoring system relies on the size and number of lesions, in addition to the percentage of the organ affected, as follows: 0, no visible lesions; 1, one small lesion apparent on slicing; 2, <5 lesions of <10 mm in diameter; 3, more than five lesions of <10 mm in diameter or one lesion >10–30 mm in diameter and/or <50% of the organ affected; 4, more than one lesion >30 mm in diameter and/or >50% of the organ affected; and 5, coalescing lesions and >70% of the organ affected. In the lungs, one extra point was awarded to animals that had pleural adhesions. All the lung lobes (left apical, left diaphragmatic, right apical, right cardiac, right accessory, and right diaphragmatic) were examined individually and the scores of these lobes were added up in order to calculate the total lung score. The head LN (retropharyngeal) and pulmonary LNs (tracheobronchial and mediastinal) were likewise examined individually, and the scores of the different LNs were added up in order to calculate the total score.

Tissue samples from the lungs and the retropharyngeal, tracheobronchial, and mediastinal LNs from 64 animals with TB lesions were used for bacteriological culture in Löwenstein-Jensen with sodium pyruvate medium (Difco, Spain), as described previously (15). Animals with TB-compatible lesions in the lungs or in the different LNs analyzed in the present study were considered as TB positive. A comparison between the P22 ELISA results and the lesion score obtained for the lungs and/or head and pulmonary LNs was then carried out.

Statistical Analysis

Wilson's 95% confidence intervals (95% CI) were calculated for the percentage of positive reactors to the different tests. ROC analysis was performed to define the optimal cut-off value (**Supplementary Material**). Quantitative values, such as E% in oral fluid samples with regard to the TBL score, were attained for the two different herds and were compared using the Mann–Whitney U-test. Moreover, the variation of quantitative values of the diagnostic techniques regarding to the TBL score was calculated using an R-squared (R^2) and interpreted as follows: 0.00–0.25 poor, 0.26–0.50 fair, 0.51–0.75 moderate, and 0.76–1.00 substantial. All the statistical tests were carried out using SPSS Statistics 25 (IBM, New York, NY, USA), and interpreted by considering a p-value of 0.05 in order to determine statistical significance.

RESULTS

With regard to the P22 ELISA carried out using oral fluid samples, a ROC curve was calculated using samples from TB-infected ($n = 64$) and TB-free ($n = 113$) animals. The optimal cut-off point was set at 100%, at which the highest Se and Sp were observed. A higher or lower cut-off point caused a loss of Se with a constant Sp, or vice versa, and it was for this reason that an E% of 100 was chosen as the cut-off point.

In the present study, 22 out of the 64 TB-infected animals attained positive results to the P22 ELISA when using oral fluids, yielding an estimated Se of 34.4% (95% CI: 22.4–45.6). All the animals from the TB-free herd tested negative to the P22 ELISA when using oral fluid samples, attaining an Sp of 100% (95% CI: 96.7–100; **Table 1**). The use of the selected cut-off point made it possible to obtain the positive predictive value [100% (95% CI: 97.4–100)], negative predictive value [77.2% (95% CI: 71.1–83.2)], and area under the curve (0.827). Nineteen out of the 22 P22 ELISA-positive goats similarly had TB-compatible lesions in their lungs, and 20 out of 22 had them in different LNs (17 out of 22 in both locations). Taking into account only the setting of 16 animals with severe lesions (lesion score over 10), the ELISA showed an Se of 75% (95% CI: 53.7–96.2). Moreover, those animals that were positive to the P22 ELISA as regards oral fluid samples had a significantly ($p = 0.018$) higher lung TBL score (**Figure 1**).

When using the serum samples, 56 out of the 64 *M. bovis*-infected goats were positive to the P22 ELISA (E% > 100), with an Se of 87.5% (77.2–93.5, 95% CI) (**Table 2**). The *M. bovis*-infected animals had a higher E% when employing the serum (median = 653.9 E%; $p < 0.0001$) than when employing the oral fluid samples (median = 66.6 E%) (**Figure 2**). Similar E% for oral fluid (median = 46.2 E%) and serum (median = 55.2 E%) samples were obtained from animals in the TB-free herd, and no significant differences were observed ($p = 0.852$). Finally, there was a very small correlation between the P22 results obtained for the oral fluid and serum samples ($R^2 = 0.032$) and between the E% results obtained for the oral fluid and the TB compatible lesions observed in the lungs of the

slaughtered goats ($R^2 = 0.142$) and the head and pulmonary LNs: retropharyngeal ($R^2 = 0.206$), tracheobronchial ($R^2 = 0.081$), and mediastinal ($R^2 = 0.116$) (**Supplementary Material**). The correlation between the oral fluid E% and the total lesion score was slightly higher ($R^2 = 0.225$).

Finally, with regard to the techniques based on cellular immune response, of the 64 goats in the TB-infected herd, 55 and 37 were considered positive reactors to the SIT test [(85.9% (95% CI: 75.3–92.4)] and the CIT test [(57.8% (95% CI: 45.6–69.1)], respectively. In this herd, 38/64 animals were positive to IGRA, with an apparent prevalence of 59.4% (95% CI: 47.1–70.5) (**Table 2**). In this respect, there was no correlation between IGRA and the total lesion score results ($R^2 = 0.004$), which was lower than the correlation observed with E% when using oral fluid samples. A poor correlation was observed between SIT and CIT tests and the total lesion score results ($R^2 = 0.042$ and 0.069, respectively) (**Supplementary Material**).

TABLE 1 | Results used to determine the sensitivity and specificity of the oral fluid P22 ELISA for diagnosis of tuberculosis in goats.

Sample type	Presence of TB-lesions	Absence of TB-lesions	Total test results
Oral fluid **ELISA test** positive	22* (TP)	0 (FP)	22 (total test positives)
Oral fluid **ELISA test** negative	42 (FN)	113** (TN)	184 (total test negatives)
Total samples analyzed	64	113	206 (total population)

*Sensitivity of the P22 ELISA was 34.4% (22/64); **Specificity of the P22 ELISA was 100% (113/113).*

DISCUSSION

In the present study, an in-house ELISA with which to detect specific antibodies against *M. bovis* in oral fluid samples was developed and evaluated for the first time in goats. The results showed a high Sp but a limited Se of the P22 ELISA for TB diagnosis using oral fluid samples from goats.

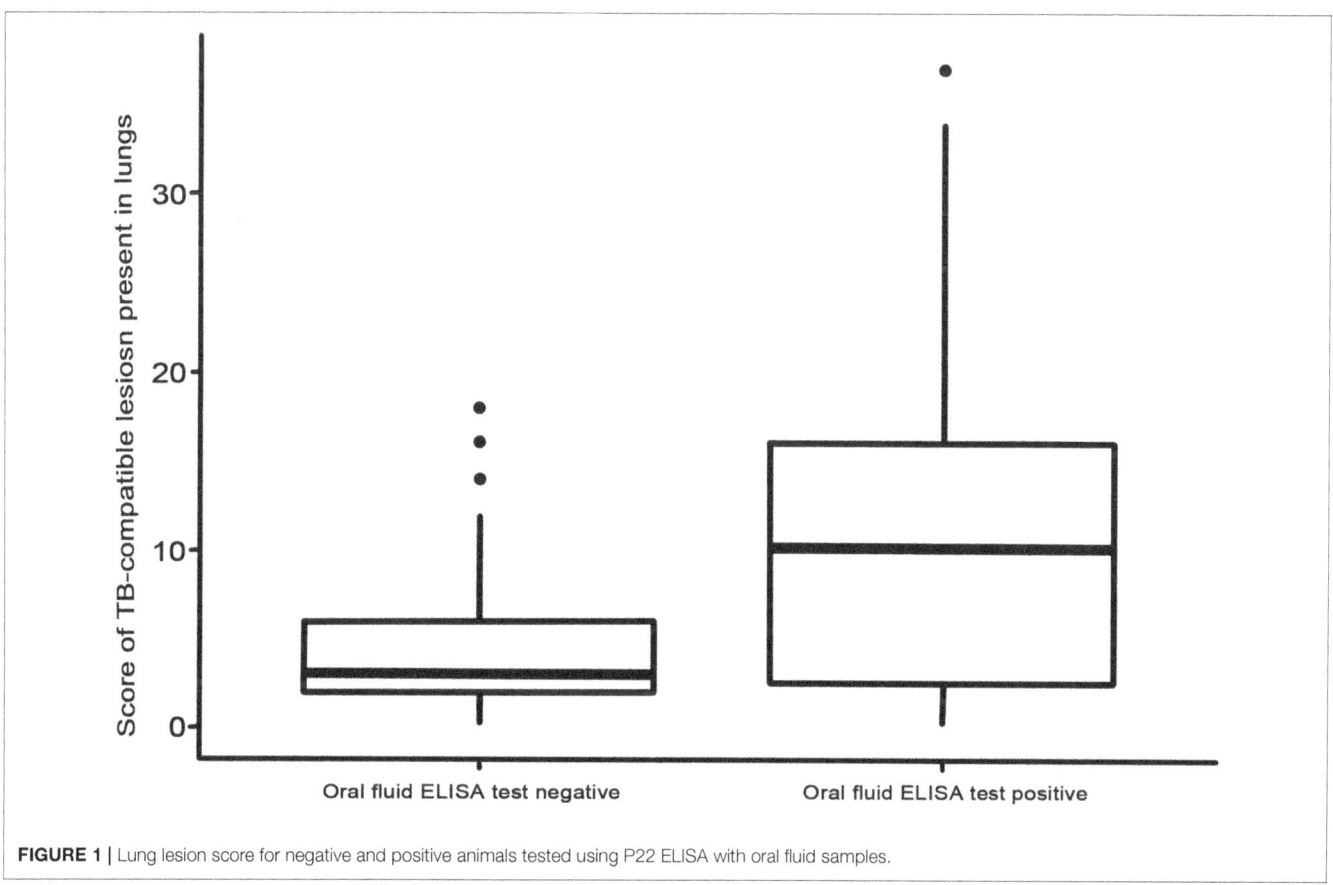

FIGURE 1 | Lung lesion score for negative and positive animals tested using P22 ELISA with oral fluid samples.

TABLE 2 | Summary of the ante-mortem tuberculosis (TB) diagnostic tests and post-mortem analysis in the goats under study.

Herd	Animals	SIT test[a]	CIT test[b]	IGRA[c]	P22 ELISA (serum)[d]	P22 ELISA (oral fluid)[d]	TB lesions in lungs	TB lesions in head and pulmonary lymph nodes
M. bovis-infected	64	55 (85.9%)	37 (57.8%)	38 (59.4%)	56 (87.5%)	22 (34.4%)	54 (84.4%)	60 (93.7%)
TB-free	113	0 (0%)	0 (0%)	0 (0%)	0 (0%)	0 (0%)	0 (0%)	0 (0%)

[a]SIT, Single intradermal tuberculin test: protocol and interpretation was performed according to Council Directive 64/432/EEC and Royal Decree RD2611/1996.
[b]CIT, Comparative intradermal tuberculin test: protocol and interpretation was performed according to Council Directive 64/432/EEC and Royal Decree RD2611/1996.
[c]IGRA, interferon-gamma release assay: an animal was considered positive to IGRA if the optical density (OD) of a sample stimulated with bovine PPD minus the OD of the aliquot stimulated with PBS (nil) was >0.05 and greater than the OD of the sample stimulated with avian PPD.
[d]P22 ELISA, an animal was considered positive to ELISA p22 when the E% value was >150 (serum) or 100 (oral fluid).

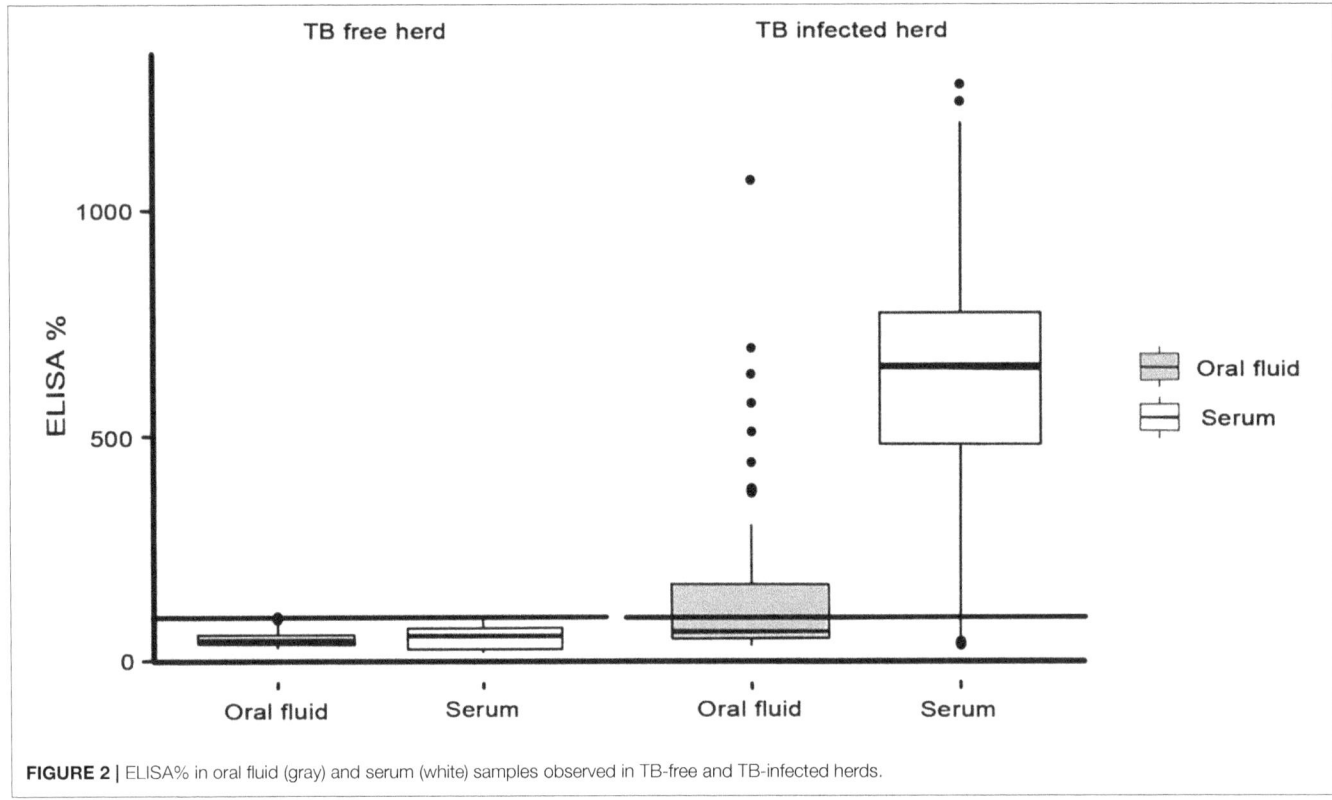

FIGURE 2 | ELISA% in oral fluid (gray) and serum (white) samples observed in TB-free and TB-infected herds.

The P22 ELISA had previously been evaluated for TB diagnosis in goats using sera and milk samples, showing promising results as regards Se and Sp (4, 8, 15). With regard to oral fluid samples for TB diagnosis, a previous study was carried out using a PPD-B-based ELISA in wild boar (13). However, to the best of the authors' knowledge, no previous studies using an ELISA for the detection of specific antibodies against TB in oral fluid samples from ruminants are available. With regard to Sp, the P22 ELISA achieved an excellent Sp of 100%, which was higher than that obtained by the serological tests described to date for the diagnosis of TB in goats using serum or milk samples (4, 7). Interference of vaccination against MAP on the diagnosis of TB in goats has been previously described in TB-free herds in other countries (30). Moreover, different studies have reported a lower Sp [58.3 (95% CI: 42.2–72.9)–96 (95% CI: 90.1–98.4)] of the P22 ELISA in MAP vaccinated goats

than in non-vaccinated goats (4, 31). The higher Sp obtained in our study [100% (95% CI: 96.7–100)] using oral fluids was related to the low Se achieved. Therefore, although both the herds studied herein were vaccinated against *M. avium* subsp. *paratuberculosis* (MAP), a cross-reaction in the TB oral fluid test owing to MAP vaccination was not demonstrated in our study using the recommended cut-off point. However, despite the optimal performance of the P22 ELISA when using serum and milk samples, the present study showed that the usefulness of oral fluid samples as regards detecting *M. bovis* infection in goats was limited, unlike that which occurred in a previous study with wild boar that reported an Se of 67.3% (13). The performance of a diagnostic test is usually evaluated by taking into account the results of a bacteriological culture that is considered the gold standard. None of the *ante-mortem* tests used to define TB infection in goats are perfect in terms of Se and Sp, and they are not, therefore, accurate indicators of the real TB status of the animals. In this respect, the results of serology were used as a reference to define the infection status in the study of wild boar, and this could have affected the accuracy of the test (13). In fact, when the Se of the P22 ELISA carried out using oral fluid samples was estimated using serum results as a gold standard, the Se was slightly higher in our study [39.3% (95% CI: 27.6–52.4) data not shown], but still lower than that reported for wild boar.

It is necessary to state that in the present study, the P22 ELISA attained a higher Se when using serum samples than when using oral fluid samples. Moreover, the Se of TB diagnostic techniques based on specific-antibody detection can be improved by using samples collected after the PPD inoculation. This phenomenon, which is denominated as the booster effect, has been reported in different species (8, 32, 33). It has been suggested that the booster effect on the antibody response is a valuable methodology by which to increase the Se of serological assays in ruminants (6, 8). Further studies with which to evaluate this booster effect in oral fluid samples are, however, required.

The Se of the antibody detection tools is generally lower than that reported when using diagnostic tools based on cellular immune response (34). However, in this work, a higher Se was obtained when using serum samples (87.5%) than when using IGRA (59.4%), SIT (85.9%), and CIT (57.8%) tests, even in the absence of the booster effect. These results support the value of serological tests as a tool for TB diagnosis in ruminants, as observed in recent studies (4, 6, 8, 9), and the importance of developing new TB diagnostic tools in order to maximize the detection of infected animals.

It is widely known that the production and concentration in the samples of the different immunoglobulin (Ig) may differ between species. In this context, the IgG concentration in the oral fluid from goats is significantly lower than that in swine (35), which may explain the differences in the Se previously stated. The IgA-antibody levels in ruminants are, on the contrary, higher than in other species, which could explain the differences observed in the diagnosis when employing IgA or IgG based-ELISAs for other infections such as Schmallenberg disease (23). Moreover, recent studies support the theory that the detection of IgA in oral fluid samples appears to be more robust and stable over time in pigs (20). Ab production in oral fluid is related to mucosal immunity, and local antigen stimulation is, therefore, of paramount importance if high levels of IgA are to be attained in that sample. This could also explain the differences observed between serum and oral fluid samples. In this respect, in the present study, a better correlation between E% in oral fluid samples and the severity of lesions was observed in the retropharyngeal LNs. These LNs are closer to the salivary glands when compared to the pulmonary LNs (mediastinal and tracheobronchial), but additional studies are required in order to confirm the potential correlation between a more severe local immune response and a higher antibody production in ruminants.

Finally, it is necessary to state that, in this study, a goat model was used to evaluate the performance of the P22 ELISA when using oral fluid samples. Previous studies have shown promising results of antibody-based platforms for the diagnosis of other diseases (e.g., FMDV or SVB) when using oral fluid samples in cattle (22, 23). The results from the present study suggest a similar or limited performance of the P22 ELISA in oral fluid samples from cattle owing to the high diagnostic pressure as a consequence of the official eradication programmes, since it is difficult to find animals in an advance stage of infection. The realization of similar studies with which to confirm this hypothesis would, nevertheless, be interesting.

In conclusion, the use of oral fluid sample biomarkers for TB diagnosis in ruminants is still far from being routinely applied and requires further validation and research. The overall results obtained from the present study suggest that employing the P22 ELISA for the detection of specific antibodies in oral fluid samples is highly specific but has a limited value as regards detecting infected animals. Nevertheless, its performance is significantly higher in the presence of severe lesions, detecting a high proportion of those animals in the herd that have these lesions.

ETHICS STATEMENT

Ethical review and approval was not required for the animal study because the animals in the present study were not considered as experimental animals. All handling and sampling procedures were performed in compliance with Spanish legislation (Royal Decree 720.7/2011). Written informed consent for participation was not obtained from the owners because the animals has an owner but he collaborates with our research center and he is aware of all the studies and publications (he prefers to be anonymous).

AUTHOR CONTRIBUTIONS

JO, JI-L, and JB wrote the manuscript and designed the figures. JO and JI-L performed the literature search. JO, JI-L, AG-B, and IA-R performed the experiments. JO, JI-L, JB, LJ, IM, IA-R, ÁR, LJ, BR, and MD interpreted the data. All the authors reviewed and approved the manuscript.

FUNDING

This study was funded by the Herramientas para alcanzar la erradicación de la tuberculosis caprina (GoaTBfree) project (PID2019-105155RB-C31) and the Spanish Government's Ministerio de Agricultura, Pesca y Alimentación. JO was supported by an FPU (Formación de Profesorado Universitario) contract-fellowship provided by the Spanish Ministerio de Ciencia, Innovación y Universidades (FPU18/05197).

ACKNOWLEDGMENTS

The authors would like to acknowledge Ana Belén Martín and Cristina Viñolo for their technical assistance.

REFERENCES

1. Brosch R, Gordon SV, Marmiesse M, Brodin P, Buchrieser C, Eiglmeier K, et al. A new evolutionary scenario for the *Mycobacterium tuberculosis* complex. *Proc Natl Acad Sci.* (2002) 99:3684–9. doi: 10.1073/pnas.052548299

2. Bezos J, Álvarez J, Romero B, Aranaz A, Juan L. Tuberculosis in goats: assessment of current *in vivo* cell-mediated and antibody-based diagnostic assays. *Vet J.* (2012) 191:161–5. doi: 10.1016/j.tvjl.2011.02.010

3. Wood PR, Corner LA, Plackett P. Development of a simple, rapid *in vitro* cellular assay for bovine tuberculosis based on the production of gamma interferon. *Res Vet Sci.* (1990) 49:46–9. doi: 10.1016/S0034-5288(18)31044-0

4. Infantes-Lorenzo JA, Moreno I, Roy A, Risalde MA, Balseiro A, de Juan L, et al. Specificity of serological test for detection of tuberculosis in cattle, goats, sheep and pigs under different epidemiological situations. *BMC Vet Res.* (2019) 15:70. doi: 10.1186/s12917-019-1814-z

5. Thomas J, Infantes-Lorenzo JA, Moreno I, Romero B, Garrido JM, Juste R, et al. A new test to detect antibodies against *Mycobacterium tuberculosis* complex in red deer serum. *Vet J.* (2019) 244:98–103. doi: 10.1016/j.tvjl.2018.12.021

6. Casal C, Infantes JA, Risalde MA, Díez-Guerrier A, Domínguez M, Moreno I, et al. Antibody detection tests improve the sensitivity of tuberculosis diagnosis in cattle. *Res Vet Sci.* (2017) 112:214–21. doi: 10.1016/j.rvsc.2017.05.012

7. O'Brien A, Whelan C, Clarke JB, Hayton A, Watt NJ, Harkiss GD. Serological analysis of tuberculosis in goats by use of the enferplex caprine TB multiplex test. *Clin Vaccine Immunol.* (2017) 24:e00518–e6. doi: 10.1128/CVI.00518-16

8. Bezos J, Roy A, Infantes-Lorenzo JA, González I, Venteo A, Romero B, et al. The use of serological tests incombination with the intradermal tuberculin test maximizes the detection of tuberculosisinfected goats. *Vet Immunol Immunopathol.* (2018) 199:43–52. doi: 10.1016/j.vetimm.2018.03.006

9. Infantes-Lorenzo JA, Gortázar C, Domínguez L, Muñoz-Mendoza M, Domínguez M, Balseiro A. Serological technique for detecting tuberculosis prevalence in sheep in Atlantic Spain. *Res in Vet Sci.* (2020) 129:96–8. doi: 10.1016/j.rvsc.2020.01.013

10. Madar R, Straka S, Baska T. Detection of antibodies in saliva–an effective auxiliary method in surveillance of infectious diseases. *Bratisl Lek Listy.* (2002) 103:38–41.

11. Prickett JR, Zimmerman JJ. The development of oral fluid-based diagnostics and applications in veterinary medicine. *Anim Health Res Rev.* (2010) 11:207–16. doi: 10.1017/S1466252310000010

12. Olsen C, Karriker L, Wang C, Binjawadagi B, Renukaradhya G, Kittawornrat A, et al. Effect of collection material and sample processing on pig oral fluid testing results. *Vet J.* (2013) 198:158. doi: 10.1016/j.tvjl.2013.06.014

13. Barasona JA, Barroso-Arévalo S, Rivera B, Gortázar C, Sánchez-Vizcaíno JM. Detection of antibodies against *Mycobacterium bovis* in oral fluid from Eurasian wild boar. *Pathogens.* (2020) 9:242. doi: 10.3390/pathogens9040242

14. Buddle BM, Wilson T, Luo D, Voges H, Linscott R, Martel E, et al. Evaluation of a commercial enzyme-linked immunosorbent assay for the diagnosis of bovine tuberculosis from milk samples from dairy cows. *CVI.* (2013) 20:1812–6. doi: 10.1128/CVI.00538-13

15. Roy A, Infantes-Lorenzo JA, Domínguez M, Moreno I, Pérez M, García N, et al. Evaluation of a new enzyme-linked immunosorbent assay for the diagnosis of tuberculosis in goat milk. *Res Vet Sci.* (2020) 128:217–23. doi: 10.1016/j.rvsc.2019.12.009

16. Kittawornrat A, Engle M, Panyasing Y, Olsen C, Schwartz K, Rice A, et al. Kinetics of the porcine reproductive and respiratory syndrome virus (PRRSV) humoral immune response in swine serum and oral fluids collected from individual boars. *BMC Vet Res.* (2013) 9:61. doi: 10.1186/1746-6148-9-61

17. Mur L, Gallardo C, Soler A, Zimmermman J, Pelayo V, Nieto R, et al. Potential use of oral fluid samples for serological diagnosis of African swine fever. *Vet Microbiol.* (2013) 165:135–9. doi: 10.1016/j.vetmic.2012.12.034

18. Schaefer R, Rech RR, Silva MC, Gava D, Ciacci-Zanella JR. Orientações para o diagnóstico de influenza em suínos. *Pesq Vet Bras.* (2013) 33:61. doi: 10.1590/S0100-736X2013000100012

19. Henao-Díaz A, Giménez-Lirola L, Magtoto R, Ji J, Zimmerman J. Evaluation of three commercial porcine reproductive and respiratory syndrome virus (PRRSV) oral fluid antibody ELISAs using samples of known status. *Res Vet Sci.* (2019) 125:113–8. doi: 10.1016/j.rvsc.2019.05.019

20. Campero LM, Schott F, Gottstein B, Deplazes P, Sidler X, Basso W. Detection of antibodies to *Toxoplasma gondii* in oral fluid from pigs. *Int J Parasitol.* (2020) 50:349–55. doi: 10.1016/j.ijpara.2019.11.002

21. Ramirez A, Wang C, Prickett JR, Pogranichniy R, Yoon K, Main R, et al. Efficient surveillance of pig populations using oral fluids. *Prev Vet Med.* (2012) 104:292. doi: 10.1016/j.prevetmed.2011.11.008

22. Archetti IL, Amadori M, Donn A, Salt J, Lodetti E. Detection of foot-and-mouth-disease virus-infected cattle by assessment of antibody-response in oropharyngeal fluids. *J Clin Microbiol.* (1995) 33:79–84. doi: 10.1128/jcm.33.1.79-84.1995

23. Lazutka J, Spakova A, Sereika V, Lelesius R, Sasnauskas K, Petraityte-Burneikiene R. Saliva as an alternative specimen for detection of Schmallenberg virus-specific antibodies in bovines. *BMC Vet Res.* (2015) 11:237. doi: 10.1186/s12917-015-0552-0

24. Bezos J, Casal C, Díez-Delgado I, Romero B, Liandris E, Álvarez J, et al. Goats challenged with different members of the *Mycobacterium tuberculosis* complex display different clinical pictures. *Vet Immunol Immunopathol.* (2015) 167:185–9. doi: 10.1016/j.vetimm.2015.07.009

25. Bezos J, Álvarez J, de Juan L, Romero B, Rodríguez S, Castellanos E, et al. Factors influencing the performance of an interferon-gamma assay for the diagnosis of tuberculosis in goats. *Vet J.* (2011) 190:131–5. doi: 10.1016/j.tvjl.2010.09.026

26. Bezos J, Casal C, Puentes E, Díez-Guerrier A, Romero B, Aguilo N, et al. Evaluation of the immunogenicity and diagnostic interference caused by *M. tuberculosis* SO₂ vaccination against tuberculosis in goats. *Res Vet Sci.* (2015) 103:73–9. doi: 10.1016/j.rvsc.2015.09.017

27. Corner LAL, Murphy D, Gormley E. *Mycobacterium bovis* infection in the Eurasian badger (Meles meles): the disease, pathogenesis, epidemiology and control. *J Comp Pathol.* (2011) 144:1–24. doi: 10.1016/j.jcpa.2010.10.003

28. Thomas J, Balseiro A, Gortázar C, Risalde MA. Diagnosis of tuberculosis in wildlife: a systematic review. *Vet Res.* (2021) 52:31. doi: 10.1186/s13567-020-00881-y

29. Vordermeier HM, Chambers MA, Cockle PJ, Whelan AO, Simmons J, Hewinson RG. Correlation of ESAT-6-specific gamma interferon production with pathology in cattle following *Mycobacterium bovis* BCG vaccination against experimental bovine tuberculosis. *Infect Immun.* (2002) 70:3026–32. doi: 10.1128/IAI.70.6.3026-3032.2002

30. Chartier C, Mercier P, Pellet MP, Vialard J. Effect of an inactivated paratuberculosis vaccine on the intradermal testing of goats for tuberculosis. *Vet J.* (2012) 191:360–3. doi: 10.1016/j.tvjl.2011.03.009

31. Roy A, Infantes-Lorenzo JA, Blázquez JC, Venteo A, Mayoral FJ, Domínguez M, et al. Temporal analysis of the interference caused by paratuberculosis vaccination on the tuberculosis diagnostic tests in goats. *Prev Vet Med.* (2018) 156:68–75. doi: 10.1016/j.prevetmed.2018.05.010

32. Bezos J, Casal C, Álvarez J, Díez-Guerrier A, Rodríguez-Bertos A, Romero B, et al. Evaluation of the performanceof cellular and serological diagnostic tests for the diagnosis of tuberculosis in an al-paca (*Vicugna pacos*) herd naturally infected with *Mycobacterium bovis*. *Prev Vet Med.* (2013) 111:304–13. doi: 10.1016/j.prevetmed.2013.05.013

33. Casal C, Díez-Guerrier A, Álvarez J, Rodríguez-Campos S, Mateos A, Linscott R, et al. Strategic use of serology for the diagnosis of bovine tuberculosis after intradermal skin testing. *Vet Microbiol.* (2014) 170:342–51. doi: 10.1016/j.vetmic.2014.02.036

34. Bezos J, Casal C, Romero B, Schroeder B, Hardegger R, Raeber AJ, et al. Current ante-mortem techniques for diagnosis of bovine tuberculosis. *Res Vet Sci.* (2014) 97(Suppl.):S44–S52. doi: 10.1016/j.rvsc.2014.04.002

35. Duncan JR, Wilkie BN, Hiestand F, Winter AJ. The serum and secretory immunoglobulins of cattle: characterization and quantitation. *J Immunol.* (1972) 108:965–76.

A Defined Antigen Skin Test for Diagnosis of Bovine Tuberculosis in Domestic Water Buffaloes (*Bubalus bubalis*)

Tarun Kumar[1], Mahavir Singh[1], Babu Lal Jangir[2], Devan Arora[3], Sreenidhi Srinivasan[4],
Devender Bidhan[5], Dipin Chander Yadav[5], Maroudam Veerasami[6], Douwe Bakker[7],
Vivek Kapur[4,8] and Naresh Jindal[9]*

[1] College of Veterinary Sciences, Lala Lajpat Rai University of Veterinary and Animal Sciences, Hisar, India, [2] Department of
Veterinary Pathology, Lala Lajpat Rai University of Veterinary and Animal Sciences, Hisar, India, [3] Haryana Pashu Vigyan
Kendra, Lala Lajpat Rai University of Veterinary and Animal Sciences, Hisar, India, [4] Huck Institutes of the Life Sciences, The
Pennsylvania State University, University Park, PA, United States, [5] Department of Livestock Production Management, Lala
Lajpat Rai University of Veterinary and Animal Sciences, Hisar, India, [6] Cisgen Biotech Discoveries Pvt. Ltd., Chennai, India,
[7] Independent Researcher, Lelystad, Netherlands, [8] Department of Animal Science, The Pennsylvania State University,
University Park, PA, United States, [9] Department of Veterinary Public Health and Epidemiology, Lala Lajpat Rai University of
Veterinary and Animal Sciences, Hisar, India

Correspondence:
Naresh Jindal
nareshjindal1@gmail.com

Bovine tuberculosis (bTB) remains endemic in domestic water buffaloes (*Bubalus bubalis*) in India and elsewhere, with limited options for control other than testing and slaughter. The prescribed tuberculin skin tests with purified protein derivative (PPD) for diagnosis of bTB preclude the use of Bacille Calmette-Guérin (BCG)-based vaccination because of the antigenic cross-reactivity of vaccine strains with *Mycobacterium bovis* and related pathogenic members of the *M. tuberculosis* complex (MTBC). For the diagnosis of bTB in domestic water buffaloes, we here assessed a recently described defined-antigen skin test (DST) that comprises overlapping peptides representing the ESAT-6, CFP-10 and Rv3615c antigens, present in disease-causing members of the MTBC but missing in BCG strains. The performance characteristics of three doses (5, 10 or 20 μg/peptide) of the DST were assessed in natural tuberculin skin test reactor (*n* = 11) and non-reactor (*n* = 35) water buffaloes at an organized dairy farm in Hisar, India, and results were compared with the single intradermal skin test (SIT) using standard bovine tuberculin (PPD-B). The results showed a dose-dependent response of DST in natural reactor water buffaloes, although the SIT induced a significantly greater ($P < 0.001$) skin test response than the highest dose of DST used. However, using a cut-off of 2 mm or greater, the 5, 10, and 20 μg DST cocktail correctly classified eight, 10 and all 11 of the SIT-positive reactors, respectively, suggesting that the 20 μg DST cocktail has a diagnostic sensitivity (Se) of 1.0 (95% CI: 0.72–1.0) identical to that of the SIT. Importantly, none of the tested DST doses induced any measurable skin induration responses in the 35 SIT-negative animals, suggesting a specificity point estimate of 1.0 (95% CI: 0.9–1.0), also identical to that of the SIT and compares favorably with that of the comparative cervical test (Se = 0.85; 95%

CI: 0.55–0.98). Overall, the results suggest that similar to tuberculin, the DST enables sensitive and specific diagnosis of bTB in water buffaloes. Future field trials to explore the utility of DST as a defined antigen replacement for tuberculin in routine surveillance programs and to enable BCG vaccination of water buffaloes are warranted.

Keywords: water buffaloes (*Bubalus bubalis*), defined antigen skin test, sensitivity, specificity, bovine tuberculosis

INTRODUCTION

Bovine tuberculosis (bTB) is a chronic inflammatory disease of cattle caused by members of the *Mycobacterium tuberculosis* complex, and in addition to being an important animal health problem, bTB also poses a significant threat to public health (1). It has been estimated that annual worldwide economic losses associated with bTB are ~USD 3 billion (2). The disease is well-controlled in high-income countries, however, bTB remains endemic in most low- and middle-income countries (LMICs), including India where bTB has significant impacts in terms of decreased productivity, increased mortality and zoonotic threat. While national control programs involving test-and-cull strategies have proven to be hugely successful in high-income countries, such approaches are often not feasible in LMICs for both social and economic reasons.

India has the largest livestock population in the world, including nearly 191 million cows and 109 million buffaloes (3). Livestock rearing is one of the most important activities in the rural areas of the country, and for many individuals, it is the only source of livelihood. Haryana, a state in northern India, has a large number (~4.3 million) of the Murrah breed of domestic water buffaloes (*Bubalus bubalis*). Indigenous buffaloes are important economically, contributing nearly 35% of the country's total milk (3). Although bTB has been well-studied in cattle generally, studies on this disease in buffalo are scarce, especially for high-producing breeds like Murrah.

A recent meta-analysis on bTB in India reported a pooled prevalence of bTB of 4.3% (95% CI: 2.7, 6.7) in buffaloes, calculated from a total of 29,037 animals tested between 1942 and 2016 (4). Without the implementation of any disease control program, this current level of endemicity is predicted to increase in the coming years, especially given the predicted intensification of dairy farming in India. Given that test-and-cull-based control programs are not implementable in India, a vaccine-based intervention strategy may be a promising solution. The Bacille Calmette-Guérin (BCG) vaccine was initially developed for control of human tuberculosis by Albert Calmette and Camille Guérin and was first used in humans in 1921 (5). While there is evidence supporting BCG-induced protection against bTB, the vaccine has not yet been licensed for use in cattle due to the presence of cross-reactive antigens that interfere with the specificity of the tuberculin skin tests recommended by the World Organisation for Animal Health (6, 7).

Recent developments in the field of bTB diagnostics have focused on fit-for-purpose tools that can reliably differentiate infected and (BCG) vaccinated animals (DIVA) in order to make implementation of BCG-based intervention strategies a possibility in LMICs. Several antigens with DIVA capability have been evaluated, of which ESAT-6, CFP-10, and Rv3615c appear to be the most promising (8, 9). These antigens have been extensively evaluated both in experimental and field conditions, and a peptide-based formulation of these antigens, henceforth referred to as the defined antigen skin test (DST), was previously evaluated for its utility in field studies in cross-bred cattle both in natural reactors and in BCG vaccinates (9, 10). Here, we assess the utility and performance of DST in buffaloes in India.

MATERIALS AND METHODS

Antigens and Peptides

The DST used in the study is comprised of *M. bovis* antigens ESAT-6, CFP-10, and Rv3615c. Peptides ($n = 13$) representing these antigens were chemically synthesized at >98% purity by GenScript USA, Inc. and USV Private Limited, India (see **Supplementary Table 1** for peptide sequences). The safety of DST has been demonstrated in *Bos taurus* subsp. *indicus* under Good Laboratory Practice (GLP) conditions in India with repeat and overdosing experiments (unpublished data). The bovine tuberculin (PPD-B) and avian tuberculin (PPD-A) were sourced from Prionics, Thermo Fisher, Schlieren, Switzerland.

Animals

To determine the performance characteristics of DST in buffaloes, skin tests were conducted in adult female Murrah buffaloes (3–5 years old) recruited from an animal farm at the Lala Lajpat Rai University of Veterinary and Animal Science (LUVAS), Hisar, Haryana, India. Recruited animals that were known bTB reactors based on prior single intradermal testing with PPD-B ($n = 11$), were housed separately from the healthy herd. Skin tests were also conducted in control naïve animals ($n = 35$) from the organized dairy farm. All animal experiments were approved by the Institutional Animal Ethics Committee (IAEC) of the institute (letter number VCC/IAEC/2590-2619 dated 27-12-2018).

Interferon-Gamma Enzyme-Linked Immunosorbent Assay

For *in vitro* stimulation of whole blood, PPD-B and PPD-A were used at a final concentration of 300 and 250 IU/ml, respectively, as per the BOVIGAM™ kit (Thermo Fisher Scientific) instructions. The DST peptide cocktail was used at $10 \mu g/ml$ in *in vitro* assays. Whole blood was collected and stimulated overnight at 37°C, 5% CO_2, with the antigens *in vitro*. BOVIGAM™ kits were used to determine IFN-γ concentrations in whole-blood culture supernatants. Results for antigen-stimulated cultures were expressed as background-corrected optical density at 450 nm (i.e., ΔOD450).

Intradermal Skin Test Procedures

Skin tests using PPD-tuberculins (PPD-A at 25,000 IU/ml and PPD-B at 30,000 IU/ml) were performed as recommended by the manufacturer (Thermo Fisher Scientific, USA), and the results were interpreted as per OIE guidelines (11). Skin thickness was measured by the same operator before administration of PPD and at 72 h post-injection. Skin test readings were measured in millimeters as per OIE-prescribed guidelines. The DST was administered in three different doses, i.e., 5, 10, and 20 μg of each peptide constituent (final injection volume = 0.1 ml), and the sites of injection were randomized. For the single intradermal test (SIT) involving only PPD-B, an increase in skin thickness of 4 mm or more was considered a positive reaction (11), whereas for DST, an increase in skin thickness of 2 mm or more was considered a positive reaction based on the studies conducted in cattle (9). For the comparative cervical test (CCT) involving injection of both PPD-A and PPD-B, a difference in increase in skin thickness between the two infection sites (B-A) is calculated. Per OIE guidelines, a measurement of >4 mm was considered positive for CCT.

Statistical Analyses

All statistical analyses were performed using Prism 8 (GraphPad Software, La Jolla, CA). Confidence intervals (CI) for the sensitivity estimates in natural reactors for DST and PPDs were calculated using the Clopper-Pearson method. For PPD-B, we calculated a one-sided CI (lower 95% CI: 76). Standard two-sided CIs were calculated for CCT, i.e., PPD (B-A) and DST using the same method with point estimates of 82% (95% CI: 48, 98).

RESULTS

Performance of the Defined Antigen Cocktail in the *in vitro* IFN-γ Release Assay

IGRAs were conducted to compare the performance of the DST peptide cocktail, composed of ESAT-6, CFP-10, and Rv3615c, with that of the PPDs (**Figure 1**). The data demonstrated that PPD-B induced a significantly greater IFN-γ response in reactor animals when compared to the DST cocktail ($P < 0.05$; mean of difference = 0.053), while there was no statistical significance in the response induced by DST vs. PPD-B minus PPD-A ($P = 0.98$). Out of 11 animals tested, nine showed IGRA positivity (IGRA cut-off > 0.1) when PPD-B alone was considered, eight were IGRA-positive by PPD-B minus PPD-A, and seven were IGRA-positive by DST; however, the differences were not statistically significant. The data suggest that the DST peptide cocktail may be used as a stimulating antigen in blood tests for diagnosis of bTB in buffaloes.

Defined Antigens Induce a Sensitive and Specific Skin Test Response

The performance of the DST was assessed in natural reactor ($n = 11$) and non-reactor ($n = 35$) buffaloes. The results showed that, when using a cut-off of 2 mm or more, the DST cocktail at 5, 10,

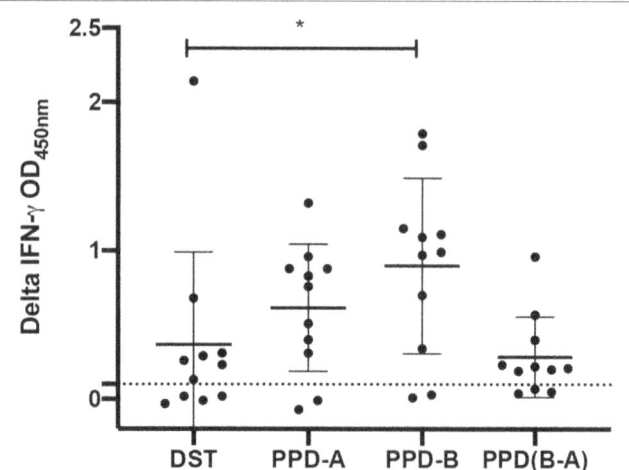

FIGURE 1 | Capacity of DST antigens to induce an *in vitro* IFN-γ response in whole blood collected from naturally infected buffaloes ($n = 11$). The background-corrected optical density (OD) values for all antigens tested are shown. The horizontal line indicates the mean (±SD), and the statistical difference between the responses was determined by using the paired *t*-test (*$P < 0.05$). The means of background-subtracted OD values for DST, PPD-A, PPD-B, and PPD(B-A) were found to be 0.37, 0.62, 0.90, and 0.29, respectively. The standard deviations for DST, PPD-A, PPD-B, and PPD(B-A) were 0.62, 0.43, 0.60, and 0.27, respectively.

and 20 μg correctly classified eight, 10 and 11 of the 11 reactors as positive, respectively (**Figure 2** and **Table 1**). The standard bovine tuberculin antigen (PPD-B), used in the SIT, induced a significantly stronger skin test response than that induced by the highest dose of DST used in this study ($P < 0.001$) and identified all 11 reactors as positive, whereas the CCT identified nine of the 11 buffaloes as reactors. Notably, none of the tested DST doses induced any measurable skin induration responses in the control group ($n = 35$).

DISCUSSION

Recent developments in the field of bTB diagnostics have centered around identifying candidate antigens for DIVA in order to enable vaccine-based interventions in LMICs. Previous studies on the use of defined skin test antigens in cattle, using a combination of ESAT-6, CFP-10, MPB70, and MPB83, concluded that these antigens are promising candidates for performing the IGRA in cattle, with the ability to differentiate between vaccinated animals and those infected with *M. bovis* (8, 12). The current study was performed to assess the performance of a recently developed peptide-based DST cocktail in Murrah buffaloes, an economically important breed of buffaloes in India. In this study, we first performed IGRAs with DST peptides at 10 μg/ml. Although PPD-B was the most sensitive in eliciting IFN-γ responses *in vitro*, there was no significant difference in the responses elicited by the DST peptides and PPD(B-A). To our knowledge, this is the first study where potential of defined skin test antigens has been demonstrated in naturally tuberculin skin test reactor domestic buffaloes. Our data demonstrated

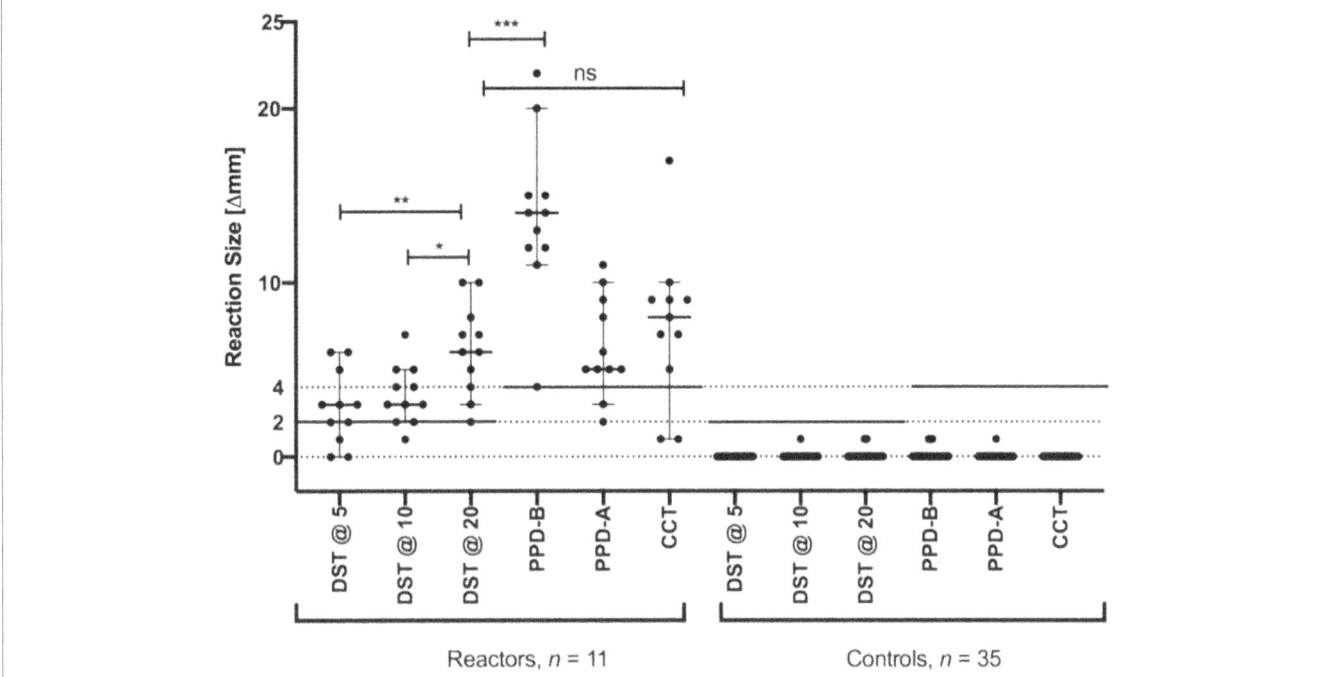

FIGURE 2 | Skin test responses for PPD-A, PPD-B and DST at three doses (5, 10, and 20 ug/ml). Responses were measured at 72 h after injection in naturally infected (n = 11) and naïve control (n = 35) buffaloes. Results are expressed as the difference in skin thickness (in millimeters) between the pre- and post-skin-test readings, with the horizontal line providing the median (±95% CI). The statistical difference between the responses was determined using analysis of variance (ANOVA) (*P < 0.05; **P < 0.01; ***P < 0.001). The solid horizontal lines at 2 and 4 mm are the cut-offs used for DST, and CCT and PPD-B, respectively. The mean skin thickness recorded for DST@5, DST@10, DST@20, PPD-B, PPD-A, and CCT in reactor buffaloes are 2.8, 3.5, 6.2, 13.8, 6.3, and 7.5 mm respectively.

TABLE 1 | Relative sensitivities of SIT, CCT, and DST at different doses.

Test[a]	Positive	Negative	Sensitivity
SIT[b]	11	0	100% (lower 95% CI: 71.5)
CCT	9	2	84.6% (95% CI: 54.5, 98.1)
DST, 5 μg	8	3	78.6% (95% CI: 49.2, 95.3)
DST, 10 μg	10	1	91.7% (95% CI: 61.5, 99.8)
DST, 20 μg[b]	11	0	100% (lower 95% CI: 71.5)

[a] The diagnostic specificity for all tests listed was found to be 100% (lower 95% CI: 71.5).
[b] The SIT and the DST with 20 μg identified all 11 natural reactors as test-positive.

that, these peptide-based antigens have promising potential for use in IGRAs as an ancillary test in concert with the skin test for distinguishing between reactor and uninfected animals. However, as this proof-of-concept study has only been performed on a small number of animals, it will be important to validate the performance of DST in a larger cohort of known infected and naïve buffaloes.

We also assessed the utility of the DST peptide cocktail as a skin test reagent in buffaloes. Of the three different doses (5, 10, and 20 μg per peptide) of DST that were compared, 20 μg/ml appeared to have the highest sensitivity, although higher concentrations may need to be tested to achieve an optimal balance between sensitivity and specificity. Most importantly, the peptide cocktail also proved to be highly

specific, as no measurable skin induration response was observed following injection into naïve uninfected buffaloes. Both SIT and the highest dose of DST were found to be 100% sensitive, identifying all 11 naturally-infected buffaloes as reactors. In this context, it is important to note that, given the high burden of environmental mycobacteria in India, PPD-B can induce non-specific responses, often leading to high rates of false-positivity with SIT. The CCT with the simultaneous injection of PPD-A helps overcome this loss of specificity associated with SIT, but only at the expense of sensitivity. The results of this study showed that the peptide-based DST provides sensitivity and specificity equivalent to that of the OIE-recommended CCT, without the need for a second injection. Moreover, DST at its highest tested dose (20 μg/ml) elicits a lower amplitude of skin test response in infected animals (6.18 ± 2.60 mm) as compared with PPD-B (13.81 ± 4.68 mm) without hindering the specificity estimate. Such exuberant non-specific PPD-B responses tend to raise concerns and limit acceptability of the SIT among farmers. In reactor buffaloes, we found that 20 μg DST produced a skin response greater than the cut-off of 2 mm in all of the animals tested. In this context, it is crucial to highlight the difference in antigen dosage that may be necessary for accurate bTB diagnosis in cattle and buffaloes. In a previous study with cross-bred cattle, pilot dose titration experiments showed that DST@10 may be the optimal dose in cross-bred cattle (9). However, here the data show that DST@20 may be better suited for bTB diagnosis in buffaloes as it identified all reactors as test-positive without compromising test Specificity. Future studies that are adequately statistically powered are required to accurately determine the antigen dosage required for diagnosis in buffaloes.

In 2019, the World Health Organization reported that over nine million people developed TB, of which ~1.5 million died (13). Only eight countries account for about two-thirds of the total reported cases of TB, with India leading the count. Moreover, some recent estimates suggest that ~9% of all human TB cases in India may be of zoonotic origin (14). Hence, it is increasingly recognized that controlling TB in the livestock population in these settings could be a major step toward attaining the ambitious End TB goal of 2035 (15). As part of these control efforts, effective methods of identifying infected animals are needed. However, there are several major limitations to the OIE-recommended tuberculin-based skin tests, including the fact that the active components in the reagent are undefined and their interference with BCG-based vaccination. In contrast, the peptide-based DST offers superior quality control and potential for DIVA has previously been demonstrated in cattle (10), and the current study indicates that the DST antigens are promising candidates for differentiating between reactor and uninfected buffaloes. Limitations of the study include the relatively small number of animals and their origin from a single dairy farm. Hence, these results will need to be verified in larger cohorts of naturally infected and naïve animals to establish more refined estimates of sensitivity and specificity of the DST in buffaloes prior to consideration for replacement of the traditional tuberculin standard. Moreover, while the DIVA capability of DST enables implementation of BCG vaccination as an intervention, the efficacy of BCG vaccination in buffaloes remains unknown. Field trials are in process to evaluate the performance of DST in larger cohorts of infected, BCG-vaccinated and naïve buffaloes, and the efficacy of BCG in buffaloes in natural transmission settings in India is being planned.

ETHICS STATEMENT

The animal study was reviewed and approved by Institutional Animal Ethics Committee, Lala Lajpat Rai University of Veterinary and Animal Sciences (LUVAS), Hisar, Haryana, India.

AUTHOR CONTRIBUTIONS

SS, VK, MV, DBa, and NJ conceptualized the study. TK, MS, BJ, DA, DBi, and DY conducted the animal experiments. MS, SS, and MV conducted the lab experiments. TK, MS, and SS analyzed the data. TK prepared the first draft. All authors contributed to the article and approved the submitted version.

FUNDING

This study was partially supported by a grant (OPP1176950) from the Bill & Melinda Gates Foundation and the U.K. Department for International Development, and the Department of Biotechnology, Government of India (BT/ADV/Bovine tuberculosis/2018 dates 29.09.2018).

REFERENCES

1. Cousins DV. Mycobacterium bovis infection and control in domestic livestock. *Revue Sci Et Tech.* (2001) 20:71–85. doi: 10.20506/rst.20.1.1263
2. Waters WR, Palmer MV, Buddle BM, Vordermeier HM. Bovine tuberculosis vaccine research: historical perspectives and recent advances. *Vaccine.* (2012) 30:2611–22. doi: 10.1016/j.vaccine.2012.02.018
3. DADF GOI. *DADF, Annual Report, 2018–19.* Department of Animal Husbandry, Dairying & Fisheries, Ministry of Agriculture, Government of India, New Delhi (2018).
4. Srinivasan S, Easterling L, Rimal B, Niu XM, Conlan AJK, Dudas P, et al. Prevalence of bovine tuberculosis in India: a systematic review and meta-analysis. *Transbound Emerg Dis.* (2018) 65:1627–40. doi: 10.1111/tbed.12915
5. Buddle BM, Vordermeier HM, Chambers MA, De Klerk-Lorist LM. Efficacy and safety of BCG vaccine for control of tuberculosis in domestic livestock and wildlife. *Front Vet Sci.* (2018) 5:259. doi: 10.3389/fvets.2018.00259
6. Chambers MA, Carter SP, Wilson GJ, Jones G, Brown E, Hewinson RG, et al. Vaccination against tuberculosis in badgers and cattle: an overview of the challenges, developments and current research priorities in Great Britain. *Vet Rec.* (2014) 175:90–6. doi: 10.1136/vr.102581
7. Vordermeier HM, Jones GJ, Buddle BM, Hewinson RG, Villarreal-Ramos B. Bovine tuberculosis in cattle: vaccines, DIVA tests, and host biomarker discovery. *Annu Rev Anim Biosci.* (2016) 4:87–109. doi: 10.1146/annurev-animal-021815-111311
8. Whelan AO, Clifford D, Upadhyay B, Breadon EL, Mcnair J, Hewinson GR, et al. Development of a skin test for bovine tuberculosis for differentiating infected from vaccinated animals. *J Clin Microbiol.* (2010) 48:3176–81. doi: 10.1128/JCM.00420-10
9. Srinivasan S, Jones G, Veerasami M, Steinbach S, Holder T, Zewude A, et al. A defined antigen skin test for the diagnosis of bovine tuberculosis. *Sci Adv.* (2019) 5:eaax4899. doi: 10.1126/sciadv.aax4899
10. Srinivasan S, Subramanian S, Shankar Balakrishnan S, Ramaiyan Selvaraju K, Manomohan V, Selladurai S, et al. A defined antigen skin test that enables implementation of BCG vaccination for control of bovine tuberculosis: proof of concept. *Front Vet Sci.* (2020) 7:391. doi: 10.3389/fvets.2020.00391
11. OIE BT. *General Disease Information Sheets.* Paris (2018).
12. Vordermeier HM, Whelan A, Cockle PJ, Farrant L, Palmer N, Hewinson RG. Use of synthetic peptides derived from the antigens ESAT-6 and CFP-10 for differential diagnosis of bovine tuberculosis in cattle. *Clin Diagn Lab Immunol.* (2001) 8:571–8. doi: 10.1128/CDLI.8.3.571-578.200
13. WHO. *Global Tuberculosis Report 2019.* (2019). Available online at: http://www.who.int/tb/publications/factsheet_global.pdf (accessed October 14, 2020).

14. Olea-Popelka F, Muwonge A, Perera A, Dean AS, Mumford E, Erlacher-Vindel E, et al. Zoonotic tuberculosis in human beings caused by Mycobacterium bovis - a call for action. *Lancet Infect Dis.* (2014) 17:e21–5. doi: 10.1016/S1473-3099(16)30139-6

15. World Health Organization. *WHO, FAO and OIE, (2017): Roadmap for Zoonotic Tuberculosis.* Geneva (2017).

Genotypic Characterization of *Mycobacterium bovis* Isolates from Dairy Cattle Diagnosed with Clinical Tuberculosis

Elizabeth Hortêncio de Melo[1], Harrison Magdinier Gomes[2]*, Philip Noel Suffys[2], Márcia Quinhones Pires Lopes[2], Raquel Lima de Figueiredo Teixeira[2], Ícaro Rodrigues dos Santos[2], Marília Masello Junqueira Franco[3], Helio Langoni[3], Antonio Carlos Paes[3], José Augusto Bastos Afonso[4] and Carla Lopes de Mendonça[4]

[1] *Programa de Pós-Graduação em Medicina Veterinária, Universidade Federal Rural de Pernambuco, Recife, Brazil,*
[2] *Laboratório de Biologia Molecular Aplicada à Micobactérias, Fundação Oswaldo Cruz, Laboratório de Biologia Molecular Aplicada à Micobactérias, Rio de Janeiro, Brazil,* [3] *Departamento de Higiene Veterinária e Saúde Pública, Faculdade de Medicina Veterinária e Zootecnia, Universidade Estadual Paulista, Botucatu, Brazil,* [4] *Clínica de Bovinos de Garanhuns, Universidade Federal Rural de Pernambuco, Garanhuns, Brazil*

*Correspondence:
Harrison Magdinier Gomes
magdinier@gmail.com

Molecular diagnosis of bovine tuberculosis plays an essential role in the epidemiological knowledge of the disease. Bovine tuberculosis caused by *Mycobacterium bovis* represents a risk to human health. This study aimed to perform the genotypic characterization of *M. bovis* isolated from bovines diagnosed as tuberculosis from dairy herds in the state of Pernambuco, Brazil. Granulomas from 30 bovines were sent for microbiological culture, and colonies compatible with *Mycobacterium* spp. were obtained in at least one culture from 17/30 granulomas. All isolates were confirmed to be *M. bovis* by *spoligotyping* and 24*loci* MIRU-VNTR typing. While *spoligotyping* characterized the isolates as SB0121, SB0295, SB0852, SB0120, and an unclassified genotype, 24*loci* MIRU-VNTR rendered two clusters of two isolates each and 13 unique profiles. *Loci* ETR-A showed higher discriminatory power, and *loci* (ETR-B, ETR-C, MIRU16, MIRU27, and QUB26) showed moderate allelic diversity. This is the first study on the genetic variability of the infectious agent cause of bovine TB in Pernambuco and demonstrates variability of strains in the state. Thus, it corroborates the importance of this microorganism as agent of bovine tuberculosis and its zoonotic potential, this epidemiological tool being a determinant in the rigor of the sanitary practices of disease control in dairy herds.

Keywords: bovine tuberculosis, dairy cattle, genotyping, *Mycobacterium bovis*, pathology, spoligotyping, MIRU-VNTR

INTRODUCTION

Bovine tuberculosis is a chronic progressive disease caused by *Mycobacterium bovis* which affects mainly cattle and buffalo but also infects other mammalian species of mammals, including humans (1). The zoonotic potential of this disease is related to the consumption of raw milk and unpasteurized derivatives, representing the main route of transmission to humans, more pronounced in rural areas. In the state of Pernambuco, a prevalence of outbreaks of 2.87 and 0.62% of infected animals was reported in 2016, with a tendency to concentrate in the Agreste region of the state and with a predominance in dairy properties (2).

The interest in nucleic acid-based diagnostic procedures increased because of the limitations of conventional testing such as lack of sensitivity and specificity of the allergic-skin test and the long period for confirming the presence of the agent by bacteriological methods (3). In addition, molecular typing methods have provided a great impetus in the molecular epidemiology studies of the *M. tuberculosis* complex including comparing mycobacterial genome sequences. Among the most used genotyping techniques for the study of the *M. tuberculosis* complex are *Spoligotyping* and Variable Number of Interspersed Repetitive Units of Mycobacteria (MIRU-VNTR) (4, 5). MIRU-VNTR has higher discriminatory power and has currently been the method of choice in the genotyping studies of *Mycobacterium* spp. and, in particular related to *M. bovis*, allows the identification of prevalent strains circulating in a herd or geographic regions (4, 5).

M. bovis infection has an impact on both animal and human health; non-etheless, scarce are the studies in the region on molecular genotyping. Given the lack of data on the contribution and nature of the *Mycobacterium tuberculosis* complex (MTBC) to bovine TB in the state of Pernambuco, we performed the genotypic characterization of Mycobacteria isolated from bovines from dairy herds in this region that were diagnosed clinically with tuberculosis, coming from dairy herds in the state of Pernambuco.

MATERIALS AND METHODS

The study included 28 bovines and two buffaloes that had been attended at the Bovine Clinic of Garanhuns/UFRPE, presenting clinical symptoms suggestive for tuberculosis. The animals were submitted to clinical examination, with information, including epidemiological, that was annotated in clinical records. Among the information present in the anamnesis provided by the owners, common to most animals, were progressive weight loss, dry cough, and decreased milk production.

According to the evolution/severity of the clinical cases and the result of the allergic-skin test, the animals were euthanized according to the current legislation (Brazil, Ministry of Agriculture, Livestock and Supply. Normative Instruction n. 19, 10 of October, 2016) and submitted for anatomopathological examination.

Fragments of organs with lesions characteristic of granulomas were collected for histopathological examination and lymph nodes with lesions for microbiological culture. The samples for bacteriology were stored in a freezer (-80°C) for further processing, while for histopathological evaluation, fragments were fixed in 10% buffered formaldehyde, processed, and stained with hematoxylin and eosin (HE). Granulomas from all 30 animals were collected and sent for microbiological culture and sample processing, and culture conditions favoring isolation of *M. bovis* were carried out following the recommendations of Franco et al. (6). Samples were minced and decontaminated according to the Petroff method, inoculated on Löwenstein–Jensen and Stonebrink medium, and incubated at 37°C for 90 days.

Nucleic acid was obtained from the cells by thermolysis. Molecular identification to the *Mycobacterium* species was performed by PCR amplification of a 1,020-bp fragment of the *gyrB* gene, as described by Chimara et al. (7) and Franco et al. (6). In the reaction, 1 µl of DNA (20 ng) and 47 µl of Master Mix ($1\times$) were used (Thermo Scientific, Waltham, MA, USA), as well as 10 pM of each of the primers MTUBf (5′ TCGGACGCGTATGCGATATC 3′) and MTUBr (5′ ACATACAGTTCGGACTTGCG 3′) [DNA Express Biotecnologia LTDA, Brazil]. The cycling profile consisted of denaturation at 95°C for 10 min, followed by 35 amplification cycles at 94°C for 1 min, 65°C for 1 min, and 72°C for 1.5 min, and a final extension at 72°C for 10 min. The amplification and fragment size were confirmed by electrophoresis in agarose gel (1%) stained with GelRed™ (Biotium, Hayward, CA, USA) using a 100-bp molecular marker (DNA Express Biotecnologia LTDA). Then, 10 µl of the amplified product was submitted for restriction fragment length polymorphism (RFLP) through digestion by restriction enzymes *RsaI*, *TaqI*, and *SacII* (Thermo Scientific, Waltham, MA, USA), following the manufacturer's recommendations. The generated fragments were separated on 2% agarose gel stained with GelRed™ using 50- and 100-bp molecular markers (DNA Express Biotecnologia LTDA). After electrophoresis, the gels were photographed in photo-documentation equipment (2UV Transilluminator UVP) and restriction patterns compared to those described by Chimara et al. (7).

Spoligotyping was performed as described by Kamerbeek et al. (4), and the amplified products underwent membrane hybridization (manufacturing *in-house*) with 43 oligonucleotides. For amplification of the DR region, 20 µM of each of primers DRa 5′ GGTTTTGGGTCTGACGAC 3′ (5′ biotinylated) and DRb (5′ CCGAGAGGGGACGGAAAC 3′), MyTaq Mix (12.5 µl), 1 µl (20 ng) genomic DNA, and ultra-pure water (9.5 µl) were submitted to PCR in a final volume of 25 µl.

MIRU-VNTR typing using a combination of 24-*loci* was performed according to Supply et al. (5). In each PCR reaction, 10 µl MyTaq Mix (Bioline®), 0.4 µl of each *primer* (20 mM), 2 µl of DNA (20 ng), and 7.2 µl of ultra-pure water were used in the final volume of 20 µl. *Mycobacterium tuberculosis* H37Rv DNA and water were used as positive and negative controls, respectively.

The genetic profile based on *spoligotyping* of each isolate was compared to those present in the international databases http://www.mbovis.org/ and http://www.pasteur-guadeloupe.fr:8081/SITVITONLINE. The 24-MIRU-VNTR patterns were compared to those present in the MIRU-VNTRplus database deposited in the application: http://www.miru-vntrplus.org/MIRU/index. The Hunter–Gaston discriminatory index (HGDI) was performed to evaluate the variability of the genotypes obtained by spoligotyping, and each of the alleles of 24-MIRU-VNTR typing.

RESULTS

The 17 animals from which *M. bovis* was isolated came from 10 municipalities in the state of Pernambuco (Alagoinha, Bom Conselho, Chã Grande, Garanhuns, Ibirajuba, Jurema, Pedra,

Pesqueira, Ribeirão, and Venturosa), which were mostly raised in the semi-intensive management system. These municipalities belong to three geographic regions of the state, namely, Southern Agreste, Central Agreste, and South Agreste. Among the animals diagnosed with the disease, females were the most affected (16/17) and 64.7% (11/17) were older than 5 years; one calf 7 months old also yielded positive culture.

The clinical examination of cattle and buffaloes revealed apathy, lack of appetite, low body mass score, seromucous nasal discharge, dry cough, dyspnea, tachypnea, polyps, crackles, and areas of silence in the lung fields. Upon evaluation of the mammary gland, two (2/17) bovines were diagnosed with hypertrophied lymph nodes: one of these presented an enlarged posterior breast of firm consistency, hyperemia and hyperthermia, and physical changes in milk in one of the teats (lumps with serum). The other bovine had an anterior breast of firm consistency but with no visible changes of the milk. During rectal examination, some animals presented nodular structures of varying sizes and hardened consistency in the region of the mesentery, serous in the rumen, and uterus.

Macroscopic observation of lesions seen during *postmortem* examination revealed that 12/17 animals (70.6%) had miliary or protruding tuberculosis, distributed mainly in the lungs, mediastinal and tracheobronchial lymph nodes, liver, and mesenteric lymph nodes and less frequently in the kidneys, spleen, and greater omentum. Among the animals with generalized tuberculosis, two cattle also showed changes in the mammary gland and the uterus, characterized by granulomatous lesions with multifocal distribution and varied sizes, with areas of calcification and abscesses.

The granulomatous nodules observed in all animals were pleomorphic and had a caseous, thick, and yellowish content, with the formation of a fibrous capsule (**Figure 1**). In buffaloes, granulomas had a more whitish color when compared to cattle (**Figure 2**). In the young calf, in addition to lung lesions, small granulomas were observed in the central nervous system and lesions compatible with meningoencephalitis.

Histopathological analysis of the lesions revealed areas of central caseous necrosis and dystrophic calcification and intense inflammatory reaction in the regions adjacent to the necrosis areas, with a predominance of epithelioid macrophages and multinucleated giant cells, like *Langhans*.

Microbiological cultivation presented growth of colonies in 17/30 (57%) samples that were confirmed to be *Mycobacterium* spp. and more specifically *M. bovis* by molecular techniques. In three samples, presence of *Trueperella pyogenes* and, in a single animal, *Nocardia* spp. was encountered. Of the 17 bacterial growths, 14 were classified by the enzymatic restriction analysis of the *gyr*B gene as *M. bovis*. However, due to the importance of bacterial isolation, recognized as a gold standard test, the 17 samples were submitted to molecular genotyping techniques by *Spoligotyping* and 24-*loci* MIRU-VNTR.

Spoligotyping revealed five spoligotypes classified as belonging to *M. bovis*, including SB0121, SB0295, SB0852, SB0120, and a *spoligotype* that was not yet present in the database (**Table 1**).

The analysis of 24-*loci* MIRU-VNTR identified 13 genetic profiles from the 17 isolates of *M. bovis* from 14 properties in the state of Pernambuco (**Table 1**).

The analysis of the discriminatory power (HGDI) of MIRU-VNTR in this study was higher, as expected, than *Spoligotyping*, respectively 0.980 and 0.713. Distribution of the isolates according to the number of alleles in each locus and the analysis of the allelic diversity of the 24-*loci* is summarized in **Table 2**. Locus ETR A showed the highest discriminatory power ($h =$ 0.69), while five *loci* (ETR B, MIRU 16, ETR C, MIRU 27, and QUB 26) were classified as moderately discriminatory with h between 0.33 and 0.58. Eight *loci* (MIRU 20, MIRU 26, Mtub 04, Mtub 29, QUB 11b, QUB 4156, Mtub 21, Mtub 39) presented low discriminatory power ($h \leq 0.27$) while 10 *loci* showed absence of allelic diversity.

Isolates one and 10 showed failures in the amplification of some *loci* that are generally attributed to possible DNA mutations or degradation (5), thus preventing the *primers* from ringing. Given these results, the respective isolates started to be analyzed only in *Spoligotyping*, obtaining significant results.

DISCUSSION

It should be noted that the state of Pernambuco occupies a prominent place in milk production in the Northeast region, and the municipality of Garanhuns and its microregion are recognized as the state's milk basin (8). Dairy cattle and buffaloes are considered more vulnerable to *M. bovis* infection, as they have a longer life expectancy, stay longer on the properties, and are subjected to the rearing semi-intensive and intensive systems, very common in the region. During milking and other common management practices, animals cohabit, therefore increasing their likelihood of contact and the transmission of tuberculosis (2, 9), considered endemic in the State of Pernambuco (2, 10). The constant transit of animals between the properties within and between neighboring municipalities, the interstate cattle trade, and the absence of an effective sanitary control of the herds are factors that contribute to the spread of the disease in the region (2, 9).

In the present study, all animals presented clinical symptoms of tuberculosis with predominating respiratory impairment. In dairy farms, female animals generally remain for longer periods depending on the reproductive period, and this could be the main reason for having observed in this study the predominance of females over the age of 5 years to be exposed to *M. bovis* when compared to young cattle (9). Non-etheless, young animals also contract the infection and develop disease, as demonstrated by *M. bovis* isolation from a 7-month-old calf. The frequency of tuberculosis in cattle aged <12 months is generally associated with the ingestion of colostrum/milk from infected cows or transplacental infection (11, 12). The most evident clinical signs were observed in the advanced stages of the disease, as described by Izael et al. (10) and Waters (13), except for the calf that manifested the disease earlier in the form of cerebral tuberculosis combined with depression and paresis of the limbs. In addition to the predominant respiratory impairment in the animals in this study, two animals showed clinical changes in the mammary gland, resulting to be similar to that described by Waters (13). This observation reinforces the potential risk of the disease to

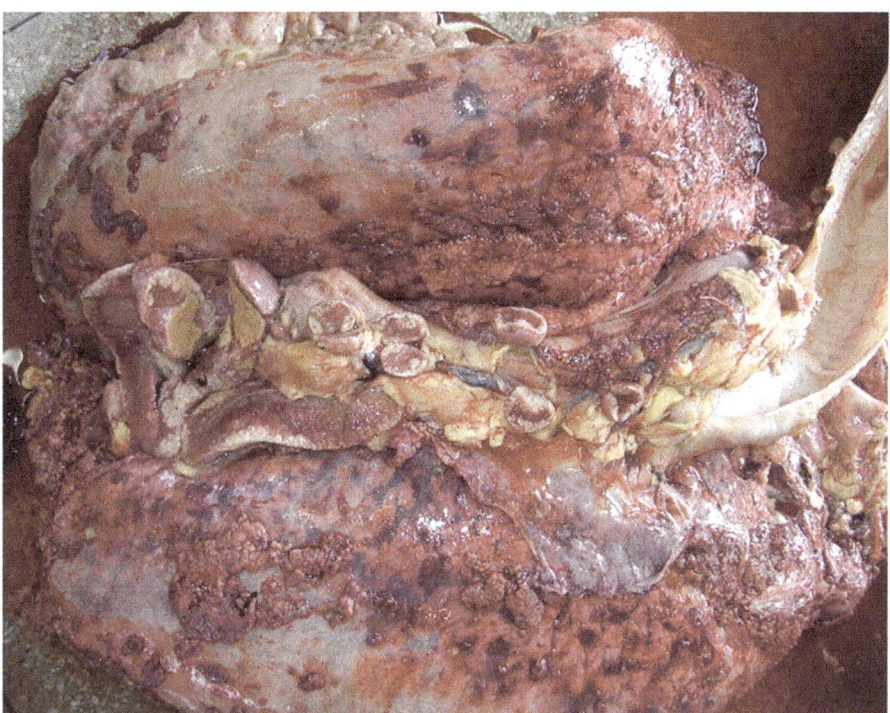

FIGURE 1 | Granulomatous lesions distributed in lung and mediastinal lymph nodes of bovines.

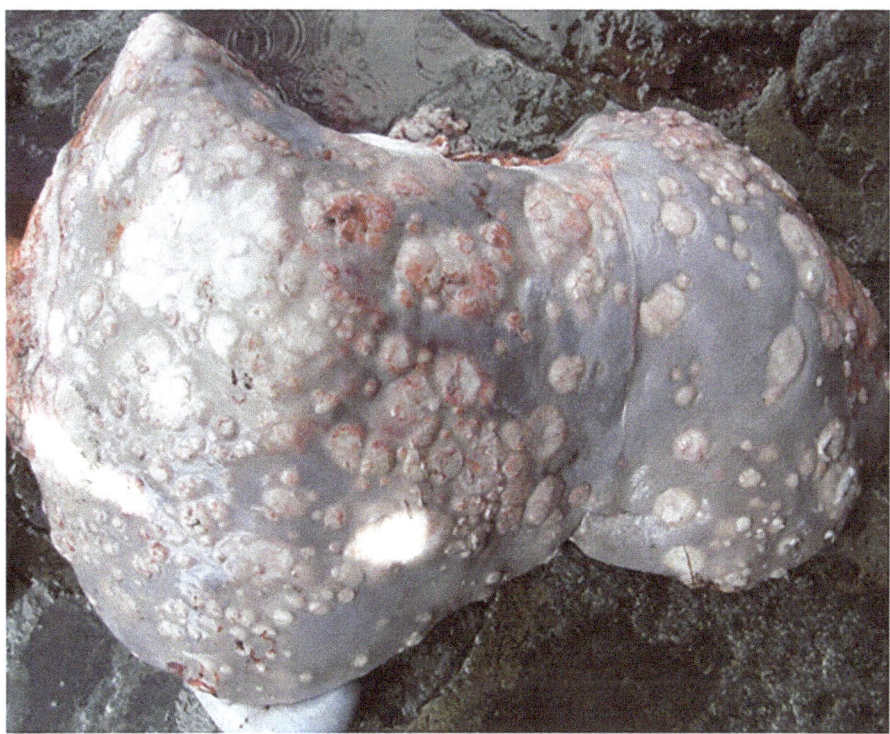

FIGURE 2 | Granulomatous lesions distributed in the liver of buffaloes.

TABLE 1 | Molecular characterization of *M. bovis* isolates from cattle in the state of pernambuco by *Spoligotyping* and MIRU-VNTR.

ID	Octal spoligotype	Cluster spoligotype	Profile of 24 MIRU-VNTR	Cluster MIRU-VNTR	SIT	Mbovis.org	Municipality
1	676773677777600	Cluster S1	2*63***313*3434253332*12	Orphan	481	SB0121	Bom conselho
5	676773677777600	Cluster S1	2263223323244142533332622	Orphan	481	SB0121	Garanhuns
6	676773677777600	Cluster S1	2263223323544342533332622	Orphan	481	SB0121	Chã grande
7	676773677777600	Cluster S1	22*32243236443425333332632	Orphan	481	SB0121	Alagoinha
9	676773677777600	Cluster S1	*2*3223323634442533332312	Orphan	481	SB0121	Pedra
10	676773677777600	Cluster S1	2*5******3*34******3*2***	Orphan	481	SB0121	Pesqueira
15	676773677777600	Cluster S1	**5322*32353434253332*12	Orphan	481	SB0121	Bom conselho
26	676773677777600	Cluster S1	2253222323534442533332512	Orphan	481	SB0121	Pesqueira
29	676773677777200	Cluster S2	2243222323534442533332112	Orphan	698	SB0295	Jurema
34	676773677777200	Cluster S2	2253222323534442513332512	Orphan	698	SB0295	Jurema
38	676773677777200	Cluster S2	2*53223323434442533332612	Orphan	698	SB0295	Ibirajuba
39	676773677777200	Cluster S2	2*43223323434442513332512	Cluster M1	698	SB0295	Ribeirão
40	676773677777200	Cluster S2	2*432233234*444251332512	Cluster M1	698	SB0295	Ribeirão
35	676773777777200	Cluster S3	2253221323234342533333512	Cluster M2	797	SB0852	Bom conselho
37	676773777777200	Cluster S3	2*53221323234342533333512	Cluster M2	797	SB0852	Bom conselho
12	676773777777600	Orphan	*1*32231342*434251332512	Orphan	482	SB0120	Garanhuns
2	New profile	Orphan	23*322331553414243332612	Orphan	New	New	Venturosa

Cluster S – cluster Spoligotyping Cluster M – cluster MIRU-VNTR.
*** Isolates that presented amplification failures in some loci.*
Order of the 24 loci of MIRU-VNTR patterns, MIRU 02–154; Mtub 04–424; ETR C–577; MIRU 04–580; MIRU 40–802; MIRU 10–960; MIRU 16–1,644; Mtub 21–1,955; MIRU 20–2059; QUB 11b-2163b; ETR A–2165; Mtub 29–2,347; Mtub 30–2,401; ETR B–2,461; MIRU 23–2,531; MIRU 24–2,687; MIRU 26–2,996; MIRU 27–3,007; Mtub 34–3,171; MIRU 31–3,192; Mtub 39 – 3,690; QUB 26 – 4052; QUB 4,156–4,156; MIRU 3–4,348.

TABLE 2 | Distribution and allele diversity (HGDI) of the 24-*loci* MIRU-VNTR.

Locus	Number of repetitions						Allele diversity HGDI
	1	2	3	4	5	6	
MIRU 02		14					0.000
Mtub 04	1	8	1				0.266
ETR C				3	7	3	0.570
MIRU 04			16				0.000
MIRU 40		15					0.000
MIRU 10		15					0.000
MIRU 16	2	3	8	1			0.571
Mtub 21	1		15				0.058
MIRU 20	2	13	1				0.275
QUB 11b			15	1	1		0.165
ETR A		4		3	6	2	0.690
Mtub 29			12	3			0.271
Mtub 30				17			0.000
ETR B	2		7	7			0.575
MIRU 23				16			0.000
MIRU 24		16					0.000
MIRU 26				1	15		0.058
MIRU 27	4		12				0.333
Mtub 34			17				0.000
MIRU 31			16				0.000
Mtub 39		15	2				0.158
QUB 26	1		1		7	5	0.582
QUB 4,156	13	2	1				0.275
MIRU 39		16					0.000

public health due to the consumption of raw milk and non-pasteurized derivatives, mainly observed in inland cities and rural areas, such as Garanhuns and the microregion (8).

The generalized form of the disease was predominant both in cattle and in the two buffaloes, with lesions that had disseminated to several organs. All animals had granulomatous injuries in the thoracic organs (lungs, pleura, tracheobronchial, and mediastinal lymph nodes), causing respiratory impairment. This result is similar to those described by Ramos et al. (14), who reported a higher prevalence of lesions compatible with tuberculosis in tracheobronchial and mediastinal lymph nodes and lungs; such typical predominance of lesions in the respiratory tract is indicative for airborne transmission. On the other hand, Alzamora Filho et al. (15) identified the most evident lesions in the lymph nodes of the head (retropharyngeal and parotid) with pulmonary parenchyma. These results corroborate with the findings of the present study, due to the typical predominance of lesions in the respiratory tract, suggesting the airway, as the main gateway for *M. bovis* in bovines. The lower occurrence of mesenteric lymph node involvement here observed was also described by Ramos et al. (14) and justified by the fact that oral route infection is secondary to the respiratory route in adult cattle.

The granulomatous lesions observed in the mammary gland and uterus common to two animals in this study reinforce the potential risk of transmission of *M. bovis* to humans due to the consumption of raw milk and its products (16, 17). On the other hand, the granulomatous lesions located in the central nervous system in young cattle are probably related to the ingestion of colostrum/milk from infected cows and can be justified by ascending infection *via* hematogenic route. This form of cerebral tuberculosis in cattle was also reported by Konradt et al. (11) and Silveira et al. (12).

The histopathological characterization of lesions present in granulomas was similar to the findings described by França et al. (18) who found in some samples a marked process of calcification with mineralization, differing from the lesions observed by Ramos et al. (14) and Silva et al. (19) who presented a more caseous aspect, suggesting that the animals that had been slaughtered were suffering from a recent infection or disease development.

The frequency of isolation of *M. bovis*, of 57%, was observed presently in animals, with clinical tuberculosis. It has been described that some factors can interfere with the success of mycobacterial isolation and in particular of *M. bovis*, including the rigorous decontamination process of samples and the chronic character of the disease that confers intense calcification of the lesions, leading to low concentrations or absence of viable bacilli (20). This might have been influenced by the low isolation of *M. bovis* in the present sampling.

Besides *Mycobacterium* spp., we also observed bacteria belonging to other genera such as *Trueperella pyogenes* and *Nocardia* spp. It is worth mentioning that some microorganisms besides these, such as *Actinomyces* spp. and *Actinobacillus* spp., are also responsible for causing granulomatous lesions similar to tuberculosis lesions (21).

In the present study, 17 isolates compatible with *Mycobacterium* spp. were subjected to molecular diagnostics by RFLP of the *gyr*B gene. However, the analysis classified only 14/17 isolates as *M. bovis*, different from the study carried out by Franco et al. (6) that obtained 100% compatibility between the isolation of *Mycobacterium* spp. and the *gyr*B analysis. The result obtained in the RFLP is probably related to factors that interfere with molecular tests, such as the presence of inhibitors of PCR reactions, low amount of viable bacilli due to chronic lesions, contaminants in the samples, and failures in extraction processing or DNA degradation (22).

Spoligotype SB0121, the most frequently encountered, was described as the most prevalent in national territory with a frequency of 29.1% in a study conducted in Latin American countries (23). The fact that we identified this *spoligotype* in the three defined geographical region studies here could be caused by the constant movement of animals, due to the practice of interstate cattle trade and also strongly suggestive for recent infections (23, 24).

The SB0295 profile was the second most prevalent *spoligotype* in this study (29%) and has been referenced in Brazil with a prevalence of 24% (23). This is similar to that in the Midwest Region of the country, being identified in 16.2% of the total isolates (25). The two isolates identified in buffaloes as SB0295 were also recorded in the Amazon region in mixed buffalo and dairy cattle breeding areas under the same management condition as reported by Carneiro et al. (26). SB0295 was identified in buffaloe isolates in Argentina, highlighting the propagation of common *M. bovis* strains among bovines and buffaloes (23).

Spoligotype SB0852 was identified in two isolates. According to the international database, SB0852 has only been registered in Italy (27), suggesting a process of natural selection of these strains between geographic locations (25) or convergent evolution (23).

Finally, two *spoligotypes* were observed in this study single isolates only, with the case for SB0120 being similar to the low frequency of occurrence in other regions of the country (6, 23, 28). The other was from a bovine that presented a *spoligotype* not present in the international database; this could be due to some microevolutionary events in the DR regions of a strain with an existing pattern (29).

In the region of development of the study, bovine tuberculosis is characterized as endemic, and the practice of commercialization and consumption of milk and fresh products increases the risk of zoonotic transmission, increasing the risk of sharing *M. bovis* isolates common among dairy cattle and the human population of the region, as previously recorded in other studies in different areas of the world. Genomic diversity in the *M. tuberculosis* complex remains a significant factor in the pathogenesis of tuberculosis, which can affect the virulence, transmissibility, host response, and drug resistance (29).

The genotyping performed in this study from the set of 24-loci MIRU-VNTR is recommended for the comparative study of *M. bovis* profiles worldwide (5). Molecular genotyping identified 13 distinct genetic profiles, suggesting a diversity of *M. bovis* within and between the regions studied and considerable higher discriminatory power as compared to *Spoligotyping*. This is according to earlier results obtained both in Brazil (25) and in other countries. This demonstrated that although a large cluster was observed by *spoligotyping* alone, there exists genetic diversity among the strains of *M. bovis* in Pernambuco, probably due to the movement of animals between different regions, states, and rural properties (23, 25).

The analysis of allelic diversity of the different MIRUs are similar to those found by Souza Filho et al. (30) and Carvalho et al. (25) and demonstrating that for this MTBC species, only six of 24 *loci* allowed good discrimination, different from *M. tuberculosis* (31). The HGDI of 24-MIRU-VNTR and *spoligotyping* in this study was 0.980 and 0.713, respectively, close to that observed by Carvalho et al. (25) with values 0.980 and 0.810 and the HGDI of 0.912 reported by Souza Filho et al. (30). Therefore, it seems that simultaneous consideration of both genotyping techniques for clustering might be more accurate for *M. bovis* transmission studies, also in the present study. However, the association between these techniques has been considered the best strategy for the molecular typing of *M. bovis* because they present better reproducibility and reliability, aiming at the analysis of strains mycobacterial (25).

This study is of great importance for the region as it is the first work carried out on molecular genotyping through the association between *Spoligotyping* and MIRU-VNTR aiming at the molecular characterization of *M. bovis* isolates and identification of circulating genotypes in the state of Pernambuco. The importance of *M. bovis* as a cause of human tuberculosis is worth mentioning, although sometimes neglected, especially in developing countries. The consumption of raw milk and dairy products and the constant exposure to reservoir animals are considered the main risk factors in the epidemiological chain of infection.

CONCLUSION

The consumption of raw milk and dairy products is a frequent habit in the region, which, together with data on the occurrence of bovine tuberculosis, increases the risk of zoonotic transmission, alerting the possibility of sharing common *M. bovis* strains between dairy cattle and the population. The genotypic characterization allowed the identification of different *M. bovis*

genotypes circulating in the state of Pernambuco, presenting both two large clusters by *spoligotyping* but evidencing considerable heterogeneity when using 24-MIRU-VNTR. Considering the diversity of genotypes obtained by combining *spoligotyping* and 24-MIRU-VNTR in the present setting, this methodology could be additive during transmission studies.

ETHICS STATEMENT

The animal study was reviewed and approved by Animal Use Ethics Committee (CEUA), of the Federal Rural University of Pernambuco accordance with COBEA and National Institute of Health Guide for Care and Use of Laboratory Animals standards.

AUTHOR CONTRIBUTIONS

EM, CM, JA, MF, HL, and AP: conducted and performed the microbiological diagnostic design of mycobacterial culture procedures. HG, PS, CM, and JA: constructed the molecular diagnostic methodology. EM, HG, PS, IS, ML, and RF: conducted and performed the molecular tests of genotyping and molecular typing. EM, CM, HG, and PS: accurately reviewed the manuscript. All authors have read and approved the final version of the manuscript.

ACKNOWLEDGMENTS

We thank the Foundation for the Support of Science and Technology of the State of Pernambuco (FACEPE) for granting the scholarship (Process n. IBPG-1461-5.05/15) and Fernando José Paganini Listoni from the Department of Veterinary Hygiene and Public Health, Faculty of Veterinary Medicine and Animal Science - UNESP - Botucatu, São Paulo, for carrying out the microbiological cultivation.

REFERENCES

1. Cousins DV, Batisda R, Cataldi A, Quse V, Redrobe S, Dow S, et al. Tuberculosis in seals caused by a novel member of the *Mycobacterium tuberculosis* complex: *Mycobacterium pinnipedii* sp. nov. *Int J Syst Evol Microbiol.* (2003) 53:1305–14. doi: 10.1099/ijs.0.02401-0

2. Lima PRB, Nascimento DL, Almeida EC, Pontual KAQ, Amaku M, Dias RA, et al. Situação epidemiológica da tuberculose bovina no estado de Pernambuco, Brasil. *Semina.* (2016) 37:3601–10. doi: 10.5433/1679-0359.2016v37n5Supl2p3601

3. Drewe JA, Smith NH. Molecular epidemiology of *Mycobacterium bovis*. In: Thoen CO, Steele JH, Kaneene JB, editors. *Zoonotic Tuberculosis: Mycobacterium Bovis and Other Pathogenic Mycobacteria.* Chichester: John Wiley (2014). p. 79–88. doi: 10.1002/9781118474310.ch7

4. Kamerbeek J, Schouls L, Kolk A, van Agterveld M, van Soolingen D, Kuijper S, et al. Simultaneous detection and strain differentiation of *Mycobacterium tuberculosis* for diagnosis and epidemiology. *J Clin Microbiol.* (1997) 35:907–14. doi: 10.1128/jcm.35.4.907-914.1997

5. Supply P, Allix C, Lesjean S, Cardoso-Oelemann M, Rüsch-Gerdes S, Willery E, et al. Proposal for standardization of optimized mycobacterial interspersed repetitive unit-variable-number tandem repeat typing of *Mycobacterium tuberculosis.* *J Clin Microbiol.* (2006) 44:4498–510. doi: 10.1128/JCM.01392-06

6. Franco MMJ, Ribeiro MG, Pavan FR, Miyata M, Heinemann MB, Filho AFS, et al. Genotyping and rifampicin and isoniazid resistance in *Mycobacterium bovis* strains isolated from the lymph nodes of slaughtered cattle. *Tuberculosis.* (2017) 104:30–7. doi: 10.1016/j.tube.2017.02.006

7. Chimara E, Ferrazoli L, Leão SC. *Mycobacterium tuberculosis* complex differentiation using *gyr*B-restriction fragment length

polymorphismanalysis. *Mem Inst Oswaldo Cruz*. (2004) 99:745–8. doi: 10.1590/S0074-02762004000700014

8. Penaforte MA Jr, Borges JM, Azevedo DS, Borges-Filho EL. Perfil dos produtores de leite do município de Garanhuns. In: de Ensino J, Extensão PE, editors. Recife: UFRPE (2009). p. 1–3. Available online at: http://www.eventosufrpe.com.br/jepex2009/cd/resumos/R1002-2.pdf. (Accessed 02 Set, 2019)

9. Veloso FP, Baumgarten KD, Mota ALAA, Ferreira F, Neto JSF, Grisi-Filho JHH, et al. Prevalence and herd-level risk factors of bovine tuberculosis in the State of Santa Catarina. *Semina*. (2016) 37:3659–72. doi: 10.5433/1679-0359.2016v37n5Supl2p3659

10. Izael MA, Silva STG, Costa NA, Souza JCA, Mendonça CL, Afonso JAB. Estudo retrospectivo da ocorrência dos casos de Tuberculose Bovina diagnosticados na Clínica de Bovinos de Garanhuns, PE de 2000 a 2009. *Cienc Anim Bras*. (2009) 1:452–7.

11. Konradt G, Bassuino DM, Bianchil MV, Bandinelli MB, Driemeier D, Pavarini SP. Neurotuberculosis in cattle in southern Brazil. *Trop Anim Health Prod*. (2016) 48:1089–94. doi: 10.1007/s11250-016-1048-z

12. Silveira AM, Nascimento EM, Konradt G, Neto EGM, Driemeier D. Galiza, GJN, et al. Tuberculosis of the central nervous system in cattle in Paraíba, Brazil. *Pesq Vet Bras*. (2018) 38:2092–8. doi: 10.1590/1678-5150-pvb-5976

13. Waters WR. Diseases of the respiratory system. In: Smith BP, editor. *Large Animal Internal Medicine*. St. Louis, MI: Elsevier (2015). p. 633-8.

14. Ramos JM, Heinemann MB, Neto JSF, Filho AFS, Cárdenas NC, Dantas AFM, et al. Isolation and identification of *Mycobacterium bovis* in bovines with positive reaction to the tuberculin test in the State of Paraíba, northeast Brazil. *Arq Inst Biol*. (2018) 85:1–7. doi: 10.1590/1808-1657000842016

15. Filho FA, Vasconcellos SEG, Gomes HM, Cavalcante MP, Suffys PN, Costa JN. Múltiplas estirpes de isolados de *Mycobacterium bovis* identificados por tipagem molecular em bovinos abatidos em matadouros-frigoríficos. *Pesq Vet Bras*. (2014) 34:103–8. doi: 10.1590/S0100-736X2014000200001

16. Cezar RDS, Silva NL, Borges JM, Santana VLA, Pinheiro JW Jr. Detection of *Mycobacterium bovis* in artesanal cheese in the state of Pernambuco, Brazil. *Int J Mycobacteriol*. (2016) 5:269–72. doi: 10.1016/j.ijmyco.2016.04.007

17. Siala M, Cassan C, Smaoui S, Kammoun S, Marouane C, Godreuil S, et al. A first insight into genetic diversity of *Mycobacterium bovis* isolated from extrapulmonary tuberculosis patients in South Tunisia assessed by Spoligotyping and MIRU-VNTR. *Plos NeglTrop Dis*. (2019) 13:1–19. doi: 10.1371/journal.pntd.0007707

18. França LR, Cruz JF, Neves VBF, Cerqueira RB. Prevalência e histopatologia de lesões sugestivas de tuberculose em carcaça de bovinos abatidos no Sudoeste da Bahia. *Rev Bras Saúde Prod Anim*. (2013) 14:721–33. doi: 10.1590/S1519-99402013000400016

19. Silva DAV, Siconelli MJL, Bürger KP, Keid LB. Comparison between tests for tuberculosis diagnosis in slaughtered bovines. *Arq Inst Biol*. (2018) 85:1–5. doi: 10.1590/1808-1657000652016

20. Ambrosio SR, Oliveira EMD, Rodriguez CAR, Neto JSF, Amaku M. Comparison of three decontamination methods for Mycobacterium bovis isolation. *Braz J Microbiol*. (2008) 39:241–4. doi: 10.1590/S1517-83822008000200008

21. Mendes RE, Schneider AF, Werlich DE, Lucca NJ, Lorenzett MP, Pilati C. Estudo anatomopatológico em tecidos condenados pelo Serviço de Inspeção Federal (SIF) por suspeita de tuberculose. *Cienc Anim Bras*. (2013) 14:448–53. doi: 10.5216/cab.v14i4.8581

22. Carel C, Nukdee K, Cantaloube S, Bonne M, Diagne CT, Laval F, et al. *Mycobacterium tuberculosis* proteins involved in mycolic acid synthesis and transport localize dynamically to the old growing pole and septum. *PLoS ONE*. (2014) 9:1–15. doi: 10.1371/journal.pone.0097148

23. Zumárraga MJ, Arriaga C, Barandiaran S, Cobos-Marín L, Waard J, Estrada-Garcia I, et al. Understanding the relationship between *Mycobacterium bovis* spoligotypes from cattle in Latin American Countries. *Res Vet Sci*. (2013) 94:9–21. doi: 10.1016/j.rvsc.2012.07.012

24. Rodríguez S, Romero B, Bezos J, Juan L, Álvarez J, Castellanos E, et al. Hight spoligotyping diversity within a *Mycobacterium bovis* population: clues to understanding the demography of the pathogen in Europe. *Vet Microbiol*. (2010) 141:89–95. doi: 10.1016/j.vetmic.2009.08.007

25. Carvalho RCT, Vasconcellos SEG, Issa MA, Filho PMS, Mota PMPC, Araújo FR, et al. Molecular typing of *Mycobacterium bovis* from cattle reared in Midwest Brazil. *PLoS ONE*. (2016) 11:1–16. doi: 10.1371/journal.pone.0162459

26. Carneiro PAM, Pasquatti TN, Takatani H, Zumárraga MJ, Marfil MJ, Barnard C, et al. Molecular characterization of *Mycobacterium bovis* infection in cattle and buffalo in Amazon Region, Brazil. *Vet Med Sci*. (2019) 6:133–41. doi: 10.1002/vms3.203

27. Boniotti MB, Goria M, Loda D, Garrone A, Benedetto A, Mondo A, et al. Molecular typing of *Mycobacterium bovis* strains isolated in Italy from 2000 to 2006 and evaluation of variable number tandem repeats for geographically optimized genotyping. *J Clin Microbiol*. (2009) 47:636–44. doi: 10.1128/JCM.01192-08

28. Parreiras PM, Andrade GI, Nascimento TF, Oelemann MC, Gomes HM, Alencar AP, et al. Spoligotyping and variable number tandem repeat analysis of *Mycobacterium bovis* isolates from cattle in Brazil. *Mem Inst Oswaldo Cruz*. (2012) 107:64–73. doi: 10.1590/S0074-02762012000100010009

29. Adesokan HK, Streicher EM, Van Helden PD, Warren RM, Cadmus SIB. Genetic diversity of *Mycobacterium tuberculosis* complex strains isolated from livestock workers and cattle in Nigeria. *PLoS ONE*. (2019) 14:1–13. doi: 10.1371/journal.pone.0211637

30. Souza Filho AF, Osório ALAR, Jorge KSG, Araújo FR, Vidal CES, Araújo CP, et al. Genetic profiles of *Mycobacterium bovis* from a cattle herd in southernmost Brazil. *Semina*. (2016) 37:3719–26. doi: 10.5433/1679-0359.2016v37n5Supl2p3719

31. Hilty M, Digimbaye C, Schelling E, Baggi F, Tanner M, Zinsstag J. Evaluation of the discriminatory power of variable number of tandem repeat (VNTR) typing of *Mycobacterium bovis* strains. *Vet Microbiol*. (2005) 109:217–22. doi: 10.1016/j.vetmic.2005.05.017

Permissions

All chapters in this book were first published by Frontiers; hereby published with permission under the Creative Commons Attribution License or equivalent. Every chapter published in this book has been scrutinized by our experts. Their significance has been extensively debated. The topics covered herein carry significant findings which will fuel the growth of the discipline. They may even be implemented as practical applications or may be referred to as a beginning point for another development.

The contributors of this book come from diverse backgrounds, making this book a truly international effort. This book will bring forth new frontiers with its revolutionizing research information and detailed analysis of the nascent developments around the world.

We would like to thank all the contributing authors for lending their expertise to make the book truly unique. They have played a crucial role in the development of this book. Without their invaluable contributions this book wouldn't have been possible. They have made vital efforts to compile up to date information on the varied aspects of this subject to make this book a valuable addition to the collection of many professionals and students.

This book was conceptualized with the vision of imparting up-to-date information and advanced data in this field. To ensure the same, a matchless editorial board was set up. Every individual on the board went through rigorous rounds of assessment to prove their worth. After which they invested a large part of their time researching and compiling the most relevant data for our readers.

The editorial board has been involved in producing this book since its inception. They have spent rigorous hours researching and exploring the diverse topics which have resulted in the successful publishing of this book. They have passed on their knowledge of decades through this book. To expedite this challenging task, the publisher supported the team at every step. A small team of assistant editors was also appointed to further simplify the editing procedure and attain best results for the readers.

Apart from the editorial board, the designing team has also invested a significant amount of their time in understanding the subject and creating the most relevant covers. They scrutinized every image to scout for the most suitable representation of the subject and create an appropriate cover for the book.

The publishing team has been an ardent support to the editorial, designing and production team. Their endless efforts to recruit the best for this project, has resulted in the accomplishment of this book. They are a veteran in the field of academics and their pool of knowledge is as vast as their experience in printing. Their expertise and guidance has proved useful at every step. Their uncompromising quality standards have made this book an exceptional effort. Their encouragement from time to time has been an inspiration for everyone.

The publisher and the editorial board hope that this book will prove to be a valuable piece of knowledge for researchers, students, practitioners and scholars across the globe.

List of Contributors

Marian Price-Carter, Geoffrey W. de Lisle and Desmond M. Collins
AgResearch, Hopkirk Research Institute, Palmerston North, New Zealand

Rudiger Brauning
AgResearch, Invermay Agricultural Centre, Mosgiel, New Zealand

Paul Livingstone
TBfree NZ, Wellington, New Zealand

Mark Neill
TBfree NZ, Christchurch, New Zealand

Jane Sinclair
TBfree NZ, Hamilton, New Zealand

Brent Paterson
TBfree NZ, Dunedin, New Zealand

Gillian Atkinson
TBfree NZ, Palmerston North, New Zealand

Garry Knowles
Aquaculture Veterinary Services Ltd., Clyde, New Zealand

Joseph Crispell
University College Dublin School of Veterinary Medicine, Dublin, Ireland

Rowland Kao
Royal (Dick) School of Veterinary Studies and Roslin Institute, University of Edinburgh, Edinburgh, United Kingdom

Tod Stuber
Diagnostic Bacteriology Laboratory, National Veterinary Services Laboratories, U.S. Department of Agriculture, Animal and Plant Health Inspection Service, Veterinary Service, Ames, IA, United States

Suelee Robbe-Austerman
Diagnostic Bacteriology Laboratory, National Veterinary Services Laboratories, U.S. Department of Agriculture, Animal and Plant Health Inspection Service, Veterinary Service, Ames, IA, United States United States Department of Agriculture: Animal and Plant Health Inspection Service, Veterinary Services, National Veterinary Services Laboratories, Ames, IA, United States

National Veterinary Services Laboratories, U.S. Department of Agriculture, Animal and Plant Health Inspection Service, Veterinary Services, Ames, IA, United States

Julian Parkhill and Simon Harris
Wellcome Sanger Institute, Wellcome Genome Campus, Cambridge, United Kingdom

James Wood
Department of Veterinary Medicine, University of Cambridge, Cambridge, United Kingdom

Malika Bouchez-Zacria
Epidemiology Unit, Paris-Sud University, Laboratory for Animal Health, French Agency for Food, Environment and Occupational Health and Safety (ANSES), Maisons-Alfort, France

Aurélie Courcoul and Benoit Durand
Epidemiology Unit, Paris-Est University, Laboratory for Animal Health, French Agency for Food, Environment and Occupational Health and Safety (ANSES), Maisons-Alfort, France

Graham Nugent, Andrew M. Gormley and Dean P. Anderson
Manaaki Whenua – Landcare Research, Lincoln, New Zealand

Kevin Crews
OSPRI, Christchurch, New Zealand
TBfree NZ, Christchurch, New Zealand

Ruth A. Little
Department of Geography, University of Sheffield, Sheffield, United Kingdom

Lucy A. Brunton
Veterinary Epidemiology, Economics and Public Health Group, Department of Pathobiology and Population Sciences, Royal Veterinary College, University of London, London, United Kingdom

Alison Prosser
Data Systems Group, Department of Epidemiological Sciences, Animal and Plant Health Agency, Weybridge, United Kingdom

Dirk U. Pfeiffer
Veterinary Epidemiology, Economics and Public Health Group, Department of Pathobiology and Population Sciences, Royal Veterinary College, University of London, London, United Kingdom
College of Veterinary Medicine and Life Sciences, City University of Hong Kong, Kowloon Tong, Hong Kong

Sara H. Downs
Epidemiology Group, Department of Epidemiological Sciences, Animal and Plant Health Agency, Weybridge, United Kingdom

Kurt C. VerCauteren and Michael J. Lavelle
National Wildlife Research Center, USDA/APHIS/ Wildlife Services, Fort Collins, CO, United States

Henry Campa III
Department of Fisheries and Wildlife, Michigan State University, East Lansing, MI, United States

Emmanouil Liandris
VISAVET Health Surveillance Center, Complutense University of Madrid, Madrid, Spain

Victor Lorente-Leal and Lucía de Juan
VISAVET Health Surveillance Center, Complutense University of Madrid, Madrid, Spain
Animal Health Department, Veterinary Faculty, Complutense University of Madrid, Madrid, Spain

Javier Bezos
VISAVET Health Surveillance Center, Complutense University of Madrid, Madrid, Spain
Animal Health Department, Veterinary Faculty, Complutense University of Madrid, Madrid, Spain

Elena Castellanos
Exosome Diagnostics Inc., Waltham, MA, United States

Christina Meiring, Paul D. van Helden and Wynand J. Goosen
Division of Molecular Biology and Human Genetics, Faculty of Medicine and Health Sciences, DST-NRF Centre of Excellence for Biomedical Tuberculosis Research, South African Medical Research Council Centre for Tuberculosis Research, Stellenbosch University, Cape Town, South Africa

Graham C. Smith and Richard J. Delahay
National Wildlife Management Centre, Animal and Plant Health Agency, York, United Kingdom

Annette Nigsch
Department of Animal Sciences, Quantitative Veterinary Epidemiology, Wageningen University, Wageningen, Netherlands

Walter Glawischnig and Zoltán Bagó
Institute for Veterinary Disease Control, Austrian Agency for Health and Food Safety, Innsbruck and Mödling, Mödling, Austria

Norbert Greber
Department for Veterinary Affairs, Office of the State Government of Vorarlberg, Bregenz, Austria

Alvaro Roy
VISAVET Health Surveillance Centre, Universidad Complutense de Madrid, Madrid, Spain

Francisco J. Salguero
Department of Pathology and Infectious Diseases, School of Veterinary Medicine, University of Surrey, Guildford, United Kingdom

Jose A. Infantes-Lorenzo
VISAVET Health Surveillance Centre, Universidad Complutense de Madrid, Madrid, Spain
Department of Pathology and Infectious Diseases, School of Veterinary Medicine, University of Surrey, Guildford, United Kingdom

Claire E. Whitehead
Camelid Veterinary Services Ltd, Reading, United Kingdom

Lucas Domínguez
VISAVET Health Surveillance Centre, Universidad Complutense de Madrid, Madrid, Spain
Departamento de Sanidad Animal, Facultad de Veterinaria, Universidad Complutense de Madrid, Madrid, Spain

Enrique Sánchez-Molano, Smaragda Tsairidou, Elizabeth Janet Glass, John Arthur Woolliams and Andrea Doeschl-Wilson
The Roslin Institute and Royal (Dick) School of Veterinary Studies, University of Edinburgh, Edinburgh, United Kingdom

Kethusegile Raphaka
The Roslin Institute and Royal (Dick) School of Veterinary Studies, University of Edinburgh, Edinburgh, United Kingdom
Department of Agricultural Research, Gaborone, Botswana

Osvaldo Anacleto
The Roslin Institute and Royal (Dick) School of Veterinary Studies, University of Edinburgh, Edinburgh, United Kingdom
Instituto de Ciências Matemáticas e de Computação, Universidade de São Paulo, São Carlos, Brazil

Georgios Banos
The Roslin Institute and Royal (Dick) School of Veterinary Studies, University of Edinburgh, Edinburgh, United Kingdom
Scotland's Rural College, Edinburgh, United Kingdom

Eamonn Gormley and Leigh A. L. Corner
School of Veterinary Medicine, University College Dublin, Dublin, Ireland

Giovanni Ghielmetti, Patricia Landolt, Ute Friedel, Roger Stephan and Sarah Schmitt
Section of Veterinary Bacteriology, Institute for Food Safety and Hygiene, University of Zurich, Zurich, Switzerland

Marina Morach
Institute for Food Safety and Hygiene, University of Zurich, Zurich, Switzerland

Sonja Hartnack
Section of Epidemiology, University of Zurich, Zurich, Switzerland

Aude Remot, Florence Carreras, Anthony Coupé, Émilie Doz-Deblauwe, Pierre Germon and Nathalie Winter
INRAE, Université de Tours, Nouzilly, France

Maria L. Boschiroli
Paris-Est University, National Reference Laboratory for Tuberculosis, Animal Health Laboratory, Anses, Maisons-Alfort, France

John A. Browne
UCD School of Agriculture and Food Science, University College Dublin, Dublin, Ireland

Quentin Marquant and Delphyne Descamps
INRAE, Université Paris-Saclay, UVSQ, Jouy-en-Josas, France

Fabienne Archer
INRAE, UMR754, Viral Infections and Comparative Pathology, IVPC, Univ Lyon, Université Claude Bernard Lyon 1, EPHE, Lyon, France

Abraham Aseffa
Armauer Hansen Research Institute, Addis Ababa, Ethiopia

Stephen V. Gordon
UCD School of Veterinary Medicine and UCD Conway Institute, University College Dublin, Dublin, Ireland

Jason E. Lombard, Tracey V. Dutcher and Cris A. Young
United States Department of Agriculture: Animal and Plant Health Inspection Service, Veterinary Services, Field Epidemiologic Investigation Services, Fort Collins, CO, United States

Elisabeth A. Patton
Wisconsin Department of Agriculture, Trade and Consumer Protection, Madison, WI, United States

Suzanne N. Gibbons-Burgener, Rachel F. Klos and Julie L. Tans-Kersten
Wisconsin Department of Health Services, Division of Public Health, Madison, WI, United States

Beth W. Carlson and Susan J. Keller
North Dakota Department of Agriculture, State Board of Animal Health, Bismarck, ND, United States

Delora J. Pritschet
North Dakota Department of Health, Bismarck, ND, United States

Susan Rollo
Texas Animal Health Commission, Austin, TX, United States

William C. Hench
United States Department of Agriculture: Animal and Plant Health Inspection Service, Veterinary Services, Ruminant Health Center, Fort Collins, CO, United States

Tyler C. Thacker, Claudia Perea and Aaron D. Lehmkuhl
United States Department of Agriculture: Animal and Plant Health Inspection Service, Veterinary Services, National Veterinary Services Laboratories, Ames, IA, United States

Paola M. Boggiatto and Mitchell V. Palmer
Infectious Bacterial Diseases Research Unit, National Animal Disease Center, Agricultural Research Service, United States Department of Agriculture, Ames, IA, United States

Carly R. Kanipe
Infectious Bacterial Diseases Research Unit, National Animal Disease Center, Agricultural Research Service, United States Department of Agriculture, Ames, IA, United States
Immunobiology Program, Iowa State University, Ames, IA, United States
Oak Ridge Institute for Science and Education (ORISE), Oak Ridge, TN, United States

Alejandro Perera Ortiz
United States Embassy, U.S. Department of Agriculture, Animal and Plant Health Inspection Service, Mexico City, Mexico
Programa de Doctorado en Ciencias Quimicobiológicas, Departamento de Inmunología, Escuela Nacional de Ciencias Biológicas, Instituto Politécnico Nacional, Ciudad de México, Mexico

Ethel Awilda García Latorre
Programa de Doctorado en Ciencias Quimicobiológicas, Departamento de Inmunología, Escuela Nacional de Ciencias Biológicas, Instituto Politécnico Nacional, Ciudad de México, Mexico

Doris M. Bravo and Tod P. Stuber
National Veterinary Services Laboratories, U.S. Department of Agriculture, Animal and Plant Health Inspection Service, Veterinary Services, Ames, IA, United States

Enrique Davalos
United States Embassy, U.S. Department of Agriculture, Animal and Plant Health Inspection Service, Mexicali, Mexico

Estela Flores Velázquez, Karen Salazar González and Erika Rosas Camacho
Dirección de Campañas Zoosanitarias de la Dirección General de Salud Animal Servicio Nacional de Sanidad, Inocuidad y Calidad Agroalimentaria, Ciudad de México, Mexico

Citlaltepetl Salinas Lara
Unidad de Investigación, Facultad de Estudios Superiores de Iztacala, Universidad Autónoma Nacional de México, Ciudad de México, Mexico

Raquel Muñiz Salazar
Laboratorio de Epidemiología y Ecología Molecular, Escuela Ciencias de la Salud, Universidad Autónoma de Baja California, Ensenada, Baja California, Mexico

Álvaro Roy, Beatriz Romero and Alberto Gómez-Buendía
VISAVET Health Surveillance Centre, Complutense University of Madrid, Madrid, Spain

Javier Ortega and Lucia de Juan
VISAVET Health Surveillance Centre, Complutense University of Madrid, Madrid, Spain
Departamento de Sanidad Animal, Facultad de Veterinaria, Universidad Complutense de Madrid, Madrid, Spain

José A. Infantes-Lorenzo, Inmaculada Moreno and Mercedes Domínguez
Unidad de Inmunología Microbiana, Centro Nacional de Microbiología, Instituto de Investigación Carlos III, Madrid, Spain

Irene Agulló-Ros
Grupo de Investigación en Sanidad Animal y Zoonosis, Departamento de Anatomía y Anatomía Patológica Comparadas, Facultad de Veterinaria, Universidad de Córdoba, Córdoba, Spain

Tarun Kumar and Mahavir Singh
College of Veterinary Sciences, Lala Lajpat Rai University of Veterinary and Animal Sciences, Hisar, India

Babu Lal Jangir
Department of Veterinary Pathology, Lala Lajpat Rai University of Veterinary and Animal Sciences, Hisar, India

Devan Arora
Haryana Pashu Vigyan Kendra, Lala Lajpat Rai University of Veterinary and Animal Sciences, Hisar, India

Sreenidhi Srinivasan
Huck Institutes of the Life Sciences, The Pennsylvania State University, University Park, PA, United States

Devender Bidhan and Dipin Chander Yadav
Department of Livestock Production Management, Lala Lajpat Rai University of Veterinary and Animal Sciences, Hisar, India

Maroudam Veerasami
Cisgen Biotech Discoveries Pvt. Ltd., Chennai, India

Douwe Bakker
Independent Researcher, Lelystad, Netherlands

Vivek Kapur
Huck Institutes of the Life Sciences, The Pennsylvania State University, University Park, PA, United States
Department of Animal Science, The Pennsylvania State University, University Park, PA, United States

Naresh Jindal
Department of Veterinary Public Health and Epidemiology, Lala Lajpat Rai University of Veterinary and Animal Sciences, Hisar, India

Elizabeth Hortêncio de Melo
Programa de Pós-Graduação em Medicina Veterinária, Universidade Federal Rural de Pernambuco, Recife, Brazil

Harrison Magdinier Gomes, Philip Noel Suffys, Márcia Quinhones Pires Lopes, Raquel Lima de Figueiredo Teixeira and Ícaro Rodrigues dos Santos
Laboratório de Biologia Molecular Aplicada à Micobactérias, Fundação Oswaldo Cruz, Laboratório de Biologia Molecular Aplicada à Micobactérias, Rio de Janeiro, Brazil

Marília Masello Junqueira Franco, Helio Langoni and Antonio Carlos Paes
Departamento de Higiene Veterinária e Saúde Pública, Faculdade de Medicina Veterinária e Zootecnia, Universidade Estadual Paulista, Botucatu, Brazil

José Augusto Bastos Afonso and Carla Lopes de Mendonça
Clínica de Bovinos de Garanhuns, Universidade Federal Rural de Pernambuco, Garanhuns, Brazil

Index

A

Alleles, 3, 123, 229-230

Alpine Pastures, 96-97, 159

Alveolar Macrophages, 163-165, 168, 173, 176-177

Animal Health, 2, 14, 27, 34, 45, 47-50, 72, 121, 133, 142, 146-147, 160-161, 163, 179-181, 184-186, 188, 201, 211, 223

Antigens, 86, 116, 120, 155, 158, 160-161, 192, 197, 216, 222-226

B

Badger-cattle, 14, 25, 88, 91

Badgers, 14-15, 17, 19-25, 27, 37-38, 47, 88-94, 99, 112, 132, 137, 139-142, 145-151, 161, 226

Biosecurity, 25, 36-39, 41-48, 60-61, 63-64, 67-68, 71

Bovine Tissue, 72-73, 76, 79, 188

Bovine Tuberculosis, 1, 6, 11-12, 14-15, 24-26, 34-38, 46-50, 57-61, 66, 68-73, 79, 81, 86-88, 93-94, 96, 111-113, 119-122, 153-155, 160-162, 164, 174, 176-180, 184, 187-188, 190, 198-199, 201, 211-213, 220-223, 226, 228, 234

Breeding Goal, 127, 129

Breeding Programmes, 127, 129, 131, 134

C

Cattle Farms, 14-21, 23-24, 47, 57-58, 66, 69, 97, 133, 142-143, 150

Cattle Herds, 14-15, 24-25, 45, 49-50, 58, 60, 93-94, 99, 133-134, 138-139, 142-143, 148-149, 151, 186

Cattle Trade, 14, 22-23, 150, 230, 233

Control Measures, 1-2, 22-24, 38-39, 44-45, 50, 53, 81, 84, 97, 99, 108, 122, 139-140, 142-143

Control Strategies, 38, 90, 92-94, 112, 121-122, 128-129, 131, 135, 140, 142-143, 145-146, 149, 209

Cut Lung Slices, 163-164, 176-177

D

Dairy Cattle, 54, 58, 121-123, 131, 133-134, 138, 178, 181-182, 185, 200-201, 204-205, 207, 209-211, 213, 228, 230, 233-234

Dairy Clusters, 203, 208, 210

Deer Numbers, 38, 41, 60, 63-67, 100, 142-143

Deer Population, 40, 60-61, 65, 97, 99-100, 108, 110, 184

Disease Control, 14, 37-40, 44-45, 48, 59, 63, 69, 81, 86, 89, 91-92, 96, 100, 127-129, 134, 137, 145-149, 159, 184, 186, 188, 198, 223, 228

Disease Elimination, 28, 90

Disease Management, 26, 37, 39, 42, 60, 67, 71, 81, 88-89, 109, 135-137, 142, 144, 188

E

Endemic Infection, 44, 108

Environmental Contamination, 82, 89, 108-109

Epidemiological Model, 121-122, 125, 127, 131, 133-134

F

Fertility Control, 89-90, 92-93, 95

Functional Potential, 190, 192-193, 196

G

Genetic Selection, 121-126, 128-132, 159, 164, 174, 178

Genetic Variation, 121-123, 127, 131-133, 178

Genotyping, 12, 25, 66, 139, 174, 228-230, 233-235

Granulomas, 78, 97, 100-103, 177, 181, 198, 201-202, 204-205, 208, 228-230, 233

Granulomatous Lesions, 78, 113, 185, 202, 208, 211, 231, 233

H

Human Activities, 137, 143

Human Dimensions, 37-38, 44, 47, 66

I

Infected Cattle, 22, 40, 49-50, 60, 63, 113, 122-123, 129, 133, 137, 144, 154, 161, 177, 182, 184-185, 190, 210, 220

Infected Farms, 14-20, 22-23

Infected Wildlife, 1, 28, 34, 36, 60, 136-137

Infection Dynamics, 96-97, 105-111, 122, 161

Infection Status, 2, 14-15, 19, 21, 23, 56, 78, 92, 94, 219

L

Lesion Score, 96, 111, 214, 216-217

Lesions, 50, 53-54, 58, 66, 69, 73-75, 77-79, 85, 87, 94, 96-97, 100-110, 112-113, 115-119, 122, 133, 136, 138-139, 141, 149, 154, 174, 177, 180-182, 184-185, 202, 204, 208-209, 211, 214-219, 229-231, 233

Livestock, 1-4, 6-12, 23-28, 31-32, 34, 36-38, 40-43, 47-48, 60-69, 71, 82, 84-86, 93, 129, 133-138, 141-145, 147, 149-151, 155, 157, 159, 176, 180-181, 185-188, 211-212, 215, 222-223, 226, 229, 235

Lung Lesions, 181, 230

Lung Tissue, 101, 163, 165-169, 171-174, 177

Lymph Nodes, 73, 89, 97, 100-103, 109-110, 116, 153-155, 161, 166, 177, 181, 185, 201, 204-205, 216, 218, 230-231, 233-234

M

Maintenance Hosts, 31, 91, 136-138, 141-142, 144

Microbiological Culture, 72-73, 75-78, 115, 228-229

Molecular Types, 14-23

Morbidity, 81, 145, 180, 212

Mortality, 28, 35, 81, 89-91, 93, 99, 136, 145, 180, 212, 223

Multinucleated Giant Cells, 173, 230

Mycobacteria, 15, 50, 56, 73-74, 76, 78-81, 97, 108-109, 111-112, 117-119, 149-151, 153-156, 158, 161, 163-164, 166-167, 171, 173-174, 176-178, 181, 187-188, 190, 196, 198-199, 201, 204, 225, 229, 234

Mycobacterial Isolation, 202, 233

Mycobacterium Caprae, 3, 12, 96-97, 111, 141, 149, 154, 160-161, 187-188

N

Neutrophils, 174-175, 177

O

Odocoileus Virginianus, 59, 61-62, 70-71, 112, 151

Oral Fluid, 214-220

P

Pastures, 14-17, 19, 21, 23, 25, 61, 63-64, 67, 93, 96-97, 155, 159, 201

Pathogenesis, 24, 93, 97, 111, 141, 148, 177, 211, 220, 233

Pathology, 12, 24, 35, 80, 96, 110, 112-114, 132, 148-149, 161, 163, 174, 177-178, 188, 190, 198, 220, 222, 228

Phenotype, 123-125, 190-191, 193, 196-198

Phylogeny, 3-4, 11, 198, 207

Pneumocytes, 163-164, 173-174

Possums, 11-12, 26-37, 94, 138-139, 146, 148

R

Resistant Sires, 121, 124-126, 129-132

Responsibilisation, 37, 39, 45

Risk Fraction, 22-23

Risk Mitigation, 37-44, 46, 62, 180

Roll-back Eradication, 26-28, 32

S

Spillover, 35, 59-60, 136, 138, 143-145, 148, 150

Spoligotyping, 2-4, 8, 15-16, 25, 75-79, 99, 148, 187, 209, 212-213, 228-230, 232-235

Stakeholders, 31, 38-39, 41-42, 44, 60, 62, 64-67, 135-147, 150, 155, 159

T

Tuberculin, 15, 24, 49-50, 58, 73-74, 86-87, 99, 111, 114-116, 120, 122, 129, 133, 142, 145, 151-152, 154, 157-161, 181, 210, 213-214, 216, 218, 220, 222-224, 226, 235

V

Value Systems, 135-137, 140, 143, 145

Virulence, 163-164, 174-175, 178, 198, 233

W

Water Buffaloes, 222-223

Wildlife Surveillance, 26, 32, 142

Z

Zoonotic Disease, 71, 122, 145, 151, 154, 180

www.ingramcontent.com/pod-product-compliance
Lightning Source LLC
Chambersburg PA
CBHW080411190526
45161CB00003B/197